ORIGINS OF THE SOCIAL MIND

ORIGINS OF
THE SOCIAL MIND

Evolutionary Psychology
and Child Development

Edited by
BRUCE J. ELLIS
DAVID F. BJORKLUND

THE GUILFORD PRESS
New York   London

© 2005 The Guilford Press
A Division of Guilford Publications, Inc.
72 Spring Street, New York, NY 10012
www.guilford.com

Printed in the United States of America

This book is printed on acid-free paper.

Last digit is print number: 9 8 7 6 5 4 3 2 1

Library of Congress Cataloging-in-Publication Data

Origins of the social mind: evolutionary psychology and child development /
edited by Bruce J. Ellis, David F. Bjorklund.
   p. cm.
  Includes bibliographical references and index.
  ISBN 1-59385-103-0 (hardcover: alk. paper)
   1. Evolutionary psychology. 2. Developmental psychology. I. Ellis,
Bruce J. II. Bjorklund, David F., 1949–
  BF711.O75 2005
  155.7—dc22

                  2004022693

ABOUT THE EDITORS

Bruce J. Ellis, PhD, spent the early years of his career at the University of Canterbury in New Zealand before taking up his current position as an Associate Professor of Family Studies and Human Development at the University of Arizona. He completed his doctoral work in evolutionary psychology at the University of Michigan and his postdoctoral work in the National Institute of Mental Health's Developmental Psychopathology Training Program at Vanderbilt University. The major focus of his research is on testing conditional adaptation models of the effects of early family environments on the timing of pubertal development and first sexual and reproductive activity. Dr. Ellis received the 1999 John F. Kennedy Center Young Scientist Award and has served on the editorial boards of *Developmental Psychology, Evolutionary Psychology, Personality and Social Psychology Review,* and *Personal Relationships.*

David F. Bjorklund, PhD, is Professor of Psychology at Florida Atlantic University, where he has taught graduate and undergraduate courses in developmental psychology since 1976. His research has focused primarily on children's cognitive development, particularly memory and strategy development. More recent interests include the adaptive nature of immaturity, deferred imitation in juvenile great apes, and evolutionary developmental psychology. Dr. Bjorklund is the author of several books, including *The Origins of Human Nature: Evolutionary Developmental Psychology* (with Anthony D. Pellegrini). He is a former Associate Editor of *Child Development* and has served on the editorial boards of the *Journal of Experimental Child Psychology, Journal of Cognition and Development, Developmental Review, Educational Psychology Review, Journal of Comparative Psychology, Developmental Psychology, Cognitive Development,* and *School Psychology Quarterly.*

CONTRIBUTORS

John Archer, PhD, Department of Psychology, University of Central Lancashire, Preston, United Kingdom

Simon Baron-Cohen, PhD, Autism Research Centre, Departments of Experimental Psychology and Psychiatry, Cambridge University, Cambridge, United Kingdom

H. Clark Barrett, PhD, Center for Behavior, Evolution and Culture; Center for Culture, Brain, and Development; and Department of Anthropology, University of California, Los Angeles, California

Jay Belsky, PhD, Institute for the Study of Children, Families and Social Issues, Birkbeck University of London, London, United Kingdom

Jesse M. Bering, PhD, Department of Psychology, University of Arkansas, Fayetteville, Arkansas

Irene Bevc, PhD, Hincks–Dellcrest Treatment Centre, Toronto, Ontario, Canada

David F. Bjorklund, PhD, Department of Psychology, Florida Atlantic University, Boca Raton, Florida

Victoria K. Burbank, PhD, Department of Anthropology, University of Western Australia, Crawley, Australia

James S. Chisholm, PhD, School of Anatomy and Human Biology, University of Western Australia, Crawley, Australia

David A. Coall, PhD candidate, School of Anatomy and Human Biology, University of Western Australia, Crawley, Australia

Bruce J. Ellis, PhD, Division of Family Studies and Human Development, University of Arizona, Tucson, Arizona

Mark V. Flinn, PhD, Departments of Anthropology and Psychological Sciences, University of Missouri, Columbia, Missouri

Frank Gemmiti, PhD candidate, School of Anatomy and Human Biology and Department of Anthropology, University of Western Australia, Crawley, Australia

David C. Geary, PhD, Department of Psychological Sciences, University of Missouri, Columbia, Missouri

Judith Rich Harris, MA, independent scholar, Middletown, New Jersey

Elizabeth M. Hill, PhD, Department of Psychology, University of Detroit–Mercy, Detroit, Michigan

Heather C. Janisse, PhD, Department of Psychology, Wayne State University, Detroit, Michigan

Brian MacWhinney, PhD, Department of Psychology, Carnegie Mellon University, Pittsburgh, Pennsylvania

Katherine Nelson, PhD, PhD Program in Psychology, City University of New York Graduate School, New York, New York

Anthony D. Pellegrini, PhD, Department of Educational Psychology, University of Minnesota–Twin Cities Campus, Minneapolis, Minnesota

David H. Rakison, PhD, Department of Psychology, Carnegie Mellon University, Pittsburgh, Pennsylvania

Justin S. Rosenberg, PhD candidate, Department of Psychology, Florida Atlantic University, Boca Raton, Florida

Nancy L. Segal, PhD, Department of Psychology, California State University, Fullerton, California

Irwin Silverman, PhD, Department of Psychology, York University, Toronto, Ontario, Canada

Peter K. Smith, PhD, Unit for School and Family Studies, Department of Psychology, Goldsmiths College, University of London, London, United Kingdom

Carol V. Ward, PhD, Department of Anthropology and Department of Pathology and Anatomical Sciences, University of Missouri, Columbia, Missouri

Glenn E. Weisfeld, PhD, Department of Psychology, Wayne State University, Detroit, Michigan

PREFACE

Evolutionary psychology has established itself as a serious discipline within the larger field of psychology. Modern evolutionary theory has been adopted by many psychologists to explain human behavior—serving as an overarching perspective, or metatheory—and we believe that this approach has been fruitful. There are now competing textbooks for college courses in evolutionary psychology, an outsider to mainstream psychology not long ago, and the topic is found in most introductory psychology textbooks as well as textbooks in developmental, cognitive, social, and personality psychology. Yet, despite being enamored with the promise of evolutionary psychology, as developmentalists we believe it has shortcomings. First, the field has paid little attention to the nature of childhood and its functions. Second, although evolutionary psychology does not ignore development, it has failed to treat it seriously in its theorizing. And, third, a close look at the basic tenets of mainstream evolutionary psychology and developmental psychology reveals contradictions that cannot be glossed over or simply "averaged" in order to successfully integrate the two. Moreover, although some scientists have written about psychological development from an evolutionary perspective (e.g., Belsky, Steinberg, & Draper, 1991; Boyce & Ellis, in press), until recently there was no overarching evolutionary perspective within developmental psychology. This shortcoming was addressed in part by the 2002 publication of David F. Bjorklund and Anthony D. Pellegrini's book *The Origins of Human Nature: Evolutionary Developmental Psychology*, which defined the field of *evolutionary developmental psychology* and provided a developmental perspective for evolutionary psychologists and an evolutionary perspective for developmental psychologists. This perspective means more than simply applying the basic precepts of evolutionary psychology to developmental phenomena; it involves a reformulation of contemporary evolutionary psychological theory, making it compatible with what we know about the processes of ontogeny.

Bjorklund and Pellegrini's book was timely, following a major symposium on the topic at the 2001 meeting of the Society for Research in Child Development and preceding special issues devoted to the topic of evolutionary developmental psychology in several journals (*Journal of Experimental Child Psychology*, 2003; the Spanish journal *Infancia*, 2003; *Human Nature*, 2002, on childhood and the evolution of the human life course; and *Learning and Individual Differences*, 2002, on the related topic of evolutionary educational psychology). However, the field is still in its infancy, and many developmental psychologists with an evolutionary perspective (or evolutionary psychologists with a developmental perspective) remain unaware that there are others who share their views, and unaware of how evolutionary thinking is being applied to research domains outside of their immediate areas of expertise. Evolutionary psychology was in a similar intellectual climate when Barkow, Cosmides, and Tooby published *The Adapted Mind* in 1992. This book presented original theoretical and review chapters from researchers working in diverse areas, all from an evolutionary psychological perspective. *The Adapted Mind* is sometimes referred to as "the Bible" of evolutionary psychology and, more than any other book, is responsible for the rapid rise of the field to academic respectability.

We hope to do something similar with this book of readings in evolutionary developmental psychology. Our contributors are respected developmental scientists, whose research on children is explicitly driven by evolutionary issues. Part I of the book contains overarching theoretical chapters that articulate the major tenets of evolutionary developmental psychology and address basic issues in the field, such as the function of childhood, gene–environment interactions, and the role of environmental risk and uncertainty in the development of reproductive strategies. Part II is composed of chapters that address classic topics in social and personality development—parent–child relationships, sibling relationships, aggression, play, incest avoidance, puberty and adolescence—from an evolutionary developmental perspective. Part III does the same for a series of topics in cognitive development: infant perception and cognition, memory, language, religious causal beliefs, understanding of animal behavior, folk knowledge, and mindreading. Taken together, these chapters provide a broad synthesis of the fields of evolutionary psychology and child development.

The contributors to this volume have followed different paths into the area of evolutionary developmental psychology, as typified by the editors of this volume. Bruce J. Ellis was trained as a canonical evolutionary psychologist in David Buss's laboratory at the University of Michigan. There he studied variation in adult mating strategies. Developmental processes were largely taken for granted and treated simply as precursors to the primary units of analysis: evolved psychological mechanisms. Ellis became dissatisfied with this approach, undertook 3 years of postdoctoral training in developmental psychopathology at Vanderbilt University, and shifted from studying adult phenotypes to developmental processes and mechanisms. His current research is largely focused on testing conditional adaptation models of the effects of early family environments on the timing of pubertal development and first sexual and reproductive activity.

David F. Bjorklund, by contrast, was trained in Peter Ornstein's laboratory as a cognitive developmental psychologist and spent most of his career studying memory and strategy development in children. His graduate training at the University of North Carolina at Chapel Hill, however, also included exposure to developmental systems theory, including the possible role that ontogeny may have played in phylogeny. He continued to read popular (and not so popular) books and articles on evolution as an avocation. When evolutionary psychology began to gain attention in the late 1980s and early 1990s, he became a quick devotee, believing he could easily meld his two academic interests. This proved more difficult than he first thought, and he spent the better part of a decade trying to resolve the seeming contradictions in the two fields and to initiate new research programs consistent with an evolutionary developmental perspective. These include such varied topics as deferred imitation in juvenile great apes, the development of children's afterlife beliefs, and sex differences in styles of play and tool use.

We are grateful to the developmental scientists who contributed chapters to this volume. Their enthusiasm for the goals of the project, hard work in bringing it to fruition, and patience in dealing with two demanding editors made this book possible. We are also indebted to the individuals who generously served as external reviewers for various chapters: Carlos Hernández Blasi, Garth Fletcher, Erika Hoff, Thomas Keenan, and Anthony Pellegrini. Finally, we would like to thank Seymour Weingarten, our editor at The Guilford Press, for his unstinting support in developing and publishing this volume. Work on *Origins of the Social Mind* was supported by an Erskine Fellowship from the University of Canterbury, which allowed two editors living on opposite sides of the world to spend a month working together in Christchurch, New Zealand.

BRUCE J. ELLIS
DAVID F. BJORKLUND

REFERENCES

Barkow, J. H., Cosmides, L., & Tooby, J. (1992). *The adapted mind*. London: Oxford University Press.

Belsky, J., Steinberg, L., & Draper, P. (1991). Childhood experience, interpersonal development, and reproductive strategy: An evolutionary theory of socialization. *Child Development, 62,* 647–670.

Bjorklund, D. F., & Pellegrini, A. D. (2002). *The origins of human nature: Evolutionary developmental psychology.* Washington, DC: American Psychological Association.

Boyce, W. T., & Ellis, B. J. (in press). Biological sensitivity to context: I. An evolutionary-developmental theory of the origins and functions of stress reactivity. *Development and Psychopathology.*

CONTENTS

Contents

II. PERSONALITY AND SOCIAL DEVELOPMENT

III. COGNITIVE DEVELOPMENT

ORIGINS OF THE SOCIAL MIND

I

CONCEPTUAL FOUNDATIONS OF EVOLUTIONARY DEVELOPMENTAL PSYCHOLOGY

Core Issues and Approaches

1

EVOLUTIONARY PSYCHOLOGY AND CHILD DEVELOPMENT

An Emerging Synthesis

DAVID F. BJORKLUND
BRUCE J. ELLIS

Evolutionary thinking has entered the mainstream of academic psychology. Yet, until recently, relatively little attention has been paid to children or development from an evolutionary psychological perspective. Evolutionary psychologists have understandably focused on adult behavior, for it is adults who reproduce, the *sine qua non* of evolutionary success. Most of the efforts of evolutionary psychologists are aimed at explaining how psychological mechanisms, selected in our environments of evolutionary adaptedness, continue to influence the behavior of contemporary people. Of special interest has been the social and sexual strategies of individuals who are already of reproductive age. At the extreme perspective, development can be viewed as an epiphenomenon—something that individuals must "do" on the way to adulthood—but that in itself has played no central role in evolution and thus has little consequence for understanding adult psychological functioning. Although this is an understandable position for an emerging discipline, the maturation of the field of evolutionary psychology has resulted in an expanded focus. There is now increasing realization that individuals must negotiate the landscapes of infancy and childhood before reaching adulthood, and that natural selection surely played as substantial a role in shaping the minds and behaviors of juveniles as it did in shaping the minds and behaviors of adults.

3

Another impediment to the integration of evolutionary and developmental psychology has been the reluctance of many developmental psychologists to embrace an evolutionary perspective. Whereas a substantial number of researchers in the areas of social, cognitive, and personality psychology have found evolutionary theory useful for interpreting their phenomena of interest or for generating new lines of research, psychologists whose specialty is describing and explaining ontogeny have been less enthusiastic. In fact, there has been some overt hostility toward evolutionary psychology by some developmentalists (see Lickliter & Honeycutt, 2003; Oyama, 2001), based mainly on the belief (incorrectly, we believe) that evolutionary psychology argues for a form of genetic determinism (behaviors are "in the genes"), which is contrary to what we know about how genes and environments interact over the course of development to produce adult form and function. At the same time, an increasing number of developmental scientists are attempting to reconcile the apparent contradictions between mainstream developmental and evolutionary psychology and to apply evolutionary thinking to obtain a clearer picture of human ontogeny (e.g., Bjorklund & Pellegrini, 2002; Boyce & Ellis, in press; Bugental, 2000; Geary, 1998; Hernández Blasi & Bjorklund, 2003; Keller, 2000). Each of the chapters in this book attempts to further these goals.

It would be disingenuous of us, however, to contend that all conceptual differences between evolutionary and developmental psychology have been resolved, that a developmental perspective has been fully incorporated into evolutionary psychology, or that developmentalists have embraced evolutionary thinking. Antagonism and misunderstanding between evolutionary and developmental psychologists persist (see commentaries to Lickliter & Honeycutt, 2003; especially Buss & Reeve, 2003, and Tooby, Cosmides, & Barrett, 2003), although we believe that many of the differences are more apparent than real (see Bjorklund, 2003).

EVOLUTIONARY CHILD PSYCHOLOGY AND EVOLUTIONARY DEVELOPMENTAL PSYCHOLOGY

As the chapters in this volume reflect, evolutionary psychologists are increasingly considering issues related to children and development, and developmental psychologists are increasingly recognizing the benefits of adopting an evolutionary perspective. On the one hand, evolutionary psychologists are applying the principles of evolutionary psychology to infants and children: What role have evolved psychological mechanisms played in adapting infants and children to their physical and social environments? In a sense, this can be considered *evolutionary child psychology*, in that the behavior of children (and infants), rather than adults, is explained in terms of the principles of evolutionary psychology (see chapters by Barrett; Harris; Rakison, this volume).

On the other hand, applying a developmental perspective to evolutionary psychology can provide a different understanding of the origins of adult phenotypes. The behaviors displayed by adults do not arise fully formed but develop over time, with different early environments often producing different adaptively patterned phenotypes (see chapters by Belsky; Chisholm, Burbank, Coall, & Gemmiti; Ellis; Silverman & Bevc, this volume, and further discussion below). For evolutionary psychologists, the distal causes of functional behavior are reliably developing (i.e., inherited) cognitive mechanisms that underwent natural selection in environments of evolutionary adaptedness. Following the tenets of the Modern Synthesis, the mechanism of inheritance is genetic. The problem then becomes, "How does information for adaptive cognition and behavior coded in the genes become realized in the organism?" The shorthand answer for most evolutionary psychologists is that genes interact with environment, producing adaptive behavior that is dependent on contexts in which the organism finds itself. This avoids the nativism of instinct theory, which holds that behavior is tightly controlled by genes. Yet it still implies (at least to some developmentalists) a form of *preformationism*, with different sets of genes coding for specific outcomes in different environments (Lickliter & Honeycutt, 2003; Oyama, 2001). What we know about ontogeny does not reflect accurately this admittedly more subtle version of genetic determinism, and we think that an explicitly *evolutionary developmental psychology* approach is needed to account for how adaptations from one generation can be transmitted and expressed in the adult phenotype of the next generation and how this influence has occurred over the course of thousands of generations (see chapters by Bjorklund & Rosenberg; Nelson; Weisfeld & Janisse, this volume).

From this perspective, evolutionary developmental psychology can be defined as

> the application of the basic principles of Darwinian evolution, particularly natural selection, to explain contemporary human development. It involves the study of the genetic and environmental mechanisms that underlie the universal development of social and cognitive competencies and the evolved epigenetic (gene–environment interactions) processes that adapt these competencies to local conditions; it assumes that not only are behaviors and cognitions that characterize adults the product of selection pressures operating over the course of evolution, but so also are characteristics of children's behaviors and minds. (Bjorklund & Pellegrini, 2002, p. 4)

The primary focus of evolutionary developmental psychology is on how nongenetic factors (in interaction with genetic factors) influence the expression of evolved psychological mechanisms over time.

Not all contributors of this volume would necessarily adopt this focus or identify themselves as evolutionary developmental psychologists, following this definition. In fact, the chapters in this volume do not reflect a homogeneous perspective. As in mainstream evolutionary psychology, there is room for contention among people who share interests in development and evolution. Yet there are some issues that differentiate scientists who examine development from an evolutionary psychological perspective from those who align themselves more exclusively with mainstream evolutionary psychology. First among them, of course, is the contention that "development matters," both in the sense that natural selection has operated on the lives of infants and children as well as on those of adults, and that an understanding of how evolved mechanisms operate to produce adult behavior must be viewed through an ontogenetic lens to reveal the full picture. Relatedly, issues of whether natural selection has served to shape children's behavior in preparation for adult life or rather to adapt them to their current environment and *not* to a future one, must be addressed (see Bjorklund, 1997; Bjorklund & Hernández Blasi, in press; Bjorklund & Pellegrini, 2002; Hernández Blasi & Bjorklund, 2003). Evolutionary developmental psychologists also examine the question of why the juvenile period is disproportionately prolonged in *Homo sapiens* compared to those of other primates.

Perhaps most centrally, an evolutionary developmental psychological approach advocates that models of *how* genes and environments interact to produce adaptations over ontogeny must go beyond the simple statements that "genes and environments interact" (see chapters by Bjorklund & Rosenberg; Belsky; Ellis; Nelson; Segal & Hill; Weisfeld & Janisse, this volume). As discussed later in this chapter, developing serious accounts of gene–environment interactions that are compatible with canonical views of both evolutionary and developmental psychology is more easily said than done. Related to this issue is the contention that children show a high degree of plasticity and adaptive sensitivity to context, and that such sensitivity not only affects developmental trajectories and children's current adaptations to their environments, but also influences various facultative "strategies" in adulthood. We examine briefly these, and related, issues in the remainder of the chapter.

ISSUES IN EVOLUTIONARY DEVELOPMENTAL PSYCHOLOGY

Deferred versus Ontogenetic Adaptations

Although there is little debate that children's cognitions and behaviors have been shaped by natural selection, it seems that natural selection has sometimes worked to prepare children for effective functioning in adulthood (*deferred adaptations*), but other times to adapt children to their immediate environment and not prepare them for future ones (*ontogenetic adaptations*) (e.g., Hernández Blasi & Bjorklund, 2003). The idea that experiences during childhood serve to prepare children for adult life is a familiar one for child developmentalists, but are there evolved adaptations that make such preparation easier? Some theorists believe so. For example, some sex differences in children's play have been proposed to prepare children for adult roles (e.g., Pellegrini & Bjorklund, 2004; Pellegrini & Smith, 1998; Smith, Chapter 11, this volume). Males and females have different self-interests, often centered around mating and parenting. Following parental investment theory (Trivers, 1972; see also Bjorklund, Yunger, & Pellegrini, 2002; Geary, 1999; chapters by Baron-Cohen; Pellegrini & Archer; Weisfeld & Janisse, this volume), males, as the less-investing sex, are more physically aggressive and compete with one another more vigorously than do females for access to mating partners. By contrast, females engage in more relational aggression and are more focused on social relationships, which are relevant to garnering support to rear their offspring to maturity. With respect to play, boys (and male mammals in general) engage in more rough-and-tumble play than girls, which some theorists have proposed serves as practice for hunting and fighting for boys. Such behavior would have conferred a selective advantage to males in ancestral environments, and likely continues to be adaptive for modern males (e.g., Geary, 1998; Pellegrini & Smith, 1998; see Pellegrini & Archer, Chapter 9, this volume; Smith, Chapter 11, this volume). Moreover, rough-and-tumble play has been hypothesized to facilitate boys' ability to encode and decode social signals (Pellegrini & Smith, 1998), which is important at all stages of social life.

Sex differences in fantasy (pretend) play are also found, with girls engaging in more play-parenting than boys, both in modern (see Geary, 1998) and traditional (see Eibl-Eibesfeldt, 1989) cultures, making it unlikely that this reflects recent Western social norms. Such play may have prepared girls for the traditional roles that women played in ancestral environments (and continue to play in most cultures today). In comparison, fantasy play in boys is more centered on dominance, aggression, and power and is often part of rough-and-tumble play. These sex differences, in both rough-and-tumble and fantasy play, may be seen as antecedents for the roles (e.g., parenting, male–male competition) children will have as adults, or would have had in the environment of evolutionary adaptedness (see Pellegrini & Bjorklund, 2004).

In general, when environmental or social conditions remain relatively stable over time, so that children's experiences provide them with reliable information about the reproductive opportunities and constraints that they are likely to encounter at adolescence and beyond, selection should favor adaptive sensitivity to context. According to *conditional adaptation models*, this sensitivity enables children to modify their phenotypes to anticipate what will likely be similar adult environments. Children have likely been "prepared" by natural selection to be sensitive to availability of resources (Ellis, Chapter 7, this volume), levels of stress (Chisholm et al., Chapter 4, this volume), and to potentially appropriate (and inappropriate) sex partners (Silverman & Bevc, Chapter 12, this volume), all of which serve not so much to adapt them to their current environment but to ones they are likely to inhabit as adults.

A concept less familiar to most child developmentalists is *ontogenetic adaptations*, which are specific to a particular time in development and do not necessarily serve to prepare children for future environments (e.g., Bjorklund, 1997; Oppenheim, 1981). Physiological mechanisms during prenatal development are readily recognized examples of ontogenetic adaptations. For example, mammals get oxygen and nutrition via the umbilical cord before birth, systems that are essential in adapting the fetus to its prenatal environment but that become obsolete once the infant leaves the protective womb of its mother. Behavioral and cognitive adaptations are less obvious but also likely exist (see Bjorklund, 1997). For example, although we listed aspects of juvenile play as reflecting deferred adaptations, other aspects may have immediate benefits, such as facilitating social relationships among peers, muscle and skeletal development, and thermoregulation (e.g., Pellegrini & Smith, 1998; Smith, Chapter 11, this volume). Similarly, aggression in children serves to establish their position in a status hierarchy and to acquire resources, each of immediate benefit (see Pellegrini & Archer, Chapter 9, this volume). As another example, Bjorklund (1987) proposed that the imitation of facial gestures observed in neonates is not conceptually similar to the imitation observed in older infants and children, as Meltzoff and Moore (1997) propose, but rather has the specific function of fostering mother–infant interaction in the early months of life and disappears when infants' social-cognitive skills improve, making such reflexive imitation superfluous. Support for this position comes from research in which rates of neonatal imitation were related to levels of mother–infant social interaction three months later (Heimann, 1989).

Natural selection may, indeed, have worked to prepare children for life in a human group, but believing this in and of itself does not tell us the precise function of any particular adaptation. One issue that should be kept in mind when contemplating evolved mechanisms in childhood is whether such adaptations serve to prepare children for life as an adult, to help them negotiate the niches of infancy and childhood, or perhaps both.

The Necessity of an Extended Childhood to Master the Complexities of Human Social Communities

Humans spend more time as pre-reproductives than any other primate (Bonner, 1988). Waiting so long before reproducing can have dire consequences for an individual (and a species), specifically, death before procreating and thus the end of one's personal genetic line. When costs are great, we assume that so also must be benefits. What can be the benefits of so extended a juvenile period in *Homo sapiens*? The simple answer is that, because of material culture, human children have much to learn to succeed as adults, and their survival is more dependent on acquired skills than any other species. We concur with this position, but what, exactly, is so complicated about human life that requires the better part of 20 years to acquire? Some have speculated that children need a prolonged childhood in order to master food-acquisition/ preparation skills or technological skills associated with tool use and manufacture (e.g., Kaplan, Hill, Lancaster, & Hurtado, 2000). Although we do not want to discount the complexity of such skills, most theorists believe that they are not so complex as to justify the length of time humans spend as pre-reproductives. Such thinking goes back at least as far as to Alfred Wallace, the codiscoverer of natural selection, who commented that hunter–gatherers were far more intelligent than they needed to be to eke out an existence on the African savannah. Most contemporary evolutionary theorists who have pondered the question argue that it is the diversity and complexity of human groups that requires an extended time to learn (e.g., Alexander, 1989; Bjorklund & Harnishfeger, 1995; Dunbar, 1998; Flinn, 1997; Geary & Flinn, 2001; Humphrey, 1976). Children require time and experience to learn how to effectively cooperate and compete with fellow conspecifics; they need to learn to "read the minds" of the people they interact with on a daily basis, to form coalitions, to know when to display certain behaviors such as aggression and sexual interest in a potential mate, and when to inhibit such urges. Because of the diversity of human cultures and traditions, such information cannot be "hardwired" into the brain in any straightforward manner; rather, it is acquired through development via the interaction between cognitive adaptations and complex human social environments over many years and a variety of contexts. This general position is made explicit by many of the authors of this volume (Baron-Cohen; Bering; Bjorklund & Rosenberg; Harris; Pellegrini & Archer; Smith) but is the central focus of the chapter by Mark Flinn and Carol Ward.

PHENOTYPIC PLASTICITY AND THE NATURE OF GENE–ENVIRONMENT INTERACTION

Over the past two decades, theory and research in evolutionary biology has begun to acknowledge that, in most species, single "best" strategies for survival and reproduction are unlikely to evolve (Gangestad & Simpson, 2000; Gross, 1996). This is because the "best" strategy varies as a function of the physical, economic, and social parameters of one's environment (Crawford & Anderson, 1989), and thus a strategy that promotes success in some environmental contexts may lead to failure in others. Selection pressures therefore tend to favor *phenotypic plasticity*, the capacity of a single genotype to produce a range of phenotypes—manifested in morphology, physiology, and/or behavior—in response to particular developmental and ecological conditions (see Pigliucci, 2001). Phenotypic plasticity is necessarily a constrained process, however, and occurs within the boundaries of genetically inherited reaction norms (see Schlichting & Pigliucci, 1998). Thus, no amount of interplay between the genes an organism carries and the physical, biological, and social environments that it experiences during ontogeny can turn a chicken into a goat. Nonetheless, there is substantial debate within the field of evolutionary developmental psychology about the nature and extent of phenotypic plasticity.

Underlying this debate, however, is consensus regarding the interactive role of genes and environments in developmental processes. Genetic and environmental influences cannot be simply partitioned. The expression of genes during development can be stimulated or inhibited by an array of internal (e.g., cytoplasmic, neural, hormonal) and external (e.g., light, gravity, temperature, social interactions) events. The phenotypic outcomes of developmental processes therefore are codetermined by the genes an organism carries and the environments that it experiences during ontogeny, and are not directly caused by either genes or environment (see Lickliter & Honeycutt, 2003).

Adaptive Phenotypic Plasticity: Conditional Adaptations

Despite this consensus, disagreement persists over the role of natural selection in shaping phenotypic plasticity. Evolutionary developmental psychologists working within the adaptationist program emphasize *adaptive* phenotypic plasticity. In this framework, the development of alternative phenotypes is conceptualized as a nonrandom process—the outcome of a structured transaction between genes and environment that was shaped by natural selection to increase the capacity and tendency of individuals to track their developmental environments and adjust their phenotypes accordingly. Along these lines, Boyce and Ellis (in press) have proposed the concept of *conditional adaptations:* "evolved mechanisms that detect and respond to specific features of childhood environments—features that have proven reliable over evolutionary time in predicting the nature of the social and physical world into which children will mature—and entrain developmental pathways that reliably matched those features during a species' natural selective history." Conditional adaptations, which reflect systematic gene–environment interactions, underpin development of contingent survival and reproductive strategies and thus enable individuals to function competently in a variety of different environments. Stated differently, natural selection promotes functional coordination between phenotypic plasticity and the range of developmental environments that were recurrently encountered during a species' evolutionary history.

Consider, for example, the caterpillar *Nemoria arizonaria*, which develops almost completely different morphologies depending upon its diet in the first three days of life (Greene, 1989, 1996). These caterpillars inhabit oak woodlands in the American Southwest and produce both spring and summer broods. Although the two broods have the same appearance when they first hatch, the spring brood feeds on oak catkins and develops the appearance of the oak's drooping flowers, whereas the summer brood feeds on oak leaves and develops the appearance of twigs. The flower morphology enables the spring brood to blend into the environment while feeding on the ubiquitous spring catkins. Likewise, the twig morph provides camouflage for the leaf-eating summer brood. If either the spring or summer broods are experimentally fed out-of-season food, they develop the corresponding out-of-season morphology and become highly vulnerable to predation. These caterpillars have therefore evolved physiological mechanisms that register features of diet in the first three days of life and activate alternative developmental pathways, which function to match the organism's morphology to its feeding ecology (Greene, 1989, 1996).

Developmental Systems Theory

By contrast, ardent proponents of *developmental systems theory* (e.g., Lickliter & Honeycutt, 2003; Moore, 2001; Oyama, 2001) have generally been critical of these kinds of adaptationist accounts, viewing the gene–environment interactionism advocated by evolutionary psychology as merely a diluted form of genetic determinism: different genes are activated depending on which environments are experienced, yielding different outcomes. There is clearly phenotypic plasticity in the adaptationist models (as advocated by the conditional adaptation perspective), but different sets of genes are still viewed as being prespecified, or *preformed,* to respond "appropriately" to specified contexts.

Developmental systems are variants of *dynamic systems* models, which explain the emergence of order in both physical (e.g., Gleick, 1987) and psychological (e.g., Kelso, 1995; Thelen & Smith, 1998; Vallacher, Read, & Nowak, 2002) systems without the need of postulating internal (e.g., homunculus; genetic instructions) or external (e.g., environment, God) agents as "directors" of developing order. Rather, "patterns and order emerge from interactions of the components of complex systems without explicit instruction either in the organism itself or from the environment" (Thelen & Smith, 1998, p. 564). With respect to ontogeny, order or structure (such as linguistic ability) is not innately specified, waiting only for the proper maturational conditions to be activated; nor is it the product of environmental shaping (e.g., learning). Rather, according to dynamic models, higher-level forms of structure emerge from the self-initiated activity of the organism in interaction with all levels of its environment. According to Lewis (2000), self-organization means that "structure does not have to be imported into a system from the outside, as presumed by learning approaches, nor preordained from within, as presumed by nativist approaches. Structure is emergent" (p. 39). By analogy, consider the formation of a rainbow. Rainbows reliably emerge when droplets of water and rays of light interact in a specific fashion, yet the design of a rainbow is not built into either water or light.

This does not imply that self-organization is sufficient to "explain" the development or evolution of adaptive function. Emerging structures must be functional if they are to survive. As Tooby et al. (2003) state: "Selection brings about a functional coordination between the stable, long-term properties of environments and the stable, cross-generationally recurrent, reliably

developing (and hence predictable or prespecifiable) properties of organisms
. . . Whenever one sees functional order, one is seeing the downstream contrivances of natural selection" (p. 862). However, natural selection does not explain how functional coordination between organisms and environments is generated. Thus, counter to Tooby et al.'s (2003) interpretation, acknowledging the central role of natural selection in the establishment of order does not obviate the need to explain the generation of structures and functions via developmental mechanisms, such as those advocated by dynamic systems models. Just as mutations produce genetic changes that can be exposed to natural selection, alterations in developmental processes produce phenotypic changes (e.g., a change in diet producing changes in size or maturational tempo) that, by placing organisms in new ecological relationships with their environments, can expose them to novel selection pressures. Thus, phenotypic plasticity can operate as a creative force in evolutionary change.

Developmental systems theorists argue against any form of preformationism, proposing that all development results from "interactions of the components of complex systems" (Thelen & Smith, 1998, p. 564) beginning at the genetic level (genes are turned on or off or express different products depending on their current biochemical environment), through the structural level (neurons generate synapses, get organized with other neurons depending on the firing of neighboring neurons), to the environmental level (neurons fire as a result of stimulation from the external world). Feedback occurs between adjacent levels (e.g., gene products influence not only the generation of structure, such as neurons, but the activity of the structures in turn influences the subsequent activity of the genes). The result is the continuous interaction between structure (e.g., genes, neurons), function (i.e., activity emanating from structures), and exogenous environmental factors at all levels of organization. No structure or function in an organism is preformed (i.e., innate), waiting only for the proper environment for its activation; rather, structure and function emerge as a result of the continuous and dynamic interaction between adjacent levels of biological and environmental organization over time. From this perspective, genes are seen not as supplying "instructions" that are carried out by cellular machinery, but as containing "information" that is expressed in a probabilistic way through dynamic interaction between genes and components in their environment.

One apt criticism of developmental systems models is that their emphasis on the emergence of structure and function via probabilistic interactions among components of complex systems makes prediction difficult, if not impossible (e.g., Tooby et al., 2003). Given the diversity of micro- and macroenvironments in which organisms live and the multitude of interactions that occur beginning with the first expression of a gene, how is it that different members of a species end up resembling one another to the extent that they do (or that any organism actually develops into adulthood)? The answer is that organisms inherit not only a species-typical genome, but also a species-typical environment, which is highly structured. For example, according to Lickliter

reliably orchestrate the ontogeny of species-typical characteristics. These structured relations produce the cognitive adaptations that are the basis of psychological explication for evolutionary psychologists, and these structured relations must still pass through the sieve of natural selection.

Ontogenetic experiences guide and constrain phenotypic development and thus directly influence how natural selection operates on organisms. Moreover, phenotypic changes resulting from modifications in developmental processes can precede changes in gene frequencies and thus expose animals to novel selection pressures (such as enabling them to inhabit new niches) that result in changes in gene frequencies. From this viewpoint, adaptationist and developmental systems perspectives are compatible, each recognizing the realities of development as a dynamic system, as well as the historical constraints that natural selection has placed on the direction that ontogeny within a species can take. As evolutionary psychologists contend, children have been prepared by evolution for certain experiences and can more readily make sense of some forms of stimulation than others. But prepared is not preformed (Bjorklund, 2003), and although not all evolutionary or developmental psychologists will agree with the integrative position we advocate here, we believe the position adequately resolves the discrepancies between extreme proponents of these two camps and reflects well our current understanding of how both development and evolution "work."

CONCLUSION

Evolutionary developmental psychology is emerging as a new field, the result of the integration of data, theory, and much thought from mainstream developmental and evolutionary psychologists. However, the resulting product in neither the average nor the sum of the two parent disciplines, but a unique perspective that nonetheless is compatible with the major tenets of both developmental and evolutionary psychology. We argue that developmental psychology can greatly benefit from taking an evolutionary perspective without falling into the "trap" of implicit nativism that some developmentalists attribute to evolutionary thinking. Similarly, we contend that evolutionary psychology can benefit from paying more explicit attention to the role of gene–environment interactions, beginning very early in life, without altering its central focus of explaining the behavior of contemporary people in terms of evolved cognitive mechanisms for solving recurrent adaptive problems faced by our ancestors. It is our contention that the study of human nature—the universal cognitive, social, emotional, and behavioral dispositions that have served to adapt our ancestors to their environments and continue to serve contemporary humans—is a worthy pursuit of psychological science. But human nature develops, and any science that ignores either the developmental or evolutionary origins of adaptive functioning is missing an important part of the picture.

REFERENCES

Alexander, R. D. (1989). Evolution of the human psyche. In P. Mellers & C. Stringer (Eds.), *The human revolution: Behavioural and biological perspectives on the origins of modern humans* (pp. 455–513). Princeton, NJ: Princeton University Press.

Bjorklund, D. F. (1987). A note on neonatal imitation. *Developmental Review, 7,* 86–92.

Bjorklund, D. F. (1997). The role of immaturity in human development. *Psychological Bulletin, 122,* 153–169.

Bjorklund, D. F. (2003). Evolutionary psychology from a developmental systems perspective: Comment on Lickliter and Honeycutt (2003). *Psychological Bulletin, 129,* 836–841.

Bjorklund, D. F., & Hernández Blasi, C. (in press). Evolutionary developmental psychology. In D. Buss (Ed.), *Evolutionary psychology handbook.* New York: Wiley.

Bjorklund, D. F., & Harnishfeger, K. K. (1995). The role of inhibition mechanisms in the evolution of human cognition and behavior. In F. N. Dempster & C. J. Brainerd (Eds.), *New perspectives on interference and inhibition in cognition* (pp. 141–173). New York: Academic Press.

Bjorklund, D. F., & Pellegrini, A. D. (2002). *The origins of human nature: Evolutionary developmental psychology.* Washington, DC: American Psychological Association.

Bjorklund, D. F., Yunger, J. L., & Pellegrini, A. D. (2002). The evolution of parenting and evolutionary approaches to childrearing. In M. Bornstein (Ed.), *Handbook of parenting* (2nd ed.), Vol. 1. The biology of parenting (pp. 3–30). Mahwah, NJ: Erlbaum.

Bonner, J. T. (1988). *The evolution of complexity by means of natural selection.* Princeton, NJ: Princeton University Press.

Boyce, W. T., & Ellis, B. J. (in press). Biological sensitivity to context: I. An evolutionary–developmental theory of the origins and functions of stress reactivity. *Development and Psychopathology.*

Bugental, D. B. (2000). Acquisition of the algorithms of social life: A domain-based approach. *Psychological Bulletin, 126,* 187–219.

Buss, D. M., & Reeve, H. K. (2003). Evolutionary psychology and developmental dynamics: Comment on Lickliter and Honeycutt (2003). *Psychological Bulletin, 129,* 848–853.

Crawford, C. B., & Anderson, J. L. (1989). Sociobiology: An environmentalist discipline? *American Psychologist, 44*(12), 1449–1459.

Dunbar, R. I. M. (1998). The social brain hypothesis. *Evolutionary Anthropology, 6,* 178–190.

Eibl-Eibesfeldt, I. (1989) *Human ethology.* New York: Aldine de Gruyter.

Flinn, M. V. (1997). Culture and the evolution of social learning. *Evolution and Human Behavior, 18,* 23–67.

Gangestad, S. W., & Simpson, J. A. (2000). The evolution of human mating: Trade-offs and strategic pluralism. *Behavioral and Brain Sciences, 23,* 573–644.

Geary, D. C. (1998). *Male, female: The evolution of human sex differences.* Washington, DC: American Psychological Association.

Geary, D. C. (1999). Evolution and developmental sex differences. *Current Directions in Psychological Science, 8,* 115–120.

Geary, D. C., & Flinn, M. V. (2001). Evolution of human parental behavior and the human family. *Parenting: Science and Practice, 1,* 5–61.

Gleick, J. (1987). *Chaos: The making of a new science.* Viking Press: New York.

Gottlieb, G. (1991). Experiential canalization of behavioral development: Results. *Developmental Psychology, 27,* 35–39.

Gottlieb, G. (1998). Normally occurring environmental and behavioral influences on gene activity: From central dogma to probabilistic epigenesist. *Psychological Review, 105,* 792–802.

Greene, E. (1989). A diet-induced developmental polymorphism in a caterpillar. *Science, 243,* 643–646.

Greene, E. (1996). Effect of light quality and larval diet on morph induction in the polymorphic caterpillar *Nemoria arizonaria (Lepidoptera: Geometridae). Biological Journal of the Linnean Society, 58*(3), 277–285.

Gross, M. R. (1996). Alternative reproductive strategies and tactics: Diversity within sexes. *Trends in Ecology and Evolution, 11,* 92–98.

Heimann, M. (1989). Neonatal imitation gaze aversion and mother–infant interaction. *Infant Behavior and Development, 12,* 495–505.

Hernández Blasi, C., & Bjorklund, D. F. (2003). Evolutionary developmental psychology: A new tool for better understanding human ontogeny. *Human Development, 46,* 259–281.

Humphrey, N. K. (1976). The social function of intellect. In P. P. G. Bateson & R. Hinde (Eds.), *Growing points in ethology* (pp. 303–317). Cambridge, England: Cambridge University Press.

Kaplan, H., Hill, K., Lancaster, J., & Hurtado, A. M. (2000). A theory of human life history evolution: Diet, intelligence, and longevity. *Evolutionary Anthropology, 9,* 156–185.

Keller, H. (2000). Human parent–child relationships from an evolutionary perspective. *American Behavioral Scientist, 43,* 957–969.

Kelso, J. A. S. (1995). *Dynamic patterns: The self-organization of brain and behavior.* Cambridge, MA: MIT Press.

Lewis, M. D. (2000). The promise of dynamic systems approaches for an integrated account of human development. *Child Development, 71,* 36–43.

Lickliter, R. (1996). Structured organisms and structured environments: Developmental systems and the construction of learning capacities. In J. Valsiner & H. G. Voss (Eds.), *The structure of learning processes* (pp. 86–107). Norwood, NJ: Ablex.

Lickliter, R., & Honeycutt, H. (2003). Developmental dynamics: Towards a biologically plausible evolutionary psychology. *Psychological Bulletin, 129,* 819–835.

Lorenz, K. (1965). *Evolution and modification of behavior.* Chicago: University of Chicago Press.

Meltzoff, M., & Moore, K. (1997). Explaining facial imitation: A theoretical model. *Early Development and Parenting, 6,* 179–192.

Moore, D. S. (2001). *The dependent gene: The fallacy of "nature vs. nurture."* New York: Freeman Books.

Oppenheim, R. W. (1981). Ontogenetic adaptations and retrogressive processes in the development of the nervous system and behavior. In K. J. Connolly & H. F. R. Prechtl (Eds.), *Maturation and development: Biological and psychological perspectives* (pp. 73–108). Philadelphia: International Medical Publications.

Oyama, S. (2001). Terms in tension: What do you do when all the good words are taken? In S. Oyama, P. E. Griffith, & R. D. Gray (Eds.), *Cycles of contingency: Developmental systems and evolution* (pp. 177–194). Cambridge, MA: MIT Press.

Pellegrini, A. D., & Bjorklund, D. F. (2004). The ontogeny and phylogeny of children's object and fantasy play. *Human Nature, 15*, 23–43.

Pellegrini, A. D., & Smith, P. K. (1998). Physical activity play: The nature and function of neglected aspect of play. *Child Development, 69*, 577–598.

Pigliucci, M. (2001). *Phenotypic plasticity: Beyond nature and nurture.* Baltimore, MD: Johns Hopkins University Press.

Schlichting, C. D., & Pigliucci, M. (1998). *Phenotypic evolution: A reaction norm perspective.* Sunderland, MA: Sinauer Associates.

Thelen, E., & Smith, L. B. (1998). Dynamic systems theories. In R. M. Lerner (Vol. Ed.), *Theoretical models of human development*, Vol. 1. In W. Damon (Gen. Ed.), *Handbook of child psychology* (pp. 563–634). New York: Wiley.

Tooby, J., & Cosmides, L. (1992). The psychological foundations of culture. In L. Cosmides, J. Tooby, & J. H. Barkow (Eds.), *The adapted mind* (pp. 19–136). New York: Oxford University Press.

Tooby, J., Cosmides, L., & Barrett, H. C. (2003). The second law of thermodynamics is the first law of psychology: Evolutionary developmental psychology and the theory of tandem, coordinated inheritances: Comment on Lickliter and Honeycutt (2003). *Psychological Bulletin, 129*, 858–865.

Trivers, R. L. (1972). Parental investment and sexual selection. In B. Campbell (Ed.), *Sexual selection and the descent of man* (pp. 136–179). New York: Aldine de Gruyter.

Vallacher, R. R., Read, S. J., & Nowak, A. (2002). The dynamical perspective in personality and social psychology. *Personality and Social Psychology Review, 6*, 265–273.

2

ONTOGENY AND EVOLUTION OF THE SOCIAL CHILD

MARK V. FLINN
CAROL V. WARD

Danny was roaming the Fond Vert area of the village with two of his closest friends on a rainy Saturday morning. They had eaten their fill of mangoes, after pelting a heavily laden tree with stones for nearly an hour, taking turns testing their skill at knocking down breakfast. Now Danny was up the cashew tree in Mr. Pascal's yard, tossing the yellow and red fruits to the smaller children below who had gathered to benefit from this kindness. Suddenly the sharp voice of his stepfather rang out from the nearby footpath. The bird-like chatter and laughter of the children immediately stopped. Danny's hand froze midway to its next prize, and with a mixed expression of surprise and fright, he turned his head to face the direction of the yell. Ordered down from the tree, Danny quickly headed home, head bowed in apparent numb submission.[1] Danny's cortisol (a stress hormone) level, measured from his saliva collected several times a day, rose from 2.2 to 3.8 µg/dl in little more than an hour. That afternoon, his secretory immunoglobulin-A levels dropped from 5.70 to 3.83 mg/dl. Three days later he had common cold symptoms: runny nose, headache, and fever. His two companions did not suffer the same fate, instead resuming their morning play, exhibiting a normal circadian decline in cortisol, and remaining healthy over the next 2 weeks.

This case example contributes to a common pattern. Children in this rural Dominican community are more than twice as likely to become ill during the week following a stressful event than children who have not recently experienced any significant stressors (Flinn & England, 2003). People everywhere appear sensitive to their social environments, often with negative consequences for their health (Cohen, Doyle, Turner, Alper, & Skoner, 2003; Maier, Watkins, & Fleschner, 1994; Marmot & Wilkinson, 1999). Mortality rates for children in orphanages and hospitals in early 20th-century America, lacking the evolutionarily normal intimacy of the family, were appalling (e.g., Chapin, 1922, p. 214). It is not lack of food or hygienic care, nor just the occurrence of traumatic events that affect child health, but the lack of social support, including parental warmth and other factors that influence emotional states (Belsky, 1997; Davidson, Jackson, & Kalin, 2001; Field, Diego, Hernandez-Reif, Schanberg, & Kuhn, 2003). Why should this be so? Why do social interactions, and a child's perceptions of them, affect physiology and morbidity? And, more generally, why is the social environment of such paramount importance in a child's world?

In Danny's village, located on the east coast of the island of Dominica, where one of us (MVF) has lived and studied over the past 16 years, most of a child's mental efforts seem focused on negotiating social relationships with parents, siblings, grandparents, cousins and other kin, friends, teachers, bus drivers, neighbors, shop owners, and so forth. Foraging for mangoes and guavas, hunting birds with catapults (i.e., "slingshots"), or even fishing in the sea from rock cliffs are relatively simple cognitive enterprises, complicated by children's conflicts with property owners and decisions about which companions to choose for garnering and sharing calories. After a few weeks of playing together, the foraging behaviors of our 9-year-old son were nearly indistinguishable from those of Danny and his other village peers. Even a novice readily acquires what initially appear to be remarkable skills. The mind of the child seems more taxed by solving social puzzles than by utilitarian concerns of collecting food.

In this chapter, we examine potential evolutionary linkages between these two most distinctive human characteristics: childhood and the social mind. We begin with a review of current theories of human life history and the family. We then evaluate the different models for the evolution of human childhood, emphasizing evidence from the fossil record. We argue that conspecific social competition was the primary selective pressure shaping the uniquely human combination of physically altricial but mentally and linguistically precocial infancy, extended childhood, and extended adolescence, enabled by extensive biparental and kin care.

EVOLUTION OF CHILDHOOD

Most of us see a picture of innocence and helplessness: a clean slate. But, in fact, what we see in the crib is the greatest mind that has ever existed, the most powerful learning machine in the universe.
—GOPNIK, MELTZOFF, AND KUHL (1999, p. 1)

The human child is a most extraordinary organism, possessed of "the greatest mind" and yet "innocent and helpless"—in effect, a larva equipped with an enormous brain. This is contrary to the general pattern among mammals: Precocial species have neonatal brain sizes twice those of comparable altricial species (Martin & MacLarnon, 1990). Even relative to other primates the human infant is unusually altricial, and highly dependent upon parents and other relatives for protection, transport, resources (e.g., food), and information (Lamb, Bornstein, & Teti, 2002). Humans, moreover, have an extended juvenile period, unlike most other altricial young, who use their protected environments to grow and mature rapidly (e.g., Ricklefs, 1983). Parental and other kin investment continues for an unusually long time, often well into adulthood and perhaps even after the death of the parents.

The selective pressures responsible for this unique suite of life-history characteristics appear central to understanding human evolution (Alexander, 1987, 1990a, 1990b, 2003; Bjorklund & Pellegrini, 2002; Blurton Jones, Hawkes, & O'Connell, 1999, 2002; Hill & Hurtado, 1996a, 1996b; Jolly, 1966, 1999; Kaplan, Hill, Lancaster, & Hurtado, 2000; Lancaster & Lancaster, 1987; Low, 2001; Mace, 2000). The delay of reproduction until almost 20 years of age, nearly double that of our hominoid relatives, the chimpanzees and gorillas (Zihlman, Bolter, & Boesch, 2004), involves prolonged exposure to extrinsic causes of mortality and longer generation intervals. What advantages of an extended childhood could have outweighed the heavy costs of reduced fecundity and late reproduction (Williams, 1966; Stearns, 1992) for our hominin[2] ancestors?

The physical growth of the child, although unusual in its temporal pattern (Bogin, 1999; Leigh, 2001), does not appear to involve especially significant challenges. The relatively slow rate of overall body growth during childhood, followed by a rapid growth spurt during puberty, may economize parental resources supporting dependent offspring. A small child requires fewer resources than a large one. Hence, delayed physical growth during childhood may have facilitated shortened birth intervals, providing a demographic advantage (Bogin & Silva, 2003).

Brain growth, however, has a different trend than overall body growth. The baby human has a large brain, with high energetic and developmental costs that use more than half (!) of its total metabolism (Holliday, 1986; Leonard & Robertson, 1994; Passmore & Durnin, 1955). Although neurogenesis is mostly completed by middle childhood, reproduction is postponed for more than a decade. What aspects of the phenotype require so much additional development? And why burden the growing child, and its caregivers, with a brain that requires so much energy for so long?

One possibility is that these anomalous patterns of brain and physical growth during human childhood are not adaptations per se, but instead are inadvertent outcomes of basic growth processes such as neoteny and heterochrony (Schultz, 1969; Gould, 1977; see also Lovejoy, 1981). Perhaps selection for an extended lifetime or increased body size involved mechanisms that could not adaptively fine-tune life history stages or growth of different parts of the phenotype. The extended juvenile period, for example, may be interpreted as an incidental outcome of selection for a longer lifespan in general. From this perspective, human childhood and the big brain were viewed in the context of major developmental processes that constrain adaptive solutions (Finlay, Darlington, & Nicastro, 2001).

The recent integration of molecular genetics with evolutionary developmental biology, however, has provided a more nuanced view of the constraints on ontogeny. Detailed knowledge of developmental mechanisms at the genetic and cellular levels (e.g., Gerhart & Kirshner, 1998) has important implications for understanding the evolution of human life histories (Finch & Sapolsky, 1999; Konner, 1991; Lovejoy, McCollum, Reno, & Rosenman, 2003). The broad scaling trends among life history events suggested by Schultz (1969) and Gould (1977), in which all phases of the lifespan remain proportional when lifespan is altered, do not accord with recent comparative analyses that indicate these more specific mechanisms result in diverse and species-specific ontogenies (Leigh, 2001; West-Eberhard, 2003). Human childhood is not likely to be an inadvertent consequence of selection for an extended lifetime or some other life history constraint (Alexander, 1987). We need a functional evolutionary explanation for this "most powerful learning machine in the universe."

THE FORAGING "PRACTICE" MODEL

Human childhood has traditionally been viewed as a period of edification: "Immatures are enabled to live a protected existence whilst they learn skills necessary for adult life" (Bowlby, 1969, p. 63). The primary question has been: What information is so important and difficult to acquire that many years are needed for its mastery? Most juvenile primates spend considerable effort playing and practicing with their physical environment and developing fighting skills (e.g., Symons, 1978; Pellegrini & Archer, Chapter 9, this volume). Compared with other primates, our motor skills do not appear especially challenging; a terrestrial environment seems more easily mastered than an arboreal one. Children may need time to acquire knowledge for tool use and complex foraging, including hunting (Darwin, 1871; Hill & Kaplan, 1999; see also Byrne, 2002a, 2002b). An extraordinarily long developmental apprenticeship is seen as useful for acquiring learned solutions to ecological problems unique to our niche (Bock, 2002). Investment in "embodied capital," via an extended childhood, has been suggested to have a fitness payoff from increased adult foraging ability (Kaplan et al., 2000).

Studies of the effects of childhood experience on subsequent adult foraging efficiency, however, do not provide clear support for the "practice" model. Ethnographic accounts of childhood have long suggested a lack of urgency or focus on training of foraging skills relative to other activities in many human societies (e.g., Chagnon, 1977; Levine, Miller, & West, 1988; Whiting & Edwards, 1988; Hirschfeld, 2002). Specific tests of the effects of childhood foraging practice on adult performance indicate little benefit from training; relatively inexperienced individuals appear to perform equal to their more experienced peers (Blurton Jones & Marlowe, 2002). Children, moreover, are capable of some types of complex foraging at an early age, suggesting that a long apprenticeship is not necessary (Bliege Bird & Bird, 2002). Previous observations of adult foraging advantage may be more appropriately interpreted as a consequence of physical size and maturity rather than from finely honed acquired skills (Bird & Bliege Bird, 2002; Blurton Jones & Marlowe, 2002). In addition to failing to support the "childhood as foraging practice" model, these studies cast further doubt on the hypothesis that physical growth is delayed to conserve parental resources, because if size is a primary determinant of foraging efficiency, then precocial early growth would seem adaptive.

Childhood as an extended "practice" period is also difficult to reconcile with the recent argument that the human brain is at least partly the evolutionary result of a Fisherian sexual selection process (Miller, 2000). From this perspective, mental abilities are viewed as a human equivalent to the peacock's tail, an ornament whose primary function is to attract mates. The development of most sexually selected ornaments and weapons (e.g., antlers, bright coloration), however, are temporally associated with sexual maturity (Andersson, 1994). For example, among many species of birds, the parts of the brain involved with the production of song are influenced by androgens released in response to the breeding season (see review in Kelley & Brenowitz, 2002). The precocial ontogeny of brain and mind during infancy and childhood seems ill suited to an ornamental courtship function during early adulthood. Why develop and maintain such a costly display so many years before (and after!) its use to attract mates? This temporal disjunction seems contrary to a Zahavian "handicap" function as well, in which apparently nonfunctional traits are maintained to illustrate sufficient genetic quality to overcome the handicap.

THE ECOLOGICAL
DOMINANCE–SOCIAL COMPLEXITY MODEL

A different approach to the problem of the evolution of human childhood involves consideration of the brain as a "social tool" (Alexander, 1971, 1989; Bjorklund & Rosenberg, Chapter 3, this volume; Brothers, 1990; Byrne & Whiten, 1988; Dunbar, 1998; Humphrey, 1976, 1983). This hypothesis suggests that many human cognitive and psychological adaptations function primarily to contend with social relationships, with ecological constraints (e.g., hunting or extractive foraging) being a more secondary source of recent evolutionary change. It appears that some human cognitive competencies, such as theory of mind and language, are most readily understood in terms of social selection pressures, although cognitive competencies for interacting with the physical (e.g., navigating) and biological world are evident as well (Geary & Huffman, 2002). The primary mental chess game shaping the distinctive changes in the neocortex (Adolphs, 2003; Allman, Hakeem, Erwin, Nimchinsky, & Hof, 2001), however, was with other intelligent hominin competitors and cooperators, not with fruits, tools, prey, or snow. Human social relationships are complex and variable. Predicting future moves of a social competitor–cooperator, and appropriate countermoves, amplified by networks of multiple relationships, shifting coalitions, and deception, make social success a difficult undertaking (Alexander, 1987, 1990a; Daly & Wilson, 1988a, 1988b; Henrich et al., 2001; Stanford, 2001; de Waal, 1982, 2001).

Indeed, the potential variety of human social puzzles is apparently infinite; no two social situations are precisely identical, nor are any two individuals ever in exactly the same social environment. Moreover, social relationships can change rapidly, requiring quick modification of strategy. Variability in these dynamics creates conditions that should favor the evolution of brain and cognitive systems above and beyond more traditional modular systems (Fodor, 1983; Tooby & Cosmides, 1995). These systems have been cast in terms of general intelligence, domain-general abilities, or executive functions that are capable of integrating and co-opting information processed by more restricted, domain-specific mechanisms (e.g., Adolphs, 2003; Geary, 2005; Hirschfeld & Gelman, 1994; cf. La Cerra & Bingham, 1998; Quartz & Sejnowski, 1999) and using mental simulations, or "scenario-building" (Alexander, 1989), to construct and rehearse potential responses to changing social conditions. These complex cognitive processes would be more capable of contending with, and producing, novelties of cultural change and individual-specific differences (Bjorklund & Rosenberg, Chapter 3, this volume; Flinn, 1997; Tomasello, 1999).

Childhood, therefore, evolved as a mechanism whereby individuals can develop these necessary social skills (Joffe, 1997). Learning, practice, and experience are imperative for social success. Social competencies require complex cognitive problem-solving abilities perhaps significantly greater than that involved with foraging skills. An extended human childhood can be directly attributed to the selection for development of a social brain that requires a lengthy ontogeny to master complex dynamic tasks such as moral reasoning (Alexander, 1987; Campbell & Muncer, 1998).

While it is widely recognized that human childhood is a learning period, there is discussion about what necessary skills are the driving force behind increased time for learning to take place. The "social tool" hypothesis to explain human intelligence was initially considered to suffer from similar limitations as the physical environment hypotheses. Comparative analyses indicated that group size and proxy measures for brain size (e.g., cranial capacity, neocortex ratios) were associated in a wide range of taxa, including primates (e.g., Kudo & Dunbar, 2001; Pawlowski, Lowen, & Dunbar, 1998; van Schaik & Deaner, 2003; see also Byrne & Corp, 2004). A major problem, however, remained unresolved: Given that hominin group size was unlikely to have been larger than that of close relatives (the other hominoids), what was qualitatively different about the hominin social environment? Of course, the most appropriate comparisons would include other species of *Homo* as well as australopithecines (Povinelli & Bering, 2002), but unfortunately these species are now extinct. Why did hominins in particular form more socially complex groups, hence creating an environment in which more sophisticated forms of social cognition (e.g., theory of mind) and general intelligence would have been favored by natural selection? Why were coalitions more important, and more cognitively taxing, for our hominin ancestors than they were for any other species in the history of life? Why did hominins evolve special cognitive abilities such as "understanding other persons as intentional agents" (Tomasello, 1999, p. 526)? Richard Alexander (1989, 1990a) suggests the following solution:

> Humans had in some unique fashion become so ecologically dominant that they in effect became their own principal hostile force of nature, explicitly in regard to evolutionary changes in the human psyche and social behavior. . . . The real challenge in the human environment throughout history that affected the evolution of the intellect was not climate, weather, food shortages, or parasites—not even predators. Rather, it was the necessity of dealing continually with our fellow humans in social circumstances that became ever more complex and unpredictable as the human line evolved. Social cleverness, especially through success in competition achieved by cooperation, becomes paramount. . . . Nothing would select more potently for increased social intelligence . . . than a within-species co-evolutionary arms race in which success depended on effectiveness in social competition. (1990a, pp. 4–7)

Alexander's scenario posits that hominins increasingly became an "ecologically dominant" species. Evidence that humans evolved into ecologically dominant predators and foragers comes from patterns of human migration and demography, as well as our variable and flexible subsistence strategies. Darwin and Wallace's (1858, p. 54) conceptualization of natural selection as a "struggle for existence" becomes in addition a *struggle with other human beings for control* of the resources that support life and allow one to reproduce. In this situation, the stage is set for a form of runaway selection, whereby the more cognitively, socially, and behaviorally sophisticated individuals are able to out maneuver and manipulate other individuals in order to gain control of resources in the local ecology, and to gain control of the behavior of other people. To the extent that access to these resources covaries with survival and reproductive outcomes—and it does in many contexts (Betzig, 1986; Chagnon, 1988; Flinn, 1986; Hed, 1987; Irons, 1979; Malthus, 1798; United Nations, 1985)—the associated sociocognitive competencies, and supporting brain systems, would be favored by natural selection.

In other words, to the extent that ecological dominance was achieved, humans became "their own principal hostile force of nature" (Alexander, 1989, p. 469) via inter- and intragroup competition and cooperation. Increasing linguistic and sociocognitive capacities were favored, because such skills allowed individuals to better anticipate and influence social interactions with other increasingly intelligent humans. This "runaway" directional selection produced greater and greater modular (e.g., language, theory of mind) and more general cognitive competencies, because success was based on relative (rather than absolute) levels of ability. Unlike static ecological challenges, the hominin social environment became an autocatalytic process, ratcheting up the selective advantage associated with the ability to anticipate the social strategies of other hominins and to simulate mentally and evaluate potential counterstrategies (Alexander, 1989). Modular competencies allowed hominins quickly and efficiently to process social information that was static, or invariant, across generations and contexts (e.g., the ability to read basic human facial expressions), whereas the more variable and, thus, less predictable features of one-on-one and coalitional social relationships favored the ability mentally to construct and manipulate a range of potential social scenarios. These more general competencies are known as working memory, attentional control, and executive functions (e.g., Baddeley, 1986; Engle, 2002; for review, see Allman, 1999; Geary, 2005). Practice during childhood for the development of social skills using these components is paramount (Bjorklund & Pellegrini, 2002) and likely to be facilitated by a protective and informative family environment.

EVOLUTION OF THE HUMAN FAMILY AS A NEST FOR THE CHILD'S SOCIAL MIND

The human family is extraordinary and unique in many respects (Alexander, 1989, 2004; Geary & Flinn, 2001; Lancaster & Lancaster, 1983). Humans are the only species to live in multimale groups with complex coalitions and extensive paternal care. Humans have concealed ovulation, altricial infants, lengthy child development, female orgasm, and menopause. These traits may be causally linked and provide important clues toward reconstructing the evolution of our (human) unusual life history.

The altricial infant is indicative of a protective environment provided by intense parenting and alloparenting in the context of kin groups (Chisholm, 1999). The human baby does not need to be physically precocial. Rather than investing in the development of locomotion, defense, and food acquisition systems that function early in ontogeny, the infant can work instead toward building a more effective adult phenotype. The brain continues rapid growth, and the corresponding cognitive competencies largely direct attention toward the social environment. Plastic neural systems adapt to the nuances of the local community, such as its language (Alexander, 1990b; Bjorklund &

Pellegrini, 2002; Bloom, 2000; Geary & Bjorklund, 2000; Geary & Huffman, 2002; Small, 1998, 2001). In contrast to the slow development of ecological skills of movement, fighting, and feeding, the human infant rapidly acquires skill with the complex communication system of human language (Pinker, 1994, 1997). The extraordinary information-transfer abilities enabled by linguistic competency provide a conduit to the knowledge available in other human minds. This emergent capability for intensive and extensive communication potentiates the social dynamics characteristic of human groups (Dunbar, 1997) and provides a new mechanism for social learning and culture. The recursive pattern recognition and abstract symbolic representation central to linguistic competencies enable the open-ended, creative, and flexible information-processing characteristic of humans—especially of children.

An extended childhood appears useful for acquiring the knowledge and practice to hone social skills and to build coalitional relationships necessary for successful negotiation of the increasingly intense social competition of adolescence and adulthood, although ecologically related play and activities (e.g., exploration of the physical environment) occur as well. The unusual scheduling of human reproductive maturity, including an "adrenarche" and a delay in direct mate competition among males (Herdt & McClintock, 2000; McClintock & Herdt, 1996) appears to extend the period of practicing social roles and extends social ontogeny.

The advantages of intensive parenting, including paternal protection and other care, require a most unusual pattern of mating relationships: moderately exclusive pair bonding in multiple-male groups. No other primate (or mammal) that lives in large, cooperative multiple-reproductive-male groups has extensive male parental care, although some protection by males is evident in baboons (Buchan, Alberts, Silk, & Altmann, 2003). The only other primates that have paternal care (e.g., indris, marmosets, tamarins, titi monkeys, night monkeys, and to a lesser extent, gibbons and gorillas) do not live in large groups. Competition for females in multiple-male groups usually results in low confidence of paternity (e.g., chimpanzees). Males forming exclusive "pair-bonds" in multiple-male groups would provide cues of nonpaternity to other males, and hence place their offspring in great danger of infanticide (Hrdy, 1999). Paternal care is most likely to be favored by natural selection in conditions where males can identify their offspring with sufficient probability to offset the costs of investment, although reciprocity with mates is also likely to be involved (Smuts, 1985; Smuts & Smuts, 1993). Humans exhibit a unique "nested family" social structure, involving complex reciprocity among males and females to restrict direct competition for mates among group members. It is difficult to imagine how this system could be maintained in the absence of another unusual human trait: concealed ovulation (Alexander & Noonan, 1979). Human groups tend to be male philopatric (males tending to remain in their natal groups), resulting in extensive male kin alliances, useful for competing against other groups of male kin (Chagnon, 1988; Wrangham & Peterson, 1996; LeBlanc, 2003). Females also have complex alliances but usually are not involved directly in the overt physical aggression characteristic of intergroup relations (Campbell, 2002; Geary & Flinn, 2002). Menopause reduces mortality risks for older women and allows them to concentrate effort on dependent children and other relatives (e.g., grandchildren) with high reproductive value (Alexander, 1974; Hawkes, 2003; cf. Hill & Hurtado, 1996b). Parents and other kin may be especially important for the child's mental development of social maps, because they can be relied upon as landmarks that provide relatively honest information. We suggest that the evolutionary significance of the human family in regard to child development is more as a nest from which social skills may be acquired than as an economic unit centered on the sexual division of labor.

THE FOSSIL RECORD

The fossil record is the single source of information we have for documenting the order and timing of acquisition of key human characteristics. For example, the discovery of the Taung skull (*Australopithecus africanus*; Dart, 1925) disproved the notion that upright, bipedal locomotion in hominin evolution was accompanied by significant brain expansion. We now have substantial data documenting that hominins were bipedal for at least 2 (Leakey, Feibel, MacDougall, & Walker, 1995; White, Suwa, & Asfaw, 1994), and perhaps as long as 4 (Brunet et al., 2002; Haile-Selassie, 2001; Senut, 2002, Senut et al., 2001), million years prior to the emergence of the genus *Homo* and the accompanying significant increases in brain size.

Paleontological data, therefore, provide a critical test of hypotheses about how and why humans evolved. We can use these data to explore associations among the evolution of childhood and other attributes such as intelligence, social dynamics, and ecology, testing the hypothesis that childhood evolved as a mechanism for developing social competency (Alexander, Hoogland, Howard, Noonan, & Sherman, 1979; Clutton-Brock, 1977; Dunbar, 1998; Foley, 1999; Plavcan, Van Schaik, & Kappeler, 1995), although definitive conclusions are difficult to achieve (Plavcan, 2000). This hypothesis is based on the argument that human intelligence evolved as a response to social competition in an ecologically dominant species (ecological dominance–social competition, or EDSC model), described in detail elsewhere (Flinn, Geary, & Ward, 2004). Specifically, we predict that evidence for prolongation of childhood should co-occur with increased intelligence and social complexity, and accompany or postdate significant changes in ecological dominance (see Bjorklund & Rosenberg, Chapter 3, this volume).

The fossil record indicates that during the past 4 million years, there has been a threefold increase in brain volume (Figure 2.1a), a significant reduction in the magnitude of the sex difference in physical size (Figure 2.1b), a disappearance of related species of hominins, and a near-doubling of the length of the developmental period (Figure 2.1c). As displayed in Figure 2.1c, in most

selective pressure for childhood itself as a stage per se. In other words, altriciality likely evolved for somewhat separate reasons from an adolescent growth spurt, and has thus appeared at different times in human evolutionary history.

The first hominin to have had relatively altricial infants was probably *Homo erectus*, roughly 1.8 mya. Female pelvic dimensions are constrained by locomotor and thermoregulatory requirements, so birth canal size in *H. erectus* was not substantially larger than in australopithecines (Begun & Walker, 1993). Adult brain sizes, however, were nearly doubled (650–900 cc in early *H. erectus* compared with 380–610 cc in *Australopithecus*; reviewed in Lee & Wolpoff, 2003). This means that in order to have appropriate neonatal proportions relative to the size of the mother's pelvic inlet, infants must have been born at a relatively small size and been relatively altricial early (Portman, 1941), likely with rapid fetal rates of postnatal brain growth (Martin, 1983). Early *Homo* individuals thus do not appear to have attained adult brain size simply by prolonging growth, given their relatively rapid rates of development (Deacon, 1997; Dean et al., 2001; Leigh, 2001; Smith, 1993). Having more altricial infants would have required more intensive parenting by the mother (see Rosenberg, 1992) and, given the decrease in sexual dimorphism occurring at this time (which may signal pair-bonding), perhaps also by the father and/ or alloparental caregivers.

Despite these ontogenetic shifts associated with the timing of birth, delayed maturation does not appear to have occurred until later in hominin evolution. Development of the dentition as a whole appears correlated with life history variables such as age at sexual maturity in primates and other mammals (e.g., Smith, 1989), and so can be used to infer the timing of important life history stages. Dental crown formation times are correlated with brain size, and therefore to life histories (e.g., Beynon, Dean, & Reid, 1991; Beynon & Dean, 1987; Bromage, 1991; but see Macho & Wood, 1995; Macho, 2001). Early *H. erectus* appears to have had relatively rapid development, similar in rate to *Australopithecus* and great apes, whereas that of modern humans is much slower (Dean et al., 2001).

Coincident with its rapid rate of development, early *H. erectus* (1.6 mya) is interpreted as having lacked a human-like adolescent growth spurt, based on the fact that the single known juvenile skeleton, KNM-WT 15000, had accelerated dental relative to postcranial skeletal development, typical of the pattern seen in humans prior to the growth spurt (Smith, 1993). There are no comprehensive data on rates of child development for hominins between 1.6 mya and 60 thousand years ago (kya), but the single Neandertal specimen examined by Dean and colleagues (2001) was modern in its dental developmental trajectory, indicating that a human-like extended childhood had occurred by this time. The apparently large brain relative to dental development observed for some Neandertal individuals (e.g., Dean, Stringer, & Bromage, 1986) may simply reflect the relatively larger adult brain in many Neandertal individuals as compared with modern humans (see Lee &

Wolpoff, 2003, for summary data). A modern human pattern of dental development was present by 800 kya (Bermudez de Castro et al., 1999), perhaps suggesting delayed maturation (Smith, 1994), but this may not imply a similar rate to modern humans (Dean et al., 2001). If it does, it might be reasonable to hypothesize that the human adolescent growth spurt was already in place by this time as well.

Longevity appears to have increased gradually from *Australopithecus* to humans with a higher proportion of individuals living to old age in the Earlyu Upper Paleolithic (Caspari & Lee, 2004). If ecological dominance reduced mortality from extrinsic causes, this would allow for selection for delayed reproduction and extended life histories (Williams, 1957). Taking all the data together, it appears that the evolution of altriciality may have begun with brain expansion, but that delayed maturation and an adolescent growth spurt may have evolved later in human evolution, perhaps as brain-size increase continued throughout the Pleistocene.

If these developmental shifts that resulted in a prolonged childhood were the result of selection for social learning, we would predict they should occur in the context of increasing social complexity. One key change in hominin social structure is the increasing stability of male–female pair-bonds and associated male coalitionary behavior. The best indicator of these behaviors in the fossil record is sexual dimorphism. Reduced body mass dimorphism is associated with both monogamy (Plavcan, 2000, 2001) and male coalitionary behavior (Pawlowski et al., 1998; Plavcan et al., 1995) in extant primates. Although the large canine-size dimorphism that characterizes all living and fossil great apes had greatly diminished in *Australopithecus* (Ward, Leakey, & Walker, 2001; Ward, Walker, & Leakey, 1999), the reduced body mass dimorphism typical of modern humans did not occur until sometime during the evolution of *H. erectus* (McHenry, 1992a, 1992b, 1994; cf. Reno, Meindl, McCollum, & Lovejoy, 2003). The body mass increase accompanying the origin of *H. erectus* suggests that female body size increased from the australopithecine condition more than did male body size. Body mass dimorphism in early *H. erectus* is difficult to estimate accurately, but disparities in size and robusticity among even early *H. erectus* crania are less than in australopithecine species, signaling a reduction in body size sexual dimorphism. By the early mid-Pleistocene, body mass dimorphism was similar to that found in modern humans (McHenry, 1994; Ruff, Trinkaus, & Holliday, 1997). The changes in social behavior accompanying the shift in mating and parenting strategies are likely to have presented novel cognitive challenges involving complex reciprocity among coalition members (Steele, 1996). Unlike gorillas, with one-male breeding groups, and chimps, with promiscuous mating and little male parental behavior, the evolving hominins were faced with the difficulties of managing increasingly exclusive pair-bonds in the midst of increasingly large coalitions of potential mate competitors.

One approach to interpreting hominin social behavior evolution would be to assume that the behavioral characteristics of the ancestor common to the australopithecine species and humans were similar to those observed in modern chimpanzees (*Pan troglodytes*) or bonobos (*Pan paniscus*) (de Waal & Lanting, 1997; Kano, 1992; Wrangham, 1999; Wrangham & Peterson, 1996; Zihlman, Cronin, Cramer, & Sarich, 1978). This is a reasonable assumption in some respects. Brain size relative to body size in chimpanzees, bonobos, australopithecines, and, presumably, the common ancestor was very similar (McHenry, 1994). However, sexual dimorphism in body weight is about 20% for chimpanzees and bonobos (Goodall, 1986; Kano, 1992). Although bonobo males are not known to show consistent coalitional aggression, male-on-male physical aggression is common and, presumably, a feature of the ancestor common to chimpanzees and bonobos (Wrangham, 1999). In any case, the degree of body mass dimorphism in chimpanzees and bonobos is considerably lower than that estimated for *A. anamensis* (Ward et al., 1999, 2001) and *A. afarensis* (McHenry, 1992b; but see Reno et al., 2003), in which males were much larger than females. The contrast suggests that the reproductive strategies of australopithecines may have differed in some respects from that of male chimpanzees or bonobos; thus, the social patterns found with chimpanzees and bonobos might not fully capture the social dynamics in australopithecines, or the selective pressures that favored larger females in the transition to *Homo*. *Australopithecus* body mass dimorphism suggests that these early hominins were polygynous, because significant mass dimorphism is not associated with monogamy in any extant primate (Plavcan, 2001). Thus, data from the hominin fossil record suggest that not only were developmental shifts resulting in the evolution of human childhood somewhat decoupled in human evolution but they also co-occurred with indicators of increasing social complexity, such as brain-size expansion and decreased sexual dimorphism. Moreover, they do not appear to be correlated with significant shifts in dietary or ecological variables (reviewed in Flinn et al., 2004).

CONCLUDING REMARKS:
CULTURE AND ONTOGENY OF THE SOCIAL MIND

Human childhood functions to create successful adults. In particular, it is a time that allows a child to master the mental processing skills necessary to negotiate the complex social and cultural interactions necessary for success as an adult. Humans are unique in the extraordinary levels of novelty that are generated by the processing of abstract mental representations. Human culture is cumulative; human cognition produces new ideas built upon the old. To a degree that far surpasses that of any other species, human mental processes must contend with a constantly changing information environment of their own creation. Cultural information may be especially dynamic, because it is a fundamental aspect of human social coalitions. Apparently arbitrary changes in cultural traits such as clothing styles, music, art, food, dialects, and so on, may reflect information "arms races" among and within coalitions. The remarkable developmental plasticity and cross-domain integration of some cognitive mechanisms may be products of selection for special sensitivity to variable social context (e.g., Boyer, 2001; Carruthers, 2000; Adolphs, 2003; Mithin, 1996). Human "culture" is not just a pool or source of information; it is an arena and theater of social manipulation and competition via cooperation. Culture is contested because it is a contest. Success at social manipulation and cooperation requires a lifetime of learning, starting at birth.

Data from comparative studies and the fossil record support the hypothesis that it is social competition that selects for intelligence in an ecologically dominant species. Dietary and ecological variables, and associated learning, do not appear to require years of learning to master and are not well correlated with changes in life history stages or indicators of cognitive sophistication in the paleontological record. The prolonged childhood of humans results from at least two separate factors; it is not the result of a single evolutionary process. It begins with the relatively early birth of altricial infants necessitated by enlargement of the brain coupled with constraints on maternal pelvic size imposed by locomotion and thermoregulatory requirements. This initial life history shift occurred early with the evolution of early *H. erectus* and initial brain-size expansion. Slower maturation rates and prolongation of a juvenile role via an adolescent growth spurt appear to have accompanied the origin of earliest *H. sapiens* later in the Pleistocene. The fossil record is too sparse to detect whether this change occurred gradually with brain expansion (Lee & Wolpoff, 2003), but we would predict that it did. Delayed maturation, therefore, may also have accompanied greater longevity (Caspari & Lee, 2004). With the origin of *Homo*, there is evidence of increased reliance on meat in the diet, but as brain size continued to expand, no clear dietary changes were evident. Diverse ecologies were encountered by the various hominin populations, indicating increased ecological dominance and flexibility. Still, the apparent lack of need for years of practice for some types of foraging casts serious doubt on ecological factors being the driving force behind intelligence (Blurton Jones & Marlowe, 2002; Bliege Bird & Bird, 2002).

Returning to the anecdotal example at the beginning of this chapter, consider the relations among stress, health, and culture. People in difficult social environments tend to be less healthy in comparison with their more fortunate peers (e.g., Flinn, 1999; Dressler & Bindon, 2000; Wilkinson, 2001; Cohen et al., 2003). Social support has reproductive consequences (e.g., Silk, Alberts, & Altmann, 2003). The obvious explanation of a better physical environment—improved housing, work conditions, nutrition, health care, and reduced exposure to pathogens and poisons—is insufficient (Marmot et al., 1991; Ellis, 1994). The specific mechanisms underlying the association between socioeconomic conditions and health are uncertain. Psychosocial stress and associated immunosuppression are possible intermediaries (Adler et al., 1994; Kiecolt-Glaser, Malarkey, Cacioppo, & Glaser, 1994). If the brain evolved as a social tool, then the expenditure of somatic resources to resolve psychosocial problems makes sense. Relationships are of paramount importance. Children elevate their stress hormone (cortisol) levels much more frequently and extensively in response to psychosocial stimuli than to challenges associated with foraging (Flinn, Quinlan, Turner, Decker, & England, 1996). The adaptive effects of the major stress hormones on neural reorganization (Huether, 1996, 1998) are consistent with the observation that children are especially sensitive to their social worlds (Flinn, 1999). "Environmental stimuli (in children mainly psychosocial challenges and demands) exert profound effects in neuronal activity through repeated or long-lasting changes in the release of transmitters and hormones which contribute, as trophic, organizing signals, to the stabilization [Norepinephrine] or destabilization [Cortisol] of neuronal networks in the developing brain" (Huether, 1998, p. 297).

Social competence is extraordinarily difficult, because the target is constantly changing and similarly equipped with theory of mind and other cognitive abilities. The sensitivity of the stress–response system to the social environment enables adaptive neural reorganization to this most salient and dynamic puzzle (Beylin & Shors, 2003). Childhood is necessary and useful for acquiring the information and practice to build and refine the mental algorithms critical for negotiating the social coalitions that are key to success in our species.

NOTES

1. From MVF field notes, July 1994.
2. "Hominin" refers to taxa more closely related to humans than to chimpanzees.

REFERENCES

Adler, N. E., Boyce, T., Chesney, M. A., Cohen, S., Folkman, S., Kahn, R. L., et al. (1994). Socioeconomic status and health. *American Psychologist, 49*, 15–24.

Adolphs, R. (2003). Cognitive neuroscience of human social behavior. *Nature Reviews, Neuroscience, 4*, 165–178.

Alexander, R. D. (1971). The search for an evolutionary philosophy of man. *Proceedings of the Royal Society of Victoria, 84*, 99–120.

Alexander, R. D. (1974). The evolution of social behavior. *Annual Review of Ecology and Systematics, 5*, 325–383.

Alexander, R. D. (1987). *The biology of moral systems.* Hawthorne, NY: Aldine de Gruyter.

Alexander, R. D. (1989). Evolution of the human psyche. In P. Mellars & C. Stringer (Eds.), *The human revolution: Behavioural and biological perspectives on the origins of modern humans* (pp. 455–513). Princeton, NJ: Princeton University Press.

Alexander, R. D. (1990a). *How did humans evolve?: Reflections on the uniquely unique species* (Museum of Zoology Special Publication No. 1). Ann Arbor: University of Michigan.

Alexander, R. D. (1990b). Epigenetic rules and Darwinian algorithms: The adaptive study of learning and development. *Ethology and Sociobiology, 11*, 1–63.

Alexander, R. D. (2004). Evolutionary selection and the nature of humanity. In V. Hosle & C. H. Illies (Eds.), *Darwinism and philosophy*. Notre Dame, IN: University of Notre Dame Press.

Alexander, R. D., Hoogland, J. L., Howard, R. D., Noonan, K. M., & Sherman, P. W. (1979). Sexual dimorphisms and breeding systems in pinnipeds, ungulates, primates, and humans. In N. A. Chagnon & W. Irons (Eds.), *Evolutionary biology and human social behavior: An anthropological perspective* (pp. 402–435). North Scituate, MA: Duxbury Press.

Alexander, R. D., & Noonan, K. M. (1979). Concealment of ovulation, parental care, and human social evolution. In N. A. Chagnon & W. Irons (Eds.), *Evolutionary biology and human social behavior: An anthropological perspective* (pp. 436–453). North Scituate, MA: Duxbury Press.

Allman, J. M. (1999). *Evolving brains*. New York: Scientific American Library.

Allman, J. M., Hakeem, A., Erwin, J. M., Nimchinsky, E., & Hof, P. (2001). The anterior cingulate cortex: The evolution of an interface between emotion and cognition. *Annals of the New York Academy of Sciences USA, 935*, 107–117.

Andersson, M. (1994). *Sexual selection*. Princeton, NJ: Princeton University Press.

Asfaw B., White T. D., Lovejoy C. O., Latimer B., Simpson S., & Suwa G. (1999). *Australopithecus garhi:* A new species of early hominid from Ethiopia. *Science, 284*, 629–635.

Baddeley, A. D. (1986). *Working memory*. Oxford, UK: Oxford University Press.

Begun, D. R., & Walker, A. (1993). The endocast. In A. Walker & R. Leakey (Eds.), *The Nariokotome* Homo erectus *skeleton* (pp. 326–358). Cambridge, MA: Harvard University Press.

Belsky, J. (1997). Attachment, mating, and parenting: An evolutionary interpretation. *Human Nature, 8*, 361–381.

Bermudez de Castro, J. M., Rosas, A., Carbonee, E., Nicolás, M. E., Rodríguez, J., & Arsuaga, J.-L. (1999). A modern human pattern of dental development in Lower Pleistocene hominids from Atapuerca-TD6 (Spain). *Proceedings of the National Academy of Sciences, 96*, 4210–4213.

Betzig, L. L. (1986). *Despotism and differential reproduction: A Darwinian view of history*. New York: Aldine.

Beylin, A. V., & Shors, T. J. (2003). Glucocorticoids are necessary for enhancing the acquisition of associative memories after acute stressful experience. *Hormones and Behavior, 43*, 1124–1131.

Beynon, A. D., & Dean, M. C. (1987). Crown formation time of a fossil hominid premolar tooth. *Archives of Oral Biology, 32*, 773–790.

Beynon, A. D., Dean, M. C., & Reid, D. J. (1991). Histological study on the chronology of the developing dentition in gorilla and orangutan. *American Journal of Physical Anthropology, 86*, 189–203.

Bird, D. W., & Bliege Bird, R. (2002). Children on the reef: Slow learning or strategic foraging? *Human Nature, 13*, 269–297.

Bjorklund, D. F., & Pellegrini A. D. (2002). *The origins of human nature: Evolutionary developmental psychology*. Washington, DC: American Psychological Association Press.

Bliege Bird, R., & Bird, D. W. (2002). Constraints of knowing or constraints of growing? *Human Nature, 13*, 239–267.

Bloom, P. (2000). *How children learn the meaning of words*. Cambridge, MA: MIT Press.

Blurton Jones, N., Hawkes, K., & O'Connell, J. F. (1999). Some current ideas about the evolution of human life history. In P. C. Lee (Ed.), *Comparative primate socioecology* (pp. 140–166). Cambridge, UK: Cambridge University Press.

Blurton Jones, N., Hawkes, K., & O'Connell, J. F. (2002). Antiquity of post-reproductive life: Are there modern impacts on hunter–gatherer postreproductive life spans? *American Journal of Human Biology, 14,* 184–205.

Blurton Jones, N., & Marlowe, F. (2002). Selection for delayed maturity: Does it take 20 years to learn to hunt and gather? *Human Nature, 13,* 199–238.

Bock, J. (2002). Learning, life history, and productivity: Children's lives in the Okavango Delta, Botswana. *Human Nature, 13,* 161–197.

Bogin, B. (1991). The evolution of human childhood. *BioScience, 40,* 16–25.

Bogin, B. (1997). Evolutionary hypotheses for human childhood. *Yearbook of Physical Anthropology, 40,* 63–89.

Bogin, B. (1999). *Patterns of human growth* (2nd ed.). Cambridge, UK: Cambridge University Press.

Bogin, B., & Silva, M. I. V. (2003). Anthropometric variation and health: A biocultural model of human growth. *Journal of Children's Health, 1*(2), 149–173.

Bowlby, J. (1969). *Attachment and loss: Vol. 1. Attachment.* London: Hogarth.

Boyer, P. (2001). *Religion explained: The evolutionary origins of religious thought.* New York: Basic Books.

Bromage, T. G. (1991). Enamel incremental periodicity in the pig-tailed macaque: A polychrome fluorescent labeling study of dental hard tissue. *American Journal of Physical Anthropology, 86,* 205–214.

Brothers, L. (1990). The social brain: A project for integrating primate behavior and neurophysiology in a new domain. *Concepts in Neuroscience, 1,* 27–51.

Brunet, M., Guy, F., Pilbeam, D., Mackaye, H. T., Likius, A., Ahounta, D., et al. (2002) A new hominid from the Upper Miocene of Chad, Central Africa. *Nature, 418,* 14–151.

Buchan, J. C., Alberts, S. C., Silk, J. B., & Altmann, J. (2003). True paternal care in a multi-male primate society. *Nature, 425,* 179–181.

Byrne, R. W. (2002a). The primate origins of human intelligence. In R. J. Sternberg & J. C. Kaufman (Eds.), *The evolution of intelligence* (pp. 79–95). Mahwah, NJ: Erlbaum.

Byrne, R. W. (2002b). Social and technical forms of primate intelligence. In F. B. M. de Waal, (Ed.), *Tree of origin: What primate behavior can tell us about human social evolution* (pp. 145–172). Cambridge, MA: Harvard University Press.

Byrne, R. W., & Corp, N. (2004). Neocortex size predicts deception rate in primates. *Proceedings of the Royal Society, B,* 2780.

Byrne, R. W., & Whiten, A. (Eds.). (1988). *Machiavellian intelligence: Social expertise and the evolution of intellect in monkeys, apes, and humans.* Oxford, UK: Oxford University Press.

Campbell, A. (2002). *A mind of her own: The evolutionary psychology of women.* London: Oxford University Press.

Campbell, A., & Muncer, S. (Eds.). (1998). *The social child.* Hove, UK: Psychology Press.

Carruthers, P. (2000). The evolution of consciousness. In P. Carruthers & A. Chamberlain (Eds.), *Evolution and the human mind* (pp. 254–275). Cambridge, UK: Cambridge University Press.

Caspari, R., & Lee, S.-H. (2004). Longevity and the evolution of modernity. *American Journal of Physical Anthropology Supplement, 41*, 73–74.

Chagnon, N. A. (1977). *Yanomamö, the fierce people* (2nd ed.). New York: Holt, Rinehart & Winston.

Chagnon, N. A. (1988). Life histories, blood revenge, and warfare in a tribal population. *Science, 239*, 985–992.

Chapin, H. D. (1922). *Heredity and child culture*. New York: Dutton.

Chisholm, J. S. (1999). *Death, hope and sex*. Cambridge, UK: Cambridge University Press.

Clutton-Brock, T. H. (1977). Sexual dimorphism, socionomic sex ratio and body weight in primates. *Nature, 269*, 797–800.

Cohen, S., Doyle, W. J., Turner, R. B., Alper, C. M., & Skoner, D. P. (2003). Emotional style and susceptibility to the common cold. *Psychosomatic Medicine, 65*, 652–657.

Daly, M., & Wilson, M. (1988a). *Homicide*. Hawthorne, NY: Aldine de Gruyter.

Daly, M., & Wilson, M. (1988b). Evolutionary social psychology and family homicide. *Science, 242*, 519–524.

Dart, R. A. (1925). *Australopithecus africanus*: The man–ape of South Africa. *Nature, 115*, 195–199.

Darwin, C. (1871). *The descent of man, and selection in relation to sex*. London: John Murray.

Darwin, C. (1877). Biographical sketch of an infant. *Mind, 2*, 285–294.

Darwin, C., & Wallace, A. (1858). On the tendency of species to form varieties, and on the perpetuation of varieties and species by natural means of selection. *Journal of the Linnean Society of London, Zoology, 3*, 45–62.

Davidson, R. J., Jackson, D. C., & Kalin, N. H. (2001). Emotion, plasticity, context, and regulation. *Psychological Bulletin, 126*, 890–906.

Deacon, T. W. (1997). What makes the human brain different? *Annual Review of Anthropology, 26*, 337–357.

Dean, M. C., Leakey, M. G., Reid, D., Schrenk, F., Schwartz, G. T., Stringer, C., et al. (2001). Growth processes in teeth distinguish modern humans from *Homo erectus* and earlier hominins. *Nature, 414*, 628–631.

Dean, M. C., Stringer, C. B., & Bromage, T. G. (1986). Age at death of the Neanderthal child from Devil's Tower, Gibraltar, and the implications for studies of general growth and development in Neanderthals. *American Journal of Physical Anthropology, 70*, 301–310.

de Waal, F. B. M. (1982). *Chimpanzee politics*. New York: Harper & Row.

de Waal, F. B. M. (2001). *The ape and the sushi master*. New York: Basic Books.

de Waal, F. B. M., & Lanting, F. (1997). *Bonobo: The forgotten ape*. Berkeley: University of California Press.

Dressler, W. W., & Bindon, J. R. (2000). The health consequences of cultural dissonance: Cultural dimensions of lifestyle, social support, and arterial blood pressure in an African American community. *American Anthropologist, 102*, 244–260.

Dunbar, R. I. M. (1997). *Gossip, grooming, and evolution of language*. Cambridge, MA: Harvard University Press.

Dunbar, R. I. M. (1998). The social brain hypothesis. *Evolutionary Anthropology, 6*, 178–190.

Ellis, L. (1994). Social status and health in humans: The nature of the relationship and its probable causes. In L. Ellis (Ed.), *Social stratification and socioeconomic inequality* (Vol. 2, pp. 123–144). Westport, CT: Praeger.

Engle, R. W. (2002). Working memory capacity as executive attention. *Current Directions in Psychological Science, 11,* 19–23.

Field, T., Diego, M., Hernandez-Reif, M., Schanberg, S., & Kuhn, C. (2003). Depressed mothers who are "good interaction" partners versus those who are withdrawn or intrusive. *Infant Behavior and Development, 26,* 238–252.

Finch, C. E., & Sapolsky, R. (1999). The evolution of Alzheimer disease, the reproductive schedule, and apoE isoforms. *Neurobiology of Aging, 20*(4), 407–428.

Finlay, B. L., Darlington, R. B., & Nicastro, N. (2001). Developmental structure in brain evolution. *Behavioral and Brain Sciences, 24,* 263–308.

Flinn, M. V. (1986). Correlates of reproductive success in a Caribbean village. *Human Ecology, 14,* 225–243.

Flinn, M. V. (1997). Culture and the evolution of social learning. *Evolution and Human Behavior, 18,* 23–67.

Flinn, M. V. (1999). Family environment, stress, and health during childhood. In C. Panter-Brick & C. Worthman (Eds.), *Hormones, health, and behavior* (pp. 105–138). Cambridge, UK: Cambridge University Press.

Flinn, M. V., & England, B. G. (2003). Childhood stress: Endocrine and immune responses to psychosocial events. In J. M. Wilce (Ed.), *Social and cultural lives of immune systems* (pp. 107–147). London: Routledge.

Flinn, M. V., Geary, D. C., & Ward, C. V. (2004). Ecological dominance, social competition, and coalitionary arms races: Why humans evolved extraordinary intelligence. *Evolution and Human Behavior, 25*(5).

Flinn M. V., Quinlan, R., Turner, M. T., Decker, S. D., & England, B. G. (1996). Male–female differences in effects of parental absence on glucocorticoid stress response. *Human Nature, 7,* 125–162.

Fodor, J. A. (1983). *The modularity of mind: An essay on faculty psychology.* Cambridge, MA: MIT Press.

Foley, R. A. (1999). Hominid behavioral evolution: Missing links in comparative primate socioecology. In P. C. Lee (Ed.), *Comparative primate socioecology* (pp. 363–386). Cambridge, UK: Cambridge University Press.

Geary, D. C. (2005). *The origin of mind: On the evolution of brain, cognition, and general intelligence.* Washington, DC: American Psychological Association.

Geary, D. C., & Bjorklund, D. F. (2000). Evolutionary developmental psychology. *Child Development, 71,* 57–65.

Geary, D. C., & Flinn, M. V. (2001). Evolution of human parental behavior and the human family. *Parenting: Science and Practice, 1,* 5–61.

Geary, D. C., & Flinn, M. V. (2002). Sex differences in behavioral and hormonal response to social threat. *Psychological Review, 109,* 745–750.

Geary, D. C., & Huffman, K. J. (2002). Brain and cognitive evolution: Forms of modularity and functions of mind. *Psychological Bulletin, 128,* 667–698.

Gerhart, J., & Kirschner, M. (1998). *Cells, embryos, and evolution.* Oxford, UK: Blackwell Science.

Goodall, J. (1986). *The chimpanzees of Gombe.* Cambridge, MA: Harvard University Press.

Gopnik, A., Meltzoff, A. N., & Kuhl, P. K. (1999). *The scientist in the crib: Minds, brains, and how children learn.* New York: Morrow.

Gould, S. J. (1977). *Ontogeny and phylogeny*. Cambridge, MA: Harvard University Press.

Haile-Selassie, Y. (2001). Late Miocene hominids from the Middle Awash, Ethiopia. *Nature, 412,* 187–191.

Hawkes, K. (2003). Grandmothers and the evolution of human longevity. *American Journal of Human Biology, 15,* 380–400.

Hed, H. M. E. (1987). Trends in opportunity for natural selection in the Swedish population during the period 1650–1980. *Human Biology, 59,* 785–797.

Henrich, J., Boyd, R., Bowles, S., Camerer, C., Fehr, E., Gintis, H., et al. (2001). Cooperation, reciprocity and punishment in fifteen small-scale societies. *American Economic Review, 91,* 73–78.

Herdt, G., & McClintock, M. K. (2000). The magical age of 10. *Archives of Sexual Behavior, 29,* 587–606.

Hill, K., & Hurtado, A. M. (1996a). *Ache life history: The ecology and demography of a foraging people.* Hawthorne, NY: Aldine de Gruyter.

Hill, K., & Hurtado, A. M. (1996b). The evolution of premature reproductive senescence and menopause in human females: An evaluation of the grandmother hypothesis. In L. Betzig (Ed.), *Human nature: A critical reader* (pp. 118–143). New York: Oxford University Press.

Hill, K., & Kaplan, H. (1999). Life history traits in humans: Theory and empirical studies. *Annual Review of Anthropology, 28,* 397–430.

Hirschfeld, L. (2002). Why don't anthropologists like children? *American Anthropologist, 104,* 611–627.

Hirschfeld, L. A., & Gelman, S. A. (1994). *Mapping the mind: Domain specificity in cognition and culture.* Cambridge, UK: Cambridge University Press.

Holliday, M. A. (1986). Body composition and energy needs during growth. In F. Falkner & J. M. Tanner (Eds.), *Human growth: A comprehensive treatise* (Vol. 2, 2nd ed., pp. 101–117). New York: Plenum Press.

Hrdy, S. B. (1999). *Mother nature: A history of mothers, infants, and natural selection.* New York: Pantheon.

Huether, G. (1996). The central adaptation syndrome: Psychosocial stress as a trigger for adaptive modifications of brain structure and brain function. *Progress in Neurobiology, 48,* 568–612

Huether, G. (1998). Stress and the adaptive self organization of neuronal connectivity during early childhood. *International Journal of Developmental Neuroscience, 16,* 297–306.

Humphrey, N. K. (1976). The social function of intellect. In P. P. G. Bateson & R. A. Hinde (Eds.), *Growing points in ethology* (pp. 303–317). New York: Cambridge University Press.

Humphrey, N. K. (1983). *Consciousness regained.* Oxford, UK: Oxford University Press.

Irons, W. (1979). Cultural and biological success. In N. A. Chagnon & W. Irons (Eds.), *Natural selection and social behavior* (pp. 257–272). North Scituate, MA: Duxbury Press.

Joffe, T. H. (1997). Social pressures have selected for an extended juvenile period in primates. *Journal of Human Evolution, 32,* 593–605.

Jolly, A. (1966). Lemur social behavior and primate intelligence. *Science, 153,* 501–506.

Jolly, A. (1999). *Lucy's legacy: Sex and intelligence in human evolution.* Cambridge, MA: Harvard University Press.

Kano, T. (1992). *The last ape: Pygmy chimpanzee behavior and ecology.* Stanford, CA: Stanford University Press.

Kaplan, H., Hill, K., Lancaster, J., & Hurtado, A. M. (2000). A theory of human life history evolution: Diet, intelligence, and longevity. *Evolutionary Anthropology, 9,* 156–185.

Kelley, D. B., & Brenowitz, E. (2002). Hormonal influences on courtship behaviors. In J. B. Becker, S. M. Breedlove, D. Crews, & M. M. McCarthy (Eds.), *Behavioral endocrinology* (2nd ed., pp. 289–330). Cambridge, MA: MIT/Bradford Press.

Kiecolt-Glaser, J. K., Malarkey, W. B., Cacioppo, J. T., & Glaser, R. (1994). Stressful personal relationships: Immune and endocrine function. In R. Glaser & J. K. Kiecolt-Glaser (Eds.), *Handbook of human stress and immunity* (pp. 301–319). New York: Academic Press.

Konner, M. (1991). Universals of behavioral development in relation to brain myelination. In K. R. Gibson & A. C. Petersen (Eds.), *Brain maturation and cognitive development: Comparative and cross-cultural perspectives* (pp. 181–223). New York: Aldine de Gruyter.

Kudo, H., & Dunbar, R. I. M. (2001). Neocortex size and social network size in primates. *Animal Behaviour, 62,* 711–722.

La Cerra, P., & Bingham, R. (1998). The adaptive nature of the human neurocognitive architecture: An alternative model. *Proceedings of the National Academy of Sciences USA, 95,* 11290–11294.

Lamb, M. E., Bornstein, M. H., & Teti, D. M. (2002). *Development in infancy* (4th ed.). Mahwah, NJ: Erlbaum.

Lancaster, J. B., & Lancaster, C. S. (1983). Parental investment: The hominid adaptation. In D. Ortner (Ed.), *How humans adapt: A biocultural odyssey* (pp. 33–65). Washington, DC: Smithsonian Press.

Lancaster, J. B., & Lancaster, C. S. (1987). The watershed: Change in parental-investment and family-formation strategies in the course of human evolution. In J. B. Lancaster, J. Altmann, A. S. Rossi, & L.R. Sherrod (Eds.), *Parenting across the life span: Biosocial dimensions* (pp. 187–205). Hawthorne, NY: Aldine de Gruyter.

Leakey, M. G., Feibel, C. S., MacDougall, I., & Walker, A. (1995). New four-million-year-old hominid species from Kanapoi and Allia Bay, Kenya. *Nature, 376,* 565–571.

LeBlanc, S. A. (2003). *Constant battles: The myth of the peaceful, noble savage.* New York: St. Martin's Press.

Lee, S. H., & Wolpoff, M. H. (2003). The pattern of evolution in Pleistocene human brain size. *Paleobiology, 29,* 186–196.

Leigh, S. R. (2001). The evolution of human growth. *Evolutionary Anthropology, 10,* 223–236.

Leonard, W. R., & Robertson, M. L. (1994). Evolutionary perspectives on human nutrition: The influence of brain and body size on diet and metabolism. *American Journal of Human Biology, 4,* 77–88.

Levine, R. A., Miller, P. M., & West, M. M. (Eds.). (1988). *Parental behavior in diverse societies* (New Directions for Child Development 40). San Francisco: Jossey-Bass.

Lovejoy, C. O. (1981). The origin of man. *Science, 211*, 341–350.

Lovejoy, C. O., McCollum, M. A., Reno, P. L., & Rosenman, B. A. (2003). Developmental biology and human evolution. *Annual Reviews of Anthropology, 32*, 85–109.

Low, B. S. (2000). *Why sex matters*. Princeton, NJ: Princeton University Press.

Mace, R. (2000). Evolutionary ecology of human life history. *Animal Behaviour, 59*, 1–10.

Macho, G. A. (2001). Primate molar crown formation times and life history evolution revisited. *American Journal of Primatology, 55*, 189–201.

Macho, G. A., & Wood, B. A. (1995). The role of time and timing in hominid dental evolution. *Evolutionary Anthropology, 4*, 1–17.

Maier, S. F., Watkins, L. R., & Fleschner, M. (1994). Psychoneuroimmunology: The interface between behavior, brain, and immunity. *American Psychologist, 49*, 1004–1007.

Malthus, T. R. (1798). *An essay on the principle of population as it affects the future improvement of society with remarks on the speculations of Mr. Godwin, M. Condorcet, and other writers*. London: Printed for J. Johnson, in St. Paul's Church-yard.

Marmot, M. G., Smith G. D., Stansfield, S., Patel, C., North, F., Head, J., et al. (1991). Health inequalities among British civil servants: The Whitehall II study. *Lancet, 337*, 1387–1393.

Marmot, M., & Wilkinson, R. G. (Eds.). (1999). *Social determinants of health*. Oxford, UK: Oxford University Press.

Martin, R. D. (1983). *Primate origins and evolution*. Princeton, NJ: Princeton University Press.

Martin, R. D., & MacLarnon, A. (1990). Reproductive patterns in primates and other mammals: The dichotomy between altricial and precocial offspring. In C. J. DeRousseau (Ed.), *Primate life history and evolution* (pp. 47–79). New York: Wiley-Liss.

McClintock, M. K., & Herdt, G. (1996). Rethinking puberty: The development of sexual attraction. *Current Directions in Psychological Science, 5*(6), 178–183.

McHenry, H. M. (1992a). Body size and proportions in early hominids. *American Journal of Physical Anthropology, 87*, 407–431.

McHenry, H. M. (1992b). How big were early hominids? *Evolutionary Anthropology, 1*, 15–20.

McHenry, H. M. (1994). Behavioral ecological implications of early hominid body size. *Journal of Human Evolution, 27*, 77–87.

Miller, G. F. (2000). *The mating mind: How sexual choice shaped the evolution of human nature*. New York: Doubleday.

Mitani, J. C., & Watts, D. (2001). Why do chimpanzees hunt and share meat? *Animal Behaviour, 61*, 915–924.

Mithen, S. J. (1996). *The prehistory of the mind: The cognitive origins of art, religion, and science*. London: Thames & Hudson.

Passmore, R., & Durnin, J. V. (1955). Human energy expenditure. *Physiological Reviews, 35*(4), 801–840.

Pawlowski, B., Lowen, C. B., & Dunbar, R. I. M. (1998). Neocortex size, social skills and mating success in primates. *Behaviour, 135*, 357–368.

Pinker, S. (1994). *The language instinct*. New York: Morrow.

Pinker, S. (1997). *How the mind works*. New York: Norton.

Plavcan, J. M. (2000). Inferring social behavior from sexual dimorphism in the fossil record. *Journal of Human Evolution, 39*, 327–344.

Plavcan J. M. (2001). Sexual dimorphism in primate evolution. *Yearbook of Physical Anthropology, 44*, 25–53.

Plavcan, J. M., Van Schaik, C. P., & Kappeler, P. M. (1995). Competition, coalitions and canine size in primates. *Journal of Human Evolution, 28*, 245–276.

Portman, A. (1941). Die Tragzeiten der Primaten und die Dauer der Schwangerschaft beim Menschen: Ein Problem der vergleichenden Biologie. *Revue Suisse de Zoologie, 48*, 511–518.

Povinelli, D. J., & Bering, J. M. (2002). The mentality of apes revisited. *Current Directions in Psychological Science, 11*, 115–119.

Quartz, S., & Sejnowski, T. (1999). Constraining constructivism: Cortical and subcortical constraints on learning in development. *Behavioral and Brain Sciences, 23*, 785–792.

Reno, P. L., Meindl, R. S., McCollum M. A., & Lovejoy, C. O. (2003). Sexual dimorphism in *Austrolopithecus afarensis* was similar to that of humans. *Proceedings of the National Academy of Sciences USA, 100*, 9404–9409.

Ricklefs, R. E. (1983). Avian postnatal development. In D. S. Farner, J. R. King, & K. C. Parkes (Eds.), *Avian biology 7* (pp. 1–83). New York: Academic Press.

Rosenberg, K. R. (1992). The evolution of modern human childbirth. *Yearbook of Physical Anthropology, 35*, 89–134.

Ruff, C. B., Trinkaus, E., & Holliday, T. W. (1997). Body mass and encephalization in Pleistocene *Homo*. *Nature, 387*, 173–176.

Schultz, A. H. (1969). *The life of primates*. New York: Universe Press.

Semaw, S., Renne, P., Harris, J. W. K., Feibel, C. S., Bernor, R. L., Fesseha, N., et al. (1997). 2.5-million-year-old stone tools from Gona, Ethiopia. *Nature, 382*, 333–336.

Senut, B., Pickford, M., Gommery, D., Mein, P., Cheboi, K., & Coppens, Y. (2001). First hominid from the Miocene (Lukeino Formation, Kenya). *Comptes Rendus de l'Academie des Sciences Paris, 332*, 137–144.

Senut, B. (2002). From apes to humans: Locomotion as a key feature for phylogeny. *Zeitschrift fur Morphologie und Anthropologie, 83*, 351–60.

Silk, J. S., Alberts, S. C., & Altmann, J. (2003). Social bonds of female baboons enhance infant survival. *Science, 302*, 1231–1234.

Small, M. F. (1998). *Our babies, ourselves*. New York: Random House.

Small, M. F. (2001). *Kids*. New York: Doubleday.

Smith, B. H. (1989). Dental development as a measure of life history in primates. *Evolution, 43*, 683–688.

Smith, B. H. (1993). The physiological age of KNM-WT15000. In A. Walker & R.E. Leakey (Eds.), *The Nariokotome* Homo erectus *skeleton* (pp. 195–220). Cambridge, MA: Harvard University Press.

Smith, B. J. (1994). Patterns of dental development in *Homo, Australopithecus, Pan* and *Gorilla*. *American Journal of Physical Anthropology, 94*, 307–325.

Smuts, B. (1985). *Sex and friendship in baboons*. New York: Aldine de Gruyter.

Smuts, B. B., & Smuts, R. W. (1993). Male aggression and sexual coercion of females in nonhuman primates and other mammals: Evidence and theoretical implications. *Advances in the Study of Behavior, 22*, 1–63.

Stanford C. B. (2001). The ape's gift: Meat-eating, meat-sharing, and human evolution. In F. B. M. de Waal (Ed.), *Tree of origin: What primate behavior can tell us about human social evolution* (pp. 95–119). Cambridge, MA: Harvard University Press.

Stearns, S. C. (1992). *The evolution of life histories.* Oxford: Oxford University Press.

Steele, J. (1996). On the evolution of temperament and dominance style in hominid groups. In J. Steele & S. Shennan (Eds.), *The archeology of human ancestry: Power, sex, and tradition* (pp. 110–134). New York: Routledge.

Symons, D. (1978). *Play and aggression: A study of rhesus monkeys.* New York: Columbia University Press.

Tomasello, M. (1999). *The cultural origins of human cognition.* Cambridge, MA: Harvard University Press.

Tooby, J., & Cosmides, L. (1995). Mapping the evolved functional organization of mind and brain. In M. S. Gazzaniga (Ed.), *The cognitive neurosciences* (pp. 1185–1197). Cambridge, MA: Bradford Books/MIT Press.

United Nations. (1985). *Socio-economic differentials in child mortality in developing countries.* New York: Author.

Van Schaik, C., & Deaner, R. (2003). Life history and cognitive evolution in primates. In F. B. M. de Waal & P. Tyack (Eds.), *Animal social complexity: Intelligence, culture and individualized societies* (pp. 5–25). Cambridge, MA: Harvard University Press.

Ward, C. V., Walker, A., & Leakey, M. G. (1999). The new hominid species *Australopithecus anamensis. Evolutionary Anthropology, 7,* 197–205.

Ward, C., Leakey, M. G., & Walker, A. (2001). Morphology of *Australopithecus anamensis* from Kanapoi and Allia Bay, Kenya. *Journal of Human Evolution, 41,* 255–368.

West-Eberhard, M. J. (2003). *Developmental plasticity and evolution.* Oxford, UK: Oxford University Press.

White, T. D., Suwa, G., & Asfaw, B. (1994). *Australopithecus ramidus,* a new species of early hominid from Aramis, Ethiopia. *Nature, 371,* 306–312.

Whiting, B. B., & Edwards, C. P. (1988). *Children of different worlds.* Cambridge, MA: Harvard University Press.

Wilkinson, R. G. (2001). *Mind the gap.* New Haven, CT: Yale University Press.

Williams, G. C. (1957). Plieotropy, natural selection, and the evolution of senescence. *Evolution, 11,* 398–411.

Williams, G. C. (1966). *Adaptation and natural selection.* Princeton, NJ: Princeton University Press.

Wrangham, R. W. (1999). Evolution of coalitionary killing. *Yearbook of Physical Anthropology, 42,* 1–30.

Wrangham, R., & Peterson, D. (1996). *Demonic males.* New York: Houghton Mifflin.

Zihlman, A., Bolter, D., & Boesch, C. (2004). Wild chimpanzee dentition and its implications for assessing life history in immature hominin fossils. *Proceedings of the National Academy of Sciences, 101*(29), 10541–10543.

Zihlman, A., Cronin, J., Cramer, D., & Sarich, V. M. (1978). Pygmy chimpanzee as a possible prototype for the common ancestor of humans, chimpanzees and gorillas. *Nature, 275,* 744–746.

3

THE ROLE OF DEVELOPMENTAL PLASTICITY IN THE EVOLUTION OF HUMAN COGNITION

Evidence from Enculturated, Juvenile Great Apes

DAVID F. BJORKLUND
JUSTIN S. ROSENBERG

H*omo sapiens* is the most educable of species. We are not the only "learning species," of course, but modern humans acquire skills and knowledge today that were unimaginable for our ancestors, and this requires a flexible cognitive system. Most contemporary cultures involve some degree of formal schooling, where children master literacy, basic mathematics, and an understanding of the inner workings of biological organisms, among other often arcane knowledge. Such knowledge and the accompanying cognitive abilities (such as reading) were not necessary for survival for our ancestors; thus, it is foolish to argue that such abilities evolved to serve the functions that they do today. Geary (1995; Chapter 19, this volume) has labeled such cognitive skills as *biologically secondary abilities* and contrasts them with *biologically primary abilities*, which were selected over the course of phylogeny for their survival value. Biologically primary abilities are universal, develop "effortlessly," and follow a typical pattern of development in all children. In contrast, biologically secondary abilities are dependent on a particular cultural milieu and often require extensive practice to master. Although the biologically primary abilities possessed by humans are often qualitatively different than those possessed by other animals (e.g., language), it is likely that only humans possess biologi-

45

cally secondary abilities, distinguishing human cognition from that displayed by most, if not all, other animals.

Biologically secondary abilities require a highly flexible, or plastic, cognitive system. This ability to modify behavior and thought may not only play an essential role in *developing* the human mind but may also have played an equally critical role in *evolving* the human mind. In this chapter, we argue that the ability of young organisms to alter their behavior in response to changes in ecological conditions provided the raw "stuff" upon which natural selection worked. From this viewpoint, mechanisms of developmental plasticity played an important role in human cognitive evolution. As most theories about how evolutionary change in a particular genetic line came about, this one is speculative. However, we conclude the chapter with research with enculturated (human-reared) apes, suggesting that patterns of results provide evidence in support of our contention that developmental plasticity in humans' ancestors contributed to the evolution of the modern human mind.

PLASTICITY

Plasticity refers to "the ability of an organism to react to an environmental input with a change in form, state, movement, or rate of activity" (West-Eberhard, 2003, p. 34). This definition can be viewed as synonymous with terms such as phenotypic plasticity, malleability, and flexibility. Primates, and humans especially, show a high degree of cognitive and behavioral plasticity from the earliest stages of development and are renowned for their ability to "bounce back" from early deleterious experiences. For example, in an early study with rhesus monkeys, Harlow, Dodsworth, and Harlow (1965) deprived subjects of social contact. These monkeys subsequently displayed abnormal social and sexual behavior. As deleterious as these effects were, Suomi and Harlow (1972) later demonstrated that by subjecting isolated monkeys to daily social contact with a younger, socially inexperienced peer, the older, socially deviant monkeys, upon reentry into the colony, behaved within the normal range.

Cognitive and behavioral plasticity is especially well documented in humans. Dramatic evidence of the reversal of the effects of early social and physical deprivation comes from institutionalization studies, in which children show recovery of social and intellectual functioning after being removed from stultifying institutions and placed in more supportive environments (e.g., O'Connor et al., 2000; Rutter et al., 1998; 2004; Skeels, 1966). There are limits to such plasticity, of course; the longer a child experiences deprivation, the less likely the reversal of the negative effects of such deprivation are apt to be. This is illustrated in a recent study by O'Connor and his colleagues (2000), who followed the course of Romanian children removed from impoverished orphanages and adopted by English parents. All children showed signs of physical, social, and intellectual deficits upon leaving the institution, but when their intelligence was assessed at age 6, most displayed normal levels. However, the degree of recovery was related to their age upon leaving the orphanage. Children who had been adopted before the age of 24 months had average to above-average IQs, comparable to those of adopted English children. Children not adopted until between the ages of 24 and 42 months had lower IQs, although still within the normal range (mean = 90). Children who were adopted early also spent more time in adopted homes than their late-adopted peers; thus, this latter group may eventually show a further increase in IQ as they spend more time in an enriching environment. Despite the numerous methodological problems associated with institutionalization studies, such findings clearly demonstrate that primates, and humans in particular, possess a substantial amount of resiliency, or developmental plasticity.

In this chapter, we argue that humans possess mechanisms of plasticity from the genetic through the behavioral and cognitive levels. In order to better understand plasticity, we must examine it from an epigenetic perspective, namely, as presented by developmental systems theory.

DEVELOPMENTAL SYSTEMS THEORY

Developmental systems theory (DST) can be thought of not so much as a theory, but rather as a theoretical perspective, or metatheory (Li, 2003; Oyama, Griffiths, & Gray, 2001; Robert, Hall, & Olson, 2001), that serves to bridge the gaps between such dichotomous concepts as nature–nurture and development–evolution. DST proponents argue against any notion of genetic determinism (i.e., the view that function or structure is "in the genes"), and instead argue that development is the continuous and bidirectional interaction between various components of the "developmental system"—including but not limited to genetic activity, structural maturation, activity emanating from structures (or function), and the environment, broadly construed.

A central concept in DST is that of *epigenesis*, defined as "an emergent process by which an organism's structure and function change from relatively undifferentiated states to increasingly specialized, differentiated forms throughout ontogeny" (Miller, 1998, p. 105). This definition is elaborated by Kuo (1976):

> We shall define behavioral epigenesis as a continuous developmental process from fertilization through birth to death, involving proliferation, diversification, and modification of behavior patterns both in space and in time, as a result of the continuous dynamic exchange of energy between the developing organism and its environment, endogenous and exogenous. The ontogenesis of behavior is a continuous stream of activities whose patterns vary or are modified in response to changes in the effective stimulation by the environment. In these epigenetic processes, at every point of energy exchange, a new relationship is established; the organism is no longer the same organism and the environment no longer the same environment as they were at the previous moment. (p. 11)

Gottlieb (1998, 2002) proposed two types of epigenesis: predetermined and probabilistic. *Predetermined epigenesis* can be thought of as a unidirectional relationship between structure and function; that is, the relationship is strictly forward feeding: genes → structural maturation → activity and experience. This view can be considered the *central dogma* of molecular biology (Gottlieb, 1998, 2002; Ho, 1998). In contrast, *probabilistic epigenesis*, which is at the heart of DST, is defined as the bidirectional relationship between structure and function. In this relationship, each level interacts with each adjacent level: genes ↔ structural maturation ↔ function.

Developmental systems theorists acknowledge that genes play a critical role in a developing system; however, their role is seen as one that is continuously and bidirectionally in interaction with the concomitant environment. If one takes such a perspective seriously, then one should expect substantial plasticity of development. Genes do not dictate any particular outcome but have their impact in interaction with the varied environments, both endogenous and exogenous to the organism, in which they find themselves. As a consequence, it should be nearly impossible to predict any specific developmental outcome. Yet despite substantial individuality, most members of a species grow up to be remarkably similar to one another. How can this be so and the tenets of DST still be valid? The answer lies in the concept of species-typical environments; that is, members of a species inherit not only a species-typical genome but also a species-typical environment, or as Lickliter (1996) states: "The organism inherits not only its genetic complement, but also the structured organization of the environment into which it is born" (p. 91). Some aspects of an organism's nongenetic inheritance are highly conservative from one generation to the next, such as gravity, oxygen, and light. Nongenetic inheritance also includes some of the cellular machinery found in the cytoplasm necessary for DNA–RNA transcription, aspects of the prenatal environment (a womb for mammals), and postnatal environment (a lactating mother for mammals). Because there is little variability from individual to individual in these species-typical environments, gene expression is similarly influenced by environmental factors for different members of a species, yielding a species-typical pattern of development.

Yet for some species, variation in environmental factors during early stages of life can have significant effects on the phenotype of the adults. For example, differences in ambient temperature during egg incubation influence sex determination in some reptiles: Above a certain temperature the embryos become female; below that temperature, they become male (Bull, 1980). Temperature presumably has it effect by activating or deactivating sets of sex-determining genes, so proposing that sex in these species is "determined" by the environment, as opposed to the genes, would be simplistic and incorrect. But such examples indicate that by alerting gene expression, variations in environments exogenous to an animal can have a great impact on the eventual phenotype (see West-Eberhard, 2003).

The developmental systems perspective requires us to rethink what is inherited from generation to generation, and, accordingly, what is involved in evolution. What evolves are not simply genes, but developmental systems. Genes are critical parts of developmental systems, but they are always expressed in an environment, and these environments (including cell cytoplasm, gravity, light, maternal nurturing) are also inherited (see Gottlieb, 1992; Oyama et al., 2001; West-Eberhard, 2003). According to Oyama (2000b),

> What is transmitted between generations is not traits, or blueprints, or symbolic representations of traits, but developmental *means* (or *resources*, or *interactants*). These means include genes, the cellular machinery necessary for their functioning, and the larger developmental context, which may include a maternal reproductive system, parental care, or other interaction with conspecifics, as well as relations with other aspects of the animate and inanimate worlds. This context, which is actually a system of partially nested contexts, changes with time, partly as a result of the developmental processes themselves. (p. 29)

That is, there are nested systems of contexts that affect development and evolution, and these systems can change over generations (although some aspects of the systems, such as gravity and light, remain largely constant). It is these systems that animals inherit; changes in the nongenetic parts of these systems affect gene expression, which in turn affect development and the phenotypic form the animal takes. At the same time, the nongenetic parts of these systems constitute important selective forces on gene frequencies.

Models of brain development acknowledge this species-typical inheritance of both biological and environmental features. For example, Greenough, Black, and Wallace (1987) proposed that specific experiences produce neural activity that in turn determines which neurons become interconnected, and which will live and which will die (see also Johnson, 1998, 2000; Nelson, 2001). The nervous systems of generations of animals have been prepared to "expect" certain types of stimulation, such as a world consisting of three-dimensional moving objects. Greenough and his colleagues referred to the processes whereby synapses are formed and maintained when an organism has species-typical experiences as *experience-expectant processes* (or *experience-expectant synaptogenesis*). For instance, merely viewing a normal world is sufficient for the visual system to develop properly. Neurons and synapses that receive species-expectant experience survive and become organized with other activated neurons, whereas those that do not receive such activation die. Thus, although the infant comes into the world prepared to develop certain abilities, these abilities are substantially influenced by experience. What is inherited seems to be a susceptibility to certain environmental experiences rather than the circuitry for detailed behaviors themselves.

Yet, despite the conservative nature of both an organism's genetic and nongenetic inheritance, DST acknowledges that there is substantial possibility for plasticity, which has important implications for understanding both development and evolution. For example, notions of "innateness" as being "in the genes," or of instinct as behavior that requires "no previous experience," must be rethought when viewed through the lens of DST. This is illustrated in research by Gottlieb on the classic phenomenon of imprinting in precocial birds (for review, see Gottlieb, 1992). Several hours after hatching, ducklings will approach the maternal call of their own species, differentiating it from the call of a related species (e.g., mallard vs. Peking duck). At first blush, this appears to be a case in which ducklings "instinctively" know the maternal call, without the benefit of previous experience. Yet these animals do have auditory experience in the egg prior to hatching; but when they are removed from their mother and incubated in isolation so that they do not even hear the peeps of their brood mates, they still reliably approach the call of a conspecific when later tested. However, when ducklings had their vocal chords treated several days prior to hatching so that they could not vocalize (a procedure that wears off several days after hatching), and were isolated from their mothers, as well as from other hatchlings, the results were different. These ducklings showed no preference and were just as likely to approach the maternal call of a chicken as that of their own species.

Such experiments demonstrate the role that species-typical experiences have on the development of what was once thought to be "instinctive" behavior. Although most ducklings in the wild can "expect" a species-typical environment consisting of a quaking mother, peeping brood mates, and their own vocalizations, making it unlikely that a mallard duck chick will form an attachment to a Rhode Island hen, such experiments demonstrate the substantial plasticity and role of experience in development, which can have profound implications for our conceptions of both ontogeny and phylogeny.

Another demonstration of the potential role of experience on the emergence of species-typical behavior comes from a recent cross-fostering study by Francis, Szegda, Campbell, Martin, and Insel (2003), who worked with two strains of mice (B6 and BALD) that show distinct behavioral patterns in open-field tests and on the Morris water maze. Single-cell B6 mice embryos were implanted in either B6 or BALD dams. After birth, half of the animals were fostered by either B6 or BALD dams. When later tested, the B6 mice who were cross-fostered to BALD dams *both* prenatally and postnatally behaved identically to BALD control mice, and significantly differently from the other B6 mice, who experienced either (or both) prenatal or postnatal cross-fostering with a B6 dam. In other words, the combination of pre- and postnatal cross-fostering produced behavior typical of the fostering species and atypical of its genetic strain. Without changing any genes, complex behavior was modified in the direction of the rearing species. One difference in the postnatal environment likely responsible, in part, for this effect is the frequency with which the B6 and BALD dams licked the pups. The B6 dams licked the pups more frequently over the first 5 postnatal days than did the BALD dams. Maternal licking has been shown to influence a pup's subsequent reaction to stress, as well as maze learning and exploratory behavior (e.g., Liu et al., 2000).

EPIGENETIC THEORIES OF EVOLUTION

Proponents of DST and probabilistic epigenesis not only look at ontogeny differently from most psychologists but also view phylogeny a bit differently. Important in such theories of evolution is an organism's ability to adjust its behavior to the local environment. *Epigenetic theories of evolution* (e.g., Ho, 1998) view a developing organism's response to environmental changes as a mechanism for phylogenetic change. From this perspective, it is the developmental plasticity of an organism that is the creative force of evolution—that generates novel behavior on which natural selection can work. According to Gottlieb (1998), "These successful phenotypes are products of individual development and thus are a consequence of the adaptability of the organism to its developmental conditions. Therefore, natural selection has preserved (favored) organisms that are adaptably responsive both behaviorally and physiologically to their developmental conditions" (p. 796).

The Baldwin Effect

The notion that ontogenetic changes can influence evolution (see Bjorklund & Pellegrini, 2002; Gottlieb, 1987, 2002; Gould, 1977) can be traced back to the revolutionary thinking of three independent theorists, all in the same year, 1896: James Mark Baldwin (1861–1934), Henry Fairfield Osborn (1857–1935), and Conway Lloyd Morgan (1852–1936). Independently, these theorists recognized that certain individuals within a population had enough "ontogenetic plasticity," so that they were able to survive immense alterations in environmental conditions and subsequently become primogenitors for new lines of descendents (see Gottlieb, 1992; Waddington, 1975). This phenomenon, known as *organic selection*, was popularized (at least among psychologists) by Baldwin (1902) and is also known as the *Baldwin effect*. According to Bering (in press),

> Baldwin's (1896) eponymous mechanism of evolutionary change involves the differential success of individual organisms within a population gaining a reproductive edge through engaging in novel behaviors. The heritability underlying such behavioral plasticity means that subsequent generations, subjected to the same environmental stressors, will similarly be more likely to propagate their genes to the next generation. These intergenerational processes of genetic expression will occur until the behavior loses much of its original plasticity in the face of recurrent environmental stressors eliciting it. That is, because the genetic potential to adapt to specific predictable conditions in the environment becomes essential for the organism's survival, the heritability for this behavioral trait drops to floor values. At this point, the behavior, which may also influence genetic expression in other domains, becomes a standardized adaptation in the species supported by specialized psychological programs. (pp. 12–13)

Although Baldwin's ideas were seen as neo-Lamarckian (Bjorklund & Pellegrini, 2002), subsequent research has provided evidence for such inheritance, initially in the 1950s by the British biologist Conrad H. Waddington (1975), and later by other researchers. Moreover, as we understand it, the Baldwin effect requires no special pleading, but can be interpreted in terms of Darwin's ideas of natural selection. Heritable variation in a trait leads to individual differences in survival/reproduction under specified environmental conditions. If those conditions are reliably present across generations, then heritable variation in that trait will be reduced, until the trait becomes universal in the population.

In a now-classic experiment, Waddington (1975) subjected pupal fruit flies (*Drosophila melanogaster*) to heat shock. In response to this treatment, some of the surviving flies developed wings that contained few or no cross-veins. Waddington subsequently bred the no-cross-vein flies and exposed the pupal flies of that second generation to heat shock as well. This produced a second generation of fruit flies that also had few or no cross-veins in their wings. After 14 generations of selective breeding, some fruit flies developed the no-cross-wing phenotype *without* the preexposure to heat shock; that is, Waddington showed that a new phenotype was eventually seen in the developing offspring, without exposure to the original activating environmental event. Waddington referred to this phenomenon as *genetic assimilation*, which he defined as "the conversion of an acquired character into an inherited one; or better, as a shift towards a greater importance of heredity in the degree to which the character is acquired or inherited" (p. 61).

Although the no-cross-vein phenotype has no apparent adaptive value, in a later study, Waddington demonstrated genetic assimilation for a more adaptive phenotype, salt tolerance. Waddington raised fruit flies on a high-salt medium and selectively bred flies that developed larger anal papillae in response, which helped the flies to excrete salt from their bodies. After 21 generations of selective breeding, this new phenotype (larger anal papillae), although initially elicited only in response to an adverse environmental condition, developed in the absence of the high-salt condition, demonstrating the epigenetic phenomenon of genetic assimilation.

Evidence of genetic assimilation has been demonstrated for a variety of species since the pioneering work of Waddington (for reviews, see Ho, 1998; Jablonka & Lamb, 1995; West-Eberhard, 2003), including mammals. For example, there is limited evidence of behavioral changes in mammals carrying over two generations. In one series of experiments, female rats that had been handled as infants (removed daily from the home cage and placed in a tin can with shavings for 3 minutes) had grandoffspring that were more active and weighed less than the grandoffspring of nonhandled rats under conditions in which the second-generation females had been permitted greater freedom to explore their environment (Denenberg & Rosenberg, 1967). In other research, Ressler (1966), using two strains of mice (C57BL and BALB), demonstrated that mice from either strain that had been raised by foster parents from the BALB strain had far better scores on four operant conditioning performance measures than C57BL-raised mice, and that this effect was maintained into the subsequent generation. Ressler wrote, "Thus, it appears that some difference in the environment provided by BALB and C57BL foster parents influences the operant performance of offspring they rear, and that this difference is at least partially replicated in the parental environment subsequently provided by these offspring and, in turn, affects the operant behavior of second generation young" (p. 267). Although the nature of the mechanisms for such multigeneration effects was not known (unobserved influences on behavior, physiology, or milk content were proposed as possibilities), these results suggested to Ressler that "a nongenetic system of inheritance based upon transmission of parental influences is potentially available to all mammals" (p. 267).

West-Eberhard (2003) has made similar proposals, suggesting that "adaptive evolution—phenotypic improvement due to selection— . . . is a two step process: first the generation of variation by development, then the screening of that variation by selection" (p. 139). West-Eberhard proposes that "new phenotypic subunits begin and evolve as products of developmental plasticity. They originate when an environmental or genetic perturbation causes a shift in gene expression, and they are consolidated under selection for improved regulation and form" (p. 129). She refers to the associated changes in gene frequency as *genetic accommodation*, and distinguishes it from genetic assimilation, which she views as more limited than the former. For example, genetic assimilation serves only to decrease (not increase) phenotypic susceptibility to environmental influences, is induced only by environmental (not genetic) perturbations, and refers only to positively (not negatively) selected traits, among others (West-Eberhard, 2003).

Mechanisms for Change

There are a number of possible mechanisms for epigenetic inheritance. One possibility is that the chances of a particular mutation increase as a result of behavioral changes in the organism or a particular condition in the environment; that is, changes in the developmental system provide a new context for genes, which increases the likelihood that they will replicate unfaithfully, producing phenotypic change in the absence of a provoking environmental event. This has been demonstrated in the bacterium *Escherichia coli* when they are deprived of amino acids, which results in not only an increased rate of the transcription of genes that promote longer survival but also an increase in the rate of mutations of those genes (Wright, 1997). Wright proposed that such "environmentally directed mutations" would permit the bacteria to alter their biochemical capabilities (e.g., becoming resistant to antibiotics), allowing them to invade new habitats. According to Jablonka (2001),

> This condition-dependent increase in mutation rate is adaptive since such targeted mutation in the relevant genes may "rescue" the cell without greatly increasing the load of mutation. It seems that through natural selection the mechanisms that allow selective control of gene expression have been coupled with mechanisms that determine the fidelity of copying, so that the inducible system that turns

genes on and off also turns the production of mutations on and off. (pp. 102–103)

Another possibility is that novel, stressful environments promote the activity of only a select set of alleles. These alleles may have been low in frequency among individuals in the prestressed environment but are associated with increased survival in the modified environment. Assuming that the once-novel environment becomes stable, after many generations of individuals possessing the beneficial alleles selectively breeding with one another, only those alleles associated with extreme values of a trait remain in the genotype. Thus, changes occur not in the production of new genes (via mutations), but in terms of the frequencies of different alleles for a particular trait, precisely as any trait can change in frequency in a population following conventional Mendelian analyses. (Of course, any single gene can have multiple effects—pleiotropy—and many different genes are likely associated with a single characteristic, making this scenario more complicated than it appears on the surface.)

Third, novel environments could activate heretofore dormant genes, or, relatedly, served to *deactivate* certain genes, the end result being similar (a different combination of genes are involved in a particular response, relative to individuals in the prestressed environment). Individuals appropriately responsive to these novel environment (i.e.., who possess genes that are activated or deactivated by environmental condition) modify their behavior, which in turn is subject to natural selection. Offspring of such individuals would presumably posses the same genes as their parents and be similarly responsive to such novel environments.

A third possible mechanism for epigenetic evolution involves nongenetic changes via *cytoplasmic inheritance*. Cytoplasmic inheritance refers to modifications that can be passed along from mothers to their offspring, not through nuclear genes, but by way of changes found in the cytoplasm of the mother's gametes (e.g., Ho, 1998; Jablonka & Lamb, 1995). For example, the asexually reproducing water flea, *Daphnia cuncullata*, grows a large protective helmet when raised in the presence of the larvae of a potential predator. The daughters, and to a lesser extent the granddaughters, also grow the helmet, even when they are raised in safe environments (Agrawal, Laforsch, & Tollrian, 1999). The mechanism for such inheritance is likely to be found in the cytoplasm and not the nuclear genes that mothers provide to their daughters (and granddaughters). In other work, Ho, Tucker, Keeley, and Saunder (1983) demonstrated cytoplasmic inheritance by selectively breeding fruit flies for the expression of the bithorax (two sets of wings) phenocopy. The novel morphology was initially expressed when embryonic flies were exposed to ether. To isolate the source of modification, Ho and her colleagues bred groups of treated males with untreated females, as well as treated females with untreated males. They reported that only the offspring of treated females expressed the bithorax phenotype. The most parsimonious interpretation of these results is that the proximate cause for the bithorax phenotype was some chemical found in the cytoplasm of the female.

There are species differences in developmental plasticity; specifically, in comparison to smaller brained animals, animals with large brains display substantial ability to learn and to modify their behavior in response to unexpected environments. According to Gottlieb (1992), it is such large-brained, behaviorally flexible species that are most likely to adapt to novel environments and are thus more likely to experience faster rates of evolution (see also McKinney, 1998; Wyles, Kunkel, & Wilson, 1983). In support of this contention, Wyles et al. reported a correlation of .97 between the rate of anatomical changes from the fossil record and the average relative brain size for different groups of animals. The larger the brain size relative to body size for a group of animals, the greater the degree of anatomical change seen in the fossil record. *Homo sapiens* had both the largest relative brain size and the fastest rate of anatomical change, followed in both categories by the hominoids (which include the lesser and great apes). According to Wyles et al., animals that acquire new skills will use them "to exploit the environment in a new way. . . . [The] nongenetic propagation of new skills and mobility in large populations will accelerate anatomical evolution by increasing the rate at which anatomical mutants of potentially high fitness are exposed to selection in new contexts" (p. 4396).

Domain-General versus Domain-Specific Mechanisms and Plasticity

The proposal that evolutionary change is motivated by the developmental flexibility of organisms seems at odds with evolutionary psychology's contention that what evolved are domain-specific mechanisms, shaped by natural selection to solve recurrent problems faced by our ancestors. Humans, like other animals, did not evolve general skills to apply to the plethora of problems (from identifying predators to mating) they faced; rather, what evolved were specific cognitive modules, each designed by natural selection to deal with a specific set of problems (e.g., Buss, 1995; Tooby & Cosmides, 1992). This does not mean that the brain is hardwired, or that learning and particular experiences are not necessary for the modules to be properly activated; but it is at odds with the degree of plasticity proposed by proponents of DST and epigenetic evolution.

However, evolutionary psychology is not monolithic, and a number of authors have proposed that there is room for both domain-specific and domain-general mechanisms in explaining human social-cognitive evolution (e.g., Bjorklund & Kipp, 1996; Flinn & Ward, Chapter 2, this volume; Geary, 2004, Chapter 19, this volume; Rakison, Chapter 13, this volume). The most relevant proposals for the current discussion are those of David Geary (2004; Geary & Huffman, 2002), who argues that not only have domain-specific information-processing modules evolved to handle recurrent problems faced by our ancestors, but so, too, have domain-general skills necessary to deal with novelty. Some aspects of an animal's environment are apt to be invariant, stable across contexts and across generations. In such situations, there would be selective pressure to develop domain-specific information-processing modules that require only species-typical environments for their proper functioning. For example, most visual abilities, although requiring experience with patterned light, develop normally in most individuals under all but the most deprived situations. Similarly, the ability to identify faces is invariant across all human environments, is critical for survival, and one might expect such an ability to be represented by modular-like information-processing mechanisms. In contrast, other aspects of an animal's environment are highly variable, both over the course of a lifetime and across generations. The complexities associated with finding food, avoiding predators, and dealing with conspecifics, in some species, would be highly variable, and an organism would be better served by developing mechanisms that are pliable, or plastic, and able to deal with the changing contingencies of an often unpredictable environment. Geary posits that evolution has shaped the emergence of such variable, domain-general cognitive abilities, as well as domain-specific abilities, and that humans' unique evolutionary history has made the selection for dealing with variability particularly strong.

The ability to deal with novelty, essentially to learn and change one's behavior based on experience, is not unique to *H. sapiens*, of course. It may benefit any long-lived species that makes its living as a generalist to be behaviorally/cognitively plastic and thus adaptable to variations in ecological conditions. Surely this describes animals such as rats, wolves, and chimpanzees, as well as humans. But Geary, along with other theorists (e.g., Alexander, 1979; Bjorklund & Harnishfeger, 1995; Humphrey, 1976), has proposed that it was the complexity of human social groups that served as a stimulus for cognitive flexibility, more so than any other single factor. However, social complexity in and of itself will not result in a cognitively flexible organism; otherwise one would expect ants, bees, and termites to be among the intellectual giants of the animal world. Other conditions are also required to result in cognitive evolution that led eventually to modern humans. Among those factors are a large brain and an extended juvenile period in which to learn the complexities of one's social group (Flinn & Ward, Chapter 2, this volume).

BIG BRAINS, AN EXTENDED JUVENILE PERIOD, SOCIAL COMPLEXITY, AND PLASTICITY

We have argued previously that it was the confluence of big brains, an extended juvenile period, and social complexity that led to the evolution of the modern human brain (Bjorklund & Bering, 2003a; Bjorklund, Cormier, & Rosenberg, 2005; Bjorklund & Pellegrini, 2002). In this section, we summarize briefly the main points of this argument and how it fits in with the larger argument for the role of developmental plasticity in human cognitive evolution.

Larger animals, on average, have bigger brains than smaller animals, simply because both brain and body develop according to allometric formulae. Brain size must therefore be evaluated in terms of body size to get an idea of how much more (or less) brain an animal has, presumably for learning and other cognitive feats (see Deacon, 1997) relative to other animals. This is determined by the *encephalization quotient* (EQ), which is a measure of the expected ratio of brain weight to body weight for a family of animals, with 1.0 being the "expected" ratio for a species (e.g., Jerison, 1973, 2002; Rilling & Insel, 1999). Thus, an EQ greater than 1.0 means that the brain weight is greater than expected for a species of that size, and conversely, an EQ of less than 1.0 would mean that a species' brain weight is less than expected, given its body weight. Although there is controversy concerning exactly how best to compute EQs, modern humans have the largest EQ of any land mammal, about 7.6. This is compared to the EQ of our closest genetic relative, chimpanzees (*Pan troglodytes*) of about 2.3 (Jerison, 1973; Rilling & Insel, 1999).

But how is it that humans have come to have such large brains? Part of the answer lies in the fact that humans have an extended juvenile period. Human neonates are born immature relative to other primates, and their brains continue to develop at a substantially rapid rate until almost the age of 3. Finlay and colleagues (Finlay & Darlington, 1995; Finlay, Darlington, & Nicastro, 2001) posit that this delayed cerebral development results in the manifestation of more neurons, as well as a greater amount of synaptic and dendritic growth. The human brain continues to gain weight (due mostly to increases in the size of neurons) well into our second decade, and associative brain neurons do not become fully myelinated until this time or later (Gibson, 1991; Yakovlev & Lecours, 1967). This delayed maturation affords humans the flexibility to make many behavioral changes and to learn the idiosyncrasies of their environment.

Although there were surely many aspects of ancient humans' environments that were variable, thus requiring an ability to learn new responses to novel situations, the social complexity of *H. sapiens*, perhaps more than any other feature, necessitated a pliable cognitive system and an extended time in which to master the ways of the social world (e.g., Alexander, 1979; Bjorklund & Harnishfeger, 1995; Geary, 2004; Humphrey, 1976). *H. sapiens* is arguably one of the most socially complex species on the planet. Although chimpanzees are undeniably highly social creatures, and as some would say, political (e.g., Byrne & Whiten, 1988; Goodall, 1986; de Waal, 1982), it is humans who have set up schools, governments, nations, and the many other sociotechnological institutions that help to separate us from the rest of the animal kingdom. We believe that over evolutionary time, selective pressures have acted upon especially *social-cognitive* abilities—those abilities related to dealing with social relationships.

An ardent supporter of the argument that human intellectual evolution stems, in large part, from our ever-burgeoning social complexity, is Robin Dunbar (1995, 1998). Dunbar proposed that large brains are not merely by-products of large bodies, but instead have coevolved with increasing group size. Dunbar put forth the *social brain hypothesis*, which "implies that constraints on group size arise from information-processing capacity of the primate brain, and that the neocortex plays a major role in this" (Dunbar, 1998, p. 184). In fact, Dunbar (1995, 1998) has shown that, for primates, the correlation between neocortex size and group size is .76. This relation, however, is mediated by rate of development. For example, Joffe (1997) examined the relationships of brain size, length of juvenile period, and social complexity among 27 different primate species, including humans, and concluded:

> An extended juvenile period has evolved in response to social pressures as evinced by the positive linear relationship between juvenile period length and social group size, and between the relative length of the juvenile period and non-visual neocortex, the main component implicated in social problem solving and cognitive memory. These social pressures have selected for an extension in the developmental stage most associated with learning. (p. 602)

The combination of large brains and an extended juvenile period would have afforded the plasticity necessary to generate individuals that display species-atypical behaviors, as predicted by epigenetic theories, which would have eventually led to evolutionary changes in the ancestors of *H. sapiens*. And because of the hypothesized role that social complexity played in shaping the human (and primate) mind, we would predict that these epigenetic effects would first be realized in the realm of social behavior.

Although aspects of epigenetic theories of evolution can be tested with infrahuman animals (e.g., Ho et al., 1983; Waddington, 1975), it is more problematic to assess such hypotheses with respect to human cognitive evolution. However, there is one extant species, closely related to humans, that has many of the characteristics hypothesized for our ancestors: large brains relative to body size, an extended juvenile period, and life in a socially complex community. We are referring, of course, to chimpanzees (*P. troglodytes* and *P. paniscus*), who last shared a common ancestor with modern humans between 5 and 7 million years ago, and who share greater than 98% of their DNA with *H. sapiens*.

There is much debate in the cognitive primatology literature over just "how much like us" chimpanzees are, with some proposing that they possess representational abilities similar to those of human children, including rudimentary theory of mind (e.g., Fouts, 1997; Goodall, 1986; de Waal, 1982); others, in contrast, argue that there is no evidence from well-controlled experiments to suggest that chimpanzees possess any representational skills on par with those observed in most 3- and 4-year-old children (e.g., Bering, in press; Povinelli & Bering, 2002). Our own view is that chimpanzees do indeed display sophisticated evidence of social learning and possess at least the *precursors* of representational abilities, which could serve as the basis for the evolution of more advanced forms of social learning, characteristic of our own species (e.g., Bjorklund & Bering, 2003a; Bjorklund et al., 2005; Bjorklund & Pellegrini, 2002). To this point, Bjorklund et al. (2005) wrote:

> If the common ancestor humans shared with chimpanzees possessed social-cognitive abilities similar to those of modern apes, it seems clear that when enhanced levels of computational power were achieved via evolutionary expansion of gross brain volume, it was in a species that was in a position to put it to good use in a complex social milieu in which sophistication in the use of both competitive and cooperative behaviors would result in clearly improved inclusive fitness. (p. 163)

Might research with these animals be able to provide some insight into human cognitive evolution and test the feasibility of epigenetic evolution in the human line?

CROSS-FOSTERING STUDIES AND THE ENCULTURATION HYPOTHESIS

Although we are aware of no transgenerational studies in primates comparable to those performed with fruit flies (cf. Waddington, 1975), there is research examining changes in a primate's behavior as a function of being raised by another species (cross-fostering). Do these animals possess the behavioral plasticity to alter their species-typical behavior to be more in line with the species with which they were raised rather than the species whose DNA they possess? If they do, this provides evidence, we argue, that primates have the behavioral flexibility to alter greatly their behavior in response to novel, early (and persistent) environments. This is the necessary (though not sufficient) requirement for epigenetic evolution as we have discussed it here. And if the rearing species is humans and the behaviors represent cognitions more in line with that of human children than that of the participants' genetic kin, it increases further the plausible role of behavioral plasticity in the evolution of human cognition.

Behavioral plasticity may produce novel phenotypes in response to many different environments, including the introduction of a new predator or prey species to an ecosystem, a change of available diet, and climatic change. But one source of environmental change that may produce drastic changes in an animal's behavior is parenting. Should mothers display species-atypical behaviors toward their infants, for whatever reason, their infants may, in turn, show a species-atypical pattern of development. Changes in parenting behavior may be an especially important source of environmental novelty for mammals, which are highly dependent on their mothers for sustenance, and especially for most primates, many of whom spend years in close proximity to their mothers.

Owren and his colleagues (Owren & Dieter, 1989; Owren, Dieter, Seyfarth, & Cheyney, 1992, 1993) conducted cross-fostering experiments between Japanese macaques and rhesus macaques (*Macaca fuscata* and *M. mulatta*, respectively). They studied the vocalizations of these monkeys and found that in cross-fostered situations, Japanese macaques continued to exhibit their species-typical vocalization (i.e., a "coo"). On the other hand, rhesus macaques that had been cross-fostered, in addition to exhibiting their species-typical vocalization (i.e., "gruff"), also displayed the "coo" vocalization of the Japanese macaque. However, exhibitions were not at the expected rate that would occur in a normal parenting situation (Owren et al., 1993). In other research, de Waal and Johanowicz (1993) assessed reconciliation behavior in a cross-fostering study with stumptail (*M. arctoides*) and rhesus (*M. mulatta*) monkeys. Reconciliation is rare in rhesus, but common in stumptail monkeys after aggressive encounters. Rhesus juveniles cohoused with stumptail monkeys showed a pattern of reconciliation more like that of their stumptail cohorts than did rhesus monkeys housed with conspecifics. The rate of reconciliation increased gradually over the 5 weeks of cohabitation and was maintained for an additional 6 weeks. Interestingly, rhesus monkeys did not alter their specific behaviors when reconciling. Stumptail monkeys frequently engage in teeth chattering and putting both hands on the hips of their partner. Cohoused rhesus monkeys did not show an increase in these behaviors, although they did show an increase in grinning during reconciliation; grinning is a species-typical behavior for rhesus monkeys. It is also worth noting that the increase in reconciliation for cohoused rhesus monkeys was not accompanied by changes in affiliative or grooming behavior. Thus, cohousing juvenile animals resulted in changes in some molar behaviors (reconciliation), but not others (affiliation and grooming), and no differences in specific (molecular) behaviors.

The most relevant studies with respect to issues of human cognitive evolution are those in which great apes (chimpanzees, orangutans, and gorillas) are reared by humans, much like human children. Will such species-atypical rearing experiences produce species-atypical behavior, perhaps more similar to that observed for human children than for mother-raised apes? This has been referred to as the *enculturation hypothesis* by Call and Tomasello (1996) who described home-raised, or *enculturated*, apes as "apes raised by humans in something like a human cultural environment (sometimes including exposure to or training in symbolic skills); the environment need not literally be a home but must include something close to daily contact with humans and their artifacts in meaningful interactions" (p. 372).

What aspects of human rearing may be of particular relevance in influencing the cognitive development of enculturated apes? From the moment they are born, human children are treated as intentional agents—that is, as if

deferred imitation in enculturated chimpanzees comes from the observations of Kellogg and Kellogg (1933) and Hayes (1951). Observations of deferred imitation occurring as young as 2 years, 11 months have been made with captive orangutans being "rehabilitated" to return to the wild (Russon, 1996), as well as with an enculturated orangutan (Miles, Mitchell, & Harper, 1996). Most of this evidence, however, lacks rigorous experimental control, thus making it uncertain whether the animals in question are truly displaying deferred imitation or perhaps acquired the behaviors through other means (e.g., operant conditioning, trial and error, local enhancement). The most convincing evidence of deferred imitation in great apes comes from controlled experimental studies that are similar to those involving human infants.

Deferred Imitation in Enculturated Apes

Modeling their deferred imitation experiments after designs used with human infants (e.g., Abravenal & Gingold, 1985; Bauer, 1997; Meltzoff, 1985, 1995), several researchers have found evidence of deferred imitation in chimpanzees (both common and pygmy, or bonobos) and, possibly, orangutans. The first published evidence of deferred imitation in enculturated apes was presented by Tomasello, Savage-Rumbaugh, and Kruger (1993) in a study that compared deferred imitation among chimpanzees (three mother-raised, and three enculturated) and human children (eight 18-month-olds and eight 30-month-olds). Of the mother-raised apes, two were bonobos (*P. paniscus*) (a 21-year-old female and a 3-year, 7-month-old female), and one was a common chimpanzee (*P. troglodytes*) (a 4-year-old male). The enculturated apes also consisted of two bonobos (a 10-year, 1-month-old male, and a 5-year-old female) and one common chimpanzee (a 4-year, 11-month-old female). The deferred imitation condition consisted of a 4-minute baseline period during which the ape was permitted to interact with the target object(s), followed by the experimenter demonstrating the target actions (e.g., making a popping noise with an oil can, turning a bar to release a vice from a table). The deferred phase began 48 hours later. The apes were again given the object(s) previously shown to them, and allowed to freely interact with them.

As expected, the enculturated chimpanzees displayed significantly greater levels of deferred imitation than the nonenculturated chimpanzees, the latter group showing floor levels of performance. However, it is interesting to note that the enculturated chimpanzees also outperformed both the 18- and 30-month-old children in deferred imitation. Tomasello and colleagues (1993) offered two possible explanations for this latter finding. First, they proposed that it is possible that this effect may be due to the age of the enculturated chimpanzees (i.e., they were, on average, over twice as old as the other participants). Concomitant with the age difference could also be a more highly developed memory system, thereby allowing the greater retention of the demonstrated actions. The second possible explanation that Tomasello et al. offered was that "the three groups (the two child groups and the enculturated chimpanzees) all have the competence to remember the model equally well, but this difference is in some 'performance' factor having to do with their understanding of the task" (p. 1702).

In a series of studies extending Tomasello et al.'s (1993) findings, Bjorklund and his colleagues (Bering, Bjorklund, & Ragan, 2000; Bjorklund, Bering, & Ragan, 2000; Bjorklund, Yunger, Bering, & Ragan, 2002; Yunger & Bjorklund, 2004) further assessed deferred imitation in enculturated apes. In the first study (Bering et al., 2000), deferred imitation of action-on-objects was assessed in three juvenile enculturated chimpanzees (*P. troglodytes*) (names, ages, and sex: Grub, 5 years, 5 months, male; Kenya, 3 years, 6 months, female; and Noelle, 2 years, 1 month, female) and three juvenile enculturated orangutans (*Pongo pygmaeus*; names, ages, and sex: Pongo, 6 years, 5 months, male; Ruby, 4 years, 7 months, female; and Christopher, 4 years, 3 months, male). All participants had been in raised in an enculturated environment since infancy, and all had had extensive contact with both human caretakers and conspecifics. To a large degree, the experiences of these animals were similar to those of human children. For example, they were heavily exposed to human artifacts, such as books, toys, and eating utensils, which they were encouraged to manipulate; they "played" with human care-takers, which involved shared–joint attention, language, and some attempts at teaching; and they slept in bed-like cages each night.

Similar to the Tomasello et al. (1993) study, the apes were first presented with the objects for a 4-minute baseline period, during which they were encouraged to interact freely with the objects. This was followed by a demon-stration phase, in which a familiar caretaker demonstrated the target behavior to the ape. Target behaviors included both simple (e.g., clapping together two cymbals) and complex (e.g., placing a plastic nail into a form board and strik-ing it with the head of a hammer) tasks. This was then followed by a 10-min-ute delay (long enough for the previous experience to be out of immediate memory), after which the deferred phase began. During this phase, the apes were re-presented with the target objects to freely interact with them. Percent-age of trials on which apes showed deferred imitation are presented for the individuals chimpanzees and orangutans in Figures 3.1 and 3.2, respectively.[1] The two older chimpanzees both displayed better than chance levels of deferred imitation, whereas Noelle, the youngest chimpanzee, displayed deferred imitation on only two of seven tasks, both simple ones. Only one of the three orangutans (Ruby) displayed deferred imitation greater than expected by chance. Although a control group of nonenculturated apes was not available for comparison, the failure of mother-raised chimpanzees and orangutans in other situations to display deferred imitation (e.g., Tomasello et al., 1993) suggests that this ability may be limited to human-reared animals.

Subsequent testing with five of the original six animals (Ruby was not available for subsequent testing) indicated continued high levels of deferred imitation for the chimpanzees but not for the orangutans (Bjorklund et al., 2000; 2002; Yunger & Bjorklund, 2004). Neither of the two remaining

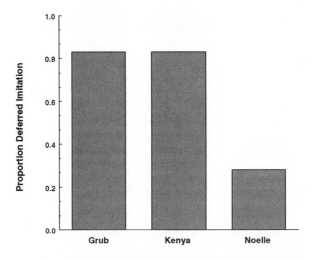

FIGURE 3.1. Proportion of tasks displaying deferred imitation for each animal: Chimpanzees. Based on data from Bering, Bjorklund, and Ragan (2000).

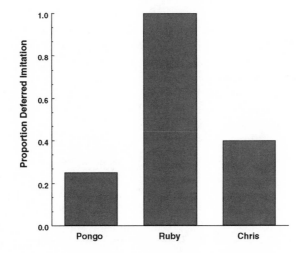

FIGURE 3.2. Proportion of tasks displaying deferred imitation for each animal: Orangutans. Based on data from Bering, Bjorklund, and Ragan (2000).

orangutans displayed deferred imitation greater than expected by chance in any subsequent testings. For the chimpanzees, levels of deferred imitation for the complex tasks were strongly associated with age ($r = .80$), whereas age and level of deferred imitation were not significantly correlated for the simple tasks ($r = .39$) (Bjorklund & Bering, 2003b). As noted earlier, even the youngest chimpanzee (2 years, 1 month at first testing) showed relatively high levels of deferred imitation on the simple tasks. This pattern of data for the chimpanzees is reminiscent of results reported for human infants, who display deferred imitation for simple behaviors as young as 6 months (Collie & Hayne, 1999), but whose ability to imitate more complicated tasks over delays increases over the second year of life (e.g., Abravanel & Gingold, 1985; Bauer, Wenner, Dropik, & Wewerka, 2000; McCall, Parke, & Kavanaugh, 1977; Meltzoff, 1985).

Although we believe that results from the studies by Tomasello et al. (1993) and those of Bjorklund and his colleagues provide good evidence for deferred imitation in enculturated chimpanzees, alternative interpretations of the results are not ruled out. It is still possible that the copying behavior observed in these animals may have been achieved via mimicry (duplication of the actions without understanding the goal of the actions) or emulation (knowledge of the general goal of the model without reproducing specific behaviors) rather than true imitation. To further reduce this likelihood, we used a generalization of imitation tasks with chimpanzees (Bjorklund et al., 2002) and orangutans (Yunger & Bjorklund, 2004). In these tasks, a model displays a behavior on a set of objects (e.g., clapping together two round, metal cymbals held by knobs), and, after a delay, the ape is given similar, but not identical items (e.g., two wooden, rectangular trowels held by handles). To display generalization of imitation, the animal must make slightly different actions on slightly different objects to produce similar results (in this case, a clapping noise). If the animals are able to display high levels of generalization of imitation, it argues against mimicry, because of the differences in behaviors that must be displayed to succeed. Similarly, because the actions and objects are similar on the two tasks (as they are in the standard deferred imitation task), it is unlikely that success can be explained as a form of emulation.

The percentage of trials on which each chimpanzee displayed generalization of imitation is presented in Figure 3.3. Also presented are independent trials of deferred imitation. As can be seen, levels of deferred imitation were higher than levels of generalization of imitation, yet each animal showed above-chance levels of generalization of imitation (Bjorklund et al., 2002). We considered this strong evidence that these juvenile, enculturated chimps (age range at testing 5 years, 9 months to 9 years, 1 month) are capable of true deferred imitation of actions on objects. Similar tests with the two orangutans indicated low levels of both deferred imitation and generalization of imitation (Yunger & Bjorklund, 2004).

We cannot make the definitive claim from these data that enculturated chimpanzees are capable of true imitation and other chimpanzees are not.

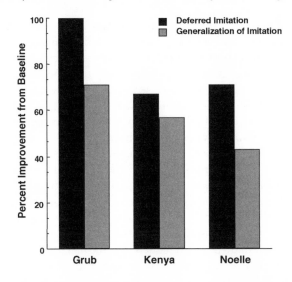

FIGURE 3.3. Percentage of deferred imitation and generalization tasks for each ape on which an improvement in performance at the deferred phase relative to baseline was observed. From Bjorklund, Yunger, Bering, and Ragan (2002). Copyright 2002 by Springer-Verlag. Reprinted by permission.

Although we believe that the generalization of imitation results reduce greatly the likelihood that mimicry or emulation is the basis for the animals' behavior, these alternatives cannot be eliminated (Call & Carpenter, 2003). And although the studies by Tomasello et al. (1993) included nonenculturated controls, the studies by Bjorklund and his colleagues did not, requiring caution in the interpretation of the findings. Nonetheless, coupled with the results of studies on referential communication with enculturated and nonenculturated apes, we believe that the results are strongly suggestive that the social-cognitive abilities of chimpanzees living in species-atypical environments are substantially changed in the direction of their foster species. What makes this particular set of findings so compelling, we believe, is that chimpanzees are humans' closest relative, and the behavior is more in line with that shown by human children than by chimpanzees raised by their mothers. Such findings, we argue, may provide insights into human cognitive evolution.

ENCULTURATED GREAT APES, DEVELOPMENTAL PLASTICITY, AND EPIGENETIC EVOLUTION

What, then, are the mechanisms underlying such "enhanced" abilities in enculturated chimpanzees? One possibility is that a history of human rearing makes chimpanzees (and to a lesser extent, orangutans) more socially responsive to humans. They learn through standard mechanisms of associative learning to attend to actions and objects of interest to humans, to follow their gaze and their pointing, and to reproduce some interesting behaviors that humans exhibit. In this scenario, enculturated apes apply their universal ape-cognition to the human social realm. Mother-raised apes have the same cognitive abilities, but because their rearing environment does not include shared–joint attention, direct teaching, or language, they have not learned to use referential pointing or to display imitative responses in the "proper" contexts (i.e., when being tested by a human experimenter). In such cases, apes have undergone a *socialization of attention* (Tomasello, 1999; see also Call & Carpenter, 2003), learning from continuous interaction with humans to attend to human behaviors that, in turn, facilitate social learning. A related possibility has been proposed by Bering (in press), which he terms the *apprenticeship hypothesis*. Apes learn that humans provide solutions to many problems, and learn to be especially attentive to human actions, which results in enhanced social-learning abilities when humans serve as models. A more radical alternative, originally proposed by Call and Tomasello (1996), is that a species-atypical rearing environment results in modification of the epigenetic course of ontogeny, producing a species-atypical pattern of development. Because of the enhanced neural and cognitive plasticity of these relatively large-brained, slow-developing animals, new social-cognitive skills emerge as a result of a substantial and consistent departure from a species-typical environment. Essentially, these chimpanzees develop a set of biologically secondary abilities, similar in form to what Geary (1995) proposed for humans. Such modifications in mental development could not occur in a species that did not possess the cognitive abilities to serve as the foundation for such change, which, we believe, chimpanzees indeed possess (Bjorklund & Bering, 2003a; Bjorklund et al., 2005).

Although we believe that the latter interpretation is more exciting, each nonetheless fits with the epigenetic theory of evolution that we advocate. The heightened degree of developmental plasticity observed in juvenile chimpanzees affords them the ability to alter their behavior in response to a species-atypical rearing environment. As a result, these animals acquire behaviors through imitation and other forms of social learning that their mother-raised peers do not. These new behaviors, had they been generated by our ancestors, would have placed the animals in new environments. This, in turn, would have exposed them to different selection pressures and, as a result, would have led to a different phylogenetic path than that experienced by animals remaining in a species-typical environment. Although we would like to provide a specific scenario of how behavioral changes associated with developmental plasticity in our ape or hominid ancestors led to the evolution of modern humans, any such scenario would be highly speculative. Nonetheless, we believe that modifications in mother–infant interactions would likely be the initiating source for such generation of species-atypical behaviors/cognitions.

What especially fascinates us is that chimpanzees are considered to be a "conservative" species, in that they likely have changed little since they last shared a common ancestor with *H. sapiens*, making them the best extant model for what our progenitors may have been like. Finding evidence that the social cognition of juvenile chimpanzees can be altered to be more in the line with that of human children, by rearing them much as human children are reared, suggests that this may have been one route for human cognitive evolution. Such an interpretation does not obviate the need for genetic mutations or for a potent role of natural selection in human evolution. But it does suggest a substantial role for developmental plasticity in generating the cognitive and behavioral novelty on which natural selection can operate, in this case, leading to the modern human mind.

NOTE

1. Behavior at both baseline and the deferred phase was classified as "target behavior" when all components of the modeled behavior were displayed, "approximation to target behavior" when significant portions of the modeled behavior were displayed (e.g., in the form board task, hitting the nail into the form board with the handle, instead of the head of the hammer, was classified as an approximation to target), or "no imitative behavior." An ape was credited with showing deferred imitation if it displayed more advanced behavior on the deferred trial than on the baseline trial (e.g., from "no imitative behavior" to "target" or "approximation to target behavior"; or from "approximation to target behavior" to "target behavior"). Trials on which an animal displayed the target behavior at baseline were eliminated from calculations, because no improvement at the deferred phase was possible.

REFERENCES

Abravanel, E., & Gingold, H. (1985). Learning via observation during the second year of life. *Developmental Psychology, 21*, 614–623.

Agrawal, A. A., Laforsch, C., & Tollrian, R. (1999) Transgenerational induction of defences in animals and plants. *Nature, 40*, 60–63.

Alexander, R. D. (1979). *Darwinism and human affairs.* Seattle: University of Washington Press.

Baldwin, J. M. (1902). *Development and evolution.* New York: Macmillan.

Bauer, P. J. (1997). Development of memory in early childhood. In N. Cowan (Ed.), *The development of memory in early childhood* (pp. 83–111). Hove, UK: Psychology Press.

Bauer, P. J. (in press). Getting explicit memory off the ground: Steps toward construction of a neuro-developmental account of changes in the first two years of life. *Developmental Review.*

Bauer, P. J., Wenner, J. A., Dropik, P. L., & Wewerka, S. S. (2000). Parameters of remembering and forgetting in the transition from infancy to early childhood. *Monographs of the Society for Research in Child Development, 65*(4, Serial No. 263).

Bering, J. M. (in press). A critical review of the "enculturation hypothesis": The effects of human rearing on great ape social cognition. *Animal Cognition.*

Bering, J. M., Bjorklund, D. F., & Ragan, P. (2000). Deferred imitation of object-related actions in human-reared juvenile chimpanzees and orangutans. *Developmental Psychobiology, 36,* 218–232.

Bjorklund, D. F., & Bering, J. M. (2003a). Big brains, slow development, and social complexity: The developmental and evolutionary origins of social cognition. In M. Brüne, H. Ribbert, & W. Schiefenhövel (Eds.), *The social brain: Evolutionary aspects of development and pathology* (pp. 133–151). New York: Wiley.

Bjorklund, D. F., & Bering, J. M. (2003b). A note on the development of deferred imitation in enculturated juvenile chimpanzees (*Pan troglodytes*). *Developmental Review, 23,* 389–412.

Bjorklund, D. F., Bering, J., & Ragan, P. (2000). A two-year longitudinal study of deferred imitation of object manipulation in an enculturated juvenile chimpanzee (*Pan troglodytes*) and orangutan (*Pongo pygmaeus*). *Developmental Psychobiology, 37,* 229–237.

Bjorklund, D. F., Cormier, C., & Rosenberg, J. S. (2005). The evolution of theory of mind: Big brains, social complexity, and inhibition. In W. Schneider, R. Schumann-Hengsteler, & B. Sodian (Eds.), *Young children's cognitive development: Interrelationships among executive functioning, working memory, verbal ability and theory of mind* (pp. 147–188). Mahwah, NJ: Erlbaum.

Bjorklund, D. F., & Harnishfeger, K. K. (1995). The role of inhibition mechanisms in the evolution of human cognition and behavior. In F. N. Dempster & C. J. Brainerd (Eds.), *New perspectives on interference and inhibition in cognition* (pp. 141–173). New York: Academic Press.

Bjorklund, D. F., & Kipp, K. (1996). Parental investment theory and gender differences in the evolution of inhibition mechanisms. *Psychological Bulletin, 120,* 163–188.

Bjorklund, D. F., & Pellegrini, A. D. (2002). *The origins of human nature: Evolutionary developmental psychology.* Washington, DC: American Psychological Association Press.

Bjorklund, D. F., Yunger, J. L., Bering, J. M., & Ragan, P. (2002). The generalization of deferred imitation in enculturated chimpanzees (*Pan troglodytes*). *Animal Cognition, 5,* 49–58.

Boesch, C., & Tomasello, M. (1998). Chimpanzee and human culture. *Current Anthropology, 39,* 591–604.

Bull, J. J. (1980). Sex determination in reptiles. *Quarterly Review of Biology, 55,* 3–21.

Buss, D. M. (1995). Evolutionary psychology: A new paradigm for psychological science. *Psychological Inquiry, 6,* 1–30.

Byrne, R.W., & Whiten, A. (Eds.). (1988). *Machiavellian intelligence: Social expertise and the evolution of intellect in monkeys, apes, and humans.* New York: Oxford University Press.

Call, J., & Carpenter, M. (2003). On imitation in apes and children. *Infancia y Aprendizaje, 24,* 325–349.

Call, J., & Tomasello, M. (1994). The production and comprehension of referential pointing by orangutans. *Journal of Comparative Psychology, 108,* 307–317.

Call, J., & Tomasello, M. (1996). The effects of humans on the cognitive development of apes. In A. E. Russon, K. A. Bard, & S. T. Parker (Eds.), *Reaching into thought: The minds of the great apes* (pp. 371–403). New York: Cambridge University Press.

Carver, L. J., & Bauer, P. J. (1999). When the event is more than the sum of its parts: Nine-month-olds' long-term ordered recall. *Memory, 7,* 147–174.

Collie, R., & Hayne, H. (1999). Deferred imitation by 6- and 9-month-old infants: More evidence for declarative memory. *Developmental Psychobiology, 35,* 83–90.

Deacon, T. W. (1997). *The symbolic species: The co-evolution of language and the brain.* New York: Norton.

Denenberg, V. H., & Rosenberg, K. M. (1967). Non-genetic transmission of information. *Nature, 216,* 549–550.

de Waal, F. B. M. (1982). *Chimpanzee politics.* London: Jonathan Cape.

de Waal, F. B. M., & Johanowicz, D. L. (1993). Modification of reconciliation behavior through social experience: An experiment with two macaque species. *Child Development, 64,* 897–908.

Dunbar, R. I. M. (1995). Neocortex size and group size in primates: A test of the hypothesis. *Journal of Human Evolution, 28,* 287–296.

Dunbar, R. I. M. (1998). The social brain hypothesis. *Evolutionary Anthropology, 6,* 178–190.

Finlay, B. L., & Darlington, R. B. (1995). Linked regularities in the development and evolution of mammalian brains. *Science, 268,* 1578–1584.

Finlay, B., L., Darlington, R. B., & Nicastro, N. (2001). Developmental structure in brain evolution. *Behavioral and Brain Sciences, 24,* 263–308.

Fouts, R. (1997). *Next of kin: What chimpanzees have taught me about who we are.* New York: Morrow.

Francis, D. D., Szegda, K., Campbell, G., Martin, W. D., & Insel, T. R. (2003). Epigenetic sources of behavioral differences in mice. *Nature Neuroscience, 6,* 445–446.

Geary, D. C. (1995). Reflections of evolution and culture in children's cognition: Implications for mathematical development and instruction. *American Psychologist, 50,* 24–37.

Geary, D. C. (2004). *The origin of mind: Evolution of brain, cognition, and general intelligence.* Washington, DC: American Psychological Association Press.

Geary, D. C., & Huffman, K. J. (2002). Brain and cognitive evolution: Forms of modularity and functions of mind. *Psychological Bulletin, 128,* 667–698.

Gibson, K. R. (1991). Myelination and behavioral development: A comparative perspective on questions of neoteny, altriciality and intelligence. In K. R. Gibson & A. C. Peterson (Eds.), *Brain maturation and cognitive development: Comparative and cross-cultural perspectives* (pp. 29–63). New York: Aldine de Gruyter.

Goodall J. (1986). *The chimpanzees of Gombe.* Cambridge, MA: Belknap Press of Harvard University.

Gottlieb, G. (1987). The developmental basis of evolutionary change. *Journal of Comparative Psychology, 101,* 262–271.

Gottlieb, G. (1992). *Individual development and evolution: The genesis of novel behavior.* New York: Oxford University Press.

Gottlieb, G. (1998). Normally occurring environmental and behavioral influences on gene activity: From central dogma to probabilistic epigenesis. *Psychological Review, 105,* 792–802.

Gottlieb, G. (2002). Developmental–behavioral initiation of evolutionary change. *Psychological Review, 109,* 211–218.

Gould, S. J. (1977). *Ontogeny and phylogeny*. Cambridge, MA: Harvard University Press.

Greenough, W. T., Black, J. E., & Wallace, C. S. (1987). Experience and brain development. *Child Development, 58,* 539–559.

Harlow, H., Dodsworth, R., & Harlow, M. (1965). Total social isolation in monkeys. *Proceedings of the National Academy of Science USA, 54,* 90–96.

Hayes, C. (1951). *The ape in our house*. New York: Harper.

Ho, M.-W. (1998). Evolution. In G. Greenberg & M. M. Haraway (Eds.), *Comparative psychology: A handbook* (pp. 107–119). New York: Garland.

Ho, M.-W., Tucker, C., Keeley, D., & Saunder, P. T. (1983). Effects of successive generations of ether treatment on penetrance and expression of the bithorax phenocopy in *Drosophila melanogaster*. *Journal of Experimental Zoology, 225,* 357–368.

Humphrey, N. K. (1976). The social function of intellect. In P. P. G. Bateson & R. Hinde (Eds.), *Growing points in ethology* (pp. 303–317). Cambridge, UK: Cambridge University Press.

Jablonka, E. (2001). The systems of inheritance. In S. Oyama, P. E. Griffiths, & R. D. Gray (Eds.), *Cycles of contingency: Developmental systems and evolution* (pp. 99–116). Cambridge, MA: MIT Press.

Jablonka, E., & Lamb, M. (1995). *Epigenetic inheritance and evolution: The Lamarckian dimension*. New York: Oxford University Press.

Jerison, H. J. (1973). *Evolution of the brain and intelligence*. New York: Academic Press.

Jerison, H. J. (2002). On theory in comparative psychology. In R. J. Sternberg & J. C. Kaufman (Eds.), *The evolution of intelligence* (pp. 251–288). Mahwah, NJ: Erlbaum.

Joffe, T. H. (1997). Social pressures have selected for an extended juvenile period in primates. *Journal of Human Evolution, 32,* 593–605.

Johnson, M. H. (1998). The neural basis of cognitive development. In W. Damon, R. Kuhn, & R. Siegler (Eds.), *Handbook of child psychology: Cognition, perception and language* (5th ed., vol. 2, pp. 1–49). New York: Wiley.

Johnson, M. H. (2000). Functional brain development in infants: Elements of an interactive specialization framework. *Child Development, 71,* 75–81.

Kellogg, W. N., & Kellogg, L. A. (1967). *The ape and the child*. New York: Hafner. (Original published in 1933)

Kuo, Z. Y. (1976). *The dynamics of behavior development: An epigenetic view*. New York: Random House.

Langer, J., Rivera, S., Schlesinger, M., & Wakeley, A. (2003). Early cognitive development: Ontogeny and phylogeny. In J. Valsiner & K. J. Connolly (Eds.), *Handbook of developmental psychology* (pp. 141–171). London: Sage.

Li, S.-C. (2003). Biocultural orchestration of developmental plasticity across levels: The interplay of biology and culture in shaping the mind and behavior across the lifespan. *Psychological Bulletin, 129,* 171–194.

Lickliter, R. (1996). Structured organisms and structured environments: Developmental systems and the construction of learning capacities. In J. Valsiner & H. G. Voss (Eds.), *The structure of learning processes* (pp. 86–107). Norwood, NJ: Ablex.

Liu, D., Diorio, J., Day, J. C., Francis, D. D., & Meany, M. J. (2000). Maternal care, hippocampal synaptogenesis and cognitive development in rats. *Nature Neuroscience, 3,* 799–806.

McCall, R. B., Parke, R. D., & Kavanaugh, R. D. (1977). Imitation of live and televised models by children one to three years of age. *Monographs of the Society for Research in Child Development, 42*(Serial No. 173).

McGrew, W. C., & Tutin, C. E. G. (1978). Evidence for a social custom in wild chimpanzees? *Man, 13,* 243–251.

McKinney, M. L. (1998). Cognitive evolution by extending brain development: On recapitulation, progress, and other heresies. In J. Langer & M. Killen (Eds.), *Piaget, evolution, and development* (pp. 9–31). Mahwah, NJ: Erlbaum.

Meltzoff, A. N. (1985). Immediate and deferred imitation in fourteen- and twenty-four-month-old infants. *Child Development, 56,* 62–72.

Meltzoff, A. N. (1995). What infant memory tells us about infantile amnesia: Long-term recall and deferred imitation. *Journal of Experimental Child Psychology, 59,* 497–515.

Meltzoff, M., & Moore, K. (1997). Explaining facial imitation: A theoretical model. *Early Development and Parenting, 6,* 179–192.

Menzel, E. (1974). A group of young chimpanzees in a one acre field. In A. M. Schrier & F. Stollnitz (Eds.), *Behavior of nonhuman primates* (pp. 83–153). San Diego: Academic Press.

Miles H. L., Mitchell R. W., & Harper S. E. (1996). Simon says: The development of imitation in an enculturated orangutan. In A. E. Russon, K. A. Bard, & S. T. Parker (Eds.), *Reaching into thought: The minds of the great apes* (pp. 278–299). New York: Cambridge University Press.

Miles, L. (1990). The cognitive foundations for reference in a signing orangutan. In S. T. Parker, & K. R. Gibson (Eds.), *"Language" and intelligence in monkeys and apes* (pp. 511–539). Cambridge, UK: Cambridge University Press.

Miller, D. B. (1998). Epigenesis. In G. Greenberg & M. M. Haraway (Eds.), *Comparative psychology: A handbook* (pp. 105–106). New York: Garland.

Nelson, C. A. (2001). Neural plasticity and human development: The role of experience in sculpting memory systems. *Developmental Science, 3,* 115–130.

O'Connor, T. G., Rutter, M., Beckett, C., Keaveny, L., Kreppner, J. M., & the English and Romanian Adoptees Study Team. (2000). The effects of global severe privation on cognitive competence: Extension and longitudinal follow-up. *Child Development, 71,* 376–390.

Owren, M. J., & Dieter, J. A. (1989). Infant cross-fostering between Japanese (*Macaca fuscata*) and rhesus macaques (*M. mulatta*) between species. *American Journal of Primatology, 18,* 245–250.

Owren, M. J. , Dieter, J. A., Seyfarth, R. M., & Cheney, D. L. (1992). "Food" calls produced by adult female rhesus (*Macaca mulatta*) and Japanese (*M. fuscata*) macaques, their normally-raised offspring, and offspring cross-fostered between species. *Behaviour, 120,* 218–231.

Owren, M. J. , Dieter, J. A., Seyfarth, R. M., & Cheney, D. L. (1993). Vocalizations of rhesus (*Macaca mulatta*) and Japanese (*M. fuscata*) macaques cross-fostered between species show evidence of only limited modification. *Developmental Psychobiology, 26,* 389–406.

Oyama, S. (2000a). *The ontogeny of information: Developmental systems and evolution* (2nd ed.). Durham, NC: Duke University Press.

Oyama, S. (2000b). *Evolution's eye: A systems view of biology–culture divide*. Durham, NC: Duke University Press.

Oyama, S., Griffiths, P. E., & Gray, R. D. (2001). *Cycles of contingency: Developmental systems and evolution*. Cambridge, MA: MIT Press.

Patterson, F. (1978). Linguistic capabilities of a lowland gorilla. In F. Peng (Ed.), *Sign language and language acquisition in man and ape* (pp. 161–201). Boulder, CO: Westview Press.

Piaget, J. (1962). *Play, dreams, and imitation in childhood*. New York: Norton.

Povinelli, D. J., & Bering, J. M. (2002). The mentality of apes revisited. *Current Directions in Psychological Science, 11*, 115–119.

Povinelli, D. J., Bering, J. M., & Giambrone, S. (2001). Chimpanzee "pointing": Another error of the argument by analogy? In S. Kita (Ed.), *Pointing: Where language, culture, and cognition meet* (pp. 35–68). Mahwah, NJ: Erlbaum.

Povinelli, D., Nelson, K., & Boysen, S. (1992). Comprehension of role reversal in chimpanzees: Evidence of empathy? *Animal Behaviour, 43*, 633–640.

Ressler, R. H. (1966). Inherited environmental influences on the operant behavior of mice. *Journal of Comparative and Physiological Psychology, 61*, 264–267.

Rilling, J. K., & Insel, T. R. (1999). The human neocortex in comparative perspective using magnetic resonance imaging. *Journal of Human Evolution, 37*, 191–223.

Robert, J. S., Hall, B. K., & Olson, W. M. (2001). Bridging the gap between developmental systems theory and evolutionary developmental biology. *Bioessays, 23*, 954–962.

Russon A. E. (1996). Imitation in everyday use: Matching and rehearsal in the spontaneous imitation of rehabilitant orangutans (*Pongo pygmaeus*). In A. E. Russon, K. A. Bard, & S. T. Parker (Eds.), *Reaching into thought: The minds of the great apes* (pp. 152–176). New York: Cambridge University Press.

Rutter, M., & the English and Romanian Adoptees Study Team. (1998). Developmental catch-up, and deficit, following adoption after severe early privation. *Journal of Child Psychology and Psychiatry, 39*, 465–476.

Rutter M., O'Connor, T. G, & the English and Romanian Adoptees (ERA) Study Team. (2004). Are there biological programming effects for psychological development?: Findings from a study of Romanian adoptees. *Developmental Psychology, 40*, 81–94.

Savage-Rumbaugh, E. S. (1986). *Ape language: From conditioned response to symbol*. New York: Columbia University Press.

Savage-Rumbaugh, E. S., McDonald, K., Sevcik, R. A., Hopkins, W. D., & Rubert, E. (1986). Spontaneous symbol acquisition and communicative use by pygmy chimpanzees (*Pan paniscus*). *Journal of Experimental Psychology: General, 115*, 211–235.

Skeels, H. M. (1966). Adult status of children with contrasting early life experiences. *Monographs of the Society for Research in Child Development, 31*(3, Serial No. 105).

Suomi, S. J., & Harlow, H. (1972). Social rehabilitation of isolate-reared monkeys. *Developmental Psychology, 6*, 487–496.

Tomasello, M. (1999). *The cultural origins of human cognition*. Cambridge, MA: Harvard University Press.

Tomasello, M., & Call, J. (1997). *Primate cognition*. New York: Oxford University Press.

Tomasello, M., Savage-Rumbaugh, S., & Kruger, A. C. (1993). Imitative learning of actions on objects by children, chimpanzees, and enculturated chimpanzees. *Child Development, 64,* 1688–1705.

Tooby, J., & Cosmides, L. (1992). The psychological foundations of culture. In J. H. Barkow, L. Cosmides, & J. Tooby (Eds.), *The adapted mind* (pp. 19–136). New York: Oxford University Press.

Waddington, C. H. (1975). *The evolution of an evolutionist.* Ithaca, NY: Cornell University.

Want, S. C., & Harris, P. L. (2001). Learning from other people's mistakes: Causal understanding in learning to use a tool. *Child Development, 72,* 431–443.

Wellman, H. M. (1990). *The child's theory of mind.* Cambridge, MA: MIT Press/Bradford Books.

West-Eberhard, M. J. (2003). *Developmental plasticity and evolution.* New York: Oxford University Press.

Whiten, A. (2000). Primate culture and social learning. *Cognitive Science, 24,* 477–508.

Wright, B. E. (1997). Does selective gene activation direct evolution? *FEBS Letters, 402,* 4–8.

Wyles, J. S., Kunkel, J. G., & Wilson, A. C. (1983). Birds, behavior and anatomical evolution. *Proceedings of the National Academy of Sciences USA, 80,* 4394–4397.

Yakovlev, P. I., & Lecours, A.-R. (1967). The myelogenetic cycles of regional maturation of the brain. In A. Minkowski (Ed.), *Regional development of the brain in early life* (pp. 3–70). Oxford, UK: Blackwell Scientific.

Yunger, J. L., & Bjorklund, D. F. (2004). An assessment of generalization of imitation in two enculturated orangutans (*Pongo pygmaeus*). *Journal of Comparative Psychology, 118,* 242–246.

4

EARLY STRESS

Perspectives from Developmental Evolutionary Ecology

James S. Chisholm
Victoria K. Burbank
David A. Coall
Frank Gemmiti

OVERVIEW

Life history theory is the developmental evolutionary ecology of life cycles. We believe that in integrating evolutionary and developmental perspectives, life history theory is poised to make important contributions to developmental and evolutionary psychology and public health. We begin with an overview of biology's adaptationist and mechanist schools to show that evolutionary theory is incomplete without a theory of development (and vice versa) and to justify our focus on the development of alternative reproductive strategies. We then review principles of life history theory and evolutionary ecology to show why environmental risk and uncertainty are expected to be major determinants of alternative reproductive strategies, and why they must be represented phenotypically to have their adaptive effect. Turning to the mechanist perspective, we briefly review arguments that the attachment process is a good candidate mechanism for entraining the development of alternative reproductive strategies contingent on early environmental risk and uncertainty. Sufficient early environmental risk and uncertainty, we contend, will be represented phenotypically during development in at least two ways: (1) subjectively, as insecure attachment and represented cognitively–affectively as insecure working models of attachment; and (2) objectively, via the psychoneuroendocrinology of early stress. We then illustrate both kinds of phenotypic (developmental) representation with evidence of associations among early stress, insecure attachment, and insecure adult attachment for both sexes, and, for women, among early stress, early menarche, and low birthweight babies. Secure attachment seems to be an effective buffer against early stress, which can have lifelong adverse effects on health. Because low birthweight is also related to poor health in adulthood, these effects can be intergenerational. We conclude that viewing life cycles as alternative reproductive strategies suggests that insecurity—in the form of insecure internal working models and/or the psychoneuroendocrine consequences of environmental risk and uncertainty—constitutes an important health concern, and that developmental evolutionary ecology may have a role in informing public health and social policy.

The word "biology" comes from the Greek *bios*, meaning "life." Evolutionary theory is our only scientific theory of life. Therefore, as Theodosius Dobzhansky famously put it, "Nothing in biology [life] makes sense except in the light of evolution" (1973). While this is self-evident and unremarkable to biologists, to some nonbiologists it is arrogant, dangerous twaddle: arrogant because they think it implies that as nonbiologists they have nothing to say about life because they have not seen the light of evolution; dangerous because of their unexamined fear that evolutionary theory is inherently racist, sexist, and genetic-determinist. In the light of modern evolutionary theory, however, there is no such implication or grounds for such fear. By modern evolutionary theory, we mean recent accounts, reemerging from an earlier tradition, that emphasize the phenotype as much as the genotype (e.g., West-Eberhard, 2003). A theory of the phenotype entails a theory of development, which, for humans, requires the full range of the life, behavioral, and social sciences. On this view, nonbiologists have a lot to say to biologists. An evolutionary theory, with a fully integrated theory of the development of the phenotype, will also finally lay to rest lingering, misguided fears that racism, sexism, and genetic determinism are inherent in evolutionary theory. Human developmental evolutionary ecology, the subject of this chapter, aims at a fully integrated evolutionary-developmental theory of human phenotypes.

ADAPTATION AND MECHANISM

There are two main perspectives in biology. The adaptationist approach focuses on what selection would be expected to favor, while the mechanist approach focuses on how organisms work (Stearns, 1982). The adaptationist approach, with roots in population genetics, works with formal (logico-mathematical) models of natural selection and its products—genes and changes in gene frequencies over generations. Adaptationists are concerned with how selection works and what is adaptive. The adaptationist approach provides the logic for all of evolutionary theory, including the concept of alternative reproductive strategies, our focus here. Exploring adaptation through the logical manipulation of symbols, however, means that adaptationists unavoidably sacrifice a degree of biological realism in order to achieve analytic precision and generality. They therefore run the risk of conflating real phenotypes with the hypothetical, symbolic genes represented in their mathematical models. Consequently, despite its unassailable logic and huge success, the adaptationist approach has sometimes neglected the development of phenotypes. In overweening adaptationism, "the organism disappeared from view, and with it went the phenotype, the ecological interactions of the phenotype with the environment that determine fitness, and the developmental interactions with the environment that produce the phenotype" (Stearns, 1982, p. 238).

Biology's mechanist approach, on the other hand, with roots in anatomy, physiology, embryology, natural history, and ethology, works with real flesh-and-blood organisms, real phenotypes. Mechanists are concerned with the phenotypic mechanisms whereby phenotypes are produced, do adaptive work, and interact with their environments in ways that affect fitness (reproductive success). The adaptationist and mechanist approaches stem from innocuous differences in interests and issues, and are in no way opposed. Adaptationists and mechanists are perfectly agreed that the ultimate cause of evolution is differential reproduction of genetically inherited variation, and that genes underlie everything an organism is or does. Mechanists, however, may be less quick to conflate phenotypic traits with hypothetical genes "for" such traits, because they are concerned with how the phenotype develops the capacity to do adaptive work and emphasize that the environment also underlies everything an organism is and does. Current mechanist thinking "emphasizes the role of the environment as an agent of *development*, not just selection, in the evolution of all forms of life" (West-Eberhard, 2003, p. 20; emphasis added).

Evolutionary epistemology (Campbell, 1974) is the branch of evolutionary theory concerned with the origin and nature of information. It views organisms (phenotypes) as matter and energy that have been organized by information. Organisms are organized by two kinds of information: old (genetic) and new (environmental). As far as individual organisms are concerned, the old (genetic) information that organizes their phenotypes is experienced afresh each generation, but it is about old environments, those of their ancestors. The new information that organizes their phenotypes is about their own environments. Organisms acquire both kinds of information during ontogeny as they are expressed or represented in their phenotypes (Bateson, 1976, 1982; Oyama, 1985, 2000; West-Eberhard, 2003). In a manner of speaking organisms are the "incorporation of the world" (Plotkin, 1994, p. ix) into living matter. To incorporate something is to take it "into the body," which makes the thing taken in an embodiment of (or about, or a representation of) some aspect of the world. "To know something," in Plotkin's words, "is to incorporate the thing known into ourselves. Not literally, of course, but the knower is changed by knowledge [information], and that change represents, even if very indirectly, the thing known" (1994, p. ix). Phylogenetically old information represented in organisms' DNA constitutes their *a priori* knowledge of the worlds into which they are born. This old information, however, is only embodied during development as the organism grows and embodies ontogenetically new information (along with matter and energy). Some genetic information, of course, is new. Occasionally, mutation and recombination provide new information, and occasionally it is adaptive. But before it can do adaptive work, it must still be embodied during development.

For phenotypic mechanisms to do adaptive work, they must be controlled: They must be focused on, directed at, or somehow about more or less specific adaptive problems; they must be "framed" (Boden, 1977). Precisely how this is accomplished is not well understood, but it has to involve representing something about ancestral and current environments phenotypically, literally embodying them in molecular, cellular, tissue, and organ system form and function. There are many kinds of information, but the kind that does adaptive work in phenotypes is "intentional" information, in the sense that it is "about" something (Dennett, 1987; Plotkin, 1994; Thompson & Derr, 2000). (In philosophy, "intention," from the Latin *intendo*, meaning "to point at," has the technical meaning of "aboutness.") Wings, for example, embody information about the environment of aerodynamics; eyes embody information about the optical environment. Each, of course, also embodies the organism's actual experience of flight and vision. We have more to say later about the phenotypic representation of adaptive problems when we suggest how information about the most generic adaptive problem is embodied during human development. But first we need to explain why this problem, environmental risk and uncertainty, is the most generic.

THE ADAPTIVE PROBLEM: ENVIRONMENTAL RISK AND UNCERTAINTY

The Assumption of Optimality: What Is Important?

The heart of evolutionary theory is the assumption of optimality, the logic of adaptation by natural selection (Parker & Maynard Smith, 1990; Seger & Stubblefield, 1996; Dennett, 1995). The optimality assumption holds that for organisms to exist, all of their direct ancestors necessarily solved the problems of staying alive, growing and developing to reproductive maturity, producing offspring and having at least one offspring do the same. Survival, growth, and development and reproduction—producing and rearing offspring—are forms of work. Doing this work successfully results in reproductive success. Thus, while fitness is measured in terms of reproductive success, it is actually work, of which survival, growth, and development and reproduction are its universal and minimum components. The work of fitness consists of "mating effort" (producing offspring, which maximizes their quantity) and "parenting effort" (rearing them, which maximizes their quality: their reproductive value or capacity for survival, growth and development, and ultimate reproduction). We know from the Second Law of Thermodynamics that doing work requires resources. At a minimum, the work of fitness requires energy, nutrients, safety or security, information, and time. The measure of fitness is inherently relative; reproductive success is never absolutely high or low (except when it is zero) but always relative to that of other individuals in a population. The result is unremitting selection for traits associated with relatively greater reproductive success. But we also know from the Second Law of Thermodynamics that resources are always limited, that entropy increases. The result is eternal conflict between life's ends and means: Unremitting selection for greater relative fitness means unremitting demand for more resources to do more fitness work. But because resources are always limited, something has to give. This is the rationale for the assumption of optimality. The assumption of optimality is the logical proposition that with limited resources and multiple adaptive problems to be solved, selection is expected to favor phenotypic mechanisms that function to allocate limited resources "wisely," which is to say, contingently, according to their probable impact on organisms' fitness under particular socioecological conditions that were recurrently encountered during their evolutionary history. Because all of the direct ancestors of all organisms that ever lived did the work of fitness with limited resources, they must have been capable of allocating these resources where they would do more good, with "good" defined as leaving descendants, which is to continue in the evolutionary game (Chisholm, 1999a).

It is important to emphasize that optimal does not mean "perfect" or "best imaginable." It means "best possible" given the information represented in existing genes, and the energy, nutrients, safety or security, information, and time available to the organism through its interactions with its environment. And what is optimal in one environment is likely to be suboptimal in another; optimality is never absolute but always contingent. The assumption of optimality means that perfection cannot exist, and that we should always think about human nature in its abundant social–cultural, ecological, and political–economical contexts. It requires that we always go beyond what is "normal," in the sense of merely common or average, and contemplate instead the adaptive significance of the full range of variability in any phenotypic trait. It therefore requires an analytic focus on the potential adaptive significance of individual differences, for if we assume that selection is inclined to favor mechanisms that produce the best possible phenotype given existing resources (energy, information, time, etc.), and if the genes and environments that construct phenotypes differ, then we have to consider the possibility that each phenotype we see is the best possible in its particular context. But at the end of the day, the assumption of optimality is just that, an assumption, a working hypothesis, and not a statement that everything actually *is* optimal, and certainly not perfect. It is a way of thinking derived from the first principles of evolutionary theory, now well grounded in formal models. These models help us think about what is naturally important. They take the general form of "under socioecological conditions x, it would be more important (optimal) for fitness to trade a reduction in y for an increase in z." We could well be wrong, of course, but so far these models have been extraordinarily productive in generating new hypotheses, and have not yet proved wrong. (Use of these models is also what most distinguishes human evolutionary ecology from evolutionary psychology [Smith, Borgerhoff Mulder, & Hill, 2001; see also Gray, Heaney, & Fairhall, 2003]).

The General Life History Problem: The Ecology of Time

Life history theory is developmental evolutionary ecology: the study of organism × environment interaction throughout development and across generations from an evolutionary perspective (Chisholm, 1999a). One of the best-grounded formal models of life history theory is that of the trade-off between current and future reproductive success. The general life history problem (Schaffer, 1983; Stearns, 1992), as the current–future trade-off is also known, is a model for predicting an organism's optimal "strategy" (it need not be conscious) for leaving descendants, on the assumption that there is a trade-off between current and future reproduction. The justification for this assumption is the logical proposition, and evidence, that above some threshold, increased reproduction in the short term (current reproduction) will decrease the number of descendants in the long term (future reproduction). The current–future trade-off (actually a continuum) can refer to within-generation reproduction (early and often vs. late and seldom) or between-generation reproduction (as many as possible in the current generation vs. as many as possible in arbitrarily distant future generations). The current–future trade-off is expected to occur when resources consumed for bearing and rearing offspring in the short term would have resulted in more descendants had they been consumed in the future, and/or when current reproduction reduces parents' capability of surviving, and thus bearing and rearing more offspring in the future. The most important implication of the current–future trade-off is that selection is no longer expected always to favor mechanisms that simply maximize the number of offspring in the short term. This is because consistently producing a small number of high-quality offspring (high reproductive value) results in more descendants in the long run than having a larger number of low-quality offspring (low reproductive value: low probability of reproducing themselves). The reason is that consistently producing a small number of high-quality offspring, generation after generation, reduces the intergenerational variance in the number of offspring. It is a logical, mathematical fact that increasing x by the multiple y through z generations (iterations) produces a larger number than increasing x through z generations by a multiple that only averages y through z generations. In simple terms, slow and steady wins the race. (Of course, fast and steady beats slow and steady, but it consumes resources at a faster rate too.) To reiterate, selection is no longer expected always to favor mechanisms that maximize the production of offspring in the current generation. It is now expected that, under certain conditions, selection will favor mechanisms that have the effect of minimizing intergenerational variance in number of offspring, for this maximizes long-term fitness or number of descendants in the future (Borgerhoff Mulder, 1992; Charnov, 1993; Gillespie, 1977; Harpending, Draper, & Pennington, 1990; Kaplan, 1994; Promislow & Harvey, 1990, 1991; Stearns, 1992).

The conditions that matter most are those of environmental risk and uncertainty, which is how evolutionary ecologists refer in general to threats to an organism's capability of leaving descendants (Charnov, 1993; Seger & Brockmann, 1987; Stearns, 1992). In risky and uncertain environments, the quantity, quality, and certainty of resources required for the work of fitness (energy, nutrients, security, time, information, etc.) are problematic, so mortality rates are high or irregular, and the most immediate adaptive problem is to have any descendants at all. Because parents in these environments lack the resources to invest in offspring, their optimal reproductive strategy (everything else being equal) is to reproduce as early and/or often as possible. Indeed, age at first reproduction seems to be the target of selection in the evolution of life history traits (Charnov, 1993; Promislow & Harvey, 1990, 1991; Stearns, 1992). Maximizing offspring quantity (current reproduction) reduces their quality, but since parents already lack the capability of making much difference in offspring quality, this is just the cost of reproduction in risky and uncertain environments. Maximizing offspring quantity maximizes the probability that some will survive and reproduce; any is better than none. It is as if adaptations for trading offspring quality for quantity in risky and uncertain environments were the phenotypic embodiment of game theory's minimax strategy of minimizing the probability of sustaining the maximum possible loss. This is the "nothing left to lose" strategy; it is the optimal strategy when the alternative is lineage extinction.

In safe and predictable environments, on the other hand, the quantity, quality, and flow of resources are at least adequate, so mortality rates are lower and steadier, survival is not such an urgent problem, and organisms can afford to produce a minimal number of high-quality offspring who, by definition, are themselves likely to survive and produce a minimal number of high-quality offspring, who, by definition, are themselves likely to do the same, and so forth. Maximizing offspring quality (future reproduction) minimizes their number, but since parents are capable of investing relatively highly in each, thereby making a difference in their reproductive value, this is just the cost of reproduction in safe and predictable environments. Maximizing offspring quality maximizes the number of descendants in arbitrarily distant future generations, or the probability of having any descendants after more generations. It is as if adaptations for trading offspring quantity for quality in safe and predictable environments were the phenotypic embodiment of game theory's maximin strategy of maximizing the probability of achieving the minimum possible (short term, one step at a time) benefit, which, as always, is just staying in the evolutionary game. This is the "bird in hand worth two in the bush" strategy; it sets the stage for a slow and steady increase in future fitness, or any fitness in a more distant future, by reducing intergenerational variance in number of offspring.

Life Cycles as Reproductive Decision Making

Evolution is not driven by differential survival or growth and development but differential fitness. Adaptations for doing the work of survival and growth and development are evolutionarily significant only to the extent that they foster reproductive success. As Bonner wrote, "Development is the inevitable result of sex and size. The single-cell stage is required for sexual reproduction, and the larger size is the result of selection for reproductive success in new niches" (1993, p. 35). Increased size conferred fitness benefits, because competition for resources put an adaptive premium on larger, more complex bodies. But the only way to get from the single-cell stage to larger, more complex and competitive bodies was through the evolution of processes for growth and development: the evolution of multicellularity (Buss, 1987). To do adaptive work, phenotypes must be focused on adaptive problems. Therefore, information about adaptive problems must be represented phenotypically, literally (if still mysteriously) embodied in molecular, cellular, tissue, and organ system form and function. This can only happen through development. On this view, development is an adaptation for reproduction, and life cycles themselves are reproductive strategies. The most pervasive adaptive problem is the general life history problem, the problem of optimizing the trade-off between current and future reproduction. Since environmental risk and uncertainty are the major determinants of the optimal current–future trade-off, we would expect selection to favor mechanisms whereby both old and new information about environmental risk and uncertainty were phenotypically embodied during development.

For an organism to adopt its optimal reproductive strategy on the basis of some environmental cue, it must be capable of perceiving the relevant cue and "choosing" the right alternative. It must be capable of perceiving, representing, and evaluating the relevant environmental information in order to "choose wisely," which is to allocate its limited resources to the most pressing adaptive problem (i.e., survival, growth and development, or producing or rearing offspring, etc.). Selection for the capability of allocating resources wisely is selection for decision making: "The last decade has seen a marked shift toward viewing organisms as 'decision makers,' selected to accurately assess the consequences of different behavioral options available to them and to express those behavioral variants that maximize their fitnesses" (Emlen, 1995, p. 8092). While many human decisions are conscious, no organism's decisions ever have to be. Organisms are hierarchies of control systems, and control systems have the inherent logical capability of decision making (e.g., Bowlby, 1969; Holland, 1992; Dennett, 1995; Thompson & Derr, 2000). For a familiar example, consider the thermostat. The thermostat "decides" to turn the heat up or down contingent on the relationship between (new) environmental information about actual room temperature and (old) information represented in its preprogrammed temperature, its set-goal. Holland notes that "we rarely think of anticipation, or prediction, as a characteristic of organisms in general, though readily ascribe it to humans. Still, a bacterium moves in the direction of a chemical gradient, implicitly predicting that food lies in that direction" (1992, p. 24). Nor are decisions limited to behavioral options: "The butterfly that mimics the foul-tasting Monarch butterfly survives because it [or natural selection] predicts that a certain wing pattern discourages predators (p. 24). "Moving in the direction of a chemical gradient" entails the bacterium's capability of "deciding" to move in that direction; "mimicking the foul-tasting Monarch" entails the butterfly's "decision" to do so. It takes two things for control systems, organic or not, to make a "decision": the capability (1) of detecting contingencies between x and y and (2) of evaluation. Natural selection endowed bacteria with the capability of detecting the contingency between direction and food, and natural selection (a control system) is itself capable of detecting the contingency between wing pattern and environment. Natural selection endowed bacteria with the capability of valuing food over its absence and natural selection itself values wing patterns associated with greater fitness.

For alternative phenotypes to be entrained contingent on an environmental cue, the organism must "choose" or "make a decision about" a developmental trajectory. This capability appeared many times in evolution (West-Eberhard, 2003). We therefore now turn to theory and evidence suggesting that the attachment process evolved as a mechanism for embodying environmental risk and uncertainty, because it enabled young humans to "choose" their optimal developmental–reproductive strategies.

THE MECHANIST SOLUTION: ATTACHMENT

Attachment: Cooperation and Conflict

In simple terms, attachment refers to the emotional attraction (value) that mothers and offspring hold for each other. As a result of this attraction, offspring are moved to seek out mothers and attempt to be close and obtain body contact, warmth, and so on, and mothers are moved to nurture offspring. Using comparative data, Gubernick (1981) showed that attachment of broadly the human sort (i.e., gradual development over months and use of the mother as a secure base and safe haven) is concentrated in mammals who had to solve two adaptive problems simultaneously: providing adequate parental investment to slow-developing infants with limited mobility, and doing so in complex, shifting, and sometimes dangerous social environments like those of many primates. One enduring source of danger, for example, has been infanticide by conspecifics other than parents, identified so far in 34 nonhuman primate species (Hrdy, 1999). The adaptive problem with slow development and limited mobility is that infants cannot readily follow their mothers or provide for themselves, so they must have alternative methods of acquiring resources. The problem with complex, shifting, and sometimes dangerous social environments is that they make it more important to identify individual adults and juveniles, and the social–emotional relations among them. Gubernick thus took issue with Bowlby's somewhat narrow view that attachment's original adaptive function was protection from predators, arguing instead that from a comparative perspective, it made more adaptive sense as a mechanism for ensuring that parental investment is directed to mothers' own young, not those of some other female. (Of course, parental investment includes protection, along with energy, nutrients, time, information, etc., but from all sorts of risk and uncertainty, not just predators.) Seen this way, the original adaptive function of attachment was cooperative, mutually beneficial to infants and mothers—as a "resource elicitation mechanism" for infants and a "maternity certainty mechanism" for mothers. Attachment is thus not for achieving love, happiness, or even subjective feelings of security, but for offspring to identify likely sources of parental investment and then to elicit them, and for mothers to identify the best recipients of their limited resources and then to invest them wisely, which is to say, contingently, according to their reproductive value or probability of providing descendants.

Cooperation, however, has its limits, for the assumption of optimality means that parents and offspring are expected to differ about what constitutes wise investment. Trivers's (1974) theory of parent–offspring conflict holds that because mother and offspring are not genetically identical, they have different fitness interest and so are expected to disagree about how much or how long the mother should invest in each offspring. The basis for this expectation is that while mothers have a 50% genetic interest in each of their offspring, so do fathers. Each offspring, therefore, has a genetic interest in both the mother's and the father's genes. In this sense, individuals are more "related to themselves" than to either parent; they cannot transmit copies of only one parent's genes into the next generation. Everything else being equal, therefore, the assumption of optimality suggests that offspring will have been selected to "want" more investment from mother than she is "willing" to provide. The end result is conflict, or politics, if you prefer. As Trivers put it, "Socialization is a process by which parents attempt to mold each offspring . . . while each offspring [is expected] to resist . . . and to attempt to mold the behavior of its parents" (1974, p. 259). Peter Marris sees the same Machiavellian potential: "The balance between assertion and compliance in a child's experience of attachment represents a fundamental learning of the nature of order and security. . . . Learning to manage the attachment relationship therefore is learning to understand order and control" (1991, p. 79). Because parent–offspring conflict flows inexorably from the logic of sexual reproduction and parental investment, it is inescapable and would constitute an enduring evolutionary "arms race" between mothers and offspring. Moreover, this arms race would

be expected to escalate if offspring evolved to require more parental investment, which is a good characterization of human evolution.

The evolutionary history of humans is one of continuing selection for patterns of growth and development that produced progressively more helpless
and dependent infants and juveniles. This is believed to have occurred for two
reasons: (1) positive feedback between sexual selection and K-selection, and
(2) the "obstetric dilemma." We begin with brief accounts of sexual selection
and K-selection, and how they interacted in human evolution, then describe
the so-called "obstetric dilemma."

Sexual selection is a form of natural selection in which the agents of selection are members of one or the other sex. It occurs when members of one sex
(usually males) compete with each other for sexual access to the other, or
when members of one sex (usually females) exercise choice about their mating
partners. In practice, it is not always easy to tell the difference, for successful
within-sex competitors are often attractive between-sex choices. Humans are
descended from hominids (8 million years ago [mya]), primates (65 mya) and
mammals generally (200 mya). As a class, mammals are characterized by substantial sex differences in parental investment, with females having been sexually selected to bear and rear offspring and males to gain sexual access to
females. All mammalian females possess anatomical and physiological adaptations for ovulation, gestation, parturition, and lactation, whereas mammalian
males tend to possess adaptations for locating females, attracting females, and
coercing or persuading other males and females into giving them their way
with females (Clutton-Brock, 1991; Trivers, 1972; Williams, 1975). This
characteristic pattern of sex differences is also widespread in primates (Hrdy
& Whitten, 1987; Wrangham, 1980), including our closest great ape relatives,
the chimpanzee and the bonobo (Wrangham, 1993). And although it is more
variable in humans than in other primates, this pattern seems to characterize
us as well (Hrdy, 1999; Lancaster, 1997; Smuts, 1992, 1995). Indeed, we
believe that the greater variability in human reproductive strategies may actually be due to an *increase* in the intensity of sexual selection during human
evolution (cf. Flinn & Ward, Chapter 2, this volume, for a contrasting perspective). The reason for this increase follows from the logic of sexual selection and parental investment theories, which Trivers realized were two sides
of the same coin: "*What governs the operation of sexual selection is the relative parental investment of the sexes in their offspring*" (1972, p. 141; original
emphasis). In effect, sex differences *are* sex differences in parental investment,
and an increase in one is expected to generate an increase in the other. Therefore, because of our particular mammalian and primate evolutionary histories
of K-selection (see below) and greater parental investment by females, any
increase in the capacity of hominid infants and juveniles to elicit or benefit
from parental investment would exert greater selection pressure on females
than on males to provide it. The resulting increased sex difference in parental
investment, in turn, would tend to increase sexual selection, driving females
and males further apart, so to speak, resulting in even greater sex differences

in reproductive strategies, with females selected to allocate even more of their limited resources to bearing and rearing offspring, and males even more to acquiring sexual access to females, in their timeless mammalian way. As females invested more time and energy in bearing and nurturing increasingly helpless and dependent infants and juveniles, they would become increasingly valuable to males as "reproductive resources," thereby increasing the marginal rate of return to males of coercing or swaying females and other males to their will in order to acquire these "resources"—for example, through an increased appetite or propensity for risk taking, impulsiveness, dominance, showing off, sexual jealousy, violence, male–male competition, and so on (e.g., Wilson & Daly, 1985; Wrangham & Peterson, 1996; Chisholm, 1999a; Hrdy, 1999; Hawkes & Bleige Bird, 2002). Everything else being equal, the more that males benefited reproductively from such tactics, the more females would have to invest in bearing and rearing children just to maintain reproduction at replacement levels.

Consider now that this anthropoid–hominid tension between male and female reproductive strategies evolved in the context of our long evolutionary history of K-selection. K-selection is a form or mode of natural selection that predominates when environments are safe and predictable, mortality rates are low and steady, and organisms die or fail to reproduce not because they are unlucky, in the wrong place at the wrong time, but because they are unfit. K-selection thus favors individuals who produce "fewer and better," more competitive offspring; K-selected species produce relatively small numbers of large, slow-developing, long-lived, big-brained, highly social offspring who acquire their relatively high reproductive value developmentally, through a great deal of parental investment. Mammals tend to be more K-selected than other classes, primates more than other orders, and humans are among the most K-selected of all species (e.g., Charnov & Berrigan, 1993; Stearns, 1992, 2000). This means that just as sexual selection was intensifying sex differences in hominid evolution, committing females to even more parental investment and males to even more "mating effort," K-selection was producing infants who developed even more slowly and required even longer and more intensive parental investment. The result would be positive feedback: The more that hominid infants required parental investment, the more females would be selected to provide it, intensifying sexual selection and sex differences even more, increasing the pressure on females to sacrifice offspring quantity for quality, requiring them to invest even more just to maintain replacement-rate reproduction.

But now consider the obstetric dilemma, which resulted in even more helpless infants who took even longer to mature, thus requiring even more and longer care. The obstetric dilemma (Washburn, 1960) was the adaptive problem of reconciling opposing selection pressures, one that narrowed the pelvis as an adaptation for bipedal locomotion and others, including K-selection, that favored intelligence and thus big brains, and thus newborns with big heads. Relative to body size, the brain size of newborn humans is 1.33 times larger than that of great apes (Bogin & Smith, 1996). The dilemma was how to accommodate ever-larger newborn crania through narrower birth canals. The solution was relatively short gestation—selection that prevented the length of gestation from increasing as much as it otherwise would have due to K-selection for slower and longer growth. Some estimates are that if human gestation were proportionately as long as it is in other primates, it would last for 21 months (Gould, 1977). With gestations perhaps only half as long as expected, it is no wonder that human infants are so helpless at birth. In solving the obstetric dilemma, however, "premature" birth aggravated the dilemma arising from positive feedback loops among K-selection, sexual selection, and parental investment: K-selected, helpless newborns requiring even more intensive care from their already overworked mothers, causing even greater sexual selection and increasing the pressure on mothers to make the trade-off between offspring quantity and quality, requiring them to invest still more just to stay in the evolutionary game. Finally, consider as well that on top of everything else, all early hominid mothers were single mothers. How could they cope? How did our species escape this arms race?

There is reason to think we escaped the way that single mothers always cope—by getting help. Help is cooperation; getting help in rearing offspring is getting "helpers at the nest," known technically as cooperative breeding. Cooperative breeding occurs in birds and mammals when biological and socioecological circumstances conspire to raise the cost of successfully rearing offspring beyond what mothers alone can provide (birds: Cockburn, 1998; mammals: Solomon & French, 1997; primates: Hrdy, 1999, 2001, 2004). Cooperative breeding works by spreading the cost of parenting more widely among those with a genetic interest in the offspring. Those with the greatest genetic interest in a child are its mother and father. (The interests of the father, however, must be devalued by the degree to which his paternity is uncertain, which is why paternity confidence and male sexual jealousy are important concerns in human evolutionary ecology.)

Phenotypic mechanisms for spreading the cost of parenting to fathers almost certainly include a range of adaptations that have the effect of supporting male–female sexual–emotional bonds or attachments. For example, consider body shape. Compared to the other great apes, humans and bonobos show relatively little sexual dimorphism in body size. But contrary to popular wisdom, this does not mean that the force of sexual selection decreased in human evolution, for unlike bonobos and the other great apes, we show a great deal of sexual dimorphism in body shape. Human males have more facial hair than females, with no plausible function other than sexual signaling. Human females are the only primate females with permanent breasts, and breast size is unrelated to capacity for lactation, either within or between species. Permanent breasts may thus have only a sexual signaling function. Bear in mind also loss of estrus, disproportionately large penis, sex during pregnancy, and the very high rate of "communicative" or nonconceptive sex (with fewer partners, too) in humans compared to nonhuman primates (e.g., Hrdy,

1999; Short, 1979; Smuts, 1995; Wrangham, 1993). Given that sucking, mouthing, stroking, hugging, cuddling, and orgasm release oxytocin, which reduces levels of the stress hormone, cortisol, and facilitates relaxation and feelings of warmth and affiliation (Carter, 1998; Insel, 2000; Uvnäs-Moberg, 1998), the evolution of human sexuality may be construed as fostering the capability for adult male–female sexual–emotional or romantic attachment. And given that the same attachment behaviors release oxytocin in infants (Gunnar, 1998), it is interesting to note that the psychobiology of infant–mother attachment is also implicated in the ontogeny of adult male–female romantic attachment (we return to this point shortly). These feelings of warmth and affiliation may have predisposed males to invest in their own off-spring, even if only indirectly, by providing resources to mothers (perhaps protection in particular [Hrdy, 1999; van Schaik & Dunbar, 1990]), thereby freeing them for more or longer direct investment. If so, increased female choice of males with a greater capability for warmth and affiliation would constitute increased sexual selection to spread the cost of parenting to males.

Increased sexual selection in the form of female choice would have provided a way out of the positive feedback between sexual selection in the form of male–male competition and K-selection. Prior to such an increase, males who were too overtly competitive and coercive may have achieved greater sexual access to females, but with their mates left to provide all the parental investment, their increasingly helpless and slow-developing children would increasingly fail to achieve their full potential reproductive value. After such an increase, females who were able to choose to mate with less overtly competitive and coercive males—those with greater capability for warmth and affiliation or sexual-romantic attachment—would have reared a higher proportion of offspring to their full potential reproductive value.

But what about offspring themselves? If cooperative breeding works by spreading the cost of parenting more widely among those with a genetic interest in the offspring, we should consider the possibility of phenotypic mechanism for spreading the cost of parenting not only from mother to father, but to offspring as well, for offspring have a greater genetic interest in themselves than they do in either parent. But how could the cost of parenting be spread to the *recipients* of parenting? After all, children cannot provide their own care; that is precisely the problem. However, they can provide for themselves, so to speak, by getting better at eliciting care, by more cleverly molding parents' (and others') behavior through their deeper understanding of order and control, thereby managing the attachment relationship (the parent–offspring arms race) in their favor. Those best at molding their parents, those with the deepest understanding of parents' intentions and the political economy of parent–offspring conflict, would tend to elicit more or longer parental investment, thereby acquiring the material and social–emotional security that by all accounts fosters survival, growth and development, and long-term reproductive success. As adults themselves, those best at molding their own parents would also tend to be good at molding not only their own offspring (thereby maintaining the parent–offspring arms race), but others as well, for as adults, they could not help but use their early experience of empathy, understanding intentions, and order and control in their "Machiavellian" attempts to mold social relations generally.

This scenario of the evolution of early learned capabilities for empathy, understanding intentions, and order and control is speculative, of course, but we think it is responsible speculation, because it is consistent with basic principles of sexual selection theory, parental investment theory, parent–offspring conflict theory, and mammalian and primate evolutionary ecology and life history, particularly the developmental evolutionary ecology of attachment. It is also consistent with an intriguing anomaly of human development: Compared to nonhuman primates, human infants are motorically and sexually altricial but cognitively and perceptually precocial, with high rates of fetal and neonatal brain growth being maintained much longer than in other primates (e.g., Bogin, 2001). Development in logicomathematical, physical, and social cognition also co-occur more in humans than nonhuman primates, thereby probably contributing to increased mutual reinforcement through crossover and integration among cognitive modes (Langer, 2000; Parker, 1996; Parker & McKinney, 1999). Slow motor development and delayed sexual maturity are hallmarks of K-selection, but precocial cognitive-perceptual development is not. On the other hand, mosaic development is phylogenetically widespread and a common source of speciation (West-Eberhard, 2003). Relatively precocial cognitive-perceptual development, especially with greater cross-modal transfer and integration, would seem to serve the adaptive function of increasing the infant's capability of managing parent–offspring conflict in its favor, eliciting more cooperation from mother, and then she from others. This may be the phylogenetic origin of the capability of developing a theory of mind (Chisholm, 2003; cf. Baron-Cohen, Chapter 18, this volume) and may even have played a role in distinguishing our species from our great ape ancestors.

Attachment as the Embodiment of Risk and Uncertainty

Bowlby realized from the start that attachment history was related to adult sexuality, but without the insights of evolutionary theory and the concept of alternative reproductive strategies, he had no way to appreciate the full significance of his clinical observation that adolescents and young adults who suffered insecure attachment histories were at increased risk for the early or impulsive display of sexual and aggressive behavior. Writing of these people in his final report to the World Heath Organization, he noted that "persistent stealing, violence, egotism, and sexual misdemeanours were among their less pleasant characteristics" (1951, p. 380). Building on the earlier work of Pat Draper and her colleagues (Draper & Harpending, 1982; Draper & Belsky, 1990), Belsky, Steinberg, and Draper (1991) were the first to provide an adaptationist model of attachment and reason for thinking that "persistent stealing, violence, egotism, and sexual misdemeanours" might represent something more than pathology. They argued that the bulk of evidence about the causes and consequences of individual differences in adult attachment and sexual behavior were consistent with their model, in which the development of reproductive strategies was contingent on attachment history, with insecure attachment adaptively biasing men and women toward so-called "mating effort" strategies and secure attachment adaptively biasing them toward "parenting effort" strategies.

Subsequently, Chisholm (1993, 1996, 1999a) reinterpreted their model in explicit evolutionary ecological and life-history theory terms. From this perspective ("developmental evolutionary ecology," as outlined above), the most generic, pervasive, and unrelenting adaptive problem is optimizing the trade-off between current and future reproduction. The major determinant of the optimal trade-off between current and future reproduction is environmental risk and uncertainty, mortality rates in particular. Because development is ultimately an adaptation for reproduction, we would expect selection to have favored developmental mechanisms for the phenotypic embodiment of both old and new information about environmental risk and uncertainty, particularly mortality rates. Children cannot directly perceive mortality statistics, but their preexisting mammalian–primate capability of forming attachments would have provided a phenotypic mechanism for gauging environmental risk and uncertainty indirectly, through their impact on parents and thus parent–child interaction. In risky and uncertain environments, mortality rates are high or unpredictable, leading to short or unpredictable lives. When death is common, so is the experience of loss: grief, anxiety, fear, and anger. Parents (and cooperating caretakers) have always been the core of their children's "environment of evolutionary adaptedness" (Bowlby, 1969, p. 50) as they transduced the impact of the larger, more complex, and potentially threatening environments into more buffered, secure versions of those environments for their children (when they could, that is). But because such buffering requires parental resources (time, energy, sleep, etc.), children are likely to experience the impact of its cost on parents as much as its benefits to them. When parents experience too much grief, anxiety, fear, and anger, they are apt to be hard-pressed to be consistently sensitive and responsive to their children's signals, thereby increasing risk for insecure attachment. On this view, buffering children against risky and uncertain environments not only protects them (when it does) but also provides them with valuable information about the environments in which they will grow and develop, and ultimately reproduce. Attachment styles may thus be adaptive in part because they embody information about local environmental risk and uncertainty, thereby making this information available for use in "decisions" about optimal developmental–reproductive strategies. Everything else being equal, in risky and uncertain environments, the optimal reproductive strategy is to reproduce early and/or often. It may be no accident that children who experience too much early risk and uncertainty are prone to insecure attachment and, as adults, to the early or impulsive display of sexual and aggressive behavior.

But how is information about environmental risk and uncertainty embodied, and how do children use it to make adaptive developmental–reproductive "decisions"? Precise answers are not readily available, but we believe existing theory and data provide some direction. To indicate what we think is a promising direction for future research, we outline some of our thinking-in-progress about the phenotypic embodiment of individual differences in the early experience of risky and uncertain environments, attachment history, and reproduction in women.

EARLY STRESS EMBODIED IN FEMALE REPRODUCTIVE STRATEGIES

The Psychoneuroendocrinology of Early Stress

From the perspective of evolutionary epistemology, information about early environmental risk and uncertainty is represented phenotypically in two ways: materially, objectively, in brain and endocrine systems; and subjectively, in thoughts and feelings about attachment. While the relationship between the two remains unclear, there is good evidence that they are correlated and related to adult reproductive function and behavior. We focus here on women, because individual differences in female reproductive strategies have major implications for maternal, child, and intergenerational and public health, and because a good deal is known about the source of these differences, including the role of attachment. With appropriate adjustment for sex differences, the same principles apply equally to male reproductive strategies.

Old information about environmental risk and uncertainty is significantly represented in the amygdala, hippocampus, corpus callosum, cerebral cortex, autonomic nervous system, and the hypothalamic–pituitary–adrenal (HPA) axis. These are highly developmentally canalized (i.e., innate) structures—processes whose evolutionary history goes back to the vertebrates. In simple terms, the amygdala embodies emotional valence: it "plays a crucial role in deciding whether a stimulus is dangerous or not" (LeDoux, 1996, p. 223). It is an evolved structure that provides the capability of experiencing fear, of valuing a stimulus as worth fearing; it represents old information that "points at" the fear experienced by ancestral owners of amygdalae. The hippocampus provides the capability of storing or representing old information about the "where and when" of stimuli that "released" the automatic or instinctive feeling of fear; it represents old information about the context of fear experienced by the ancestral owners of hippocampi. Fear of falling provides a ready example: In highly schematic terms, it is as if the child's vestibular (motion perception) system automatically represents the sensation of falling. This new information about the infant's current environment (that of falling) is then somehow matched with old information about ancestral falls that is somehow represented in its hippocampus. When this match between old and new information is made, it activates the autonomic nervous system and the "fight–flight" response, releasing a flood of catecholamine hormones and subjective feelings of fear, the amygdala's automatic evaluation of falling as "bad." Together, the amygdala and hippocampus help solve the problem of using information about value (security: approach; fear, insecurity: avoid) in an adaptive way. This is the problem of making useful connections between new information about the organism's current environment and old information about value, with "useful" defined in terms of the past fitness implications of the new information (e.g., Aggleton, 1992; LeDoux, 1996; Panksepp, 1998). The fight–flight response to immediate threat has obvious fitness benefits, but there is more to life than short-term survival, and the body cannot sustain high levels of arousal for long. This is where the HPA axis comes in. Its primary function is homeostatic, to return arousal levels to baseline, thereby protecting against the deleterious effects of prolonged exposure to fast-acting catecholamines through the release of glucocorticoid hormones, of which cortisol is foremost in humans. The HPA axis is functioning at birth, if not before (Gunnar & Cheatham, 2003). Chronic environmental risk and uncertainty chronically activate the fight–flight response, causing chronic activation of the HPA axis and risk for permanently abnormal (high or low) levels of cortisol (Boyce & Ellis, in press). Chronically unresponsive parenting and insecure attachment are also associated with altered cortisol profiles in infants (Blunt Bugental, Martorell, & Barraza, 2003; Gunnar, 2000; Gunnar, Brodersen, Nachmias, Buss, & Rigatuso, 1996; Gunnar & Donzella, 2002). Mark Flinn and his colleagues (Flinn, Quinlan, Turner, Decker, & England, 1996) found too that children of single mothers who lacked adequate support from kin had cortisol profiles significantly different from children of mothers with husbands and/or support from kin. On the other hand, as mentioned, warm, response-contingent parenting releases oxytocin in the infant, which reduces cortisol levels and promotes feelings of relaxation, warmth, and affiliation (Carter, 1998; Insel, 2000; Uvnäs-Moberg, 1998).

When children experience enough safety and predictability, and/or enough warm, response-contingent parenting and concomitant cortisol-reducing oxytocin, their neuroendocrine systems automatically make connections between old representations of security (good) and new representations of their current environments that are resistant to change. When they do not experience enough safety, predictability, or warm, response-contingent stimulation, they make more connections between old representations of fear or insecurity (bad) and their current environments. From the perspective of evolutionary epistemology, these connections have the adaptive function of enabling children to construct cognitive–emotional representations of themselves and others, and thereby to predict the future—their own and attachment figures' behavior. Bowlby (1969) referred to such representations as "internal working models" of attachment. Constructing such models requires the cognitive–perceptual capability of the child to detect contingencies between his or her own behavior and that of the attachment figure. Detecting contingencies "releases" pleasant feelings, as evidenced by heightened attention and smiles, which motivate children to seek more contingencies. It is therefore simultaneously cognitive–emotional and rewarding–motivating. It is as if there were innate (reliably developing) connections between old information about good (security) and bad (insecurity) represented in the amygdala, and old information about contingency–detection represented in the hippocampus. This innate information control system enables the formation of new connections between old information about value (good, security: approach) and new information about the child's current environment, people (and objects) that are contingently responsive to him or her. Because people with the greatest interest in a child provide the most, the warmest and most consistent response-contingent stimulation, the child automatically attaches feelings of value to them (Csibra, Gergeley, Biro, Koos & Brockbank, 1999; Gergely & Watson, 1999; Watson, 2001).

These findings illustrate the role of parents' interest in modulating children's arousal, which is the whole adaptive point of parental investment: buffering them against environmental risk and uncertainty. When parents (or others) are able and willing to demonstrate their interest by providing sufficiently positive, warm, and responsive parental investment, there will be few objective representations of environmental risk and uncertainty in their children's psychoneuroendocrinology (amygdala, hippocampus, autonomic nervous system, HPA axis, etc.), and they will construct more secure subjective representations of attachment relations because their perceptions of response–contingency literally feel good, and because of their empirically based assumption or expectation that because they are treated well, parents must believe they are worth treating well, and therefore intend to treat them well in the future. Everything else being equal, in safe and predictable environments, the optimal reproductive strategy is to maximize future reproduction, which entails the phenotypic representation of environmental security and predictability. But when parents are unable to provide sufficient buffering, more of the risk and uncertainty of their larger environments will filter through them to become represented objectively, in their children's psychoneuroendocrinology, and subjectively, in the form of insecure internal working models. The same will happen if parents are unwilling to provide sufficient buffering— which they might because of parent–offspring conflict, "preferring" instead to invest in offspring quantity rather than the quality of any one offspring. Either way, under conditions of chronic risk and uncertainty, the optimal strategy (*ceteris paribus*) is to maximize current reproduction. If girls growing up in risky and uncertain environments are inclined to "persistent stealing, violence, egotism, and sexual misdemeanours" as adults, it may be because, from the perspective of the current–future trade-off, they have nothing left to lose. While we cannot know about the relationship between the actual content of infants' internal working models and their neuroendocrinology, and the relationship between infant attachment and adult attachment is complex and difficult to quantify, there is reason to believe that women (and men) with insecure attachment histories are inclined to the early and/or impulsive expression of sexual-romantic behavior (Belsky et al., 1991; Buunk, 1997; Feeney, 1999;

Grossmann, Grossmann, Winter, & Zimmerman, 2002; Hazan & Shaver, 1987; Hazan & Zeifman, 1999; Roisman, Madsen, Hennighausen, Sroufe, & Collins, 2001; Sharpsteen & Kirkpatrick, 1997).

Having outlined how early environmental risk and uncertainty may be represented in women's psychoneuroendocrinology, we now examine in more detail some of the biological, psychological, and public health correlates and consequences of the early and/or impulsive expression of sexual-romantic behavior.

The Cost of Maximizing Current Reproduction

Adaptations for survival and growth and development evolved because they had the effect of enabling complex organisms to reproduce. Having reached reproductive maturity, the organism is in a position to reallocate limited resources from survival and growth and development to reproduction. Consequently, age at first reproduction, the apparent target of selection on life history traits, is affected by the countless organism × environment interactions that brought it to reproductive maturity; it is an "overdetermined" or "packaged" trait. For women, age at first reproduction is proximally contingent on age at menarche and age at first sexual intercourse, both of which are affected by the old information represented in their genes and the new information about their environments, and matter and energy, as they are embodied during development. The variance in age at menarche attributed to genetic factors ranges between 10% (Johnston, 1974) and 74% (Kaprio et al., 1995), which suggests that it is highly environmentally labile, as would be expected if it were part of an adaptively contingent alternative reproductive strategy. Age at menarche is also affected by the environment, being delayed when the flow of material resources is inadequate or uncertain, resulting in poor health and nutrition (Ellison, 1990). This makes adaptive sense, because women in poor condition are less capable of producing and rearing children; their own and their infants' reproductive value would be compromised by even trying. However, evidence is accumulating that, given adequate health and nutrition, age at menarche is also affected by the inadequate or uncertain flow of social–emotional resources, being accelerated under conditions of chronic early stress or insecurity and concomitant chronic activation of the HPA axis (see reviews in Chisholm, 1999a; Worthman, 1999; see also Ellis, Chapter 7, this volume). This makes another kind of adaptive sense, because the subjective experience of chronic early stress (insecurity, fear, anger) is the phenotypic embodiment of the kind of environmental risk and uncertainty characterized by high or unpredictable mortality—the circumstances in which avoiding lineage extinction is the most urgent adaptive problem. Evidence for these two kinds of environmental influences on age at menarche suggests an adaptively contingent response hierarchy: Everything else being equal, women who lack the energy and nutrients to conceive, gestate, and lactate should not get pregnant until conditions improve, regardless of their social–emotional environments;

women who have adequate material resources but face risky and uncertain social–emotional environments should get pregnant as early and/or often as possible to maximize current reproduction.

The other proximal determinant of women's age at first reproduction, age at first sexual intercourse, is also affected by genes and environment. One way that genetic factors affect age at first intercourse is via their influence on the psychoneuroendocrinology of age at menarche, which is usually correlated with age at first sex (and would have been more highly correlated in our mammalian–primate–hominid evolutionary past) (e.g., Bernard, 1975; Cvetkovich, Grote, Lieberman, & Miller, 1978; Phinney, Jensen, Olsen, & Cundick, 1990; Udry & Cliquet, 1982). Genetic factors probably also affect age at first sex via their influence on women's libido, which, barring male, peer, or family coercion, is likely to be a factor in women's choice to have sex at a given age. But whatever the genetic influences on age at first sex may be, there is abundant evidence that early or impulsive sexual activity ("sexual misdemeanours," in Bowlby's rather Victorian phrase) is associated with early environmental risk and uncertainty, including poverty or inequality (Mott, Fondell, Hu, Kowaelski-Jones, & Menaghan, 1996; Miller et al., 1997), divorce or family instability (Ellis et al., 2003; Wyatt, Durvasula, Gutherie, LeFranc, & Forge, 1999), including insecure adult attachment (Chisholm, Quinlivan, Petersen, & Coall, 2005), and sexual abuse (Boyer & Fine, 1992; Fiscella, Kitzman, Cole, Sidora, & Olds, 1998; additional references in Chisholm, 1999a). Finally, to the extent that the phenotypic embodiment of early risk and uncertainty includes negative internal working models of attachment relations, which amount to insecurity or anxiety about the future, it is interesting to note that women who report early first sex also report shorter expected lifespans (Chisholm, 1999b; Chisholm et al., 2005). If insecure internal working models represent the embodiment of environmental risk and uncertainty, of which high or unpredictable mortality rates are the most important consequence, this would make adaptive sense.

Chronic environmental risk and uncertainty are bad for health, because they result in chronic HPA axis activation and chronically altered cortisol levels, which can have long-term deleterious effects on health, including diabetes, cardiovascular disease, immune system dysfunction, obesity, neuronal cell death (especially in the hippocampus, thus leading to memory dysfunction), anxiety and depression, and increased risk for addictions of all sorts (e.g., Heim, Owens, Plotsky, & Nemeroff, 1997; McEwen, 1995; McEwen & Seeman, 1999; Meaney, 2001; Sapolsky, 1992; Sapolsky, Romero, & Munck, 2000). From our perspective, however, these conditions do not represent pathology as much as costs of reproduction in risky and uncertain environments; that is, while they certainly are not good or adaptive, such impairments may be the unavoidable trade-offs of maximizing current reproduction in the face of inadequate or uncertain resources. This possibility arises for two reasons: First, trade-offs are entailed by the assumption of optimality. Evolution is an impersonal force of living nature that results in the continuation, with modification, of life forms; it "cares" about health and well-being only to the extent that they are associated with reproductive success. In principle, this is why all organisms senesce and die; organisms are not designed to live healthy, happy, and long lives, but to reproduce. Second, maximizing current reproduction is, in principle, the optimal reproductive strategy in the face of chronic risk and uncertainty, which result in chronic activation of the HPA axis.

While the evidence as yet is only suggestive, chronic activation of the HPA axis has, in turn, been implicated in early activation of the hypothalamic–pituitary–gonadal (HPG) axis (Herman-Giddens, Sandler, & Friedman, 1988; Trickett & Putnam, 1993), which controls pubertal development. Cortisol levels increase with Tanner stages of pubertal development (Netherton, Goodyer, Tamplin, & Herbert, 2004) and indeed begin their ascent a year before menarche itself (Legro, Lin, Demers, & Lloyd, 2003). The direction of effects here is not clear, of course, but early-maturing women also tend to have a higher body mass index (i.e., heavier and shorter) than on-time women (Wellens et al., 1994; Merzenich, Boeing, & Wahrendorf, 1993) and higher estrogen levels (Apter, 1996; Apter, Cacciatore, Alfthan, & Stenman 1989), both of which are positively associated with cortisol (Kiess et al., 1995; Vamvakopoulos & Chrousos, 1993). In addition, to the extent that age at first intercourse is associated with age at menarche (see earlier discussion), it is interesting to note that women reporting earlier first intercourse had attenuated cortisol responses (smaller increase and faster recovery) to a standardized stressor than women who were older at first sex (Brody, 2002). Likewise, young women who had been sexually abused within the previous couple of months showed significantly lower cortisol compared to matched controls (King, Mandansky, King, Fletcher, & Brewer, 2001). And to the extent that early menarche is frequently associated with conduct disorders or antisocial behavior (Caspi & Moffitt, 1991; Ge, Brody, Conger, Simmons, & Murry, 2002), it is also interesting to note that low cortisol indicates low autonomic nervous system arousal and predicts antisocial behavior up to a year later (Pajer, Gardner, Kirillova, & Vanyukov, 2001; Susman & Pajer, 2004).

The proposition that HPA activity is associated with early menarche or sexual behavior may at first seem paradoxical, for it is well known that HPA activity suppresses HPG activity (Chrousos & Gold, 1992; Susman, 1997). But from the perspective of developmental evolutionary ecology, this is not paradoxical in principle. As we have seen, development is ultimately for reproduction, and the adaptive function of developmental plasticity is to maximize the probability that adults will reproduce in the environments into which they were born. This entails phenotypic mechanisms for entraining the adult's optimal reproductive strategy contingent on environmental cues, especially about risk and uncertainty. We would therefore expect the timing of such cues to make a difference in their effects on the adult phenotype. For instance, Virginia Vitzthum (2001) notes that when healthy, well-nourished Western women take up vigorous exercise, they frequently stop menstruating, whereas chronically malnourished women in developing countries who have been doing hard labor all their lives frequently have completed family sizes of six, eight, or more. She interprets this apparent paradox in terms of life-history theory and the well-known physiological process of acclimatization: Western women are highly reactive to exercise precisely because they have acclimatized to good nutrition and health during development; chronically malnourished, hard-laboring women have acclimatized to marginal and uncertain resources. Susman and Pajer (2004) reach the same conclusion about acclimatization to chronic psychosocial stress:

> Under these chronically fearful and challenging conditions, individuals adapt by attenuation or down regulation of arousal so as to avoid chronic arousal and excessive energy expenditure. Such energy expenditure related to chronic arousal would otherwise lead to traumatic stress disorder and cardiovascular and immune system pathophysiology. Thus, as an adaptive strategy in early develop-ment, the stress response system/arousal system does not respond in a typical way to novelty and challenges. (p. 21)

Boyce and Ellis (in press) make analogous arguments about acclimatization to psychosocial stress but propose as well a more complex model in which high neuroendocrine reactivity to stress in adults is U-shaped, contingent on both innate, temperamental differences in reactivity, and high and low levels of early stress, with the majority, the low responders, at the bottom of the U, having experienced more or less equal amounts of early stress and support or buffering against stress.

If chronic early environmental risk and uncertainty entail chronic activa-tion of the HPA axis, which in turn entails early activation of the HPG axis, we may have a mechanism for entraining the optimal reproductive strategy under conditions of environmental risk and uncertainty, namely, reproducing as early and/or often as possible. This may help to explain why girls experi-encing higher levels of psychosocial stress have earlier menarche than other girls. It does not end there, though, for women with early menarche seem to be at higher risk for delivering low birthweight babies (Scholl et al., 1989; Chisholm, 1999a; Coall & Chisholm, 2003). Low birthweight, in turn, is a risk factor for infant and child mortality, and a wide range of adult diseases (Henricksen, 1999; Phillips, 1998; Barker, 1999; Wahlbeck et al., 2001).

CONCLUSIONS: EVOLUTION, DEVELOPMENT, INEQUALITY, AND HEALTH

Evolution is the control system whereby living forms continue, with modifica-tion, through time. This requires reproduction: Evolution continues because all of the direct ancestors of all organisms that ever lived reproduced, and enough of their descendants have done the same. Modification occurs through the embodiment of old (and occasionally new, mutated, or recombined) genetic information and new environmental information in new phenotypes during development. Along with embodied matter and energy, this information enabled enough organisms to solve the adaptive problems required for leaving descendants. The most generic, consistently important adaptive problem is predicting the future in order to optimize the trade-off between current and future reproduction. Because the optimal current–future trade-off is contingent on environmental risk and uncertainty, and death (or other failure to reproduce) is the most important consequence of environmental risk and uncertainty, the most important new environmental information to be embodied is about mortality rates. The only way that information about mortality rates can be represented phenotypically is indirectly, through the effects of its causes, correlates, and consequences. One way these effects are represented is in ancient neuroendocrine mechanisms that evaluate stimuli as good (approach) or bad (avoid) and prepare the organism for dealing with good or bad futures. When too many evaluations of "bad" have to be made, the organism begins to pay the price of allocating too many scarce resources merely to survival, thus trading off growth, development, mating, and/or parenting. Because parenting—and therefore parent–offspring conflict—became increasingly important in mammalian, primate, and especially human evolution, there would seem to have been a corresponding increase in selection on human juveniles to elicit and prolong parental investment, with the attachment process providing a plausible mechanism via the capability to develop or construct more sophisticated internal working models, theory of mind, and politics: "understanding order and control" in attachment relations. Because the whole adaptive point of parental investment is buffering offspring from environmental risk and uncertainty, the effect of risky and uncertain environments on parents could not help but be transduced to offspring through the attachment process, resulting in the embodiment of risk and uncertainty in the form of insecure internal working models.

Finally, it is crystal clear that inequality is a major source of risk and uncertainty in the modern world, because it leads to ill-health, shortened lives, and many other attenuated human capabilities (e.g., Farmer, 2003; Kawachi & Kennedy 2003; Nussbaum, 1995; Sen, 1990, 1992, 1993; Wilkinson, 1996; Chisholm & Burbank, 2001). To our way of thinking, inequality is not just individual or group differences in access to energy, nutrients, security, information, time, and so on, but inequality in achieving what these resources are for: the capability of doing the work of fitness. From the perspective of developmental evolutionary ecology, resources have value to the extent that organisms are capable of converting them into fitness, thereby continuing in the evolutionary game. In the face of chronic inequality (risk and uncertainty), the optimal reproductive strategy is to maximize current reproduction, because this enables people to just "have a life" (and any descendants). But at what cost? People everywhere naturally value health over illness and pleasure over pain. If people are capable of having a "good life," with maximum security and predictability, then evolutionary theory suggests that reducing inequality may be the best way to continue. Such use of our only scientific theory of life is the premise and promise of evolutionary public health.

REFERENCES

Aggleton, J. P. (1992). *The amygdala.* New York: Wiley.

Apter, D. L. (1996). Hormonal events during female puberty in relation to breast cancer risk. *European Journal of Cancer Prevention, 5,* 476–482.

Apter, D. L., Cacciatore, B., Alfthan, H., & Stenman, U. H. (1989). Serum luteinizing hormone concentrations increase 100-fold in females from 7 years to adulthood, as measured by time-resolved immunofluorometric assay. *Journal of Clinical and Endocrinological Metabolism, 68,* 53–57.

Barker, D. J. P. (1999). Fetal origins of coronary heart disease. *Acta Paediatrica Supplement, 422,* 78–82.

Bateson, P. P. G. (1976). Rules and reciprocity in behavioural development. In P. Bateson & R. Hinde (Eds.), *Growing points in ethology* (pp. 401–421). Cambridge, UK: Cambridge University Press.

Bateson, P. P. G. (1982). Behavioural development and evolutionary processes. In King's College Sociobiology Study Group (Ed.). *Current problems in sociobiology* (pp. 133–151). Cambridge, UK: Cambridge University Press.

Belsky, J., Steinberg, L., & Draper, P. (1991). Childhood experience, interpersonal development, and reproductive strategy: An evolutionary theory of socialization. *Child Development, 62,* 647–670.

Bernard, J. M. (1975). Adolescence and socialization for motherhood. In S. Dragastin & G. Elder (Eds.), *Adolescence in the life cycle* (pp. 227–252). New York: Wiley.

Blunt Bugental, D., Martorell, G. A., & Barraza, V. (2003). Hormonal costs of subtle forms of infant maltreatment. *Hormones and Behavior, 43,* 237–244.

Boden, M. A. (1977). *Artificial intelligence and natural man.* Hassocks, UK: Harvester Press.

Bogin, B. A. (2001). *The growth of humanity.* New York: Wiley-Liss.

Bogin, B. A., & Smith, B. H. (1996). Evolution of the human life cycle. *American Journal of Human Biology, 8,* 703–716.

Bonner, J. T. (1993). *Life cycles.* Princeton, NJ: Princeton University Press.

Borgerhoff Mulder, M. (1992). Reproductive decisions. In E. Smith & B. Winterhalder (Eds.), *Evolutionary ecology and human behavior* (pp. 339–374). Hawthorne, NY: Aldine de Gruyter.

Bowlby, J. (1951). Maternal care and mental health. *Bulletin of the World Health Organization, 3,* 355–534.

Bowlby, J. (1969). *Attachment.* New York: Basic Books.

Boyce, W. T., & Ellis, B. J. (in press). Biological sensitivity to context: I. An evolutionary–developmental theory of the origins and functions of stress reactivity. *Development and Psychopathology.*

Boyer, D. K., & Fine, D. (1992). Sexual abuse as a factor in adolescent pregnancy and child maltreatment. *Family Planning Perspectives, 24,* 4–11.

Brody, S. (2002). Age at first intercourse is inversely related to female cortisol reactivity. *Psychoneuroendocrinology, 27,* 933–943.

Buss, L. W. (1987). *The evolution of individuality*. Princeton, NJ: Princeton University Press.

Buunk, B. P. (1997). Personality, birth order and attachment styles as related to various types of jealousy. *Personality and Individual Differences, 23*, 997–1006.

Campbell, D. T. (1974). Evolutionary epistemology. In P. Schlipp (Ed.), *The philosophy of Karl Popper* (Vol. XIV, pp. 413–463). La Salle, IL: Open Court.

Carter, C. S. (1998). Neuroendocrine perspectives on social attachment and love. *Psychoneuroendocrinology, 23*, 779–818.

Caspi, A., & Moffitt, T. E. (1991). Individual differences are accentuated during periods of social change: The case of girls at puberty. *Journal of Personality and Social Psychology, 61*, 157–168.

Charnov, E. L. (1993). *Life history invariants*. New York: Oxford University Press.

Charnov, E. L., & Berrigan, D. (1993). Why do female primates have such long lifespans and so few babies? *Evolutionary Anthropology, 1*, 191–194.

Chisholm, J. S. (1993). Death, hope and sex: Life history theory and the development of reproductive strategies. *Current Anthropology, 34*, 1–24.

Chisholm, J. S. (1996). The evolutionary ecology of attachment organization. *Human Nature, 7*, 1–37.

Chisholm, J. S (1999a). *Death, hope and sex: Steps to an evolutionary ecology of mind and morality*. New York: Cambridge University Press.

Chisholm, J. S. (1999b). Attachment and time preference: Relations between early stress and sexual behavior in a sample of American university women. *Human Nature, 10*, 51–83.

Chisholm, J. S. (2003). Uncertainty, contingency and attachment: A life history theory of theory of mind. In K. Sterelny & J. Fitness (Eds.), *From mating to mentality: Evaluating evolutionary psychology* (pp. 125–155). New York: Psychology Press.

Chisholm, J. S., & Burbank, V. K. (2001). Evolution and inequality. *International Journal of Epidemiology, 30*, 206–211.

Chisholm, J. S., Quinlivan, J. A., Petersen, R. W., & Coall, D. A. (2005). Early stress predicts age at menarche and first birth, adult attachment and expected lifespan. Manuscript submitted for publication.

Chrousos, G. P., & Gold, P. W. (1992). The concept of stress and stress system disorders. *Journal of the American Medical Association, 267*, 1244–1252.

Clutton-Brock, T. H. (1991). *The evolution of parental care*. Princeton, NJ: Princeton University Press.

Coall, D. A., & Chisholm, J. S. (2003). Evolutionary perspectives on pregnancy: Maternal age at menarche and infant birth weight. *Social Science and Medicine, 57*, 1771–1781.

Cockburn, A. (1998). Evolution of helping behavior in cooperatively breeding birds. *Annual Review of Ecology and Systematics, 29*, 141–177.

Csibra, G., Gergeley, G. Biró, S., Koós, O., & Brockbank, M. (1999). Goal attribution without agency cues: The perception of "pure reason" in infancy. *Cognition, 72*, 237–267.

Cvetkovich, G. S., Grote, B. M., Lieberman, E., & Miller, W. M. (1978). Sex role development and teenage fertility-related behavior. *Adolescence, 13*, 231–236.

Dennett, D. (1987). *The intentional stance*. Cambridge, MA: MIT Press/Bradford.

Dennett, D. C. (1995). *Darwin's dangerous idea*. New York: Simon & Schuster.

Dobzhansky, T. (1973). Nothing in biology makes sense except in the light of evolution. *American Biology Teacher, 35*, 125–129.

Draper, P., & Belsky, J. (1990). Personality development in evolutionary perspective. *Journal of Personality, 58,* 141–161.

Draper, P., & Harpending, H. C. (1982). Father absence and reproductive strategy: An evolutionary perspective. *Journal of Anthropological Research, 38,* 255–273.

Ellis, B. J., Bates, J. E., Dodge, K. A., Fergusson, D. M., Horwood, L. J., Petit, G. S., et al. (2003). Does father absence place daughters at special risk for early sexual activity and teenage pregnancy? *Child Development, 74,* 801–821.

Ellison, P. T. (1990). Human ovarian function and reproductive ecology: New hypotheses. *American Anthropologist, 92,* 933–952.

Emlen, S. T. (1995). An evolutionary theory of the family. *Proceedings of the National Academy of Science USA, 92,* 8092–8099.

Farmer, P. (2003). *Pathologies of power: Health, human rights, and the new war on the poor.* Berkeley: University of California Press.

Feeney, J. A. (1999). Adult romantic attachment and couple relationships. In J. Cassidy & P. Shaver (Eds.), *Handbook of attachment: Theory, research, and clinical applications* (pp. 355–377). New York: Guilford Press.

Fiscella, K., Kitzman, H. J., Cole, R. E., Sidora, K. J., & Olds, D. (1998). Does child abuse predict adolescent pregnancy? *Pediatrics, 101,* 620–624.

Flinn, M. V., Quinlan, R. J., Turner, M. T., Decker, S. A., & England, B. G. (1996). Male–female differences in effects of parental absence on glucocorticoid stress response. *Human Nature, 7,* 125–162.

Ge, X., Brody, G. H., Conger, R. Simmons, R. L., & Murry, V. M. (2002). Contextual amplification of pubertal transitional effects on African American children's problem behaviors. *Developmental Psychology, 38,* 42–54.

Gergely, G., & Watson, J. S. (1999). Early social–emotional development: Contingency perception and the social-biofeedback model. In P. Rochat (Ed.), *Early social cognition: Understanding others in the first months of life* (pp. 101–137). Mahwah, NJ: Erlbaum.

Gillespie, J. H. (1977). Natural selection for variances in offspring number: A new evolutionary principle. *American Naturalist, 111,* 1010–1041.

Gould, S. J. (1977). *Ontogeny and phylogeny.* Cambridge, MA: Harvard/Belknap Press.

Gray, R. D., Heaney, M., & Fairhall, S. (2003). Evolutionary psychology and the challenge of adaptive explanation. In K. Sterelny & J. Fitness (Eds.), *From mating to mentality: Evaluating evolutionary psychology* (pp. 247–269). New York: Psychology Press.

Grossmann, K. E., Grossmann, K., Winter, M., & Zimmermann, P. (2002). Attachment relationships and appraisal of partnership: From early experience of sensitive support to later relationship representation. In L. Pulkkinen & A. Caspi (Eds.), *Paths to successful development: Personality in the life course* (pp. 73–105). New York: Cambridge University Press.

Gubernick, D. J. (1981). Parent and infant attachment in mammals. In D. Gubernick & P. Klopfer (Eds.), *Parental care in mammals* (pp. 243–305). New York: Plenum Press.

Gunnar, M. R. (1998). Quality of early care and buffering of neuroendocrine stress reactions: Potential effects on the developing human brain. *Preventive Medicine, 27,* 208–211.

Gunnar, M. R. (2000). Early adversity and the development of stress reactivity and regulation. In C. Nelson (Ed.), *The effects of adversity on neurobehavioral devel-*

opment: Minnesota Symposium on Child Psychology (Vol. 31, pp. 163–200). Mahwah, NJ: Erlbaum.

Gunnar, M. R., & Cheatham, C. L. (2003). Brain and behavior interfaces: Stress and the developing brain. *Infant Mental Health Journal, 24*, 195–211.

Gunnar, M. R., & Donzella, B. (2002). Social regulation of the LHPA axis in early human development. *Psychoneuroendocrinology, 27*, 199–220.

Gunnar, M. R., Brodersen, L., Nachmias, M., Buss, K. A., & Rigatuso, J. (1996). Stress reactivity and attachment security. *Developmental Psychobiology, 29*, 191–204.

Harpending, H. C., Draper, P., & Pennington, R. L. (1990). Culture, evolution, parental care and mortality. In A. Swedlund & G. Armelagos (Eds.), *Disease in populations in transition* (pp. 251–225). South Hadley, MA: Bergin & Garvey.

Hawkes, K., & Bleige Bird, R. L. (2002). Showing off, handicap signalling and the evolution of men's work. *Evolutionary Anthropology, 11*, 58–67.

Hazan, C., & Shaver, P. R. (1987). Romantic love conceptualized as an attachment process. *Journal of Personality and Social Psychology, 52*, 511–524.

Hazan, C., & Zeifman, D. M. 1999. Pair bonds as attachments: Evaluating the evidence. In J. Cassidy & P. R. Shaver (Eds.), *Handbook of attachment: Theory, research, and clinical applications* (pp. 336–354). New York: Guilford Press.

Heim, C., Owens, M. J., Plotsky, P. M., & Nemeroff, C. B. (1997). The role of early adverse life events in the etiology of depression and posttraumatic stress disorder: Focus on corticotropin releasing factor. *Annals of the New York Academy of Science, 821*, 194–207.

Henricksen, T. B. (1999). Foetal nutrition, foetal growth restriction and health in later life. *Acta Paediatrica Supplement, 429*, 4–8.

Herman-Giddens, M. E., Sandler, A. D., & Friedman, N. E. (1988). Sexual precocity in girls: An association with sexual abuse? *American Journal of Diseases of Children, 142*, 431–433.

Holland, J. H. (1992). Complex adaptive systems. *Daedalus, 121*, 17–30.

Hrdy, S. B. (1999). *Mother nature: Maternal instincts and how they shape the human species.* New York: Pantheon.

Hrdy, S. B. (2001). The optimal number of fathers: Evolution, demography and history in the shaping of female mate preferences. *Annals of the New York Academy of Sciences, 907*, 75–96.

Hrdy, S. B. (2004). Comes the child before man: How cooperative breeding and prolonged post-weaning dependence shaped hominid potentials. In B. Hewlett & M. Lamb (Eds.), *Culture and ecology of hunter–gatherer children* (pp. 65–91). Hawthorne, NY: Aldine de Gruyter.

Hrdy, S. B., & Whitten, P. L. (1987). Patterning of sexual activity. In B. B. Smuts, D. L. Cheney, R. M. Seyfarth, & R. W. Wrangham (Eds.), *Primate societies* (pp. 370–384). Chicago: University of Chicago Press.

Insel, T. R. (2000). Toward a neurobiology of attachment. *Review of General Psychology, 4*, 176–185.

Johnston, F. (1974). Control of age at menarche. *Human Biology, 46*, 159–171.

Kaplan, H. S. (1994). Evolutionary and wealth flows theories of fertility: Empirical tests and new models. *Population and Development Review, 20*, 753–791.

Kaprio, J., Rimpela, A., Winter, T., Viken, R. J., Rimpela, M., & Rose, R. J. (1995). Common genetic influences on BMI and age at menarche. *Human Biology, 67*, 739–753.

Kawachi, I., & Kennedy, B. A. (2003). *The health of nations: Why inequality is harmful to your health*. New York: New Press.

Kiess, W., Meidert, A., Dressendorfer, R. A., Schriever, K., Kessler, U., Konig, A., Schwarz, H. P., & Strasburger, C. J. (1995). Salivary cortisol levels throughout childhood and adolescence: Relation with age, pubertal stage, and weight. *Pediatric Research*, *37*(4, Pt. 1), 502–550.

King, J. A., Mandansky, D., King, M., Fletcher, K., & Brewer, J. (2001). Early sexual abuse and low cortisol. *Psychiatry and Clinical Neurosciences*, *55*, 71–74.

Lancaster, J. B. (1997). The evolutionary history of human parental investment in relation to population growth and social stratification. In P. Gowaty (Ed.), *Feminism and evolutionary biology: Boundaries, intersections and frontiers* (pp. 466–488). New York: Chapman & Hall.

Langer, J. (2000). The heterochronic evolution of primate cognitive development. In S. T. Parker, J. Langer, & M. L. McKinney (Eds.), *Biology, brains and behavior* (pp. 215–236). Santa Fe, NM: School of American Research Press.

LeDoux, J. E. (1996). *The emotional brain*. New York: Simon & Schuster.

Legro, R. S., Lin, H. M., Demers, L. M., & Lloyd, T. (2003). Urinary free cortisol in adolescent Caucasian females during perimenarche. *Journal of Endocrinology and Metabolism*, *88*, 215–219.

Marris, P. (1991). The social construction of uncertainty. In C. M. Parkes, J. Stevenson-Hinde, & P. Marris (Eds.), *Attachment across the life cycle* (pp. 77–90). London: Routledge.

McEwen, B. S. (1995). Stressful experience, brain and emotions: Developmental, genetic and hormonal influences. In M. Gazzaniga (Ed.), *The cognitive neurosciences* (pp. 1117–1135). Cambridge, MA: MIT Press.

McEwen, B. S., & Seeman, T. (1999). Protective and damaging effects of mediators of stress. In N. E. Adler, M. Marmot, B. S. McEwen, & J. Stewart (Eds.), *Socioeconomic status and health in industrialized nations* (pp. 30–47). New York: New York Academy of Science.

Meaney, M. J. (2001). Maternal care, gene expression and the transmission of individual differences in stress reactivity across generations. *Annual Review of Neuroscience*, *24*, 1161–1192.

Merzenich, H., Boeing, H., & Wahrendorf, J. (1993). Dietary fat and sports activity as determinants for age at menarche. *American Journal of Epidemiology*, *138*, 217–224.

Miller, B. C., Norton, M. C., Curtis, T., Hill, E. J., Schvaneveldt, P., & Young, M. (1997). The timing of sexual intercourse among adolescents: Family peer and other antecedents. *Youth and Society*, *29*, 54–83.

Mott, F. L., Fondell, M. M., Hu, P. N., Kowaleski-Jones, L., & Menaghan, E. G. (1996). The determinants of first sex by age 14 in a high-risk adolescent population. *Family Planning Perspectives*, *28*, 13–18.

Netherton, C. M., Goodyer, I. M., Tamplin, A., & Herbert J. (2004). Salivary cortisol and dehydroepiandrosterone in relation to puberty and gender. *Psychoneuroendocrinology*, *29*, 125–40

Nussbaum, M. C. (1995). Human capabilities, female human beings. In M. C. Nussbaum & J. Glover (Eds.), *Women, culture and development: A study of human capabilities* (pp. 61–104). Oxford, UK: Clarendon Press.

Oyama, S. (1985). *The ontogeny of information*. New York: Cambridge University Press.

Oyama, S. (2000). *Evolution's eye: A systems view of the biology–culture divide*. Durham, NC: Duke University Press.

Pajer, K. A., Gardner, W., Kirillova, G. P., & Vanyukov, M. M. (2001). Sex differences in cortisol level and neurobehavioral disinhibition in children of substance abusers. *Journal of Child and Adolescent Substance Abuse, 10*, 65–72.

Panksepp, J. (1998). *Affective neuroscience: The foundation of human and animal emotions*. New York: Oxford University Press.

Parker, G. A., & Maynard Smith, J. (1990). Optimality theory in evolutionary biology. *Nature, 348*, 27–33.

Parker, S. T. (1996). Using cladistic analysis of comparative data to reconstruct the evolution of cognitive development in hominids. In E. Martins (Ed.), *Phylogenies and the comparative method in animal behaviour* (pp. 361–399). New York: Oxford University Press.

Parker, S. T., & McKinney, M. L. (1999). *Origins of intelligence: The evolution of cognitive development in monkeys, apes and humans*. Baltimore: Johns Hopkins University Press.

Phillips, D. L. (1998). Birth weight and the future development of diabetes: A review of the evidence. *Child: Care Health and Development, 22*, 37–53.

Phinney, V. G., Jensen, L. C., Olsen, J. A., & Cundick, B. P. (1990). The relationship between early development and psychosexual behaviors in adolescent females. *Adolescence, 25*, 321–332.

Plotkin, H. C. (1994). *Darwin machines and the nature of knowledge*. Cambridge, MA: Harvard University Press.

Promislow, D. E., & Harvey, P. H. (1990). Living fast and dying young: A comparative analysis of life-history variation in mammals. *Journal of the Zoological Society of London, 220*, 417–437.

Promislow, D. E., & Harvey, P. H. (1991). Mortality rates and the evolution of mammal life histories. *Acta Oecologica, 12*, 94–101.

Roisman, G. I., Madsen, S. D., Hennighausen, K. H., Sroufe, L. A., & Collins, W. A. (2001). The coherence of dyadic behavior across parent–child and romantic relationships as mediated by the internalized representation of experience. *Attachment and Human Development, 3*, 156–172.

Sapolsky, R. M. (1992). *Stress, the aging brain and the mechanisms of neuron death*. Cambridge, MA: MIT Press.

Sapolsky, R. M., Romero, L. M., & Munck, A. U. (2000). How do glucocorticoids influence stress responses?: Integrating permissive, suppressive, stimulatory and preparative actions. *Endocrine Reviews, 21*, 55–89.

Schaffer, W. M. (1983). The application of optimal control theory to the general life history problem. *American Naturalist, 121*, 418–431.

Scholl, T. O., Hediger, M. L., Vasilenko, P., Ances, I. G., Smith, W. K., & Salmon, R. W. (1989). Effects of early maturation on fetal growth. *Annals of Human Biology, 16*, 335–345.

Seger, J., & Brockmann, H. J. (1987). What is bet-hedging? In P. H. Harvey & L. Partridge (Eds.), *Oxford surveys in evolutionary biology* (Vol. 4, pp. 182–211). Oxford, UK: Oxford University Press.

Seger, J., & Stubblefield, J. W. (1996). Optimization and adaptation. In M. Rose & G. Lauder (Eds.), *Adaptation* (pp. 93–123). New York: Academic Press.

Sen, A. K. (1990). More than a 100 million women are missing. *New York Review of Books, 37*, 61–66.

Sen, A. K. (1992). *Inequality reexamined*. New York: Russell Sage Foundation.

Sen, A. K. (1993, May). The economics of life and death. *Scientific American*, pp. 40–47.

Sharpsteen, D. J., & Kirkpatrick, L. A. (1997). Romantic jealousy and adult romantic attachment. *Journal of Personality and Social Psychology, 72*, 627–640.

Short, R. V. (1979). Sexual selection and its component parts: Somatic and genital selection as illustrated by man and the great apes. *Advances in the Study of Behavior, 9*, 131–158.

Smith, E. A., Borgerhoff Mulder, M., & Hill, K. (2001). Controversies in the evolutionary social sciences: A guide for the perplexed. *Trends in Ecology and Evolution, 16*, 128–135.

Smuts, B. B. (1992). Male aggression against women: An evolutionary perspective. *Human Nature, 3*, 1–44.

Smuts, B. B. (1995). The evolutionary origin of patriarchy. *Human Nature, 6*, 1–32.

Solomon, N. G., & French, J. A. (Eds.). (1997). *Cooperative breeding in mammals*. Cambridge, UK: Cambridge University Press.

Stearns, S. C. (1982). The role of development in the evolution of life histories. In J. Bonner (Ed.), *Evolution and development* (pp. 237–258). New York: Springer-Verlag.

Stearns, S. C. (1992). *The evolution of life histories*. New York: Oxford University Press.

Stearns, S. C. (2000). Life history evolution: Successes, limitations and prospects. *Naturwissenschaften, 87*, 476–486.

Susman, E. J. (1997). Modeling developmental complexity in adolescence: Hormones and behavior in context. *Journal of Research on Adolescence, 7*, 283–306.

Susman, E. J., & Pajer, K. (2004). Biology–behavior integration and antisocial behavior in girls. In M. Putallaz & K. L. Bierman (Eds.), *Aggression, antisocial behavior, and violence among girls: A developmental perspective* (pp. 23–47). New York: Guilford Press.

Thompson, N. S., & Derr, P. G. (2000). Intentionality is the mark of the vital. In F. Tonneau & N. S. Thompson (Eds.), *Perspectives in ethology: Vol. 13. Evolution, culture, and behavior* (pp. 213–229). New York: Plenum Press.

Trickett, P. K., & Putnam, F. W. (1993). Impact of child sexual abuse on females: Toward a developmental, psychobiological integration. *Psychological Science, 4*, 81–87.

Trivers, R. L. (1972). Parental investment and sexual selection. In B. G. Campbell (Ed.), *Sexual selection and the descent of man* (pp. 136–179). Chicago: Aldine.

Trivers, R. L. (1974). Parent–offspring conflict. *American Zoologist, 14*, 249–262.

Udry, J. R., & Cliquet, R. L. (1982). A cross-cultural examination of the relationship between ages at menarche, marriage, and first birth. *Demography, 19*, 53–63.

Uvnäs-Moberg, K. (1998). Oxytocin may mediate the benefits of positive social interactions and emotions. *Psychoneuroendocrinology, 23*, 819–835.

Vamvakopoulos, N. C., & Chrousos, G. P. (1993). Evidence of direct estrogenic regulation of human corticotropin-releasing hormone gene expression: Potential implications for the sexual dimophism of the stress response and immune/inflammatory reaction. *Journal of Clinical Investigation, 92*, 1896–902.

van Schaik, C. P., & Dunbar, R. I. M. (1990). The evolution of monogamy in large primates: A new hypothesis and some crucial tests. *Behaviour, 32*, 31–62.

Vitzthum, V. J. (2001). Why not so great is still good enough. In P. T. Ellison (Ed.),

Reproductive ecology and human evolution (pp. 179–202). New York: Aldine de Gruyter.

Wahlbeck, K., Forsen, T., Osmond, C., Barker, D. J., & Eriksson, J.G. (2001). Association of schizophrenia with low maternal body mass index, small size at birth and thinness during childhood. *Archives of General Psychiatry, 58,* 48–52.

Washburn, S. L. (1960). Tools and human evolution. *Scientific American, 203,* 36–43.

Watson, J. S. (2001). Contingency perception and misperception in infancy: Some potential implications for attachment. *Bulletin of the Menninger Clinic, 65,* 296–320.

Wellens, R., Malina, R. M., Roche, A. F., Chumlea, W. C., Guo, S., & Siervogel, R. M. (1994). Body size and fatness in young adults in relation to age at menarche. *American Journal of Human Biology, 4,* 783–787.

West-Eberhard, M. J. (2003). *Developmental plasticity and evolution.* New York: Oxford University Press.

Wilkinson, R. G. (1996). *Unhealthy societies: The afflictions of inequality.* London: Routledge.

Williams, G. C. (1975). *Sex and evolution.* Princeton, NJ: Princeton University Press.

Wilson, M. I., & Daly, M. (1985). Competitiveness, risk-taking and violence: The young male syndrome. *Ethology and Sociobiology, 6,* 59–73.

Worthman, C. M. (1999). Evolutionary perspectives on the onset of puberty. In W. Trevathan, E. O. Smith, & J. J. McKenna (Eds.), *Evolutionary medicine* (pp. 135–163). Oxford, UK: Oxford University Press.

Wrangham, R. W. (1980). An ecological model of female-bonded groups. *Behaviour, 75,* 262–300.

Wrangham, R. W. (1993). The evolution of sexuality in chimpanzees and bonobos. *Human Nature, 4,* 47–79.

Wrangham, R. W., & Peterson, D. (1996). *Demonic males: Apes and the origin of human violence.* Boston: Houghton Mifflin.

Wyatt, G. E., Durvasula, R. S., Guthrie, D., LeFranc, E., & Forge, N. (1999). Correlates of first intercourse among women in Jamaica. *Archives of Sexual Behavior, 28,* 139–157.

5

DEVELOPMENTAL BEHAVIORAL GENETICS AND EVOLUTIONARY PSYCHOLOGY

Tying the Theoretical and Empirical Threads

NANCY L. SEGAL
ELIZABETH M. HILL

OVERVIEW

Our aim in this chapter is to fulfill two goals. The first is to show how behavioral–genetic methods can be used to test evolutionary-based hypotheses concerning human behavioral and physical development. The second is to show how evolutionary reasoning informs developmental behavioral genetics (DBG). Following an overview and comparison of these disciplines, available twin and adoption methods are reviewed, followed by a description of new views of phenotypic development and plasticity, as well as illustrative research examples from the relevant literature. The chapter concludes with a summary of current knowledge and assessment of future approaches and directions.

Brief Overview of Developmental Behavioral Genetics

Behavioral genetics lies at the juncture of psychology and genetics. It is concerned with the inherited transmission of behavioral traits and sources of variation underlying those traits within populations. Variation can be organized into two broad classes: genetic and environmental. Genetic variance can be further organized into additive and nonadditive effects. Additive genetic effects, which occur when genes "add up" in accordance with gene dosage, are transmitted across generations and cause members of the same family to be more similar to each other. Nonadditive effects, which occur when genes interact either at the same or at different loci, generally are not transmitted across generations and do not run in families. Full siblings occasionally share nonadditive traits, because they have a 25% chance of inheriting the same genes from each parent. Monozygotic (MZ) twins are the only pair of relatives who share all sources of genetic variance. Environmental variance can be either shared or nonshared. Shared environments make family members alike, whereas nonshared environments make family members different. Research shows that for most measured behavioral traits, the greatest source of environmental variance is nonshared (Plomin, DeFries, McClearn, & McGuffin, 2001).

Estimates of genetic and environmental effects are valid only for a specific population at one point in time, not for any individual. Specifically, these estimates express the extent to which members of a population differ due to genetic or environmental differences between them. For example, genetic estimates of personality traits are about 50%. This does not mean that one-half of an individual's personality is due to their genes and the other half is due to their experiences; its refers only to differences at the population level. Furthermore, these estimates may characterize only a particular population, measured at a particular time and with a particular instrument; changes in any of these may affect the result. It is also important to appreciate that for traits influenced by many genes, such as intelligence, variation in one of those genes may be affected by the genetic background of the individual (Nijhout, 2003).

DBG is concerned with two types of change in physical and behavioral traits during development. The first type concerns changes in heritability (the extent to which individual differences in measured traits are associated with genetic differences) during development. Such changes may occur as different genetic and environmental systems become active during the lifespan; as we grow and develop, some genes get switched on at particular times (e.g., at adolescence, when secondary sexual development occurs) and some experiences become more important (e.g., the greater independence of adolescents vs. children in selecting their friends and activities). In addition, heritability increases when environments among individuals are more alike, because environmental homogeneity causes individual differences to become more closely tied to genetic differences. Conversely, heritability decreases when environments become more different among people, because environmental heterogeneity causes individual differences to become more closely tied to people's varying experiences. The second type concerns change in age-to-age genetic correlations, specifically, the extent to which genetic effects at one age are correlated with genetic effects expressed at another age.

The development of general intelligence illustrates both types of change. IQ heritability appears to increase with age, from approximately 20% in infancy to 60% in adulthood (McClearn et al., 1997). This is evident in the stability of MZ twin correlations, the decline in dizygotic (DZ) twin correlations, and the absence of similarity in adoptive siblings as they approach adolescence (Segal, 2000a). Thus, shared environments appear to affect intelligence when children are young and living at home, but become less significant as individuals age and seek environments more compatible with their genetic proclivities. It is also possible that, with development, more genes relevant to intelligence become active. With respect to the second type of developmental change, there is evidence that genetic effects on intelligence at early ages are also expressed at later ages (Plomin, 1990).

Some criticisms of DBG have come from individuals working within a developmental systems theory framework. Developmental systems theory views development as proceeding in a bidirectional manner across hierarchical, multiple levels: genetic activity, neural activity, behavior, and environment (Gottleib, 1995; also see Bjorklund & Pellegrini, 2002). It rejects the population approach (i.e., partitioning of genetic and environmental effects on behavioral traits), arguing that it is deterministic and neglects developmental processes. These criticisms have, however, been rebutted by Scarr (1995), who points out that behavior geneticists clearly recognize the probabilistic nature of gene–behavior relationships. Furthermore, she notes that estimating probable genetic and environmental outcomes on behavioral traits can yield valuable information about population problems, without denying the fact that atypical settings may be associated with atypical consequences in individual cases.

Brief Overview of Evolutionary Psychology

In contrast with behavioral genetics, *evolutionary psychology* (EP) focuses on species uniformities, especially the origins and functions of adaptations affecting different behavioral patterns and strategies. It is mostly concerned with ultimate behavioral explanations (explanations emphasizing behavioral functions in terms of survival and reproduction), as compared with proximal explanations (explanations emphasizing immediate causal events associated with behavior), although both are of interest (Mealey, 2000). Four central themes have been identified: to understand why the mind is designed as it is; to determine how the mind is organized; to understand the different parts and mechanisms of the mind; and to elucidate the ways in which environments interact with the mind to yield different behaviors (Buss, 1999).

EP tests hypotheses and questions derived from evolutionary-based theories, such as Hamilton's (1964) kin selection theory. Kin selection theory, which explains altruism with reference to the relative genetic relatedness of the interactants, is especially relevant to the material reviewed in this chapter. Hamilton reasoned that natural selection will favor alleles predisposing individuals to act in ways favoring transmission of those alleles into future generations. (Alleles are different forms of a gene, such as brown or blue for eye color.) Nepotism, in which alleles influence individuals to favor related individuals who are likely to carry replicas of these alleles, is an indirect means by which these alleles can be preserved. Dawkins (1989) cautions that people do not consciously compute the benefits and losses associated with engaging in altruistic acts; instead, they are influenced by their genes to act in ways that are consistent with such computations.

EP offers a new level of understanding for studies of behavioral phenomena, but is not intended to replace alternative theories (Crawford, 1998). For example, psychodynamic interpretations of MZ twins' close social relationship emphasize their similar appearance as possibly interfering with their developing identity and sense of self (Siemon & Adelman, 1986). It is further argued that their physical identity is responsible for their similar treatment by others. EP would regard these events as proximal mechanisms; indeed, the psychodynamic literature offers a rich source of proximal events from which to choose. However, EP would consider the twins' genetic identity as possibly underlying their similar behaviors and their perceptions of those similarities. These perceptions may, in fact, trigger the feelings of social attraction observed between MZ twins at all stages of development, even MZ twins reared apart (Segal, Hershberger, & Arad, 2003).

Behavioral genetics and evolutionary psychology have generally progressed with little contact between them. However, some investigators have identified shared interests and are encouraging collaborative efforts. The next section summarizes areas of commonality between them.

Behavioral Genetics and Evolutionary Psychology: A New Partnership?

Behavioral genetics and EP have shared concerns despite their historical, methodological, and conceptual differences (Mealey, 2001). These commonalities have been variously documented over the years by Freedman (1968), Buss (1987, 1990), Crawford and Anderson (1989), Belsky, Steinberg and Draper (1991), Segal (1993, 1997a), Bailey (1997), Segal and MacDonald (1998), Buss and Greiling (1999), and Mealey (2001). Main themes are that (1) evolutionary biology provides behavioral genetics with an additional theoretical perspective for interpretation of findings, and (2) behavioral genetics offers powerful methods for testing hypotheses generated by evolutionary biology.

Mealey's (2001) overview may be the best recent treatment of themes common to behavioral genetics and EP. Joint efforts can illuminate a range of developmental issues, especially those concerning kinship. She notes that, for evolutionary psychologists, "kinship, via the effect of inclusive fitness, constitutes a core construct of relevance to all social interaction" (p. 23). Behavioral geneticists rely on kinship to unravel genetic and environmental influences underlying development, although only developmental social geneticists focus specifically on social interaction as the unit of analysis (e.g., see Scott, 1977;

Hahn, 1990). Regardless, kinship is central to individuals' developmental life histories, so it is of interest to members of numerous social science disciplines.

Mealey outlines several goals toward which behavioral genetics and EP may jointly aspire. Among them is the task of determining how adaptive and nonadaptive trait variations map onto life history strategies. Life history strategies are organized systems of rules and decisions that guide how individuals allocate time and resources to reproduction, growth, and survival over the life course (Crawford & Anderson, 1989). A number of research approaches to specific problems are suggested. For example, studying MZ twins raised apart can show how rearing influences may trigger different psychological processes in genetically identical individuals. Another possibility (the "bullet approach") involves finding MZ twins who differ in traits of interest, then examining their lives retrospectively to identify key experiential differences and perceptions of these differences.

Several relevant studies are summarized below, following a review of twin types and twin methods.

TWIN, FAMILY, AND ADOPTION METHODS

Types of Twins

Monozygotic (MZ) and Dizygotic (DZ)

MZ (or identical) twins occur when a fertilized egg, or zygote, divides during the first 2 weeks of gestation. MZ co-twins share 100% of their genes, but various sources of influence can alter genetic identity and phenotypic expression (see Segal, 2000a, and references therein). For example, differences in X chromosome inactivation—the random "shutting down" of one of the two X chromosomes in each cell nucleus of human females—can lead to MZ female twin discordance for X-linked traits, such as color-blindness and fragile X syndrome. This process occurs 6 to 8 days after an egg is fertilized. If the fertilized egg divides before this time to produce MZ female twins, it is possible that one twin will have more paternally derived X chromosomes active and the co-twin will have more maternally derived X chromosomes active. Nondisjunction (the failure of chromosomes to separate properly during cell division) can produce MZ twins discordant for Down syndrome (trisomy 21) or Turner syndrome (X0). Relatively delayed zygotic division (occurring after the eighth postconceptional day) has been associated with anatomical and physical reversals (e.g., opposite handedness or hair whorl) in approximately 25% of MZ twins. Physical and behavioral differences between MZ twins have also been linked with chorion type (Prescott, Johnson, & McArdle, 1999), unequal fetal blood supply (Machin & Still, 1996), and birth order (Boggess & Chisholm, 1997).

DZ (or fraternal) twins result from the separate fertilization of two eggs by two spermatozoa. DZ twins thus share 50% of their genes on average, by descent, as do nontwin siblings. Furthermore, DZ twins may be same-sex or opposite-sex. DZ twins' behavioral and physical differences are explained by genetic and environmental differences between them.

Twinning rates have escalated considerably in recent years. The number of twins (MZ and DZ combined born to women between 40 and 44 years of age) increased by 63% in the years 1980–1997 (Martin & Park, 1999). This change has been explained chiefly with reference to new assisted reproductive technologies that are currently available (Hecht & Magoon, 1998). Less well known is the fact that assisted reproductive technologies have also increased the MZ twinning rate (albeit less markedly), perhaps by altering the early environment of the developing embryo (Hecht, 1995). British and Belgian laboratories have reported increases of 1 and 1.2%, as compared with the population rate of 0.4% (Edwards, Mettler, & Walters, 1986; Derom, Vlietinck, Derom, Van den Berghe, & Thiery, 1987; also see Hecht, 1995).

Twin variants

MZ twins vary in their degree of similarity, as indicated earlier. Some studies comparing two-chorion and one-chorion MZ twins have reported greater resemblance between one-chorion than between two-chorion twins in some cognitive and personality measures (see Sokol et al., 1995, and references therein). In addition, MZ twins vary with respect to their degree of physical similarity. Such pairs would be potentially interesting to evolutionary researchers examining perceptions of resemblance as indicators of genetic relatedness, which possibly affect social relatedness. For example, resemblance in physical traits offers information, albeit approximate, as to genetic relatedness. MZ twins who differ physically may feel lower levels of social closeness to one another than MZ twins who look more physically alike. Twins raised apart are of considerable value to behavioral genetics investigators, because they provide direct estimates of heritability in the absence of selective placement. This is because the extent of their resemblance to one another only reflects the effects of their shared genes. They are also valuable to evolutionary researchers, as discussed below.

Virtual twins (VTs) are unrelated children of the same age who have been reared together since infancy (Segal, 2000b). They may be composed of two adopted children or one adopted child and one biological child in the family. Thus, they are the perfect complement to MZ twins reared apart, because they replicate the twin situation, but without the genetic link. VTs offer a direct estimate of the effects of shared environmental influences on behavior.

Variant forms of DZ twinning include superfecundation (conception of DZ twins following separate coital acts during the same menstrual cycle) and superfetation (multiple conceptions separated by 3–4 weeks; see Segal, 2000a). Some superfecundated twins do not share a father, a circumstance that may prompt custody suits (Ambach, Parson, & Brezinka, 2000). These events are presumably rare, but lack of detection and documentation may mask their true frequency. The presence of DZ co-twins with different fathers in twin study samples could spuriously inflate heritability estimates (such superfetated twins share one-fourth of their genes, on average). Additional discussion of unusual forms of MZ and DZ twinning is provided in Segal (2000a).

Determination of Twin Type

Correct classification of twin type is an essential step in the research process, because misclassification yields misleading estimates of genetic and environmental influences on phenotypes (Segal, 2000a). Comparative analysis of co-twins' multiple blood group systems provides accurate results, especially when combined with physical measures (Lykken, 1978). Researchers are now relying increasingly on DNA profile analysis as a more accurate and less expensive procedure (Richards et al., 1993). However, physical resemblance questionnaires can be reliably substituted for laboratory methods if the latter are precluded (Segal, 2000a).

Twin and Adoption Designs

MZ–DZ Twin Comparisons

The classic twin design compares trait resemblance between MZ and DZ co-twins. Greater MZ than DZ twin resemblance demonstrates genetic influence on the trait(s) in question. A fundamental assumption in twin research is that trait-relevant environmental influences function similarly for MZ and DZ twins. This concept has been challenged by some critics, yet there is little evidence of meaningful links between twins' treatment and their behavioral outcomes (Hettema, Neale, & Kendler, 1995).

Several variants of the classic twin design are potentially useful to evolutionary developmental studies. The MZ half-sib method includes MZ twins who are married with children (Segal, 1997a, 2000a). Twin aunts (or twin uncles) in these families are "genetic parents" to their nieces and nephews; nieces and nephews are "genetic children" to their twin aunts and uncles. Social relations between these unusual adult–child pairs can be compared to those within DZ twin families in which customary relationships are maintained. For example, it is possible to test the hypothesis that MZ twin aunts (or uncles) would provide greater care for and invest greater effort in their nieces and nephews relative to DZ twins aunts (or uncles). A study examining this issue is currently in progress at the Twin Studies Center at California State University, Fullerton.

Co-twin control involves providing different training or experiences to MZ co-twins to assess the effects of the intervention by controlling the genotype. Natural co-twin control studies appraise the consequences of accidents, illness, or other unusual events that affect one twin but not the other. Evolutionary researchers could use this design to explore the roots of differential parental favoritism or abuse. To our knowledge, such a study has never been undertaken.

Twins as couples designs compare the social-interactional events and outcomes of MZ and DZ twins in collaborative situations. Thus, the focus of analysis is the pair rather than the individual twins, as in the classic method. This design offers insights into how the genetic backgrounds of the interactants contribute to joint social behaviors. The prediction is that individuals with similar genotypes (MZ twins) will be more cooperative, and individuals with dissimilar genotypes (DZ twins) will be more competitive.

DZ twin designs, especially those including superfecundated pairs, would be welcome in evolutionary analyses of behavioral consequences of genetic and social relatedness. Several studies have indicated that DZ pairs with fewer shared blood groups showed reduced behavioral similarity and greater uncertainty over twin type than pairs with greater numbers of blood groups in common (Bock, Vandenberg, Bramble, & Pearson, 1970; Dumont-Driscoll & Rose, 1983). The hypothesis that superfecundated twins should show lower levels of altruism and social attraction than ordinary DZ twins could be tested.

Adoption Designs

Twins reared apart are valuable research subjects in a range of evolutionary-based studies, including research on life history strategies and tactics (Crawford & Anderson, 1989), reproductive variables (Mealey & Segal, 1993), and social relatedness (Segal et al., 2003). Reared apart MZ twins who occupy different birth order positions in their respective families could offer new perspectives on Sulloway's (1996) hypothesis that firstborns are more traditional and laterborns are more rebellious (Segal & MacDonald, 1998). Specifically, it would be of interest to know if co-twins' genetically based personality traits were influenced in predictable ways.

Virtual twins are an informative comparison group for assessing the effects of genetic relatedness, rearing, and familiarity on social relations. This is particularly true when the pair is composed of a biological child and an adoptee, and there are other biological children in the family, because it becomes possible to compare the social affiliation between biological siblings who differ in age with unrelated same-age siblings whose rearing situation is similar to that of twins. Evolutionary reasoning would predict greater affiliation between related than between unrelated siblings. Assessment of sib–sib and parent–child relations would be informative in such families, in comparison with corresponding relationships from ordinary intact families.

ILLUSTRATIVE EXAMPLES OF RESEARCH USING AN EVOLUTIONARY APPROACH TO BEHAVIOR GENETICS

This section reviews selected studies whose approaches, designs, and findings reflect the combined efforts of behavioral genetics and EP. Domains include physical maturation, social relations, and other behaviors.

Physical Growth and Development

Age at Puberty

Evolutionary-based studies have consistently shown an association between father absence and pubertal timing in daughters (Ellis, McFayden-Ketchum, Dodge, Petit, & Bates, 1999; Ellis & Garber, 2000). The explanation, based on work by Belsky et al. (1991), is that early rearing affects reproductive strategies in ways that would have been adaptive, in a reproductive sense, across the range of human environments. Children from families with high stress and/or limited resources (e.g., father absence) would be expected to show accelerated developmental rates.

Twin and family studies have posed some challenge to this interpretation. Rowe (2000) showed genetic effects for both age at menarche (.44) and timing of puberty (.40), as well as a negligible shared environmental contribution. Thus, fathers' genetically based behaviors may be transmitted to their daughters. Some recent supporting evidence comes from Comings, Muhleman, Johnson, and MacMurray (2002), who showed a family association between the short alleles of the androgen receptor (AR) gene and behaviors such as aggression, impulsivity, number of sexual partners, father absence, and age at menarche. Resolution might come from studies of MZ twins reared apart, whose different life experiences could affect their pubertal timing. Farber (1981) reported a mean difference of 9.3 months in age at menarche for 28 pairs of MZ female twins reared apart, greater than the typical 2.8–3.5 month difference for MZ twins reared together (see Treolar & Martin, 1990). It is therefore possible that specific rearing factors may have affected menarche in the separated twins. (See further discussion in Ellis, Chapter 7, this volume.)

Mealey and Segal (1993) used the rare group of MZ twins reared apart to further explore variables related to reproductive success. They found greater genetic influence on reproduction-related behaviors in males than in females. This outcome was, however, directly related only to childhood health. A subsequent twin study found greater genetic influence on age at first intercourse among males than among females (Dunne et al., 1997). This finding was, however, restricted to a younger cohort for whom social constraints on sexual behavior were more relaxed than those applicable to an older cohort. Even though male reproductive potential exceeds female reproductive potential, unsuccessful daughters are more likely than unsuccessful sons to produce some offspring (Mealey, 2000).

Fluctuating Asymmetry

Fluctuating asymmetry (FA) refers to the body's deviation from perfect consistency of form or bilateral symmetry (Thornhill & Gangestad, 1999). These small, random deviations occur in traits that are genetically coded as symmetrical, but which are formed imprecisely because of various developmental stressors (Parsons, 1990). Increased FA, as measured by greater left–right differences in physical attributes (e.g., wrist width, foot breadth, or facial width), suggests greater developmental instability associated with stressful environmental and biological factors, such as susceptibility to toxins or infections. FA has been of interest to evolutionary psychologists with respect to its associations with reproductively relevant traits. Researchers have found, for example, that females prefer the body scents of more symmetrical males, although this was not true for male preferences (Thornhill & Gangestad, 1999). Individuals with lower FA have also been shown to have higher IQ scores (Furlow, Armijo-Prewitt, Gangestad, & Thornhill, 1997).

Disentangling the effects of FA from other indicators of physical attractiveness (e.g., age and hair color) has been problematic. The co-twin control design, borrowed from behavioral genetics and used by Mealey, Bridgstock, and Townsend (1999), was a way to resolve this difficulty. Photographs of Australian MZ twins were used to construct left–left and right–right composite pictures. Twenty-five male and 38 female judges rated each composite on physical similarity and physical attractiveness scales. Zygosity of the twins was determined by blood group analysis. Interestingly, lower FA twins were perceived to be more attractive than their relatively higher FA co-twins. This finding is important, because it shows that an environmentally induced trait can affect perceptions of a fitness-related trait (i.e., attractiveness) in genetically identical individuals.

A subset of twins in this sample was later used to assess whether more symmetrical co-twins believed they were treated preferentially by their parents, from childhood to age 16 (Mealey, 2002). Twenty-five of the MZ pairs completed the Parental Bonding Instrument (PBI), developed by Parker, Tupling, and Brown (1979). Meaningful patterns were not detected in these data. However, one item ("made me feel I wasn't wanted") showed a significant effect, albeit not in the predicted direction. Specifically, *more* symmetrical twins felt less wanted than did their less symmetrical co-twins. This finding, while of interest, could have occurred by chance, so it warrants further study.

Mealey proposed that parental discrimination of twins might not rely on their relative facial symmetry. She also noted that FA in childhood may differ from FA during adolescence, due to significant growth periods. She further proposed that sufficient parental resources in this sample may allow investment in co-twins perceived to be the less healthy in the pair, rather than higher investment in healthier twins, which would be expected when resources are scarce. In other words, parents who are relatively well off can risk investing their time and effort in children who may be less likely to thrive than their siblings. The small sample size urges cautious interpretation.

Cooperation, Competition, and Altruism

Cooperation, competition, and altruism have been of considerable interest to evolutionary psychologists. Twin studies present an elegant method for testing hypotheses derived from kin selection theory, because of the differential genetic relatedness of MZ and DZ twins. Kin selection theory predicts that individuals should direct greater care and cooperation toward close genetic relatives, as compared with more distant genetic relatives or unrelated individuals. Twin studies are a good way to test this class of predictions because the individuals are the same age and were raised in the same family. Most studies of twin relations have used the twins-as-couples design.

Joint Puzzle Solving

Previous work by (Segal, 1993, 1997a) demonstrated greater cooperation between 6- to 11-year-old MZ than DZ twins on joint puzzle solving. All sequences were filmed and scored by judges for selected behaviors (e.g., positioning of the puzzle, facial expressivity). Elaboration of this work used the ratings of three independent judges (Segal, 2002). Perceptions of individuals unfamiliar with the twins bear on the question of whether individuals respond to, or create, MZ and DZ twins' differential levels of behavioral resemblance and affectional ties.

Judges rated each film according to six dimensions: mutuality, nature of interactions, behavioral accommodation, role division, involvement, and contribution. Helmert contrasts were used to test hypotheses regarding twin group differences. MZ pairs scored significantly higher than DZ pairs on mutuality, cooperation, accommodation, involvement, and contribution, and lower on role division. These findings, and the previous analyses, indicate that individuals respond to, rather than create, MZ and DZ twins' differing interactional styles.

"Pseudotwin Pairs"

The following study applied a developmental social-genetic approach to an evolutionary question: Does previous experience with a familiar or unfamiliar genotype affect later social interactions? This question has been addressed by Scott's (1977) seminal work on social behavior in dogs. It had already been shown that similar genotypes cooperate more than dissimilar genotypes, consistent with evolutionary predictions. However, Scott was interested in how experience with genetically similar and dissimilar others might modify joint behavior. He showed that early rearing with a dog of a different breed was associated with increased cooperation during later interactions with either the same or a different breed interactant. However, rearing with a dog from the same breed was associated with reduced cooperation with an unfamiliar interactant. It may be that early experience with different individuals encourages greater behavioral flexibility during subsequent interactions. In contrast, early experience with only similar individuals may reduce behavioral flexibility. Based on Scott's findings with different dog breeds, twins were used to test the hypothesis that unfamiliar MZ pairs would display less cooperation than unfamiliar DZ pairs. Cooperative behavior between unfamiliar male and female pairs was also compared (Segal, 1997a; Segal, Connelly, & Topolski, 1996).

The sample included 14 MZ twin pairs (4 male and 10 female) and 16 same-sex DZ twin pairs (6 male and 10 female), ranging in age from 8.0 to 11.7 years. The twins were organized into 30 unfamiliar "pseudopairs" by placing each MZ and DZ co-twin with a twin from a different MZ or DZ pair. Partners were matched for age, sex, and IQ. Each new set was videotaped while completing two puzzles. Contrary to expectation, social-interactional differences between unfamiliar MZ and DZ sets were not detected. However, female–female sets showed significantly higher levels of cooperation, mutuality, and accommodation than male–male sets. Twins in the age range and social classes represented may experience sufficient diversity in their social experiences, allowing cooperative interactions with unfamiliar partners.

Prisoner's Dilemma

The Prisoner's Dilemma (PD) is a non-zero-sum game. This means that the total amount that can be gained is variable; both players may win or lose (Principia Cybernetica, 1993). The structure of the game comes from the situation of collaborators facing a choice of confessing to a crime without knowing what the other will do. There are four possible outcomes: mutual cooperation, mutual competition, defect by player 1, and defect by player 2. This game offers meaningful opportunities to assess cooperation and trust between players. PD has been administered to children, adolescents, and adults, with gender, ethnicity, social status, and familiarity manipulated by investigators. The first genetically informative experiment, using a twins-as-couples design, was reported by Segal and Hershberger (1999) using adolescent and adult twins. Evolutionary reasoning predicted that MZ twins would show more frequent cooperative choices than DZ twins.

Participants were 59 MZ twin pairs and 37 DZ same-sex twin pairs, who ranged in age from 10.92 to 82.67 years. Co-twins played one game consisting of 100 consecutive trials for which they were given immediate feedback on choices and points earned. They were advised to focus on their own personal gain.

Multivariate analysis of variance revealed an overall significant effect from zygosity, with significant univariate effects from cooperative and competitive choices. The direction of the differences demonstrated greater cooperation among MZ twin pairs, as expected. The effects of sex approached statistical significance, while the sex × zygosity interaction was nonsignificant. Furthermore, mutual cooperation increased across the 100 trials for MZ twins but decreased across trials for DZ twins. It was striking that despite MZ twins' more frequent cooperation, they continued to make more competitive than cooperative choices. This may suggest greater restraint of selfishness or competition by MZ than by DZ twins (Axelrod & Hamilton, 1981; Charlesworth, 1996). Specifically, MZ pairs may cooperate more than DZ pairs by competing less. Another way to think about it is that MZ twin individuals show self-interest but are also interested in their co-twin's welfare.

Simultaneous Cooperation and Reciprocal Altruism

Loh and Elliott (1998) compared cooperation and competition between MZ and DZ twins, 7.6 to 9.7 years old, in Singapore, under two conditions: (1) simultaneous cooperation (SCO), in which reward distribution was equal between players; and (2) reciprocal altruism (RA), in which equality of reward distribution was uncertain. Behavior was assessed during a marble-pull game in which players pulled a device delivering marbles to individually assigned cups. However, if players worked against each other, then the marble would not enter either cup.

A significant zygosity × condition effect was found. In the SCO condition, MZ twins competed, whereas DZ twins cooperated. The reverse was true in the RA condition. It was suggested that within-pair MZ dominance relations may be unstable, because partners may change roles; as such, reward equality offers opportunities for "dominance testing," given the low relationship risk (Loh & Elliott, 1998, p. 408). However, when reward equality was uncertain, MZ twins behaved as though equality was a "necessary result" rather than a goal (p. 408). In contrast, DZ twins showed inequality in intrapair relations, yet did not need to compete in the SCO situation, in which reward quality was guaranteed. DZ twins would be expected to be more competitive in situations that did not ensure equality in outcome. Interestingly, in this study, DZ twins ended up with fairly equal rewards after playing many competitive rounds. The main contribution of this study is that MZ and DZ twin relations can be affected by context and condition. MZ and DZ twins' different behavioral motivations make sense with reference to their degree of genetic overlap and condition. Such an experiment has never been tried with twins reared apart and reunited, but it would be of interest in terms of whether, and how, common rearing affected the twin relationship. Based on previous studies, it is expected that outcomes would be the same as for ordinary twins.

Other Domains

Many behavioral domains have benefited from applying (or considering) behavioral genetics and evolutionary perspectives conjointly, but space allows only a selected sampling of this work. Behaviors considered elsewhere include intelligence (Bouchard, Lykken, McGue, Segal, & Tellegen, 1990), personality (Segal & MacDonald, 1998), psychopathology (Gottesman, 1991; Mealey, 1995), sexual orientation (Bailey, Kirk, Zhu, Dunne, & Martin, 2000), infant social behavior and temperament (Freedman, 1974; Plomin, & Rowe, 1979), parenting (Mann, 1992; Perusse, Neale, Heath, & Eaves, 1994), happiness (Lykken, 1999), bereavement (Segal & Blozis, 2002; Segal, Sussman, Marelich, Mearns, & Blozis, 2002), marital status (Trumbetta & Gottesman, 1997), and mate selection (Lykken & Tellegen, 1993).

A NEW PARADIGM FOR UNDERSTANDING THE PHENOTYPE?: DEVELOPMENTAL ISSUES

Individual Differences: A Closer Look

Under what conditions would one expect individual differences to reflect random variation or noise around an ideal optimum, or to be contingent on the environment? If we can determine when individual differences are meaningful (i.e., related to "fitness"), we could then analyze their adaptive significance. Buss and Greiling (1999) discuss *adaptive* individual differences. They classify individual differences as adaptive, maladaptive, or neutral. Evolutionary sources of adaptive individual differences would include frequency-dependent selection and early environmental calibration of an environmentally sensitive mechanism. Frequency-dependent selection can maintain two variants in a population when a strategy is only successful if it is present in low frequency. In dimensions that may be important for fitness and reproduction, additional variation among individuals may exist because of plasticity during development. Genetic and environmental underpinnings of individual differences would vary for these two types of mechanisms.

Thus, individual differences within a population may or may not be related to adaptation, and may or may not be primarily the result of genetic differences. A basic problem for evolutionary-oriented behavior geneticists will be to distinguish adaptive individual differences arising from frequency-dependent selection from those arising from early environmental calibration of an environmentally sensitive mechanism. Assistance will be needed from evolutionary biologists studying possible developmental responses to heterogeneous environments (Schlichting & Pigliucci, 1998).

The evolutionary approach brings another challenge to behavior geneticists, which arises from viewing the phenotype as the target of natural selection. Characteristics of greatest interest are those that are subject to selection (or can be convincingly traced to characteristics that were subject to selection in our ancestral environment, or traced through a comparative method to characteristics of other mammals that are subject to selection). After defining the phenotype, we must determine what selective forces are at work, in order to understand the evolutionary significance of individual differences.

For example, sex differences and gender roles are a primary focus of evolutionary psychologists, but they are not central to theory in behavior genetics. In this case, evolutionary theory can be informative. Lalumière, Quinsey, and Craig (1996) made the prediction that males will show a larger variance component due to nonshared environment than would females, because males are subject to more intrasexual competition and also employ more alternate life-history strategies. Characteristics of the reproductive life course vary among species and among individuals within a species. Various authors have differentiated two fairly distinct patterns in human reproductive life histories, called "short-term" and "long-term" mating strategies (reviewed in Buss & Schmidt, 1993). Whereas a short-term strategy appears weighted toward mating competition, a long-term strategy appears to use more effort on parental investment. Life history theory attempts to explain variation in life history characteristics, such as age at maturation, size at birth, or average number of offspring (Roff, 1992; Stearns, 1992). Men and women differ on average in their expression of these two strategies, but variation within sexes also occurs (Low, 2000).

In general, the variance in reproductive success (defined as lineage persistence, having children who themselves survive and reproduce) is more variable among men than among women. Hence, intrasexual competition is expected to be stronger among males than among females. Lalumière et al. (1996) made the prediction that males will show a larger variance component due to nonshared environment than would females, because intrasexual competition would lead males to compete more with their own brothers than females would compete with their sisters. They assume that several different but equally rich niches are available in a heterogeneous environment, but some specialization is required to exploit them fully. If sibling competition is associated with nonshared environmental variance, then any factor that increases sibling competition or conflict would covary with this variance component.

Thus, considerations from EP predict that males would show a larger nonshared environment effect than females in aspects of the phenotype relevant to reproductive life-history strategies. Cleveland, Udry, and Chantala (2001) examined components of variance in sex-typed behaviors for adolescent males and females. The sample included sibling pairs of varied relatedness. For males, 25% of the variance was attributed to genetic sources (G), 0% to shared environment (SE), and 75% to nonshared environment and measurement error (NSE). For females, proportions were 38% G, 0% SE, and 62% NSE, a nonshared effect that is smaller than for males, supporting our prediction. In another analysis of the same adolescent sample, focusing on depressed mood and several other variables, the best fitting model used separate parameters for males and females. A higher proportion of variance was found for nonshared environment for males; for depressed mood, the NSE proportions were .69 for males, .51 for females (Jacobson & Rowe, 1999). Alcohol consumption, specifically use, abuse, and dependence, is a behavioral outcome that has been modeled separately for males and females (Prescott,

Aggen, & Kendler, 1999). While the differences are not large, models for males consistently have a larger proportion of variance estimated for NSE (e.g., .44 for males, .34 for females; Prescott et al., 1999).

In summary, evolutionary-oriented behavioral geneticists face numerous questions: What is the phenotype of interest? Is the variation adaptive? How does selection act? If the variation is adaptive, how do individual differences arise during development? Current research in development has revitalized our understanding of epigenesis and its role in development. Development is seen as a process through which adaptive calibration can occur, fine-tuning the phenotype to the environment. In parallel, behavior-genetic analyses need to be sufficiently fine-grained to examine complex changes over time. Some investigators are currently developing appropriate analytical models (e.g., see Neale & McArdle; McArdle & Hamagami, 2003).

Interaction of Persons and Environments through Ontogeny

Human ontogeny may never be penetrable using behavior-genetic or developmental systems paradigms. The sequential character of development is complex, and behavior-genetic observational (rather than experimental) methods often capture one dimension of a phenotype at one time point. Even at single time points, interactions between genes and environment are rarely analyzed. Genotype (G) × environment (E) interaction occurs when a given genotype is associated with a different phenotype, depending on the environment experienced throughout development. Examples of genotype G × E interactions are not commonly found in the behavior-genetics literature. It may be that they rarely exist, or that our experimental methods and sample sizes lack sufficient statistical power to detect them (Wahlsten, 1990). In a rare example, data on twin pairs reared apart was used to estimate G × E effects on risk of becoming a regular smoker, suggesting that as much as 25% of the risk may derive from the interaction between genotype and shared environment (Health et al., 2002).

Another behavior genetic study examined G × E interaction by comparing families grouped by environment. Rowe, Jacobson, and Van den Oord (1999) reported differential heritability for verbal IQ among adolescents, depending upon environment. Specifically, a sample of almost 2000 sibling pairs (twins, full and half siblings, and cousins living together) was divided into groups based on parental education level. Variance components were then estimated for each group. Heritability of verbal IQ was higher among families with more education, while the effect of shared environment increased for families with less education. The authors interpreted these findings as supporting the idea that genetic variation can be expressed to a greater degree when the environment is benign.

Two recent studies illustrate the promise of using designs testing G × E interactions between specific genetic markers and a specific environmental factor (Caspi et al., 2002, 2003). A longitudinal study of over 500 male children, studied from birth to early adulthood, examined the outcomes of antisocial behavior (Caspi et al., 2002) and depression (Caspi et al., 2003). The frequency of antisocial behavior in young adulthood was compared across groups defined according to childhood abuse (no maltreatment, probable, and severe) and genotype of a marker of monoamine oxidase (high activity, low activity) (Caspi et al., 2002). An extensive literature has shown that this marker is associated with antisocial behavior; it is a functional polymorphism that affects the levels of various neurotransmitters. The effect of childhood maltreatment on antisocial behavior was shown in both marker groups, but the relationship was much stronger with one form of the marker than the other. Genetic liability to childhood abuse thus differed. Those with one form of the marker showed high levels of antisocial behavior only when they experienced childhood maltreatment. Those with the other form of the marker were less responsive to maltreatment, implying that there may be a protective effect of higher monoamine oxidase activity. The analysis of depression frequency used a similar design, comparing groups defined by their genotype on a functional marker of the serotonin transporter and the degree of recent stressful experiences (Caspi et al., 2003). The predictor variables were similarly well chosen; pharmacological therapies for depression affect serotonergic neurotransmission, and the role of stressful life events in depression is accepted. Again, an interaction between gene and environment was found, in which the probability of depression was increased as the number of recent stressful events increased, but the slope of the increase varied greatly by genotype. Reasons for this variation in response to experience are uncertain. Perhaps some alleles allow adaptive variation in susceptibility to environmental influence. Evolutionary researchers could address such possibilities through comparative studies of the appearance of new alleles across related species.

Gene–environment correlations are ubiquitous in behavior-genetic studies. That is to say, because individuals (with different genotypes) are not randomly distributed across environments affecting their development, certain genotypes will be associated with certain environmental factors (Plomin et al., 2001). Three types of genotype–environment correlation have been described: passive, evocative, and active (Plomin, DeFries, & Loehlin, 1977; Scarr & McCartney, 1983). Each type represents a different nonrandom relationship between genes and environments. The *passive* genotype–environment correlation describes a situation in which children inherit genotypes that are associated with their family environments. The *evocative* genotype–environment correlation describes a situation in which a child with a given genotype elicits certain responses from others. The *active* genotype–environment correlation describes a situation in which an individual seeks or creates environments compatible with his or her genotypic predispositions.

The importance of genotype–environment correlation was shown in a recent family study, the Nonshared Environment and Adolescent Development (NEAD) study, which focused extensively on nonshared environmental effects on behavior (Reiss, Niederheiser, Hetherington, & Plomin, 2000). Its aim was to determine how siblings experienced different family environments, in terms of family process. Along with twins, the sample included full siblings who had not experienced a divorce, and full siblings, half-siblings, and genetically unrelated siblings in stepfamilies. Measures were obtained using self-reports by multiple informants, as well as videotapes of interactions between family members. The main conclusions were that (1) parent–child relationships are central to adolescent development, but primarily because of shared genes (as discussed below), (2) child genetic factors evoke particular social responses from parents and siblings, and (3) nonshared, unique factors are very complex (Reiss et al., 2000). None of the differential parenting and sibling experience measures were independent of genetic differences. The most striking finding was the importance of gene–environment correlations, which were very prevalent (e.g., adolescent antisocial behavior was correlated with parents' harsh punishment level).

Thus, development of individual differences in adjustment is conceived as a complex sequential process. In this process, family relationships are responsive to heritable traits in developing children, and these traits evoke characteristic responses from parents and other family members. These responses then continue to influence the child's behavior, and certain transactions in families are seen as necessary for full expression of certain behaviors (Reiss et al., 2000). The correlation between adolescent antisocial behavior and parental behavior provides a good example. Reiss et al. analyzed child and parent effects at two points in time (cross-lagged correlations). Parent effects initiated at time 1 (early to mid-adolescence) by child factors, such as irritability or troublesome behavior, appear to explain much of the association at time 2 (three years later) between parental negativity and adolescent antisocial behavior. Parental reactions at time 1 may be protective (by increased positivitity and monitoring) or exacerbating (by increased negativity). They summarized the probable developmental sequence as (1) a genetic factor affects a precursor of antisocial behavior, (2) parents respond to the precursor, and (3) the parental response further shapes the precursor behavior into a fully developed characteristic. While they make the interpretation of genetic effects more difficult, gene–environment correlations and interactions may represent the basic processes of ontogeny. Understanding the interplay between genes and environments over time is a major task for evolutionary developmental psychology.

CONCLUSIONS

Current State of Knowledge

Both behavioral genetics and evolutionary psychology have now entered the mainstream of developmental research. Both remain controversial, most likely because both have been misunderstood. Both are concerned with genetic aspects of behavior, yet neither embraces the view (as some critics have claimed) that behavior is strictly determined by the genes. Both disciplines remain highly focused on salient environmental influences that modify genetic expression. For example, behavioral geneticists are interested in identifying experiential factors causing some MZ twins to differ in intelligence, personality, and psychopathology. Evolutionary psychologists are interested in how life events may modify developmental pathways, such as the effects of father absence on sexuality, as discussed in this chapter.

Most researchers endorse the view that understanding behavior is enhanced through interdisciplinary efforts, although many continue to conduct their research from a single theoretical perspective. Behavioral genetics and EP are interdisciplinary fields, in and of themselves, since both rely heavily on input from psychologists, biologists, anthropologists, and geneticists. They have, however, relied less often on input from each other. The studies reviewed in this chapter were intended to illustrate what can be accomplished in developmental areas via the joint efforts of both disciplines. Our hope was also to excite the imaginations of researchers by suggesting new designs and approaches that can enrich ongoing projects.

The Human Genome Project has recently revealed that humans possess 30,000 genes, less than the anticipated number (Pennisi, 2003). Nevertheless, associating specific genetic factors with specific behaviors, and identifying critical environmental effects, remain daunting future tasks. Breakthroughs from the Human Genome Project should allow new ways to explore familiar phenotypes, as well as behaviors that have not yet been examined.

Future Directions

Understanding the Human Phenotype

Nature via Nurture: Genes, Experience and What Makes Us Human is the title of a recent book by the well-known science writer, Matt Ridley (2003). In it, he explains what has become increasingly obvious to behavioral science researchers, as well as countless parents, namely, that the nature-versus-nurture debate is outmoded. No one has yet isolated a phenotype that is solely the product of genes or environments. We learn from Ridley that the debate has been recast as "nature via nurture"—the idea that genetic factors are expressed by affecting the nature and impact of our experiences during development. ("Nature via nurture" was first used by Bouchard et al., 1990, in their analysis of monozygotic reared-apart [MZA] twins' IQ scores.) More recently, Bouchard observed that children's behaviors may drive their parents' rearing practices, suggesting "nurture via nature" as another appropriate term for the sequential interaction of genes and experience in behavioral development (Bouchard, 1997). This phrase also captures the concept of *reactive gene–environment correlation*, the idea that parental treatment is largely fashioned by children's genetically influenced personalities, talents, and temperaments.

Understanding the Human Developmental Environment

It is becoming more apparent that genetic regulation of complex traits varies during development. Traditional biometric–genetic analyses analyses cannot be easily applied to epigenetic processes that involve emergent properties of gene–environment systems that develop in stages (McClearn, 1993). Human longitudinal studies, such as NEAD, are beginning to provide evidence that the genetic factors associated with adolescent adjustment are different for early and late adolescence (as shown by cross correlations at two time points). In parallel, behavior-genetic analyses need to be sufficiently fine-grained to examine complex changes over time. Some investigators are currently developing appropriate analytical models (e.g., see Neale & McArdle, 2000; McArdle & Hamagami, 2003). Observational studies with humans (no matter how multivariate) may never yield a fully accurate picture of how genetic and environmental factors function during development, however. Studying epigenetic processes in development and the interaction of genes and environments, via experimental studies, can be done more easily with nonhumans given the greater controls over genotype and environment.

In recent commentaries and reviews, Panksepp (Panksepp, Moskal, Panksepp, & Kroes, 2002; Panksepp & Pankesepp, 2000) promotes a comparative approach to understanding behavior he calls "neuroevolutionary psychobiology." He advocates research using gene microarray technology to characterize gene expression patterns. To understand fundamental features of the human mind, he suggests that research focus on highly conserved emotional and motivational brain systems that are homologous among mammals. Through evolution, higher mental processes were integrated with more primitive motivational and emotional systems. Panksepp describes a multidisciplinary approach that triangulates between behavior genetic studies of heritability and individual genes, molecular studies of context, and differential gene expression and traditional psychobiological studies of brain–behavior relationships (Panksepp et al., 2002). For example, the role of social loss in depression risk can be fruitfully studied in other social mammals given the similarity among mammals in neural circuits subserving separation distress and in behavioral responses to separation (Panksepp et al., 2002). Psychobiological experiments on the neural consequences of separation, complemented by molecular genetic studies, could be triangulated with human observational or epidemiological studies focused on social loss and depression risk, and eventually including specific genes. The studies of Caspi et al. (2002, 2003), described earlier, represent progress in this direction.

Echoing the commentary of Panksepp et al. (2000, 2002), Bateson (2003) has envisioned a new horizon of behavioral biology with movement between levels, from molecular biology and neurosciences up to behavior, and back. Since completely controlled experimental studies are virtually impossible with humans, researchers should use nonhuman research far more than is currently done. While higher cognitive processes could not be studied, many motivational and emotional phenotypes (using inbred mouse strains and other standard animal models) could be examined. Evolutionary oriented behavior geneticists could use animal research to better describe patterns of development (epigenesis, GE correlations, G × E interactions) in various phenotypic dimensions.

Refinement of Twin and Adoption Methodology

The classic MZ–DZ twin comparison has undergone considerable refinement over the years. Twins, when used in conjunction with full-siblings, half-siblings, and stepsiblings, allow powerful insights into developmental processes, often challenging traditional beliefs about behavior. For example, a recent study showed stronger feelings of closeness and familiarity among reunited MZ than among DZ twin pairs, mirroring what one finds in twins reared together (Segal et al., 2003). More revealing, twins felt closer and more familiar toward their newly found twin than to their nonbiological sibling with whom they were raised. Mechanisms underlying this finding remain to be identified, yet the finding itself suggests that correlates of genetic relatedness play key roles in our social relationships. Another advance is that sophisticated quantitative techniques, by including multiple kinships (i.e., twins, siblings, parents, and offspring) in single studies (Eaves et al., 1999), allow sensitive partitioning of genetic and environmental effects on behavior. Access to large numbers of twins has been facilitated by the establishment of national registries around the world (see Segal, 2003).

VTs (discussed earlier) have recently entered the behavioral-genetics arena and are about to make their way into the EP realm. Analyses thus far indicate modest effects of shared environments on intellectual resemblance (Segal, 2000b). In a combined VT–twin analysis, a shared environmental component for body mass index (BMI) was demonstrated (Segal & Allison, 2002). It was concluded that prior studies may have underestimated shared environmental influences on BMI, because the designs lacked the power or ability to detect them. Now, in an ongoing developmental study of peer and sibling effects, social relations will be compared among MZ twins, DZ twins, VTs, and best friends. The goal of this research is to test kinship-genetic predictions of greater cooperation and affiliation between close genetic relatives (MZ twins), compared with less closely related genetic relatives (DZ twins) and unrelated individuals (VTs). Best-friend pairs will provide an informative contrast with VTs; individuals in both pairs are unrelated genetically, but best friends choose to be together, whereas VTs do not.

Molecular Genetic Analyses

A great deal has been written about the effects of molecular genetic analysis and the fruits of the Human Genome Project on developmental research. Three areas have been identified: uncovering continuities and discontinuities in development, discerning the meaning of abnormal behavioral patterns, and understanding gene–environment associations (Plomin, 1998). Comparing MZ twins discordant for behavioral problems and major psychopathologies can tell us a great deal about these issues. DZ twins are well–suited to gene-mapping approaches, because they are matched in age and share family experiences (Lyons & Bar, 2001). Additional discussion of related concepts is available in Plomin, DeFries, Craig, and McGuffin (2003).

Gene–behavior associations at the molecular level are also likely to advance cooperative efforts in behavioral genetics and EP. Parental favoritism has so far been understood with respect to perceived similarities between parents and children; however, specific genes shared by some parent–child pairs may underlie these preferences. Using DZ same-sex twins would offer good tests of such behavior given the controls for age and gender. Specifically, parents who perceived greater behavioral and/or physical similarity to one DZ twin may direct benefits toward that child that are not given to the other; parents may not be aware of, or even acknowledge, these acts. Child abuse by parents could be similarly examined. It should be possible to identify families with twins in which abuse has occurred, to see if parents selectively direct abuse toward DZ co-twins perceived to show less resemblance to them, or whom they judge to be less healthy or attractive than their twin sibling.

Unusual Research Designs

The possibility of human cloning has been omnipresent since the birth of Dolly the lamb in 1996. Human cloning suggests a range of intriguing experiments that would engage the interests of behavioral geneticists and evolutionary psychologists. Exposure of the same genotype to different experiences would be one way to identify the range of resulting behaviors, as well as life history strategies and tactics (see Dennenberg, 2002). Other informative experiments might compare social relatedness between cloned parent–child pairs with ordinary parent–child pairs. It would not be unexpected to find increased closeness and understanding between such couples, similar to what has been found for MZ twins (Segal, 1997b, 2002).

It is, of course, unlikely that human cloning will occur in the very near future. It does, however, urge us to consider available human models that might mimic cloning situations. A televised segment of four mother–daughter pairs who look and behave very similarly is relevant in this regard (Segal, 1997b). They described an unusual closeness between them. Until human cloning comes to pass, perhaps we could focus on gathering additional such cases to enrich our understanding of the fabric of human social relations.

Summary

This chapter has two aims: first, to show how behavioral–genetic methods can be used to test evolutionary-based hypotheses concerning human behavioral and physical development, and second, to show how evolutionary reasoning can inform developmental behavioral genetics. Behavioral genetics and evolutionary psychology have shared concerns despite their historical, methodological, and conceptual differences. EP provides behavioral genetics with an additional theoretical perspective for interpretation of findings, and behavioral genetics offers powerful methods for testing hypotheses generated by EP. Evolutionary-oriented behavior geneticists can target thorny questions, such as distinguishing adaptive individual differences from developmental noise. Where adaptive variation is shown, researchers can proceed to determine how individual differences arise during development.

Both EP and behavior genetics converge on an appreciation of development as an interaction of persons and environments through ontogeny. The sequential character of phenotypic development is complex, involving gene–environment correlations and interactions as basic processes. Understanding the interplay between genes and environments over time is a major task for evolutionary developmental psychology. In order to advance the field in this direction, we recommend that future work include more use of experimental studies of nonhuman animals, more use of refined family and sibling designs to augment the classic MZ–DZ twin comparison, and more research on gene–behavior associations, using molecular genetics.

ACKNOWLEDGMENTS

Preparation of this chapter was supported, in part, by an American Fellowship (2003-04) from the American Association for University Women (to Nancy L. Segal), National Institute of Mental Health Grant No. R01 MH63351, and a California State University Senior Faculty Research Award. Some of the ideas in this chapter were presented by Elizabeth M. Hill at the Theory Construction and Research Methodology Workshop of the National Council on Family Relations, Houston, Texas, November, 2002.

REFERENCES

Ambach, E., Parson, W., & Brezinka, C. (2000). Superfecundation and dual paternity in a twin pregnancy ending with placental abruption. *Journal of Forensic Sciences, 45*, 181–183.

Axelrod, R., & Hamilton, W.D. (1981). The evolution of cooperation. *Science, 211*, 1390–1396.

Bailey, J. M. (1997). Are genetically based individual differences compatible with species-wide adaptations? In N. L. Segal, G. E. Weisfeld, & C. C. Weisfeld (Eds.), *Uniting psychology and biology: Integrative perspectives on human development* (pp. 81–100). Washington, DC: American Psychological Association Press.

Bailey, J. M., Kirk, K. M., Zhu, G., Dunne, M. P., & Martin, N. G. (2000). Do individual differences in sociosexuality represent genetic or environmentally contingent strategies?: Evidence from the Australian Twin Registry. *Journal of Personality and Social Psychology, 78*, 537–545.

Bateson, P. (2003). The promise of behavioural biology. *Animal Behavior, 65,* 11–17.

Belsky, J., Steinberg, L., & Draper, P. (1991). Childhood experience, interpersonal development, and reproductive strategy: An evolutionary theory of socialization. *Child Development, 62,* 647–670.

Bjorklund, D. F., & Pellegrini, A. D. (2002). *The origins of human nature: Evolutionary developmental psychology.* Washington, DC: American Psychological Association Press.

Bock, R. D., Vandenberg, S. G., Bramble, W., & Pearson, W. (1970). A behavioral correlate of blood-group discordance in dizygotic twins. *Behavior Genetics, 1,* 89–98.

Boggess, K. A., & Chisholm, C. A. (1997). Delivery of the nonvertex second twin: A review of the literature. *Obstetrics and Gynecology Survey, 52,* 728–735.

Bouchard, T. J., Jr. (1997). The genetics of personality. In K. Blum & E. P. Noble (Eds.), *Handbook of psychiatric genetics* (pp. 273–296). Boca Raton, FL: CRC Press.

Bouchard, T. J., Jr., Lykken, D. T., McGue, M., Segal, N. L., & Tellegen, A. (1990). Sources of human psychological differences: The Minnesota Study of Twins Reared Apart. *Science, 250,* 223–228.

Buss, D. M. (1987). Evolutionary hypotheses and behavioral genetic methods: Hopes for a union of two disparate disciplines. *Behavioral and Brain Sciences, 10,* 20.

Buss, D. M. (1990). Toward a biologically informed psychology of personality. *Journal of Personality, 58,* 1–16.

Buss, D. M. (1999). *Evolutionary psychology, The new science of the mind.* Needham Heights, MA: Allyn & Bacon.

Buss, D. M., & Greiling, H. (1999). Adaptive individual differences. *Journal of Personality, 67,* 209–243.

Buss, D. M., & Schmitt, D. P. (1993). Sexual strategies theory: An evolutionary perspective on human mating. *Psychological Review, 100,* 204–232.

Caspi, A., McClay, J., Moffit, T. E., Mill, J., Martin, J., Craig, I. W., et al. (2002). Role of genotype in the cycle of violence in maltreated children. *Science, 297,* 851–854.

Caspi, A., Sugden, K., Moffitt, T. E., Taylor, A., Craig, I. W., Harrington, H., et al. (2003). Influence of life stress on depression: Moderation by a polymorphism in the 5-HTT gene. *Science, 301,* 386–389.

Charlesworth, W. R. (1996). Cooperation and competition: Contributions to an evolutionary and developmental model. *International Journal of Behavioral Development, 19,* 25–39.

Cleveland, H. H., Udry, J. R., & Chantala, K. (2001). Environmental and genetic influences on sex-typed behaviors and attitudes of male and female adolescents. *Personality and Social Psychology Bulletin, 27,* 1587–1598.

Comings, D. E., Muhleman, D., Johnson, J. P., & MacMurray, J. P. (2002). Parent-daughter transmission of the androgen receptor gene as an explanation of the effect of father absence on age at menarche. *Child Development, 73,* 1046–1051.

Crawford, C. (1998). The theory of evolution in the study of human behavior: An introduction and overview. In C. Crawford & D. L. Krebs (Eds.) *Handbook of evolutionary psychology* (pp. 3–41). Mahwah, NJ: Erlbaum.

Crawford, C. B., & Anderson, J. L. (1989). Sociobiology: An environmentalist discipline? *American Psychologist, 44,* 1449–1459.

Dawkins, R. (1989). *The selfish gene* (2nd ed.). Oxford, UK: Oxford University Press.

Derom, C., Vlietinck, R, Derom, R., Van den Berghe, H., & Thiery, M. (1987).

Increased monozygotic twinning rate after ovulation induction. *Lancet, 2,* 1236–1238.

Dennenberg, V. H. (2002). Cloning: A tool for behavioral research. *APS Observer, 15,* 11.

Dumont-Driscoll, M., & Rose, R. J. (1983). Testing the twin model: Is perceived similarity due to genetic identity? *Behavior Genetics, 13,* 531–532.

Dunne, M. P., Martin, N. G., Statham, D. J., Slutske, W. S., Dinwiddie, S H., Bucholz, K. K., et al. (1997). Genetic and environmental contributions to variance in age at first sexual intercourse. *Psychological Science, 8,* 211–216.

Eaves, L. J., Heath, A., Martin, N., Maes, H. Neale, M., Kendler, K., et al. (1999). Comparing the biological and cultural inheritance of personality and social attitudes in the Virginia 30,000 study of twins and their relatives. *Twin Research, 2,* 62–80.

Edwards, R. G., Mettler, L., & Walters, D. E. (1986). Identical twins and *in vitro* fertilization. *Journal of In Vitro Fertilization and Embryo Transfer, 3,* 114–117.

Ellis, B. J., McFayden-Ketchum, S., Dodge, K. A., Petit, G. S., & Bates, J. E. (1999). Quality of early family relationships and individual differences in the timing of pubertal maturation in girls: A longitudinal test of an evolutionary model. *Journal of Personality and Social Psychology, 77,* 387–401.

Ellis, B. J., & Garber, J. (2000). Psychosocial antecedents of variation in girls' pubertal timing: Maternal depression, stepfather presence, and marital and family stress. *Child Development, 71,* 485–501.

Farber, S. L. (1981). *Identical twins reared apart.* New York: Basic Books.

Freedman, D. G. (1968). An evolutionary framework for behavioral research. In S. G. Vandenberg (Ed.), *Progress in human behavior genetics* (pp. 1–6). Baltimore: Johns Hopkins University Press.

Freedman, D. G. (1974). *Human infancy: An evolutionary perspective.* Hillsdale, NJ: Erlbaum.

Furlow, B. F., Armijo-Prewitt, T., Gangestad, S., & Thornhill, R. (1997). Fluctuating asymmetry and psychometric intelligence. *Proceedings of the Royal Society of London, B264,* 823–829.

Gottesman, I. I. (1991). *Schizophrenia genesis: The origins of madness.* New York: Freeman.

Gottlieb, G. (1995). Some conceptual deficiencies in "developmental" behavior genetics. *Human Development, 38,* 131–141.

Hahn, M. E. (1990). Approaches to the study of genetic influence on developing social behaviors. In M. E. Hahn, J. K. Hewitt, N. D. Henderson, & R. H. Benno (Eds.), *Developmental behavior genetics: Neural, biometrical and evolutionary approaches* (pp. 60–80). New York: Oxford University Press.

Hamilton, W. D. (1964). The genetical evolution of human behaviour. *Journal of Theoretical Biology, 7,* 1–52.

Health, A. C., Todorov, A. A., Nelson, E. C., Madden, P. A., Bucholz, K. K., & Martin, N. G. (2002). Gene–environment interaction effects on behavioral variation and risk of complex disorders: The example of alcoholism and other psychiatric disorders. *Twin Research, 5,* 30–37.

Hecht, B. R. (1995). The impact of assisted reproductive technology on the incidence of multiple gestation. In L. G. Keith, E. Papiernik, D. M. Keith, & B. Luke (Eds.), *Multiple pregnancy: Epidemiology, gestation and perinatal outcome* (pp. 175–190). New York: Parthenon.

Hecht, B. R., & Magoon, M. W. (1998). Can the epidemic of iatrogenic multiples be conquered? *Clinical Obstetrics and Gynecology, 41*, 126–137.

Hettema, J. M., Neale, M. C., & Kendler, K. S. (1995). Physical similarity and the equal-environment assumption in twin studies of psychiatric disorders. *Behavior Genetics, 25*, 327–335.

Jacobson, K. C., & Rowe, D. C. (1999). Genetic and environmental influences on the relationships between family connectedness, school connectedness, and adolescent depressed mood: Sex differences. *Developmental Psychology, 35*, 926–939.

Lalumière, M. L., Quinsey, V. L., & Craig, W. M. (1996). Why children in the same family are so different from one another. *Human Nature, 7*, 281–290.

Loh, C. Y., & Elliott, J. M. (1998). Cooperation and competition as a function of zygosity in 7- to 9-year-old twins. *Evolution and Human Behavior, 19*, 397–411.

Low, B. (2000). *Why sex matters: A Darwinian look at human behavior*. Princeton, NJ: Princeton University Press.

Lyons, M. J., & Bar, J. L. (2001). Is there a role for twin studies in the molecular genetics era? *Harvard Review of Psychiatry, 9*, 318–323.

Lykken, D. T. (1978). The diagnosis of zygosity in twins. *Behavior Genetics, 8*, 437–473.

Lykken, D. T. (1999). *Happiness: What studies on twins show us about nature, nurture, and the happiness set point*. New York: Golden Books.

Lykken, D. T., & Tellegen, A. (1993). Is human mating adventitious of the result of lawful choice? A twin study of mate selection. *Journal of Personality and Social Psychology, 65*, 56–68.

Machin, G. A., & Still, L. K. (1996). The twin–twin transfusion syndrome: Vascular anatomy of monochorionic placentas and their clinical outcomes. In L. G. Keith, E. Papiernik, D. M. Keith, & B. Luke (Eds.), *Multiple pregnancy: Epidemiology, gestation and perinatal outcome* (pp. 367–394). New York: Parthenon.

Mann, J. (1992). Nurturance or negligence: Maternal psychology and behavioral preference among preterm twins. In J. H. Barkow, L. Cosmides, & J. Tooby (Eds.), *The adapted mind: Evolutionary psychology and the evolution of culture* (pp. 367–390). New York: Oxford University Press.

Martin, J. A., & Park, M. M. (1999). Trends in twin and triplet births: 1980–97. *National Vital Statistics Reports, 47*, 1–17.

McArdle, J. J., & Hamagami, F. (2003). Structural equation models for evaluating dynamic concepts within longitudinal analyses. *Behavior Genetics, 33*, 137–159.

McClearn, G. E. (1993). Genetics, systems, and alcohol. *Behavior Genetics, 23*, 223–230.

McClearn, G. E., Johansson, B., Berg, S., Pedersen, N. L., Ahern, F., Petrill, S. A., et al. (1997). Substantial genetic influence on cognitive abilities in twins 80 or more years old. *Science, 276*, 1560–1563.

Mealey, L. (1995). The sociobiology of sociopathy: An integrated evolutionary model. *Behavioral and Brain Sciences, 18*, 523–599.

Mealey, L. (2000). *Sex differences: Developmental and evolutionary strategies*. New York: Academic Press.

Mealey, L. (2001). Kinship: The tie that binds (disciplines). In H. R. Holcomb, III (Ed.), *Conceptual challenges in evolutionary psychology: Innovative research strategies* (pp. 19–38). Dordrecht, the Netherlands: Kluwer.

Mealey, L. (2002, June). *Do parents show favoritism for their symmetric children?* Paper presented at the meeting of the Human Behavior and Evolutionary Society (HBES), New Brunswick, NJ.

Mealey, L., Bridgstock, R., & Townsend, G. C. (1999). Symmetry and perceived facial attractiveness: A monozygotic co-twin comparison. *Journal of Personality and Social Psychology, 76*, 157–165.

Mealey, L., & Segal, N. L. (1993). Heritable and environmental variables affect reproduction-related behaviors, but not ultimate reproductive success. *Personality and Individual Differences, 14*, 783–794.

Neale, M. C., & McArdle, J. J. (2000). Structured latent growth curves for twin data. *Twin Research, 3*, 165–177.

Nijhout, N. F. (2003). The importance of context in genetics. *Scientific American, 91*, 416–423.

Panksepp, J., & Panksepp, J. B. (2000). The seven sins of evolutionary psychology. *Evolution and Cognition, 6*, 108–131.

Panksepp, J., Moskal, J. R., Panksepp, J. B., & Kroes, R. A. (2002). Comparative approaches in evolutionary psychology: Molecular neuroscience meets the mind. *Neuroendocrinology Letters, 23*(Suppl. 4), 105–115.

Parker, G., Tupling, H., & Brown, L. (1979). A parental bonding instrument. *British Journal of Medical Psychology, 52*, 1–10.

Parsons, P. A. (1990). Fluctuating asymmetry: An epigenetic measure of stress. *Biological Review, 65*, 131–145.

Pennisi, E. (2003). Reaching their goal early, sequencing labs celebrate. *Science, 300*, 409.

Perusse, D., Neale, M. C., Heath, A. C., & Eaves, L. J. (1994). Human parental behavior: Evidence for genetic influence and potential implication for gene–culture transmission. *Behavior Genetics, 24*, 327–335.

Plomin, R. (1990). *Nature and nurture.* Pacific Grove, CA: Brooks/Cole.

Plomin, R. (1998). Child development, molecular genetics, and what to do with genes once they are found. *Child Development, 69*, 1223–1242.

Plomin, R., DeFries, J. C., Craig, I. W., & McGuffin, P. (2003). *Behavioral genetics in the postgenomic era.* Washington, DC: American Psychological Association Books.

Plomin, R., DeFries, J. C., & Loehlin, J. C. (1977). Genotype–environment interaction and correlation in the analysis of human behavior. *Psychological Bulletin, 84*, 309–322.

Plomin, R., DeFries, J. C., McClearn, G. E., & McGuffin, P. (2001). *Behavioral genetics* (4th ed.). New York: Worth.

Plomin, R., & Rowe, D. C. (1979). Genetic and environmental etiology of social behavior in infancy. *Developmental Psychology, 15*, 62–72.

Plomin, R., & Rutter, M. (1998). Child development, molecular genetics, and what to do with genes once they are found. *Child Development, 69*, 1223–1242.

Prescott, C. A., Aggen, S. H., & Kendler, K. S. (1999). Sex differences in the sources of genetic liability to alcohol abuse and dependence in a population-based sample of U.S. twins. *Alcoholism: Clinical and Experimental Research, 23*, 1136–1144.

Prescott, C. A., Johnson, R. C., & McArdle, J. J. (1999). Chorion type as a possible influence on the results and interpretation of twin study data. *Twin Research, 2*, 244–249.

Principia Cybernetica. (1993). *Zero sum games.* Available online at: *http:llpespmc1.vub.ac.be/ZESUGAM.html*

Reiss, D., Niederheiser, J. M., Hetherington, E. M., & Plomin, R. (2000). *The Relationship Code: Deciphering genetic and social influences on adolescent development*. Cambridge, MA: Harvard University Press.

Richards, B., Skoletsky, J., Shuber, A. P., Balfour, R., Stern, R. C., Dorkin, H. L., et al. (1993). Multiplex PCR amplification from the CFTR gene using DNA prepared from buccal brushes/swabs. *Human Molecular Genetics, 2*, 159–163.

Ridley, M. (2003). *Nature via nurture: Genes, experience and what makes us human*. London: HarperCollins.

Roff, D. A. (1992). *The evolution of life histories: Theory and analysis*. New York: Chapman & Hall.

Rowe, D. C. (2000). Environmental and genetic influences on pubertal development: Evolutionary life history traits? In J. L. Rodgers, D. C. Rowe, & W. B. Miller (Eds.), *Genetic influences on human fertility and sexuality: Recent empirical and theoretical findings* (pp. 147–168). Boston: Kluwer.

Rowe, D. C., Jacobson, K. C., & Van den Oord, E. J. C. G. (1999). Genetic and environmental influences on vocabulary IQ: Parental education level as moderator. *Child Development, 70*, 1151–1162.

Scarr, S. (1995). Commentary. *Human Development, 38*, 154–158.

Scarr, S., & McCartney, K. (1983). How people make their own environments: A theory of genotype — environment effects. *Child Development, 54*, 424–435.

Schlichting, C. D., & Pigliucci, M. (1998). *Phenotypic evolution: A reaction norm perspective*. Sunderland, MA: Sinauer.

Scott, J. P. (1977). Social genetics. *Behavior Genetics, 7*, 327–346.

Segal, N. L. (1993). Twin, sibling and adoption methods: Tests of evolutionary hypotheses. *American Psychologist, 48*, 943–956.

Segal, N. L. (1997a). Twin research perspective on human development. In N. L. Segal, G. E. Weisfeld, & C. C. Weisfeld (Eds.), *Uniting psychology and biology: Integrative perspectives on human development* (pp. 145–173). Washington, DC: American Psychological Association Press.

Segal, N. L. (1997b). Behavioral aspects of intergenerational cloning: What twins tell us. *Jurimetrics, 38*, 57–67

Segal, N. L. (2000a). *Entwined lives: Twins and what they tell us about human behavior*. New York: Plume.

Segal, N. L. (2000b). Virtual twins: New findings on within-family environmental influences on intelligence. *Journal of Educational Psychology, 92*, 442–448.

Segal, N. L. (2002). Human cloning: A twin-research perspective. *Hastings Law Journal, 53*, 1073–1084.

Segal, N. L. (2003). Spotlights (Reared apart twin researchers); research sampling; literature, politics, photography and athletics. *Twin Research, 6*, 72–81.

Segal, N. L., & Allison, D. B. (2002). Twins and virtual twins: Bases of relative body weight revisited. *International Journal of Obesity, 26*, 437–441.

Segal, N. L., & Blozis, S. A. (2002). Psychobiological and evolutionary perspectives on coping and health characteristics following loss: A twin study. *Twin Research, 5*, 175–187.

Segal, N. L., Connelly, S. L., & Topoloski, T. D. (1996). Twin children with unfamiliar partners: Genotypic and gender influences on cooperation. *Journal of Child Psychology and Psychiatry, 37*, 731–735.

Segal, N. L., & Hershberger, S. L. (1999). Cooperation and competition in adolescent twins: Findings from a prisoner's dilemma game. *Evolution and Human Behavior, 20*, 29–51.

Segal, N. L., Hershberger, N. L., & Arad, S. (2003). Meeting one's twin: Perceived social closeness and familiarity. *Evolutionary Psychology, 1*, 70–95.

Segal, N. L., & MacDonald, K. B. (1998). Behavior genetics and evolutionary psychology: A unified perspective. *Human Biology* [Special issue: J. Gilger & S. L. Hershberger, Eds.,. *Advances in human behavioral genetics: A synthesis of quantitative and molecular approaches]*, 70, 159–184.

Segal, N. L., Sussman, L. S., Marelich, W. D., Mearns, J., & Blozis, S. A. (2002). Monozygotic and dizygotic twins' retrospective and current bereavement-related behaviors: An evolutionary perspective. *Twin Research, 5*, 188–195.

Siemon, M., & Adelman, M. B. (1986). Communicating the relational shift: Separation among adult twins. *American Journal of Psychotherapy 40*, 96–109.

Sokol, D. K., Moore, C. A., Rose, R. J., Williams, C. J., Reed, T., & Christian, J. C. (1995). Intrapair differences in personality and cognitive ability among young monozygotic twins distinguished by chorion type. *Behavior Genetics, 25*, 457–466.

Stearns, S. (1992). *The evolution of life histories*. Oxford, UK: Oxford University Press.

Stewart, E. A. (2000). *Exploring twins: Towards a social analysis of twinship*. London: Macmillan.

Sulloway, F. J. (1996). *Born to rebel: Birth order, family dynamics, and creative lives*. New York: Pantheon.

Thornhill, R., & Gangestad, S. W. (1999). The scent of symmetry: A human sex pheromone that signals fitness? *Evolution and Human Behavior, 20*, 175–201.

Treolar, S. A., & Martin, N. G. (1990). Age at menarche as a fitness trait: Nonadditive genetic variance detected in a large twin sample. *American Journal of Human Genetics, 47*, 137–148.

Trumbetta, S. L., & Gottesman, I. I. (1997). Pair-bonding deconstructed by twin studies of marital status: What is normative? In N. L. Segal, G. E. Weisfeld, & C. C. Weisfeld (Eds.), *Uniting psychology and biology: Integrative perspectives on human development* (pp. 485–491). Washington, DC: American Psychological Association Press.

Wahlsten, D. (1990). Insensitivity of the analysis of variance to heredity-environment interaction. *Behavioral and Brain Sciences, 13*, 109–161.

II

PERSONALITY AND
SOCIAL DEVELOPMENT

6

DIFFERENTIAL SUSCEPTIBILITY TO REARING INFLUENCE

An Evolutionary Hypothesis and Some Evidence

JAY BELSKY

If readers of this volume were polled as to whether they believe that all children are equally susceptible to rearing influence, be that influence cast in terms of parental behavior or child care experience, to cite but two broad domains of putative influence, it seems unlikely that most respondents would answer in the affirmative; that is, upon reflecting on what should be a central issue in the study of rearing effects, most developmentalists would probably contend that children vary in whether or not, or at least the degree to which, they are affected by particular styles of parenting or other aspects of child rearing. Yet if one reads through the voluminous literature on the influence of parenting, the effects of child care, or even the role of peers in shaping individual differences in development, it is rare to find work that systematically examines what is referred to in this chapter as the "differential susceptibility hypothesis," that is, the notion that children vary in their susceptibility to rearing influence (but see Kendler & Eaves, 1986, for a related argument pertaining to psychiatric illness).

In fact, even though it is true that for decades now scholars have written about gene–environment interaction (Plomin, 1986) or organismic specificity (Wachs & Gandour, 1983), it remains the case that there is little theory that addresses the issue of differential susceptibility. Moreover, a case can be made that Wachs and Gandour's organismic-specificity hypothesis, which asserts that different features of the environment will affect different children differently, has stimulated little research outside its proponent's own laboratory (and that much of the evidence they have amassed in support of it suffers from post hoc interpretation), and that gene–environment interactions are often posed more as hypotheses by the more environmentally inclined to discount behavior-genetic explanations of behavior than as ideas that serve to guide much empirical inquiry in human development (for a recent and outstanding exception, see Caspi et al., 2002).

In light of this state of developmental affairs, my purpose in this chapter is to reintroduce the notion that children likely vary in their susceptibility to rearing influence (see also Boyce & Ellis, in press). In what follows, I outline evolutionary reasoning that leads me to theorize that children should vary in their susceptibility to rearing, particularly children growing up in the same family, and review some recent evidence emanating from my own work and that of others, that is consistent with this reasoning. To be noted in advance is that the findings summarized are presented only in illustration of the more general concept being proposed, and that all the research cited pertains to between-family differences in children's susceptibility, not to within-family variation. Despite these limitations, the work reviewed, some of it reported here for the first time, provides compelling evidence to support the claim that more intensive effort should be devoted to discerning for which children, which child-rearing experiences prove most influential.

One implication of the arguments advanced is that if it is the case that children do, indeed, vary in their susceptibility to rearing influence, then most studies to date that fail to examine the prospect of differential susceptibility both over- and underestimate the effects of rearing experience. More specifically, by failing to distinguish between children who are more and less susceptible to a particular aspect of rearing, be it exposure to authoritarian parenting or poor-quality child care, coefficients of association linking rearing and child functioning probably overestimate the effects of rearing on children who are rather unsusceptible and underestimate them in the case of children who are highly susceptible. In other words, the proverbial .3 correlation that so routinely emerges between a rearing variable and a child development outcome may be the result of zero-order associations in the case of nonsusceptible children being averaged together with .5 or larger associations in the case of highly susceptible children. Should this in fact be so, implications for intervention would be profound.

AN EVOLUTIONARY ARGUMENT

From the perspective of evolutionary biology, all life is designed for the replication of genes in future generations. Organisms are defined as being successful, in fact, when they achieve high levels of reproductive fitness and, by definition, natural selection shapes organisms in the service of this core "goal" of life. Although it is certainly the case that humans differ from many other living things in myriad ways, it is incontestable that humans also have been shaped by natural selection and thus possess many features that in the ancestral past, even if not in the present, promoted reproductive fitness.

Time is a core component in the process of evolution, because it is over time that natural selection "sculpts" organisms in ways that maintain or enhance their reproductive fitness. A truism about time is that the future is fundamentally uncertain, so it remains the case that what in the past might have proved to be adaptive could, some time in the future, prove otherwise. This reality, of course, is what the process of natural selection is all about. Physical and physiological features or behaviors of an organism that once may have contributed to its reproductive success but no longer do so become susceptible to elimination by natural selection. This is most likely to occur when the feature in question undermines reproductive success in the changed ecology and least likely when the changed ecology merely renders the once adaptive feature neutral in terms of its fitness consequences (vestigial traits, e.g., the human tailbone).

Because natural selection designs living things to disperse genes successfully in future generations, and because the future is invariably uncertain at least to some degree, in the ancestral environments in which human behavior and development evolved, parents could not have known completely—at a conscious or unconscious level—what psychological and behavioral developments in their progeny would most positively influence reproductive fitness. The same is certainly true in the modern era. Consider in this regard the killing fields of Cambodia, in which intellectuals were among the first singled out for elimination, and the recent wars and resulting refugee crises in the Balkans. In all likelihood, parents of many Cambodian victims encouraged the very intellectual curiosity and educational attainment that subsequently had such unintended dire consequences for their grown children. Just as surely many Kosovoans living in Marshall Tito's Yugoslavia taught their children to befriend neighbors whose ethnic origins differed from their own, perhaps never imagining that such trust and openness might discourage their grown children from abandoning their homes, thereby leaving them in the path of genocidal Serbian forces. Similar analysis could, of course, be applied to Jews residing in Germany and much of Europe prior to the World War II—and just as surely to many peoples through much of human history, both recorded and unknown.

In light of the fact that parents could, inadvertently, direct children down what would become developmental blind alleys that proved to undermine rather than enhance reproductive (and social) success in our ancestral past (as well as in the present), it seems plausible that nature would have designed a strategy to reduce the costs of such "mistakes in guidance." One solution to the problem of the future rewarding developmental outcomes quite inconsistent with those fostered by parental rearing would involve the "hedging of bets" in just the same way that a financial investor does. Rather than committing all resources to a savings account, an equity fund, or even a mattress, most investment advisors recommend diversification. Diversification reduces the costs associated with making a bet regarding return on an investment that, ultimately, turns out to be misguided. Only part of one's investment portfolio thus ends up at risk, rather than all one's financial resources.

If one conceptualizes children as investments that are supposed to have reproductive payoffs (i.e., produce grandchildren, great grandchildren, etc.), as they surely are when viewed from a biological and evolutionary standpoint, then a sensible strategy for reducing the risk of no payoff in a world plagued by uncertainty would also involve diversification. Thus, if the direction that parents consciously or unconsciously endeavored to shape their children proved to carry costs because the anticipated developmental outcomes did not produce the benefits anticipated, the reproductive fitness of parents would likely be somewhat protected were it the case that their children were not equally susceptible to their efforts to shape them. Indeed, only the child or children who were reactive and responsive to their parents' socialization efforts would pay the cost of such "misdirection," whereas those who were less susceptible to rearing (i.e., less "plastic," more "fixed") would probably be less likely to suffer the consequences of such "misdirection." Of course, at other times and in other circumstances, it would surely be those offspring who followed their parents' lead who would flourish, in which case the less plastic children might not achieve the same levels of success, including reproductive success, as their siblings (unless, of course, their "fixed" attributes proved to fit the future world extremely well).

It must be understood that the notion that the reproductive fitness of parents would be enhanced, on average, via diversification of progeny and, thereby, the hedging of bets (about the future environments children will encounter) in no way implies a conscious or deliberative strategy on the part of the parent. All that is implied from an evolutionary perspective is that in bearing and rearing children who differ in their traits and even susceptibility to rearing influence, parents would be functioning—biologically and socially—*as if* they were consciously deliberating differential payoffs of different actions and their consequences. Nevertheless, it seems worth entertaining the possibility that, eventually, parents could come to appreciate which children are more or less susceptible to their efforts to socialize them—in the broadest sense of the term. A possibly added benefit of bearing children who vary in their susceptibility to rearing could then derive from recognition and appreciation in such differences, especially if parents then differentially endeavored to influence their offspring, investing more time and effort in those more susceptible to their efforts, and less time and effort in those less susceptible. In other words, should parents develop awareness of when their parental investment was most likely to pay off and adjust their investment accordingly, they could possibly further increase their ultimate reproductive success, if only by not squandering energy and effort in rearing offspring unlikely to benefit directly from it.

In summary, evolutionary thinking leads to the proposal that natural selection has designed into humans variation in susceptibility to rearing influence, and that such variation makes especial sense when viewed from a within-family perspective. By bearing children who vary in their susceptibility to rearing, parents—through no conscious effort or awareness—hedge their bets that the manner in which they desire their children to develop will prove reproductively successful. Thus, we should expect children in the same family to vary in terms of their susceptibility to parental influence. Were this so, it might account, in part, for why shared environmental influences are so lacking in much behavior-genetic work, whereas nonshared environmental effects are so ubiquitous (Plomin & Daniels, 1987). After all, shared environmental effects emerge when children in the same family are influenced *in the same way and to the same degree* by common rearing experiences. The evolutionary reasoning just outlined suggests that such effects should be the exception rather than the rule, as they appear to be.

The preceding argument is based on the potential fitness benefits that parents derive from bearing and rearing offspring who vary in their susceptibility to rearing influences. In view of the fact that parents and children do not share 100% of their genes, and thus do not have identical reproductive interests, it must be acknowledged that just because parents might benefit from diversifying their offspring in the manner under consideration does not necessarily mean that children themselves would benefit. Because the course of natural selection will be scripted by fitness consequences for parents and children alike, the implications of differential susceptibility to rearing need to be considered from the standpoint of children as well.

Because children who share the same parents share as much genetic material with each other, on average, as does each child with each parent (i.e., 50%), it would seem that, in the same way and to the same extent, that parents would benefit from bearing and rearing offspring who vary in their susceptibility to rearing experience, so would children benefit by differing from their siblings in terms of their susceptibility to rearing. To appreciate this, direct and indirect fitness benefits must be distinguished. Whereas direct reproductive benefits accrue from the reproduction of self, children, grandchildren, and other direct descendants, indirect reproductive benefits accrue from the enhanced fitness of, in this case, siblings, nieces and nephews, and their direct descendants (i.e., inclusive fitness). Thus, a child highly susceptible to a particular rearing experience would not only stand to benefit *directly* should exposure to that rearing experience promote what proved to be a fitness-enhancing development, but the same child would stand to benefit *indirectly* should that same rearing experience ultimately prove to be reproductively counterproductive if the child in question had a sibling who proved unaffected by the rearing experience. Conversely, a child highly unsusceptible to a particular rearing experience would stand to benefit *indirectly* if that same rearing experience carried fitness benefits for a susceptible sibling. In the

same way, then, that parents hedge their bets on the uncertain future by bearing offspring who vary in their susceptibility to rearing experience, siblings
would stand to benefit—as if they, too, had hedged their bets—in a sibship
that comprised individuals varying in their susceptibility to rearing influence.

The fact that parents and children alike would seem to benefit from the
diversification of offspring in terms of their susceptibility to rearing influence
raises the prospect that no role need be played at all by natural selection in the
process described, because random variation resulting from the sexual recombination of parental genomes could accomplish the same outcome. At the
present time, there seems to be limited theoretical grounds for deciding
whether differential susceptibility to rearing could simply be an inadvertent
by-product of the reshuffling of parents' genomes each time they reproduce
rather than an adaptive consequence of natural selection. The fact, however,
that genetic moderation of environmentally induced reproductive strategies
has been identified in nonhuman species (Alcock, 2001), and that new human
evidence to be presented later in this chapter chronicles genetic differences in
susceptibility to child maltreatment in relation to subsequent development of
antisocial behavior (Caspi et al., 2002), provides grounds for at least entertaining the prospect that differential susceptibility is not simply a by-product
of (blind) sexual recombination but of natural selection.

Another important theoretical issue—on which this entire chapter rests—
is probably also beyond resolution at this time. And it has to do with the presumption that, even if only for some, what happens in the family (at least at
the hands of parents) matters at all when viewed from the perspective of evolutionary theory. Harris (Chapter 10, this volume, p. 254, emphasis added)
argues that

> experiences within the family in the first 5 or 10 years of life *might* be a poor indi-
> cator of the conditions one will have to face outside the family in adulthood,
> which means that basing one's lifelong behavioral strategy on these experiences
> *could* be a serious mistake. As Tooby and Cosmides (1990) pointed out, there is a
> cost involved in locking in a behavioral strategy too early: "The individual is sub-
> sequently committed to pursuing that strategy, even *if* it finds itself in situations
> where that strategy is radically inappropriate" (pp. 46–47).

Relatedly, Trivers (1985) argued that while offspring may have no choice but
to comply with their parents' wishes during their years of dependence upon
them, they should not allow themselves to be permanently molded by parental
rearing behavior, because doing so would ultimately lower their inclusive fitness. Persuaded by such argument, Harris (Chapter 10, this volume, p. 254)
concluded that "evolution would be unlikely to produce a mechanism that
caused long-term selection of behavioral strategies to be based on experiences
within the family."

However persuasive this argument might first appear to the evolutionary
and biologically minded, three things should be noted. First, not all evolution-

ary theorists view the developmental consequences of family experiences in the same way as do Harris (Chapter 10, this volume), Tooby and Cosmides (1990), and Trivers (1985). Geary and Flinn (2001, p. 25), for example, have counterargued that "the complexity of social dynamics places a premium on parental behavior that fosters and enables the developmental acquisition of socio-competitive and other competencies." Second, evidence recently reported by Caspi et al. (2002) pertaining to a very specific—and anticipated—gene–environment interaction would clearly seem to contradict Harris (see below), at least in terms of the broad-sweeping nature of her conclusions regarding (the lack of enduring) parental influence on *all* aspects of behavioral development manifest outside of the family in the case of *all* children in *all* families.

The third point to be made in response to the notion that it would be counterproductive, at least from an evolutionary perspective, for experiences in the family during childhood to shape behavior outside of the family later in life is that arguments in favor of this position seem to be based on the undocumented and probably undocumentable assumption that the local ecologies in which early human behavior evolved were so changeable that any developments in the individual fostered by family experiences in childhood would, necessarily, poorly prepare the child for reproductive success in adulthood. Careful consideration of the meaning of the terms "might," "could," and "if" in the quotes cited two paragraphs earlier importantly qualify the meaning of the statements made by Harris (Chapter 10, this volume) and by Tooby and Cosmides (1990), however, in that they underscore the point that family influences that are maintained into adulthood *would not necessarily* be reproductively counterproductive. Indeed, all one has to do is posit that local ecological conditions were tolerably stable across adjacent generations in at least some of the environments of evolutionary adaptation to make a plausible case for why it would make biological sense for a child's development to be susceptible to influence by those who have more in common genetically with the child than anyone else, other than a sibling, and thus why susceptibility to parental influence might be adaptive in the first place (Belsky, in press). Under such conditions, it would seem eminently plausible that parental effects could and perhaps would dovetail with the conditions that progeny faced when reproductively mature, resulting in parental influences fostering reproductive success rather than undermining it, as Harris (Chapter 10, this volume), Trivers (1985), and Tooby and Cosmides (1990) apparently presume would generally be the case.

In fact, when considered from this perspective, one might critique Harris's (Chapter 10, this volume) emphasis on the importance of nonkin and especially peers in shaping personality development and reproductive success. After all, because parents and children have so much more in common genetically than do peers, it would seem to make much more biological sense for children's personality development and reproductive success to be shaped by parents than by peers. Ultimately, however, there seems to be no good reason to pit the family and the peer group against one another, at least on theoretical grounds. A wiser theoretical formulation might be to acknowledge that both sources of influence could shape personality development, reproductive strategy and, thereby, reproductive success. In fact, even though the perspective advanced in this chapter is that children are differentially susceptible to rearing experience, it is certainly conceivable—perhaps even likely—that things are far more complicated than that. For some individuals, it may be, as Harris argues, peers who exert the most developmental impact; for others, it might be parents; for others, it could be neither; and for still others, it could be both.

Throughout this chapter, my working hypothesis is that not only do children vary in their susceptibility to rearing influence, and that such variation is a by-product of natural selection, but also that such variation is a (primary) function of the genotype. Having said that, however, it should be acknowledged that differential susceptibility to rearing could arise, at least in theory, from some kind of environmental factor or experience. Boyce and Ellis (in press), for example, argue that variation in "biological sensitivity to context" (i.e., biological reactivity to environmental stimuli) demarcates variation in susceptibility to rearing experience, and that such differential reactivity is itself partially environmentally determined. Prenatal experiences, for example, that elevate intrauterine cortisol levels could establish reactivity thresholds to future environmental inputs, thereby producing organisms that are differentially responsive to objectively identical experience.

Not only does this point of view seem eminently reasonable, but there seems to be no obvious reason why variation in susceptibility to rearing could not be both born and made—other than the tendency of the human mind to create dichotomies, and all too often false ones at that. Conceivably, those individuals whose genes predispose them to be susceptible to rearing experiences—broadly conceived—could be experientially induced, perhaps *in utero*, perhaps following birth, to become nonresponsive to rearing, far less responsive (than would otherwise be the case), or even hypersusceptible. But could intra- or extrauterine experiences transform an unsusceptible genotype into a (more) susceptible phenotype? Comparative evidence reviewed by Boyce and Ellis (in press) certainly indicates that this is at least possible.

EMPIRICAL EVIDENCE

However attractive the preceding conceptualization of differential susceptibility to rearing influence may be, whether conceptualized as genetically or experientially determined, or as a product of natural selection or the mere reshuffling of parental genes, it is not unreasonable to wonder whether we can move beyond theoretical formulation and ask, fundamentally, whether any data do indeed indicate that children vary in their susceptibility to rearing. Three sets of evidence are considered. The first derives from behavior-genetic studies that do not directly measure environmental processes, and thus only indirectly suggests differential susceptibility to rearing influence. The second body of evidence derives from nongenetically informed investigations that directly measure—and sometimes manipulate—rearing experience and thus provide more direct evidence that children vary in their susceptibility to rearing influence. Finally, the third set of evidence is quite unique, coming from a single and recently reported study that directly measured genes and rearing experience.

Behavior-Genetic Studies

Although it has been documented repeatedly that much behavioral development is heritable, with heritability estimates averaging about 50% for almost all phenomena measured (see Segal & Hill, Chapter 5, this volume), one thing that remains unclear from much of this research is whether different parts of a distribution of a measured outcome are equally or differentially the result of genotypic influences; that is, does the 50% figure reflect the fact that about half of every individual's behavior is genetically determined, or that very high—or low, or even intermediate—levels of the behavior in question are inherited, but that other levels of the same behavior are much less a product of genotypic influences?

The fact that heritability may not be the same across the spectrum of a measured behavioral phenomenon is intriguingly suggested by a series of investigations addressing this very issue (Deater-Deckard, Reiss, Hetherington, & Plomin, 1997; Price, Simonoff, Waldman, Asherson, & Plomin, 2001). For example, several studies indicate that it is low IQ rather than IQ in the normal (or very high) range that is most heritable (Detterman, Thompson, & Plomin, 1990; Horn, Loehlin, & Willerman, 1979; Volger & DeFries, 1983). The fact that still other research suggests, quite the contrary, that it is high IQ rather than normal (or low) IQ that is most heritable (Bailey & Horn, 1986; Bailey & Revelle, 1991; Jensen, 1987), does not mitigate the important point that a heritability estimate does not indicate where in the distribution inheritance exerts its influence.

In the case of psychopathology, for example, one might presume that it is extremely high levels of externalizing or internalizing behavior problems that are most likely to reflect biologically based and inherited influences, rather than environmental ones (McGuffin, Owen, O'Donova, Thapar, & Gottesman, 1994; but see Scarr, 1993, for the opposite view). Yet when Rende, Plomin, Reiss, and Hetherington (1993) addressed this very issue with respect to depression in adolescents, in a sample consisting of more than 700 pairs of teenage siblings participating in a combined twin and stepfamily study, they found just the opposite: True environmental influences played a disproportionate role at the high end of the depression distribution and genetic forces at the lower end, leading the authors to conclude that "environmental factors which affect both siblings may contribute greatly to the etiology of extreme depressive symptomology" but "not to individual differences" (p. 1395). And this was true in both nondivorced and stepfamilies. In a related study using the same sample, somewhat similar, though not as strong, results emerged when the focus of interest was externalizing and internalizing problem behavior, with the data documenting somewhat lower heritability at very high levels of these problems (Deater-Deckard et al., 1997). Interestingly, the case seems rather different for language development in early childhood, with greater heritability for language disability (i.e., extremely low scores) than for language ability throughout the normal range (Price et al., 2001). In summary, by documenting differential heritabilities across different parts of a distribution of scores on measures of IQ, depression, externalizing problems, and linguistic functioning, results from these behavior-genetic studies indirectly indicate that nonheritable, environmental influences will vary as well across the very same distribution of scores. This fact is perfectly consistent with the notion that individuals vary in their susceptibility to rearing influence.

Nongenetically Informed Studies Directly Assessing Rearing Experiences

Investigations to be cited that directly measure processes of rearing and provide evidence consistent with the notion that children vary in their susceptibility to rearing influence reveal—perhaps somewhat surprisingly—that it may be infants with negative and perhaps even difficult temperaments who are especially susceptible to rearing influence, at least with respect to developmental outcomes involving self-control and the development of behavior problems. Some of the work to be cited was carried out in direct response to my earlier theorizing about differential susceptibility to rearing (Belsky, 1997a, 1997b) and, where that is the case, this will be noted; in other cases, the work was independent of any such theorizing. Consideration of pertinent developmental data begins with a study of primates before proceeding to research on human infants, toddlers, and preschoolers.

The primate evidence derives from Suomi's (1997) studies of rhesus macaques selectively bred so as to vary in their fearfulness and proclivity to become anxious. When highly anxious, "uptight" monkeys and their far less anxious counterparts were cross-fostered to highly skilled or average foster mothers, dramatic rearing effects emerged, but only in the case of the highly anxious monkey. Whereas uptight infants foster-reared to average mothers exhibited expected deficits in early exploration patterns and exaggerated biobehavioral responses to minor environmental perturbations, these same high-reactive infants actually appeared to be behaviorally precocious when cross-fostered to especially nurturant females. Indeed, these latter infants, physically separated from their mother at an earlier point in development, locomoted and explored their environment more and displayed less behavioral disturbance during weaning than not only the high-reactive infants cross-fostered to average mothers but also even the average infants reared by either type of foster mother.

Follow-up investigation of these selectively bred and differentially foster-reared monkeys when they were moved into larger social groups at 6 months of age revealed additional evidence of differential susceptibility to rearing influence, marked by seemingly positive outcomes for the uptight monkeys reared by particularly competent foster mothers. These individuals became especially adept at recruiting and retaining other group members as allies in response to agonistic encounters and, perhaps as a consequence, they subsequently rose to and maintained top positions in the group's dominance hierarchy. In contrast, temperamentally similar, high-reactive individuals cross-fostered to control mothers tended to drop to and remain at the bottom of the same dominance hierarchy. Importantly, no such rearing effects were evident among the average infants. In other words, the range of reaction of the uptight monkeys in response to these contrasting rearing conditions greatly exceeded that of their average-reactive counterparts subjected to the same variation in rearing regimens. Suomi (1995) speculated that uptight monkeys excel under supportive rearing conditions because they spend lots of time looking rather than doing and thus learn a great deal about what it takes to succeed in the group.

With respect to humans, the first work to be considered comes from a series of studies carried out by Kochanska (1993) testing the hypothesis that more fearful, inhibited and negatively emotional (i.e., "uptight"?) children 26–41 months of age would be more affected by maternal discipline and socialization than would less negative ones when it came to the development of self-control. Results of analyses designed to determine whether maternal child-rearing strategy—particularly the extent to which mothers relied upon gentle guidance versus forceful control—differentially predicted children's functioning revealed that the apparent effect of mothering varied dramatically across more and less negatively reactive children. With respect to children refraining from playing with off-limits toys in the lab when no adults were present, maternal behavior explained only 1% of the variance in the case the low fearful/anxious children, but a significant 23% in the case of the highly fearful children. With respect to the maternal report of children's proclivity to follow rules, maternal gentle discipline that deemphasized power assertion accounted for 4% of the variance in the case of the low fearful/anxious children but a significant 18% in the case of the highly fearful and anxious children.

In a subsequent study, Kochanska, Mordhorst, and Reschly (1997) sought to determine whether these differential effects of mothering discerned during the toddler years were evident as early as the first year of life. Thus, in a second investigation, 8 to 10-month-olds were observed in a situation in which it was mother's responsibility to keep the child from touching and playing with a highly attractive toy. The behavior to be explained in this work was the child's probability of complying with a maternal directive not to touch the toy in the 5-second period following each maternal prohibition. Once again, Kochanska et al. found that maternal discpline predicted the restraint of the more negative and fearful children but not of the less negative and less fearful children. In fact, in the case of the 25% most negatively emotional infants, maternal discipline explained a significant 41% of the variance in children's restraint; the corresponding figure in the case of the 25% least negative children was an insignificant 2% of the variance. In contrast to Suomi's (1995) observational-learning analysis of why uptight monkeys proved so susceptible to rearing, Kochanska (1995, 1997) accounted for her findings in terms of Dienstbier's (1984) hypothesis that anxious children are more responsive to socialization because they more readily and intensely experience internal discomfort when they transgress or are caught transgressing. Needless to say, these divergent accounts are by no means mutually exclusive.

One of the limitations of the aformentioned work of Kochanska is its cross-sectional design, with parenting, temperament, and children's self-control being measured at roughly the same point in time. Several more recent studies redress this limitation while specifically testing the *a priori* proposition that infants with more negative temperaments may be more susceptible to rearing influence, at least insofar as the development of self-control and/or problem behavior is concerned. One investigation carried out in Israel focused upon difficult infant temperament, measured via maternal reports and observed negativity, synchrony in mother–infant interaction during face-to-face exchanges when infants were 9 months of age, and self-control at age 2, as measured by compliance with maternal cleanup requests and capacity to refrain from eating candy until receiving permission (Feldman, Greenbaum, & Yirmiya, 1999). Just as expected on the basis of preliminary theorizing by Belsky (1997a, 1997b), mutually synchronous mother–infant interaction predicted greater self-control more strongly in the case of children who had had difficult temperament as infants ($r[18] = .65$) than in the case of infants who did not ($r[18] = .25$).

Recent research by Morrell and Murray (2003) raises the prospect that the process of differential susceptibility to rearing influence on self-control-related developmental outcomes may also be operative within the first year of life, at least if one considers marked infant distress and irritability, labeled "emotional and behavioral dysregulation" (EBD) in the study, as an index of (lack of) self-control. This is because Morrell and Murray found that observed EBD at 4 months of age interacted with observed coercive parenting measured at the same time in predicting EBD 5 months later. Although the investigators did not provide clear indication that the predictive link between early coercive parenting and later EBD was stronger for infants who evinced higher rather than lower levels of EBD at 4 months of age, given the manner in which they reported their results, this would seem to be exactly the likely origin of the detected statistical interaction.

Perhaps a more compelling test of the differential susceptibility to rearing hypothesis comes from a longitudinal study carried out Belsky, Hsieh, and Crnic (1998) as part of a larger investigation of some 125 working- and middle-class Caucasian families rearing firstborn sons. In this research, infant negative emotionality was measured at 1 year of age, relying upon a variety of observational procedures, as well as parental reports. Mothering and fathering were observed and rated during the course of eight home visits conducted across the second and third year of the child's life. Positive parenting reflected the extent to which mothers or fathers were positively affectionate and sensitive in interacting with the child. Negative parenting reflected the extent to which the parent was hostile, irritable, and intrusive in controlling the child.

With measures of positive and negative mothering and fathering in hand, Belsky et al. (1998) sought to predict two separate developmental outcomes when children were 36 months of age: how shy, inhibited, and reticent the child was during a series of laboratory procedures and the extent to which mothers and fathers reported the child as having externalizing behavior problems involving aggression and noncompliance. Just as in the work of Suomi (1995), Kochanska (1997), and Feldman et al. (1999) we, too, found that variance accounted for by parenting in predicting children's functioning was noticeably greater for children who had been highly negative as infants than for those scoring below the median on negative emotionality (14 vs. 4% for externalizing problems; 27 vs. 4% for inhibition).

Results from the Belsky et al. (1998) study pertaining to the prediction of inhibition were replicated recently in a longitudinal investigation of children's wariness upon starting school. Using data obtained at age 15 months on infant inhibition–wariness–negativity and maternal sensitivity (measured in different situations), Early and associates (2002) tested the hypothesis that the effect of maternal sensitivity on wariness during the first months of kindergarten would vary as a function of early inhibition–wariness–negativity. And consistent with other research, this is exactly what they found: Whereas higher levels of maternal sensitivity significantly predicted lower levels of inhibition during the first month of school in the case of children classified as wary–inhibited–negative in infancy, even after controlling for early wariness, children's wariness during the transition to kindergarten was not predicted by earlier maternal sensitivity in the case of children not so classified as infants.

Rubin, Burgess, Dwyer, and Hastings (2003) also present evidence that, at the least, seems not inconsistent with findings pertaining to the differential susceptibility hypothesis reviewed through this point. In their research, 2-year-olds' anger proneness in the face of frustration (caused by not being able to obtain a toy in a plastic container) and inability to manage impulses (as reflected in failure to refrain from touching crayons when instructed to do so) interacted, once aggregated into a composite measure of "behavioral–emotional dysregulation" (i.e., emotional negativity?), with observational measurements of negative mothering (i.e., hostile affect + intrusive controlling behavior) in predicting externalizing problems at age 4. Although Rubin et al. plotted this interaction so as to illuminate how high versus moderate versus low levels of maternal negativity moderated the predictive power of behavioral–emotional dysregulation, the significant interaction detected is just the one predicted—indeed, by this time, anticipated—on the basis of other work under consideration. Thus, there is every reason to presume that had the interaction been plotted in reverse, with parenting moderating the predictive power of toddler dysregulation (rather than the other way around), the Rubin et al. research would have revealed evidence consistent with the differential susceptibility hypothesis, namely, that the apparent influence of early maternal negativity on later externalizing problems was restricted to, or at least most pronounced in, the case of children who at age 2 evinced high levels of anger and an inability to manage their impulses. Of course, this cannot be known for certain. Furthermore, it remains unclear whether the moderating role of child temperament in this instance reflects the moderating role of an inborn and genetically determined feature of behavioral development or of a behavioral inclination that is itself a product of earlier socialization. From the standpoint of the proposition that children vary in their susceptibility to rearing, and that highly negative children are more susceptible than others, at least with respect to self-control-related developmental outcomes, this does not matter. But to the extent that one wants to distinguish between the point of view advanced in this chapter—that differential susceptibility is principally, even if not exclusively, a heritable feature of individual—and that advanced by Boyce and Ellis (in press) highlighting the experiential determinants of "biological sensitivity to context," then it does.

This same issue of the origins of high and low negative emotionality must be kept in mind when considering the pattern of findings that emerged when Deater-Decker and Dodge (1997) examined the behavior problems of children in middle childhood in response to my preliminary theorizing about differential susceptibility to rearing influence (Belsky, 1997a). These investigators took advantage of retrospective maternal reports of infant temperament obtained just before children entered kindergarten and concurrent measures of parental use of harsh discipline to manage children, in order to predict children's externalizing problems during their first 6 years of schooling. More specifically, they examined the mean correlation between maternal harsh discipline prior to kindergarten entry and externalizing problems during each of the first 6 years of school, separately for children who were and were not retrospectively characterized (at the point of entering kindergarten) as having highly persistent temperaments as infants. Consistent with previous findings, they found that children who as infants were described as highly resistant to intrusion and persistent in pursuing forbidden activities—that is, negatively reactive to efforts to control them—were apparently more affected by the discipline they received than were other children. Thus, the children who as infants were characterized as being hyperresistant to control were more likely to show many or few externalizing problems depending upon the degree to which they experienced harsh punishment than were children who were less negatively responsive to efforts to control them. In other words, the effect of harsh punishment on externalizing problems presumed by many developmentalists to exert a general effect on all children seemed restricted to a subset of children.

One of the things especially intriguing about all this recent evidence suggesting that it may well be highly negative infants/toddlers who are particularly susceptible to rearing influence is that it accords nicely with some work on the theorized role of maternal sensitive responsiveness in promoting infant attachment security. One well-cited study is that reported more than two decades ago by Crockenberg (1981), designed to test the hypothesis that the availability of social support to a mother would enhance her capacity to be sensitively responsive to her infant and, thereby, to facilitate the development of a secure rather than insecure attachment. In this work, Crockenberg did indeed find that social support was predictive of infant attachment security but only, quite intriguingly, in the case of highly irritable infants. Once again we see, then, that it is highly negative infants who may be particularly susceptible to rearing influence, in this case benefiting from the social support afforded their mothers.

This effect of maternal care on infant–mother attachment security has been extensively studied by developmentalists. To my knowledge, however, no one has specifically addressed the question of whether, as the work of Crockenberg (1981) might now be read to indicate, it is highly negative infants who are most affected by the quality of care they receive when it comes to explaining why some infants develop secure and others insecure attachments. Is it possible that this could explain why the theorized and repeatedly discerned relation between quality of mothering and attachment security turns out to be more modest in magnitude than might be anticipated? In 1987, Goldsmith and Alansky reported a meta-analysis of the then-available literature and chronicled a reliable effect size of 0.16 with respect to the impact of mothering on infant attachment security. More recently, in an update of that meta-analysis, this time involving more than 4,000 infants and their mothers drawn from 66 investigations, De Wolff and van IJzendoorn (1997) chronicled an effect size of 0.22.

This moderate relation between maternal sensitive responsiveness and infant attachment security derived from correlational studies is highlighted here because it contrasts so markedly with the findings of perhaps the most carefully conducted study to date examining the effect of sensitive mothering on attachment security. In this Dutch work, Van den Boom (1994) randomly assigned 50 lower class mothers to an experimental group that received an intervention geared toward promoting maternal sensitivity, and 50 other mothers to a control group that did not receive any such intervention. Not only did the intervention enhance, as was intended, the sensitivity of mothers to their infants' positive and negative emotional cues, as measured by home observations of maternal behavior when infants were 9 months of age, but it also affected, as anticipated, infant attachment security, as measured 3 months later. In fact, whereas only 22% of the infants in the control group were classified as securely attached at 12 months of age, the corresponding figure in the case of the experimental mothers, whose mothering had been enhanced, was 300% greater—66%.

Why are these rather dramatic results of this carefully controlled experiment, which clearly chronicles a causal effect of mothering on attachment security, so at odds with the more modest effects discerned in the two meta-analyses of correlational studies? In light of the arguments advanced in this chapter, it seems especially notable that the answer to this question might well have something to do with the unique nature of the sample that van den Boom studied—a small detail intentionally omitted up to this point. Purposefully, this Dutch investigator preselected her sample to consist of infants who were highly irritable as newborns! Indeed, in order to be included in either the experimental or control condition, infants had to score high in irritability on two separate assessments of neonatal behavior carried out within the early days of life. Although there can be no certainty that it was the heightened irritability of the Dutch infants that made them so susceptible to improvements in maternal sensitive responsivenes, this interpretation certainly seems credible in light of all the results summarized through this point. Indeed, when these Dutch data are considered in the context of all the evidence presented, there would seem to be grounds to conclude that children do seemingly vary in their susceptibility to rearing influence, and that one factor determining whether they are likely to be affected by care that is more versus less nurturant is their temperament and especially their proneness to negative emotions.

In an attempt to provide a further test of this specific hypothesis in preparation of this chapter, I drew upon data gathered as part of the National Institute of Child Health and Human Development (NICHD) Study of Early Child Care (with the assistance of R. Pasco Fearon), specifically those data dealing with (1) infant negative mood measured by means of maternal report when children were 6 months of age, (2) maternal sensitivity assessed during the course of semistructured observations of mother–infant interaction videotaped when children were 6, 15, 24, and 36 months of age, (3) extensive observational assessments at these same four times of measurement of the quality of child care in the case of children in some kind of child care arrangement for more than 10 hours per week when these data collections were scheduled, and (4) maternal reports of problem behavior and emotional adjustment obtained when children were 3 years of age (see NICHD Early Child Care Research Network, 1998, for description of all measurements). After dividing the sample in terms of those infants described by mothers as relatively more emotionally negative (i.e., above the median) and those described as relatively less emotionally negative (i.e., below the median) in their mood on the questionnaire measure of temperament at 6 months of age, structural equation modeling was used to determine, in two separate sets of analyses, whether the effect of two separate latent constructs of rearing environment differentially predicted a latent construct of maternally reported problem behavior measured at 3 years of age (and also comprised of multiple indicators). In one set of analyses involving 1,075 cases (i.e., irrespective of child care experience) for whom maternal sensitivity was observationally measured at all four measurement occasions, maternal sensitivity was the rearing feature investigated. In a second set of analyses involving 335 children whose quality of child care was observationally measured at each of four separate times of measurement, quality of observed nonmaternal child care was the rearing feature investigated. The quality-of-care measure reflected the extent to which the nonmaternal caregiver(s) provided attentive, warm, responsive, and stimulating care to the child.

To test differential rearing hypotheses, the sample was split into two equal groups at the median of infant temperament-negativity and the same model fitted for both groups using linear structural relationships (LISREL VIII; Jöreskog & Sorböm, 1993). Covariance matrices were used throughout and parameter estimates and test statistics were derived using maximum likelihood estimation. Cross-group constraints forced all parameter estimates to be the same for both groups. A second model was then estimated that was identical to this constrained two-group model except that the structural term between the rearing latent variable and the behavior problem latent variable was free to vary between the two groups (all other constraints remained the same). The difference in χ^2 (on 1 degree of freedom) between the two models thus represents the improvement in model fit when the path between rearing and behavior problems is estimated separately for each group and hence the associated significance assesses the null hypothesis that the effect of rearing on outcome is equal for infants who are low and high on temperamental negativity.

As predicted, and consistent with the evidence already summarized from many other investigations, the changes in fit between the two nested models were significant for both maternal sensitivity ($\chi^2[1] = 7.25$, $p < .01$) and quality of child care ($\chi^2[1] = 4.42$, $p = .036$). The final models, in which the structural terms between the latent variables were estimated separately for each group, are shown in Figure 6.1, with their respective standardized parameter estimates. Considering maternal sensitivity first, it should be noted that despite the significant difference in the magnitude of the structural path between sensitivity and behavior problems, z tests revealed a significant negative path both for infants who scored above the median on temperamental negativity ($z = 6.80$, $p < .001$) and for those who scored below ($z = 3.62$, $p < .001$). Of importance, however, is that, just as anticipated on the basis of past work, the path was stronger in the case of children who scored high in negativity as infants. It should be noted that, overall, the final unconstrained model departed significantly from the observed covariance matrix ($\chi^2[61] = 200.4$, $p < .001$), but as several authors have pointed out (e.g., Bollen, 1989; Loehlin, 1998), given large samples, statistically significant departures from the model may not necessarily be substantively important. Goodness-of-fit

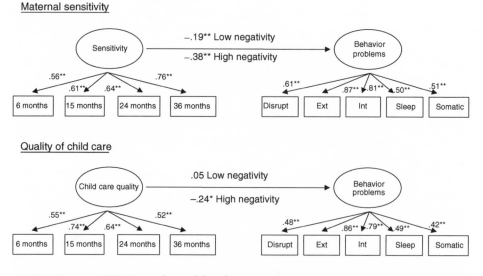

FIGURE 6.1. LISREL path models of maternal sensitivity–child care quality and 36-month behavior problems with standardized maximum likelihood parameter estimates. Structural paths estimated separately for high and low infant negativity; $n = 1,075$ for maternal sensitivity and 336 for quality of child care. ** $p < .01$; * $p < .05$.

indices (GFIs) revealed acceptable levels of model fit (LISREL GFI = .96 and root-mean-square error of approximation (RMSEA) = .046). In the main, results were similar when quality of child care served as predictor. In this case, however, the path between quality-of-care and behavior problems was only significant for the group of highly negative infants (high negativity: $z = 2.45$, $p = .014$; low negativity: $z = .53$, $p = .60$; overall model fit: $\chi^2(61) = 83.7$, $p = .01$; GFI = .95, RMSEA = .037).

Beyond the research reviewed through this point highlighting the seemingly especial susceptibility to rearing of highly negative infants, at least with respect to self-control-related developmental outcomes (and perhaps IQ), it is noteworthy that several recent studies of children at older ages highlight the fact that it is the combination of problems with emotional–behavioral control and poor rearing environments that, in particular, forecast continued problems with self-regulation, as evinced by high levels of externalizing behavior problems. Consider in this regard Morris and associates' (2002) recent report showing that it was first and second graders scoring high in irritable distress for whom harsh and hostile mothering predicted externalizing problem behavior reported by teachers. Whereas the slope of the regression line linking problematic parenting with problem behavior was .31 ($p < .05$) in the case of children scoring high on irritable distress, it was an insignificant .06 in the case of other children. Studying similarly aged children, Denham and associates (2000) reported that the beneficial effects of proactive parenting (i.e., supportive presence, clear limit setting) and the adverse effects of parental anger on externalizing problems at age 7 and/or 9 were most pronounced in the case of children who scored high on externalizing problems (i.e., disobedient, aggressive, angry) at an earlier time of measurement (i.e., mean age = 55 months), even after controlling for problem behavior at the initial measurement occasion. Consider, as a final example of such work, Stoolmiller's (2001) research showing that a synergistic interaction between (retrospectively reported) child manageability problems during early childhood (e.g., temper tantrums, excessive crying, disobedience) and parent disciplinary tactics when children were 10 years of age characterized growth rates from grade 4 through 8 in teacher-reported externalizing behavior problems among boys. More specifically, problematic discipline practices (e.g., scolding, yelling, threating, being inconsistent) observed during the course of visits to children's homes predicted increasing antisocial behavior on the part of sons only in the case of those who scored high on unmanageability during their first 5 years of life.

With the exception of the first set of data reviewed, namely, that collected by Suomi (1997) on monkeys, all the evidence considered through this point could be regarded as compromised by virtue of its correlational nature; that is, the research conducted by Kochanska (1993, 1995, 1997; Kochanska et al., 1997), Feldman et al. (1999), and Deater-Decker and Dodge (1997); that cited in the immediately preceding paragraph; as well as that conducted by myself (Belsky et al., 1998; and herein) examined statistical associations between some rearing experience and some developmental outcome, usually dealing with self-control, separately for children who could be described, in general terms, as more and less negatively emotional. The possibility remains, as a result, that relations detected between experience and development could be a function of some unmeasured, third variable, a situation unlikely to explain the results of Suomi's (1997) experimental work with monkeys, in which infants were randomly assigned to varying rearing conditions, as well as being bred for different styles of emotional reactivity.

Blair (2002) recently reported a study that in some respects mirrors Suomi's (1997) more powerful experimental design using human infants in illuminating the differential susceptibility to rearing of more and less negatively emotional infants, though selective breeding was not employed to create different geno- and phenotypes. Drawing upon data collected as part of the Infant Health and Development Program (1990), in which low-birthweight, premature infants from economically disadvantaged homes were randomly assigned to experimental and control treatment conditions, Blair (2002) tested Belsky's (1997a, 1997b) proposition that an enriched rearing experience comprised of educational day care in the second and third year of life, combined with home visiting and parent support over the child's first 3 years, would differentially impact children with varying temperaments. As predicted, infants who were highly negatively emotional and assigned to the early-intervention treatment experimental group scored substantially lower on externalizing problems when 3 years of age than did similarly tempered infants randomly assigned to the control group, with no such treatment effect proving detectable in the case of other infants. Intriguingly, exactly the same results emerged when the outcome in question was retarded cognitive functioning (i.e., IQ < 75), with highly negative infants assigned to the experimental intervention being five times less likely to score at or below 75 on an IQ test at age 3 than their negatively emotional counterparts assigned to the control condition; no such experimental effects emerged in the case of infants scoring low on negative emotionality.

A Study Directly Measuring Genes and Rearing Experience

Perhaps the most intriguing evidence to emerge recently that can be interpreted in terms of differential susceptibility to rearing was reported by Caspi and associates (2002), who directly (and prospectively) measured, as part of a long-term investigation of a New Zealand birth cohort, (1) the exposure of boys to any of a variety of forms of child maltreatment while growing up, and (2) a functional polymorphism in the gene encoding the neurotransmitter-metabolizing enzyme monoamine oxidase A (MAOA). The MAOA gene is located on the X chromosome and encodes the MAOA enzyme, which metabolizes neurotransmitters such as norepinephrine, serotonin, and dopamine, rendering them inactive. Significantly, this particular gene was selected for investigation, because genetic deficiencies in MAOA activity have been linked with aggression in mice and humans.

In view of evidence that the effect of child maltreatment on antisocial behavior, including criminality, in adulthood is rather variable, Caspi et al. (2002) hypothesized—and found—that the gene in question moderated the effect of maltreatment on antisocial behavior in adulthood; that is, it was principally children with one form of the gene—that associated with low MAOA activity—who proved more violence prone than would otherwise have been expected when subject to child maltreatment. For those children with the alternative version of the gene (i.e., that associated with high MAOA activity), a far lesser effect of child maltreatment emerged. In other words, one version of the gene resulted in boys being especially adversely affected by problematic child rearing, whereas the other version of the gene apparently led them to be relatively (even if not completely) impervious to the effects of child maltreatment, or at least the effect of child maltreatment on antisocial behavior.

What is not clear from this work, but would be fascinating to know in view of the research reviewed in the preceding section of this chapter, is whether the boys with the gene apparently marking susceptibility to child maltreatment, at least in the case of antisocial behavior, were also highly negatively emotional as infants. Unfortunately, because members of the New Zealand sample's behavioral development was not assessed until they were 3 years of age, this is impossible to determine. It is, of course, a hypothesis worth pursuing in other work, because the Caspi et al. (2002) data, in conjunction with much other research considered in this chapter, raises the possibility that supportive rearing environments disproportionately benefit and unsupportive rearing environments disproportionately harm the development of highly negative infants because they possess a particular version of the MAOA gene investigated by Caspi and colleagues.

CONCLUSIONS

Evolutionary theorizing led me to entertain the possibility that children, especially within a family, should vary in their susceptibility to rearing influence, because this would be an important way through which parents could hedge their (unconscious) reproductive bets in the face of an ever-present uncertain future. Whereas it would make sense to produce some children who are fixed strategists, perhaps entirely immune to socialization efforts, who would thrive in particular contexts that fit their proclivities, it would also make sense to produce some who are more plastic, capable of fitting and thriving in a variety of niches depending upon the rearing conditions they encountered while growing up. Ultimately, however, it may not be best to think in terms of discrete fixed and plastic types but rather a continuum of plasticity.

Relatedly, it may make more sense to think of differential susceptibility to rearing in domain-specific rather than domain-general terms. Rather than conceptualizing some children as more or less susceptible to rearing influence *in general*, it may be most useful to think of children as varying in their susceptibility *with respect to particular developmental outcomes*. Thus, whereas one child might be highly susceptible to music instruction (perhaps because of a highly sensitive auditory system), he or she might be far less susceptible to parental influence with respect to the development of conscience, with the reverse being true of another child. Similarly, it remains conceivable that whereas children with certain versions of the MAOA gene studied by Caspi et al. (2002) are more susceptible to the adverse effects of child maltreatment on antisocial behavior, it could be children with other versions of this gene—or of other genes—who are more susceptible to the effects of child maltreatment on attention, reading, emotional security, or a host of other developmental outcomes that are influenced by problematic child rearing. Indeed, not inconsistent with this possibility are the results a second study by Caspi et al. (2003) showing that variation in the serotonin transporter (5-HTT) gene moderated the effect of child maltreatment on lifetime susceptibility to major depression, with certain versions of this polymorphism being associated with substantially elevated risk of depression when individuals had experienced maltreatment, but other versions being associated with much lower rates of depression, even when individuals shared the same child rearing history (i.e., victims of child maltreatment).

However reasonable this domain-specific conceptualization appears, work by Boyce and associates (1995) raises the prospect that susceptibility to influence may be more domain-general rather than domain-specific. That may be so because these health researchers found, consistent with virtually all the data cited in this chapter, that exposure to high and low levels of psychological stress predicted high and low levels of physical illness only in the case of high psychobiologically reactive (3 to 5-year-old) children, leading the investigators to conclude "that only a subset of individuals may be susceptible to the health-altering effects of stressors and adversity" (p. 411). Clearly, a challenge for the future is to discover how domain-general versus domain-specific differential susceptibility to rearing influence proves to be.

ACKNOWLEDGMENTS

Work on this chapter was supported by a cooperative agreement with the National Institute of Child Health and Human Development (U10-HD25420). I wish to express appreciation to all collaborating investigators of the NICHD Study of Early Child Care.

REFERENCES

Alcock, J. (2001). *The triumph of sociobiology*. Oxford, UK: Oxford University Press.

Bailey, J. M., & Horn, J. (1986). A source of variance in IQ unique to the lower-scoring monozygotic (MS) cotwin. *Behavior Genetics, 16*, 509–516.

Bailey, J. M., & Revelle, W. (1991). Increased heritability for lower IQ levels? *Behavior Genetics, 21*, 397–404.

Belsky, J. (1997a). Variation in susceptibility to rearing influence: An evolutionary argument. *Psychological Inquiry, 8*, 182–186.

Belsky, J. (1997b). Theory testing, effect-size evaluation, and differential susceptibility to rearing influence: The case of mothering and attachment. *Child Development, 64*, 598–600.

Belsky, J. (in press). The developmental and evolutionary psychology of intergenerational transmission of attachment. In L. Ahnert & C. S. Carter (Eds.), *Attachment and bonding*. Cambridge, MA: MIT Press.

Belsky, J., Hsieh, K., & Crnic, K. (1998). Mothering, fathering, and infant negativity as antecedents of boys' externalizing problems and inhibition at age 3: Differential susceptibility to rearing influence? *Development and Psychopathology, 10*, 301–319.

Blair, C. (2002). Early intervention for low birth weight preterm infants: The role of negative emotionality in the specification of effects. *Development and Psychopathology, 14*, 311–332.

Bollen, K. A. (1989). *Structural equations with latent variables* (Vol. 14). New York: Wiley.

Boyce, W., Chesney, M., Alkon, A., Tschann, J., Adams, S., Chesterman, B., et al. (1995). Psychobiological reactivity to stress and childhood respiratory illnesses: Results from two prospective studies. *Psychosomatic Medicine, 57*, 411–422.

Boyce, W. T., & Ellis, B. J. (in press). Biological sensitivity to context: I. An evolutionary–developmental theory of the origins and functions of stress reactivity. *Development and Psychopathology.*

Caspi, A., McClay, J., Moffitt, T., Mill, J., Martin, J., Craig, I., et al. (2002). Role of genotype in the cycle of violence in maltreated children. *Science, 297,* 851–854.

Caspi, A., Sugden, K., Moffitt, T. E., Taylor, A., Craig, I. W., Harrington, H., et al. (2003). Influence of life stress on depression: Moderation by a polymorphism in the 5 HTT gene. *Science, 301,* 386–389.

Crockenberg, S. (1981). Infant irritability, mother responsiveness, and social support influences on the security of infant–mother attachment. *Child Development, 52,* 857–865.

Deater-Deckard, K., & Dodge, K. (1997). Spare the rod, spoil the authors: Emerging themes in research on parenting. *Psychological Inquiry, 8,* 230–235.

Deater-Deckard, K., Reiss, D., Hetherington, E. M., & Plomin, R. (1997). Dimensions and disorders of adolescent adjustment: A quantitative genetic analysis of unselected samples and selected extremes. *Journal of Child Psychology and Psychiatry, 38,* 515–525.

Denham, S., Workman, E., Cole, P., Weissbrod, C., Kendziora, K., & Zahn-Waxler, C. (2000). Prediction of externalizing behavior problems from early to middle childhood: The role of parental socialization and emotion expression. *Development and Psychopathology, 12,* 23–45.

De Wolff, M., & van IJzendoorn, M. (1997). Sensitivity and attachment: A meta-analysis on parental antecedents of infant attachment. *Child Development, 68,* 571–591.

Detterman, D., Thompson, L., & Plomin, R. (1990). Differences in heritability across groups differing in ability. *Behavior Genetics, 20,* 369–384.

Dienstbier, R. (1984). The role of emotion in moral socialization. In C. Izard, J. Kagan, & R. Zajore (Eds.), *Emotions, cognitions, and behaviors* (pp. 484–513). New York: Cambridge University Press.

Early, D., Rimm-Kaufman, S., Cox, M., Saluja, G., Pianta, R., Bradley, R., et al. (2002). Maternal sensitivity and child wariness in the transition to kindergarten. *Parenting: Science and Practice, 2,* 355–377.

Feldman, R., Greenbaum, C., & Yirmiya, N. (1999). Mother–infant affect synchrony as an antecedent of the emergence of self-control. *Developmental Psychology, 35,* 223–231.

Geary, D. C., & Flinn, M. V. (2001). Evolution of human parental behavior and the human family. *Parenting: Science and Practice, 1,* 5–61.

Goldsmith, H., & Alansky, J. (1987). Maternal and infant predictors of attachment. *Journal of Consulting and Clinical Psychology, 55,* 805–816.

Horn, J., Loehlin, J., & Willerman, L. (1979). Intellectual resemblance among adoptive and biological relatives. *Behavior Genetics, 9,* 177–207.

Infant Health and Development Program. (1990). Enhancing the outcomes of low-birth-weight, premature infants. *Journal of the American Medical Association, 263,* 3035–3042.

Jensen, A. (1987, June). *Twins: The puzzle of non-genetic variance.* Paper presented at the 17th Annual Meeting of the Behavior Genetics Association, Minneapolis, MN.

Jöreskog, K. G., & Sörbom, D. (1993). *LISREL VIII: User's reference guide.* Chicago: Scientific Software International.

Kendler, K., & Eaves, L. (1986). Models for the joint effect of genotype and environment on liability to psychiatric illness. *American Journal of Psychiatry, 14,* 279–289.

Kochanska, G. (1993).Toward a synthesis of parental socialization and child temperament in early development of conscience. *Child Development, 64,* 325–347.

Kochanska, G. (1995). Children's temperament, mother's discipline and security of attachment: Multiple pathways to emerging internalization. *Child Development, 66,* 597–615.

Kochanska, G. (1997). Multiple pathways to conscience for children with different temperaments: From toddlerhood to age 5. *Developmental Psychology, 33,* 228–240.

Kochanska, G., Mordhorst, M., & Reschly, A. (1997, April 5). *Child temperament and maternal discipline as contributors to emerging restraint in infancy.* Paper presented at the biennial meetings of the Society for Research in Child Development, Washington, DC.

Loehlin, J. C. (1998). *Latent variable models: An introduction to factor, path, and structural analysis* (3rd ed., Vol. 11). Mahwah, NJ: Erlbaum.

McGuffin, P., Owen, M., O'Donova, M., Thapar, A., & Gottesman, I. (1994). *Seminars in psychiatric genetics.* London: Gaskell.

Morrell, J., & Murray, L. (2003). Parenting and the development of conduct disorder and hyperactive symptoms in childhood: A prospective longitudinal study from 2 months to 8 years. *Journal of Child Psychology and Psychiatry, 44,* 489–508.

Morris, A., Silk, J., Steinberg, L., Sessa, F., Avenevoli, S., & Essex, M. (2002). Temperamental vulnerability and negative parenting as interactings predictors of child adjustment. *Journal of Marriage and the Family, 64,* 461–471.

NICHD Early Child Care Research Network. (1998). Early child care and self-control, compliance, and problem behavior at 24 and 36 months. *Child Development, 69,* 1145–1170.

Plomin, R. (1986). *Development, genetics, and psychology.* Hillsdale, NJ: Erlbaum.

Plomin, R., & Daniels, D. (1987). Why are children in the same family so different from each other? *Behavioral and Brain Sciences, 10,* 1–16.

Price,T. S., Simonoff, E., Waldman, I., Asherson, P., & Plomin, R. (2001). Hyperactivity in pre-school children is highly heritable. *Journal of the American Academy of Child and Adolescent Psychiatry, 40*(12), 1362–1364.

Rende, R., Plomin, R., Reiss, D., & Hetherington, E. M. (1993). Genetic and environmental influences on depressive symptomology in adolescence. *Journal of Child Psychology and Psychiatry, 34,* 1387–1398.

Rubin, K., Burgess, K., Dwyer, K., & Hastings, P. (2003). Predicting preschoolers' externalising behaviors from toddler temperament, conflict, and maternal negativity. *Developmental Psychology, 39,* 164–176.

Stoolmiller, M. (2001). Synergistic interaction of child manageability problems and parent-discipline tactics in predicting future growth in externalizing behavior for boys. *Developmental Psychology, 37,* 814–825.

Scarr, S. (1993). Biological and cultural diversity: The legacy of Darwin for development. *Child Development, 64,* 1333–1353.

Suomi, S. (1995). Influence of attachment theory on ethological studies of biobehavioral development in nonhuman primates. In S. Goldberg, R. Muir, & J. Kerr (Eds.), *Attachment theory: Social, developmental and clinical perspectives* (pp. 185–202). Hillsdale, NJ: Analytic Press.

Suomi, S. (1997). Early determinants of behaviour: Evidence from primate studies. *British Medical Bulletin, 53,* 170–184.

Tooby, J., & Cosmides, L. (1990). On the universality of human nature and the uniqueness of the individual: The role of genetics and adaptation. *Journal of Personality, 58,* 17–67.

Trivers, R. (1985). *Social evolution.* Menlo Park, CA: Benjamin/Cummings.

Van den Boom, D. (1994). The influence of temperament and mothering on attachment and exploration: An experimental manipulation of sensitive responsiveness among lower-class mothers and irritable infants. *Child Development, 65,* 1457–1477.

Volger, G., & DeFries, J. (1983). Linearity of offspring–parent regression for general cognitive ability. *Behavior Genetics, 13,* 355–360.

Wachs, T., & Gandour, M. (1983). Temperament, environment, and six-month cognitive-intellectual development: A test of the organismic-specificity hypothesis. *International Journal of Behavioral Development, 6,* 135–152.

7

DETERMINANTS OF PUBERTAL TIMING

An Evolutionary Developmental Approach

BRUCE J. ELLIS

Pubertal maturation is a dynamic biological process—punctuated by visible changes in stature, body composition, and secondary sexual characteristics— that culminates in the transition from the prereproductive to the reproductive phase of the human life cycle. The timing of this transition is variable and has substantial social and biological implications. An extensive body of research now indicates that early pubertal maturation in girls is associated with a variety of negative health and psychosocial outcomes in Western societies. In particular, early-maturing girls are at greater risk later in life for unhealthy weight gain (e.g., Adair & Gordon-Larsen, 2001; Wellens et al., 1992), breast cancer (e.g., Sellers et al., 1992; Kelsey, Gammon, & John, 1993), and a variety of other cancers of the reproductive system (e.g., Marshall et al., 1998; McPherson, Sellers, Potter, Bostick, & Folsom, 1996; Wu et al., 1988); have higher rates of teenage pregnancy, spontaneous abortion and stillbirths, and low birthweight babies (Ellis, 2004); and tend to show more disturbances in body image, to report more emotional problems, such as depression and anxiety, and to engage in more problem behaviors, such as aggression and substance abuse (e.g., Caspi & Moffitt, 1991; Dick, Rose, Viken, & Kaprio, 2000; Graber, Lewinsohn, Seeley, & Brooks-Gunn, 1997; Ge, Conger, & Elder, 1996). Given this sobering array of outcomes, it is critical to understand the life experiences and pathways that place girls at increased risk for early pubertal maturation.

Life history theory (Charnov, 1993; Roff, 1992; Stearns, 1992) provides a metatheoretical framework for the study of timing of pubertal maturation from an evolutionary developmental perspective. It attempts to explain the timing of reproductive development and events across the lifespan in terms of evolved strategies for distributing metabolic resources between the competing demands of growth, maintenance, and reproduction. Life history theory constitutes a set of widely held basic assumptions that have shaped how evolutionary scientists generate and test middle-level theories of pubertal timing. In this chapter, I review four middle-level theories—energetics theory, stress-suppression theory, psychosocial acceleration theory, and paternal investment theory. Each applies the basic assumptions of life history theory to the question of environmental influences on timing of pubertal maturation in girls. These middle-level theories are consistent with and subsumed by life history theory but have not been directly deduced from it (i.e., the middle-level theories are inductions rather than deductions from the metatheory). Each middle-level theory reviewed in this chapter provides a different translation of the higher-order principles of life history theory into specific hypotheses and predictions that are tested in research. The current review demonstrates how these theories compete to achieve the best operationalization of the core logic of life history theory as it applies to variation in pubertal timing (see Ketelaar & Ellis, 2000, for further discussion of metatheoretical research programs).

For both theoretical and empirical reasons, the focus of this chapter is on girls' rather than boys' sexual development. First, at a theoretical level, the life history approach to pubertal timing pivots around the trade-off between allocation of resources to physical growth and production of offspring. Because this trade-off is particularly relevant to females (given their direct somatic investment in production and nurturing of offspring), life history theory has been applied more broadly and successfully to the question of female than male pubertal timing. Second, at an empirical level, there is a clear and easily assessed marker of female but not male pubertal timing: age at menarche. Consequently, vastly more research has been conducted on timing of pubertal development in females than in males. A review of antecedents of male pubertal timing is not feasible at this time, given the current state of theory and data.

SOURCES OF VARIATION IN PUBERTAL TIMING

Individual differences in the timing of pubertal development are influenced by both genes and environment. Behavior-genetic modeling has been used to partition sources of variance in pubertal timing into genetic and environmental components. Almost all behavior-genetic research has employed a single indicator of pubertal timing: age at menarche. Menarche occurs late in the maturation of the hypothalamic–pituitary–gonadal (HPG) axis and is commonly used as a marker of attainment of pubertal status. Large behavior-genetic studies employing twin designs in Australia, Great Britain, Finland, Norway, and the United States have converged on the conclusion that genotypic effects account for 50–80% of the variation in menarcheal timing and that the remaining variance is attributable to nonshared environmental effects and measurement error (Golden, 1981; Kaprio et al., 1995; Rowe, 2002; Treloar & Martin, 1990; van den Akker, Stein, Neale, & Murray, 1987).[1] Complementing these behavior-genetic analyses are recent molecular-genetic investigations, which have begun to identify allelic variation associated with timing of development of secondary sexual characteristics (Kadlubar et al., 2003) and age at menarche (e.g., Comings, Muhleman, Johnson, & MacMurray, 2002; Stavrou, Zois, Ioannidis, & Tsatsoulis, 2002), although specific genetic determinants are still largely unknown. Some researchers have interpreted the absence of shared environmental effects in behavior-genetic studies as evidence that the shared experiences of siblings do not increase similarity in pubertal timing (see Bailey, Kirk, Zhu, Dunne, & Martin, 2000; Comings et al., 2002; Rowe, 2000a, 2000b). Given the apparent absence of shared environmental effects, one might ask whether evolutionary models specifying psychosocial influences on pubertal timing are necessarily wrong.

I contend that the answer to this question is "No," for several reasons (see especially Ellis, 2004). First, heritability is a population statistic that indexes the degree to which individual differences in genes account for individual differences in an observed trait in a given environmental context. Heritability estimates can change dramatically when social or physical environments change (e.g., Dunne et al., 1997; Rowe, Jacobson, & Van den Oord, 1999; Turkheimer, Haley, Waldron, D'Onofrio, & Gottesman, 2003). Indeed, Chasiotis, Scheffer, Restmeier, and Keller (1998), analyzing German data, have shown that heritability of age of menarche is highly context-specific. Second, both Kaprio et al. (1995) and Treloar and Martin (1990) found that at least half of the genetic variance in age of menarche was nonadditive (i.e., genetic variance that does not cause parents and offspring to be more similar). Nonadditive genetic variance (whether detected or undetected) inflates heritability and deflates shared environmentality estimates in standard twin designs (Grayson, 1989). Third, alternatives to standard twin designs have produced clear evidence of shared environmental influence on age of menarche. Farber (1981), for example, reported that monozygotic twins (MZ) reared together were most similar in menarcheal age (average difference = 2.8 months), followed by MZ twins reared apart (average difference = 9.3 months), followed by dizygotic (DZ) twins reared together (average difference = 12.0 months). That MZ twins reared apart were most similar in menarcheal timing to DZ twins reared together suggests that individual differences in age of menarche are influenced by the degree to which girls share common environments (as well as common genes). Fourth, the types of environmental influences posited by psychosocial models of pubertal timing are likely to have a nonshared component because their effects are not equivalent across siblings in the same home. Finally, it has been well-documented that the timing of pubertal maturation in girls is sensitive to a variety of external factors, such as exercise, nutrition, and stress (e.g., Parent et al., 2003).

In conclusion, genotypic effects on timing of pubertal development are probabilistic and are best conceptualized as coding for a "reaction norm"; that is, genotypes are capable of producing a range of phenotypic expressions, and actual timing of puberty is an emergent property of the genotype and the environment in which it occurs. This reaction norm perspective (see especially Stearns & Koella, 1986) potentially reconciles behavior-genetic and psychosocial models of variation in pubertal timing.

THE LIFE HISTORY APPROACH TO TIMING OF PUBERTAL DEVELOPMENT

The key units of analysis in life history theory (Charnov, 1993; Roff, 1992; Stearns, 1992) are life history traits: the suite of maturational and reproductive characteristics that define the life course (e.g., age at weaning, age at sexual maturity, adult body size, time to first reproduction, interbirth interval, and litter size). Life history theory attempts to explain variation in life history traits in terms of evolved trade-offs in distribution of metabolic resources to competing life functions: growth, maintenance, and reproduction. These trade-offs are inevitable because metabolic resources are finite, and time and energy used for one purpose cannot be used for another. For example, resources spent on growth and development (e.g., later age at sexual maturity, larger adult body size, and increased social quality and competitiveness) cannot be spent on current production of offspring; thus, the benefits of a prolonged childhood are traded off against the costs of delayed reproduction. Life history theory posits the existence of phenotypic mechanisms that actually make these trade-offs by selecting between or "making decisions" about alternative ways of distributing resources (Chisholm, 1999). Natural selection favors mechanisms that, in response to ecological conditions, trade-off resources between growth, maintenance, and reproduction in ways that recurrently enhanced inclusive fitness during a species' evolutionary history. (See Chisholm, Burbank, Coall, & Gemmiti, Chapter 4, this volume, for a more extensive explication of life history theory.)

Given the mix of fitness costs and benefits associated with different timing of reproductive development, selection should *not* favor phenotypic mechanisms that systematically bias allocation of resources toward either growth, maintenance, or reproduction. Rather, consistent with the reaction norm perspective discussed earlier, selection can be expected to favor adaptive developmental plasticity of mechanisms (within genetic capacities and constraints) in response to particular ecological conditions (Belsky, Steinberg, & Draper, 1991; Boyce & Ellis, in press; Chisholm, 1996; Ellison, 2001).[2] Anatomical, physiological, endocrine, and/or developmental mechanisms that track slow, more pervasive changes in the environment often take the form of *conditional adaptations:* "evolved mechanisms that detect and respond to specific features of childhood environments—features that have proven reliable over evolutionary time in predicting the nature of the social and physical world into which children will mature—and entrain developmental pathways that reliably matched those features during a species' natural selective history" (Boyce & Ellis, in press). Conditional adaptations, which reflect systematic gene–environment interactions, underpin development of contingent survival and reproductive strategies and thus enable individuals to function competently in a variety of different environments. Consistent with this perspective, many, if not most, organisms are capable of altering their life histories in response to their environment (Kaplan & Lancaster, 2003). From a life history perspective, conditional adaptations should be engineered to monitor evolutionarily relevant features of one's environment as a basis for contingently allocating resources to survival, growth, development, and reproduction. These resources should be allocated in nonrandom ways that, during a species' evolutionary history, recurrently optimized trade-offs between current and future reproduction, and between number and fitness of offspring (see Chisholm, 1996, 1999).

A central question in life history theory is: When should individuals reach sexual maturity? That is, when should individuals stop converting surplus energy into growth and begin converting it into reproduction? And most critically, what are the relevant developmental experiences and environmental cues that bias individuals toward relatively early versus late reproductive development? Competing answers to this question have been proposed in the life history literature, as reviewed below.

THE ENERGETICS THEORY OF TIMING OF PUBERTAL DEVELOPMENT

Drawing on life history theory, various evolutionary biologists and psychologists (e.g., MacDonald, 1999; Miller, 1994; Surbey, 1998) have argued that in K-selected species (those characterized by high-investment/low-fertility reproductive strategies, such as humans) there should be a negative correlation between resource scarcity and speed of sexual maturation. These theorists posit that members of the human species, under conditions of chronic low energy availability, are primed to delay maturation and reproductive viability until predictably better times (see also Wasser & Barash, 1983). The core argument is that natural selection has favored physiological mechanisms that track variation in resource availability and adjust physical development to match that variation. Consistently good conditions in early and middle childhood signal to the individual that accelerated development and early reproduction are sustainable. Conversely, conditions of resource scarcity cause the individual to reserve energy for maintenance and survival (rather than growth or reproduction). As Ellison (2001, pp. 133–134) suggests:

The adjustment of growth trajectories to chronic ecological conditions is an example of developmental plasticity that is itself assumed to be adaptive. An individual growing up under conditions of chronically low energy availability may be better off growing slowly and being smaller as an adult. Slower growth will divert less energy from maintenance functions. Smaller adult size will also result in lower average metabolic rate and lower maintenance costs.

This theory, linking chronic resource availability to timing of pubertal development, is henceforth referred to as *energetics theory*.

Energetics theory yields the core hypothesis (Hypothesis 1) that children who experience chronically poor nutritional environments will grow slowly, experience late pubertal development, and achieve relatively small adult size, whereas children who experience chronically rich nutritional environments will grow quickly, experience early pubertal development (relative to their genetic potential), and achieve relatively large adult size. Food availability is critical because surplus metabolic energy—the extent to which energy production exceeds maintenance costs—can be harvested by animals and converted into growth and reproduction. The greater the surplus, the greater the capacity for both growth and reproduction. Data from developing countries have consistently supported Hypothesis 1: Children who experience chronically poor nutritional environments, whether assessed indirectly through socioeconomic status (SES) (e.g., Foster, Menken, Chowdhury, & Trussell, 1986; Abioye-Kutyei et al., 1997) or directly in dietary studies (e.g., Khan, Schroeder, Martorell, Haas, & Rivera, 1996; Qamra, Mehta, & Deodhar, 1991), tend to experience relatively late pubertal development. The necessary condition for delayed puberty, however, appears to be sustained nutritional deprivation; the level of dietary variation found in modern Western societies does not appear to meet these conditions (with the exception of high-fiber diets) (e.g., de Ridder et al., 1991; Meyer, Moisan, Marcoux, & Bouchard, 1990).

These data are consistent with the secular trend (beginning at least 170 years ago in England) toward earlier onset of pubertal development, as well as faster tempo of pubertal development (de Muinck Keizer-Schrama & Mul, 2001; Worthman, 1999), in association with general improvements in health and nutrition accompanying modernization (Tanner, 1990). Specifically, age of menarche in Europe dropped from approximately 17 to 13 years of age between 1830 and 1960 (Eveleth & Tanner, 1990). The secular trend has been most intense within lower SES groups (e.g., Abioye-Kiteyi et al., 1997; Veronesi & Gueresi, 1994), where living conditions have improved most dramatically over time. Effects of SES on girls' pubertal timing are generally absent, however, in countries where lower SES groups do not suffer from systematic malnutrition and disease (e.g., Moffitt, Caspi, Belsky, & Silva, 1992; Surbey, 1990).

According to energetics theory, early maturing girls have more surplus energy. Indeed, Ellison (1990) posits that timing of pubertal maturation serves as a kind of "bioassay" of the chronic qualities of the environment, particularly energy availability, encountered during childhood. According to Ellison (1990, 1996, 2001), girls use this bioassay to establish a lifetime set-point for baseline levels of adult ovarian function and reproductive effort, as evidenced by substantial integrity in ovarian function across the reproductive lifespan. In total, girls who experience earlier sexual development are in better physiological condition and have more metabolic resources to devote to reproduction. A second hypothesis (Hypothesis 2) derived from energetics theory, therefore, is that girls who experience relatively early sexual maturation have higher reproductive capacity than their later-maturing peers (see also Udry, 1979; Voland, 1998).

To evaluate the "reproductive capacity hypothesis," it is useful to decompose reproductive capacity into more specific, measurable indicators and to contrast early and late maturing girls on these measures. According to the reproductive capacity hypothesis, earlier maturing girls should have higher ovarian functioning (e.g., growth and maturation of follicles, production of ovarian steroid hormones), higher fecundity (the probability of becoming pregnant when reproductively cycling and engaging in sexual intercourse), higher fertility (number of offspring), greater lactational capacity, better pregnancy outcomes (i.e., lower rates of spontaneous abortions, stillbirths, congenital abnormalities, prematurity, low birthweight, and retardation in offspring), and greater fitness of offspring. There are reasonably well-developed literatures on the relations between age of menarche and ovarian functioning, fetal wastage (spontaneous abortions and stillbirths), fetal growth, and fecundity. Although there is evidence that earlier age at menarche is associated with higher levels of ovarian hormonal functioning, as reviewed by Ellis (2004), there is no consistent evidence that earlier pubertal maturation translates into higher reproductive functioning. Compared with girls whose age at menarche is in the average range for their population, early-maturing girls do not have shorter latencies between menarche and regular menstrual cycling, are not more successful at maintaining pregnancies that culminate in live birth, are not more successful at promoting fetal growth, and are not more fecund or reproductively successful.

As suggested in the preceding discussion of life history theory, timing of pubertal maturation (whether early or late) represents a trade-off in distribution of metabolic resources toward different possible reproductive strategies. Early reproductive development tends to bias allocation of resources toward short-term (current) reproduction and greater number of offspring, whereas later reproductive development tends to bias resources toward long-term (future) reproduction and greater fitness of offspring. Although earlier pubertal development in girls predicts earlier age at first sex and reproduction (e.g., Bingham, Miller, & Adams, 1990; Udry & Cliquet, 1982), girls whose pubertal development is in the normative range for their population are no less fertile or fecund than their earlier maturing peers. Most important, earlier developing girls may be sacrificing offspring quality, as suggested by the literatures on fetal wastage and fetal growth (Ellis, 2004). In summary, early pubertal development is not an indicator of high reproductive capacity. Rather, consistent with life history theory, it can be conceptualized as an important component of a reproductive strategy that is biased toward current reproduction and offspring number.

PSYCHOSOCIAL MODELS OF PUBERTAL TIMING:
I. STRESS-SUPPRESSION THEORY

The energetics theory of pubertal timing, positing that resource scarcity delays pubertal development, has been applied more broadly to encompass psychosocial stressors. According to this expanded version of the theory, adverse physical or social conditions, whether experienced as chronically low energy availability or psychosocial stress, should cause animals in K-selected species to delay pubertal development and reproduction until predictably better times (MacDonald, 1999; Miller, 1994). This theory, linking both physical and social stressors to timing of pubertal development, is henceforth referred to as *stress-suppression theory*.

Stress-suppression theory has been supported by neurophysiological research linking stress to suppression of the HPG axis. When activation of these stress response systems is of sufficient duration and magnitude, the functioning of the HPG axis can be suppressed at several levels, including decreased gonadotropin-releasing hormone (GnRH) pulsatility, disrupted GnRH surge secretion, decrease in pituitary responsiveness to GnRH, and alteration of stimulatory effects of gonadotropins on sex steroid production (e.g., Dobson, Ghuman, Prabhakar, & Smith, 2003; Rivier & Rivest, 1991; cf. Ferin, 1999, who reviews primate research indicating a paradoxical increase in gonadotropin in response to stress during the mid- to late-follicular phase of the menstrual cycle). Linkages between the stress response systems and the HPG axis thus provide a clearly articulated mechanism through which psychosocial stress could delay pubertal development. In humans, these linkages are supported by a substantial body of research indicating that energetic stress, and some research suggesting that psychosocial stress, can induce reproductive dysfunction in women (e.g., Ellison, 2001; Ferin, 1999; Marcus, Loucks, & Berga, 2001; Nappi & Facchinetti, 2003).

Human and nonhuman primate research investigating the stress-suppression hypothesis, however, has examined the effects of stress on ovarian functioning in mature females. No published experimental work has manipulated psychosocial stress in immature female primates and then followed those animals prospectively to determine downstream effects on timing of pubertal development. To my knowledge, relevant experimental research in large mammals has only been conducted on pigs. This applied agricultural research has assessed the impact of management stressors (i.e., mixing with unfamiliar conspecifics, relocation to new pens, truck transport) on attainment of puberty in gilts. Contrary to the stress-suppression hypothesis, management stressors, either on their own or in combination with boar contact, generally stimulate earlier pubertal development in gilts (Hughes, Philip, & Siswadi, 1997, and references therein). Gilts raised in total confinement systems, however, tend to experience delayed puberty (Thompson & Savage, 1978).

Controlled human experimentation, of course, does not exist. But some relevant information has been obtained by analyzing timing of pubertal development under conditions of war. A number of studies have been conducted in relation to World War II. These investigations examined median ages at menarche in given regions before, during, and after the war. In Europe, the Soviet Union, and Japan, the secular trend toward earlier pubertal development was already well under way by the time of World War II. In Belgium (Wellens, Malina, Beunen, & Lefevre, 1990), Finland (Kantero & Widholm, 1971), France (Olivier & Devigne, 1983), Germany (Tanner, 1962), Japan (Hoel, Wakabayashi, & Pike, 1983), the Netherlands (van Noord & Kaaks, 1991), and Russia (Bielicki, 1986), this trend was reversed during the period of World War II. There can be little doubt that adverse conditions associated with the war delayed pubertal development. This research, however, does not enable determination of the specific conditions that caused this delay. There were many confounding stressors—food rationing, changes in dietary composition, increased physical activity, suffering from cold, prevalence of disease, physical injury, as well as psychological trauma—any of which could have plausibly contributed to the temporary reversal in the secular trend.

In summary, although connections between the stress response systems and the HPG axis provide a plausible mechanism through which psychosocial stress could delay pubertal development, there is little evidence that psychosocial stress actually does delay puberty. The data on changes in pubertal timing during periods of war are interesting but confounded. Most critical, as reviewed below, the hypothesis that psychosocial stress delays human pubertal development runs counter to the results of most longitudinal research on this topic. In total, the current empirical literature does not support expanding energetics theory into a more general stress-suppression theory of pubertal timing that encompasses psychosocial stressors (Ellis, 2004). Admittedly, relevant research is scant, often indirect, and mostly nonexperimental. The point is not that these limited investigations disconfirm the hypothesis that psychosocial stress inhibits pubertal development, but rather that almost no extant research has supported it.

PSYCHOSOCIAL MODELS OF PUBERTAL TIMING: II. PSYCHOSOCIAL ACCELERATION THEORY

As discussed earlier, life history theory comprises a broad set of theoretical principles that can be used to derive a number of more specific theoretical models. In some cases, these derivative models provide competing perspectives on a common question. In contrast to the stress-suppression theory presented earlier, an alternative set of life history models focuses on the role of familial and ecological stressors in provoking early onset of pubertal development and reproduction (Belsky et al., 1991; Chisholm, 1993, 1996, 1999; Wilson & Daly, 1997).

Belsky et al. (1991) were the first to propose a life history model of the role of psychosocial stressors in accelerating timing of puberty in girls. Indeed, they regarded the proposition of a linkage between psychosocial experiences early in life and pubertal timing as a unique and "uncanny" prediction distinguishing their "evolutionary theory of socialization" from more traditional theories of socialization, as well as from mainstream thinking about determinants of pubertal timing. Belsky et al. posited that "a principal evolutionary function of early experience—the first 5–7 years of life—is to induce in the child an understanding of the availability and predictability of resources (broadly defined) in the environment, of the trustworthiness of others, and of the enduringness of close interpersonal relationships, all of which will affect how the developing person apportions reproductive effort" (p. 650). Drawing on the concept of sensitive-period learning of reproductive strategies, Belsky et al. theorized that humans have evolved to be sensitive to specific features of their early childhood environments, and that exposure to different environments biases children toward the development of different reproductive strategies. Children whose experiences in and around their families of origin are characterized by relatively high levels of stress (e.g., scarcity or instability of resources, father absence, negative and coercive family relationships, lack of positive and supportive family relationships) are hypothesized to develop in a manner that speeds rates of pubertal maturation, accelerates sexual activity, and orients the individual toward relatively unstable pair-bonds and lower levels of parental investment. In contrast, children whose experiences in and around their families are characterized by relatively high levels of support and stability are hypothesized to develop in the opposite manner (Belsky et al., 1991).

In essence, Belsky et al. (1991) proposed that the context of early rearing "sets" the person's reproductive strategy in a way that was likely to have functioned adaptively in that context in the environments in which humans evolved. Over the course of our natural selective history, ancestral females growing up in adverse family environments may have reliably increased their reproductive success by accelerating physical maturation and beginning sexual activity and reproduction at a relatively early age, without the expectation that paternal investment in child rearing would be forthcoming, and without the precondition of a close, enduring relationship with a mate (Belsky et al., 1991). A shortened reproductive time table in this context may have increased the probability of having at least some offspring that survive and reproduce. As Chisholm (1996) suggests, "When young mammals encounter conditions that are not favorable for survival—i.e., the conditions of environmental risk and uncertainty indexed by emotional stress during development—it will generally be adaptive for them to reproduce early" (p. 21).

Although the stress-suppression theory posits that environmental stress and uncertainty should result in later pubertal development and lower fertility, Chisholm (1996, 1999) proposes that this should only be the case when parents have the capacity to shape conditions in ways that significantly enhance the health, competitiveness, and eventual reproductive success of their offspring. When parents lack this capacity, allocation of resources should be biased toward reproducing early and often. One element of this accelerated reproductive strategy is to shorten the time before sexual maturity (i.e., accelerate pubertal development). As Chisholm (1999, pp. 57–58) has stated:

> From the perspective of life history theory (and contrary to a great deal of "common sense") when parents' resources are limited it is *not* necessarily adaptive or rational for them to have fewer offspring so as to be able to invest more in each one. In other words, even when mortality rates are not high the optimal strategy for parents who lack the material or social resources (e.g., power, prestige) to *make a difference* in their children's reproductive value (e.g., health, education, employment or marriage prospects, competence as parents . . .) may well be to *increase* fertility (to maximize current reproduction) while reducing investment in each child (which tends to decrease future reproduction). . . . The "non-intuitive message" here (as Monique Borgerhoff Mulder [1992:350] described this apparent paradox) is that when the flow of resources is chronically low or unpredictable—which is when we might otherwise expect parents to be most solicitous of their offspring—it may in fact be (or have been) evolutionarily adaptive for parents to "hedge their bets" against lineage extinction by *reducing* parental investment and allocating their limited resources not to parenting effort (or even, beyond some threshold, to their *own* health and longevity), but to *offspring production* instead.

In summary, low-quality parental investment may signal an environment where variations in parental care and resources are not closely linked to variation in reproductive success. Under these conditions, the developing child should accelerate reproductive maturation. This theory, linking psychosocial stress to earlier puberty, is henceforth referred to as *psychosocial acceleration theory*.

Psychosocial acceleration theory posits that warm, cohesive family environments slow down pubertal development, whereas degraded, conflictual family environments accelerate it. Empirical research to date has provided reasonable, though incomplete, support for the theory (Ellis, 2004). On the one hand, there is converging evidence from a number of methodologically sound studies that greater parent–child warmth and cohesion is associated with later pubertal development (e.g., Ellis, McFadyen-Ketchum, Dodge, Pettit, & Bates, 1999; Graber, Brooks-Gunn, & Warren, 1995). This research also suggests that greater frequency of parent–child interactions predicts later puberty. On the other hand, the proposed accelerating effect of parent–child conflict and coercion on pubertal development is yet to be clearly established (cf. Moffitt et al., Silva, 1992; Ellis et al., 1999).

PSYCHOSOCIAL MODELS OF PUBERTAL TIMING:
III. PATERNAL INVESTMENT THEORY

The *paternal investment theory* of the timing of pubertal development is a variant of psychosocial acceleration theory and is based, fundamentally, on the theorizing of Draper and Harpending (1982, 1988). These authors hypothesized that the developmental pathways underlying variation in daughters' reproductive strategies are especially sensitive to the father's role in the family and the mother's sexual attitudes and behavior in early childhood. Both psychosocial acceleration theory and paternal investment theory specify relevant developmental experiences and psychosocial cues that bias individuals toward earlier versus later sexual development. But in specifying those experiences and cues, psychosocial acceleration theory focuses on a multiplicity of qualities and features of the family ecology (including quality of father–daughter relationships and father absence) as they relate to the child's overall experiences of stress versus support. By contrast, paternal investment theory focuses specifically on the father's role in the family and the mother's sexual attitudes and behavior toward men. In other words, paternal investment theory, as formulated by Ellis (2004), posits a unique and central role for quality of paternal investment in regulation of daughters' sexual development, separate from the effects of other dimensions of psychosocial stress and support in the child's environment. Paternal investment theory is not inconsistent with psychosocial acceleration theory, given that the narrow set of predictions generated by paternal investment theory are almost fully subsumed by the broader set of predictions generated by psychosocial acceleration theory. Rather, paternal investment theory narrows the focus of psychosocial acceleration theory and moves it closer to its roots in Draper and Harpending (1982).

In all regions of the world, and across all social and economic systems, mothers invest more time and energy in the direct care of children than do fathers (Geary, 2000). Although mothers (and sometimes their female kin) form the primary foundation of parental care in all societies, the contribution of fathers to the family is—and presumably always has been—widely variable. In his review of the evolution and proximate expression of human paternal investment, Geary (2000) proposed (1) that over human evolutionary history, fathers' investment in families tended to improve but was not essential to the survival and fitness of children, and (2) that selection consequently favored a mixed paternal strategy, with different men varying in the extent to which they allocated resources to care and provisioning of children. Under these conditions, selection should favor psychological mechanisms in females that are especially attuned to variation in the willingness and ability of males to invest in families.

Consistent with this logic and drawing on the concept of sensitive-period learning of reproductive strategies, paternal investment theory posits that girls detect and internally encode information specifically about the quality of paternal investment during approximately the first 5 years of life as a basis for

(1) calibrating the development of neurophysiological systems involved in timing of pubertal maturation and (2) calibrating development of related motivational systems that make certain types of sexual behavior more or less likely in adolescence.

Relevant cues to paternal investment are provided by both fathers and mothers. Perhaps the most important cue is father presence versus absence (i.e., the extent to which women rear their children with or without consistent help from the man who is father to the children). Other important cues may include frequency of father–daughter interactions, levels of cohesion and conflict in father–daughter relationships, the quality and stability of the father–mother relationship, the mother's attitudes toward men, the mother's sexual and repartnering behavior, and the daughter's exposure to her mother's boyfriends and to stepfathers.

Paternal investment theory posits that early experiences associated with low-quality paternal investment function to entrain the development of reproductive strategies that are matched to that social milieu—a milieu in which male parental investment is relatively unreliable and/or not closely linked to variation in reproductive success. Girls in this context are predicted to develop in a manner that accelerates pubertal maturation and onset of sexual activity and orients the individual toward relatively unstable pair-bonds. As Belsky et al. (1991) suggest, in environments where paternal investment is not important, "a young woman who waits for the right man to help rear her children may lose valuable reproductive opportunities at a time when her health and physical capability are at their peak and when her mother and senior female kin are young enough to be effective surrogates" (p. 653).

Conversely, early experiences associated with high-quality paternal investment are hypothesized to entrain development of reproductive strategies to match that social milieu—a milieu in which male parental investment is reliable and forthcoming, and in which variations in offspring quality are sensitive to provision of paternal care and resources. Girls in this context are predicted to develop in a manner that slows pubertal maturation, delays onset of sexual activity and reproduction, and increases reticence in forming sexual relationships. Under these conditions, a longer prereproductive developmental period enables daughters to practice and refine sociocompetitive competencies (Geary & Flinn, 2001) and facilitates formation of relatively long-term pair-bonds with reliable and nurturant mates.

Paternal investment theory provides the foundation for a series of predictions about the role for fathers and other adult males in regulation of girls' pubertal timing. Although the theory began with a focus on father absence versus presence, it has since been elaborated to include multiple dimensions of paternal investment (e.g., the dimensional quality of paternal involvement in father-present homes, the quality of father–mother relationships, the effects of father figures) and specifically conceptualizes father-effects as distinct from the more general effects of familial and ecological stress. Paternal investment theory has now been tested in a number of investigations and has received provisional empirical support. In well-nourished populations, girls from father-absent homes tend to experience earlier pubertal development than do girls from father-present homes (e.g., Quinlan, 2003; Moffitt et al., 1992), and the earlier father-absence occurs, the greater the effect (e.g., Moffitt et al., 1992; Surbey, 1990; Quinlan, 2003). There is also initial longitudinal evidence that, within father-present homes, higher levels of paternal caretaking and involvement are associated with later pubertal development in daughters (Ellis et al., 1999). The possibility that father figures accelerate girls' pubertal timing is intriguing but in need of further theoretical development and empirical testing (see Ellis, 2004). Finally, there is consistent evidence that quality of paternal investment uniquely predicts timing of pubertal development in daughters, independent of other aspects of the family ecology (e.g., Ellis et al., 1999; Ellis & Garber, 2000; Moffitt et al., 1992).

CRITICISMS OF PSYCHOSOCIAL ACCELERATION AND PATERNAL INVESTMENT THEORIES

Psychosocial acceleration and paternal investment theories have been challenged in the literature on a number of grounds (see Ellis, 2004). The most compelling empirical critique has been offered by behavior geneticists. Theoretical critiques have come from within the fields of evolutionary psychology and biology.

The Behavior Genetic Critique

An important limitation of all of the human research on antecedents of pubertal timing reviewed in this chapter is that it is not genetically informative. The psychosocial models of pubertal timing presented herein rest on the concept of conditional reproductive strategies; that is, they emphasize environmentally triggered processes that shunt individuals toward given reproductive strategies. An alternative explanation, however, is that individual differences in pubertal timing and associated characteristics represent heritable reproductive strategies that result from genetic differences. Consider the following two related possibilities.

First, girls who mature earlier tend to exhibit earlier onset of sexual activity and earlier age of first marriage and first birth. This covariation may occur because early pubertal timing results in precocious sexual and reproductive behavior or because pubertal, sexual, and reproductive timing are genetically correlated traits (Rowe, 2002). Accelerated reproduction in turn is associated with increased probability of divorce and lower quality paternal investment (e.g., Amato, 1996; Bennett, Bloom, & Miller, 1995). Because mothers who are early maturers tend to have daughters who are early maturers (see Sources of Variation in Pubertal Timing), the correlation between family environments and timing of pubertal maturation in girls may be spurious; that is, it may be due simply to genetic transmission of pubertal timing and associated characteristics (e.g., Belsky et al., 1991; Kim & Smith, 1998; Rowe, 2000a; Surbey, 1990).

The correlational methods used by researchers to examine relations between social environments and pubertal timing cannot rule out this alternative explanation; indeed, Moffitt et al. (1992) embraced just this interpretation upon reporting linkages between early experience and pubertal timing. However, many researchers have incorporated control variables into their analyses to account, at least in part, for possible genetic influences. These controls have included the child's initial level of pubertal development (Graber et al., 1995; Steinberg, 1988; N. B. Ellis, 1991), the mother's age at menarche (Campbell & Udry, 1995; Graber et al., 1995; Kim & Smith, 1998a; Surbey, 1990), the mother's sexual and reproductive history (Ellis & Garber, 2000; Kim & Smith, 1998; Quinlan, 2003), and the daughters' physical characteristics, such as weight, percentage of body fat, and biliac diameter (e.g., Campbell & Udry, 1995; Graber et al., 1995; Moffitt et al., 1992). In most cases, the observed relations between family environment and pubertal timing have not been meaningfully altered by inclusion of these control variables. Nonetheless, genetically controlled research designs that incorporate environmental measures are greatly needed, because we cannot be certain by any means that the controls implemented to date fully take into account biological inheritance.

Second, Comings et al. (2002) have proposed a more specific version of the genetic transmission theory based on a variant of the X-linked androgen receptor gene. According to Comings et al., fathers carry X-linked genes that are associated with aggression and impulsivity, sexual promiscuity, and associated patterns of marital conflict and dissolution. These genes are transmitted to daughters, in whom they are associated with paternal absence, earlier age at menarche, and precocious sexual activity. Comings et al. found support for this theory in two clinical samples (males hospitalized for substance abuse, female outpatient volunteers for a weight control program). Jorm, Christensen, Rodgers, Jacomb, and Easteal (2004), however, found no support for the theory in two epidemiological studies using general population samples. Further research is needed to reconcile these contradictory results, because the current balance of evidence does not yet permit evaluation of the X-linked genetic transmission theory.

Finally, Belsky (2000) suggests that the environmental and genetic transmission models could both be right, but that each applies to only a subset of the population. Specifically, covariation between childhood experiences and timing of puberty may be primarily genetic for some individuals but not for others. In an extensive review of the literature, Belsky (Chapter 6, this volume) has documented wide variation between children in the extent to which they are affected by particular styles of parenting or other aspects of childrearing (see also Boyce & Ellis, in press). Such variation appears to have a substantial genetic basis (see Caspi et al., 2002, 2003).

Indeed, Caspi et al. have argued that the very reason why molecular-genetic studies, such as those reported above by Comings et al. (2002) and Jorm et al. (2004), so often prove inconsistent in their findings is because gene–environment interactions are likely to be widespread, and sampling from different populations may well lead to different proportions of cases that are and are not susceptible to a particular environmental experience. In summary, the psychosocial acceleration and paternal investment theories of pubertal timing may only apply to those subsets of the population that are genetically susceptible to rearing influences.

An Evolutionary Theoretical Critique

The psychosocial acceleration and paternal investment theories of pubertal timing have also been challenged on conceptual grounds (Bailey et al., 2000; Rowe, 2000a, 2000b). This challenge concerns the evolutionary logic underlying early experiential calibration of reproductive strategies. Bailey et al. (2000, p. 538) suggest that paternal investment theory necessitates several rather strong assumptions about ancestral social environments:

> First, in ancestral environments, frequent shifts must have occurred between high and low paternal investment mating systems (respectively, "Dads" and "Cads" [Wilson, 1994]). Such shifts would be necessary for the evolution of such a complex, contingent adaptation. Second, although frequent shifts must have occurred within populations over time, in general, fathers' behavior must have been a reliable indicator of paternal investment at daughter's age of reproduction; cross-generational changes in mating system would disrupt father–daughter signaling. Third, within ancestral breeding populations, men would have needed to be rather homogenous in their sexual strategies (nearly all "Dads" or all "Cads"). Otherwise, there would be little benefit to a daughter drawing inferences about the likelihood of paternal investment from her father's behavior.

This critique has been further articulated by Kanazawa (2001, p. 330):

> Assume that 50% of men in a society comprises "cads" and the other 50% "dads" (Draper and Harpending, 1982, 1988). Further assume that there is no inherited tendency for girls to mate with one kind or the other; daughters of women who mated with cads are no more likely to mate with cads than those of women who mated with dads. . . . In this situation, if girls from father-absent homes experience early puberty and adopt a more promiscuous reproductive strategy (mating without long-term commitment), then their strategy will be just as likely to be maladaptive as to be adaptive because they will be just as likely to mate with a dad as with a cad. The same is true of girls from father-present homes. If they delay their puberty and avoid sexual promiscuity, their strategy will be just as likely to be maladaptive as to be adaptive because they will be just as likely to mate with a cad as with a dad. Under such circumstances, any evolved tendency to take cues from the mating situations of their mothers, as is posited by the model, will not be selected.

These critiques contend that it would be maladaptive for girls to use child-hood exposures to fathers' and mothers' reproductive strategies as a basis for calibrating development of their own reproductive strategies unless there is homogeneity within populations.

Developmental plasticity is necessarily a constrained process. Although it would seem advantageous for individuals to respond to environmental changes quickly, appropriately, and with maximal flexibility throughout their lives, high levels of responsiveness are not always either possible or desirable. Instead, for many phenotypic characteristics, individuals have been selected to register particular features of their childhood environments as a basis for entraining relevant developmental pathways (e.g., Boyce & Ellis, in press; Chisholm, 1999; Shonkoff & Phillips, 2000; West-Eberhard, 2003). As discussed in Boyce and Ellis (in press), there are several reasons to expect early entrainment. I only reiterate one of those reasons here: Many complex adaptations are "built" during development and cannot be easily rebuilt when environments fluctuate. For example, age at menarche is influenced by programmed patterns of gonadotropin release that are established *in utero*, when androgen concentrations imprint the fetal HPG axis, and are subsequently modified by fat accumulation during childhood (Cooper, Kuh, Egger, Wadsworth, & Barker, 1996; Koziel & Jankowska, 2002).

The core issue raised by the preceding critiques, however, is whether fathers' and mothers' reproductive strategies provide children with reliable information about the reproductive opportunities and constraints that they are likely to encounter in adulthood. As extensively reviewed by Chisholm (1999), the answer to this question is almost certainly "yes." Familial and ecological conditions in childhood prepare individuals for the sociosexual niche that they are likely to inhabit in adulthood (Belsky et al., 1991). This preparation occurs internally through personality development and externally through intergenerational transmission of social and economic resources. These transmissions affect the reproductive opportunities and constraints in nonrandom ways, moving children into greater alignment with their parents.

Kanazawa (2001) has studied empirically the nature of information transmitted by parental reproductive strategies. His starting assumption was that father presence versus absence and quality of paternal investment experienced by girls in the home function as microlevel indicators of the degree of monogamy versus polygyny in the society at large. Kanazawa conducted cross-cultural analyses in which he coded for either simultaneous polygyny (pervasiveness of polygyny in legally polygynous societies) or serial polygyny (annual divorce rates in legally monogamous societies). These indices were then correlated with mean age at menarche in each society, after controlling for race, year of study, and population measures of health and welfare (per capita GDP [gross domestic product] and female literacy rates). Consistent with paternal investment theory, Kanazawa found that menarche occurred earlier in societies characterized by higher levels of simultaneous or serial polygyny. These data are consistent with the proposition that female pubertal timing is responsive to parental reproductive strategies, and that these strategies (contrary to Kanazawa's own criticism quoted earlier) provide reliable cues to the macrolevel mating systems into which children will mature. Moreover, quality of parental resources and investment prepares children more specifically for their likely position in those mating systems.

CONCLUSIONS

What is the nature of environmental influences on timing of pubertal maturation in girls? If that question had been asked 15 years ago, before the application of life history theory to human sexual development, the answer would have been very different from the one presented in this chapter. The answer provided in a 1988 review, for example, included weight and body mass, intensity and duration of exercise, nutrition, physical illness, number of children in the family, and altitude (Brooks-Gunn, 1988). The notion that social experiences influence something as biological and presumably genetic as pubertal timing was not taken seriously, especially among psychologically minded students of human development. That changed with the publication of psychosocial acceleration theory by Belsky et al. in 1991, which advanced uncanny predictions about relations between family processes and pubertal timing. That theorizing stimulated the major body of research and theory reviewed in this chapter. Life history theory provided the framework, missing from previous developmental theories, for conceptualizing psychosocial influences on timing of pubertal development.

A key direction for future research involves untangling the effects of physical and socioemotional stressor on timing of puberty. Hulanicka's (1999; Hulanicka, Gronkiewicz, & Koniarek, 2001) research on Polish schoolgirls is especially informative in this regard. Within the same samples, poverty was found to forecast later pubertal development, while family dysfunction predicted earlier development. These data suggest that physical and socioemotional stressors have independent (and perhaps countervailing) effects on pubertal timing. Coall and Chisholm (2003) have proposed that the effects of physical and socioemotional stressors on pubertal timing are hierarchically ordered, whereby pubertal timing is contingent first on health and nutrition and, when these are adequate, second on socioemotional conditions.

Much remains to be learned about the effects of family environments on pubertal timing. Most critical is the need for genetically controlled research designs that incorporate environmental measures. Neurophysiological studies that test for intervening mechanisms are also greatly needed. Finally, more careful attention must be paid to the nature of psychosocial effects on pubertal timing (e.g., sensitive periods, effects of chronic vs. acute exposure to stressors, curvilinear relations, and interactions between socioemotional and physical stressors). Despite these complexities, it is my hope that this review leads to new knowledge about the causes of pubertal timing in girls, and that this knowledge is ultimately helpful in predicting and controlling the pubertal transition.

NOTES

1. It is important to note that only the United States (Rowe, 2000a) and Finnish (Kaprio et al., 1995) studies assessed menarcheal age during adolescence. In contrast to the heritability data on age at menarche, subsequent analyses on Finnish twin cohorts yielded approximately equal heritability (.40) and shared environmentality (.45) estimates for overall levels of pubertal development in 12-year-old girls (as indexed by the Pubertal Development Scale). By age 14, however, estimated heritability increased to .70, and shared environmentality decreased to .02 (Dick, Rose, Pulkkinen, & Kaprio, 2001).
2. Although selection can be expected to favor adaptive developmental plasticity, this does not imply that all individuals are equally plastic. As reviewed by Belsky (Chapter 6, this volume) and Boyce and Ellis (in press), some individuals are more susceptible to rearing influences than others. This issue is addressed in greater detail below (see Criticisms of Psychosocial Acceleration and Paternal Investment Theories).

REFERENCES

Abioye-Kuteyi, E. A., Ojofeitimi, E. O., Aina, O. I., Kio, F., Aluko, Y., & Mosuro, O. (1997). The influence of socioeconomic and nutritional status on menarche in Nigerian school girls. *Nutrition and Health*, 11, 185–195.

Adair, L. S., & Gordon-Larsen, P. (2001). Maturational timing and overweight prevalence in US adolescent girls. *American Journal of Public Health*, 91, 642–644.

Amato, P. R. (1996). Explaining the intergenerational transmission of divorce. *Journal of Marriage and the Family*, 58, 628–640.

Bailey, J. M., Kirk, K. M., Zhu, G., Dunne, M. P., & Martin, N. G. (2000). Do individual differences in sociosexuality represent genetic or environmentally contingent strategies?: Evidence from the Australian twin registry. *Journal of Personality and Social Psychology*, 78, 537–545.

Belsky, J. (2000). Conditional and alternative reproductive strategies: Individual differences in susceptibility to rearing experiences. In J. L. Rodgers, D. C. Rowe, & W. B. Miller (Eds.), *Genetic influences on human fertility and sexuality: Theoretical and empirical contributions from the biological and behavioral sciences* (pp. 127–145). Boston: Kluwer Academic.

Belsky, J., Steinberg, L., & Draper, P. (1991). Childhood experience, interpersonal development, and reproductive strategy: An evolutionary theory of socialization. *Child Development*, 62, 647–670.

Bennett, N. G., Bloom, D. E., & Miller, C. K. (1995). The influence of nonmarital childbearing on the formation of first marriages. *Demography*, 32, 47–62.

Bielicki, T. (1986). Physical growth as a measure of the economic well-being of populations: The twentieth century. In F. Falkner & J. M. Tanner (Eds.), *Human growth* (2nd ed., pp. 283–305). New York: Plenum Press.

Bingham, C. R., Miller, B. C., & Adams, G. R. (1990). Correlates of age at first sexual intercourse in a national sample of young women. *Journal of Adolescent Research, 5,* 18–33.

Boyce, W. T., & Ellis, B. J. (in press). Biological sensitivity to context: I. An evolutionary–developmental theory of the origins and functions of stress reactivity. *Development and Psychopathology.*

Brooks-Gunn, J. (1988). Antecedents and consequences of variations in girls' maturational timing. *Journal of Adolescent Health Care, 9,* 365–373.

Campbell, B. C., & Udry, J. R. (1995). Stress and age at menarche of mothers and daughters. *Journal of Biosocial Science, 27,* 127–134.

Caspi, A., & Moffitt, T. E. (1991). Individual differences are accentuated during periods of social change: The sample case of girls at puberty. *Journal of Personality and Social Psychology, 61,* 157–168.

Caspi, A., McClay, J., Moffitt, T. E., Mill, J., Martin, J., Craig, I. W., et al. (2002). Role of genotype in the cycle of violence in maltreated children. *Science, 297*(5582), 851–854.

Caspi, A., Sugden, K., Moffitt, T. E., Taylor, A., Craig, I. W., Harrington, H., et al. (2003). Influence of life stress on depression: Moderation by a polymorphism in the 5-HTT gene. *Science, 301*(5631), 386–389.

Charnov, E. L. (1993). *Life history invariants.* Oxford, UK: Oxford University Press.

Chisholm, J. S. (1993). Death, hope, and sex: Life-history theory and the development of reproductive strategies. *Current Anthropology, 34,* 1–24.

Chisholm, J. S. (1996). The evolutionary ecology of attachment organization. *Human Nature, 7,* 1–38.

Chisholm, J. S. (1999). *Death, hope and sex: Steps to an evolutionary ecology of mind and morality.* New York: Cambridge University Press.

Coall, D. A., & Chisholm, J. S. (2003). Evolutionary perspectives on pregnancy: Maternal age at menarche and infant birth weight. *Social Science and Medicine, 57,* 1771–1781.

Comings, D. E., Muhleman, D., Johnson, J. P., & MacMurray, J. P. (2002). Parent–daughter transmission of the androgen receptor gene as an explanation of the effect of father absence on age of menarche. *Child Development, 73,* 1046–1051.

Cooper, C., Kuh, D., Egger, P., Wadsworth, M., & Barker, D. (1996). Childhood growth and age at menarche. *British Journal of Obstetrics and Gynaecology, 103,* 814–817.

de Muinck Keizer-Schrama, S. M. P. F., & Mul, D. (2001). Trends in pubertal development in Europe. *Human Reproduction Update, 7,* 287–291.

de Ridder, C. M., Thijssen, J. H., Van 't Veer, P., van Duuren, R., Bruning, P. F., Zonderland, M. L., et al. (1991). Dietary habits, sexual maturation, and plasma hormones in pubertal girls: A longitudinal study. *American Journal of Clinical Nutrition, 54,* 805–813.

Dick, D. M., Rose, R. J., Pulkkinen, L., & Kaprio, J. (2001). Measuring puberty and understanding its impact: A longitudinal study of adolescent twins. *Journal of Youth and Adolescence, 30,* 385–400.

Dick, D. M., Rose, R. J., Viken, R. J., & Kaprio, J. (2000). Pubertal timing and substance use: Associations between and within families across late adolescence. *Developmental Psychology, 36,* 180–189.

Dobson, H., Ghuman, S., Prabhakar, S., & Smith, R. (2003). A conceptual model of the influence of stress on female reproduction. *Reproduction, 125,* 151–163.

Draper, P., & Harpending, H. (1982). Father absence and reproductive strategy: An evolutionary perspective. *Journal of Anthropological Research, 38,* 255–273.

Draper, P., & Harpending, H. (1988). A sociobiological perspective on the development of human reproductive strategies. In K. B. MacDonald (Ed.), *Sociobiological perspectives on human development* (pp. 340–372). New York: Springer-Verlag.

Dunne, M. P., Martin, N. G., Statham, D. J., Slutske, W. S., Dinwiddie, S. H., Bucholz, K. K., et al. (1997). Genetic and environmental contributions to variance in age at first sexual intercourse. *Psychological Science, 8,* 211–216.

Eveleth, P. B., & Tanner, J. M. (1990). *World-wide variation in human growth* (2nd ed.). Cambridge, UK: Cambridge University Press.

Ellis, B. J. (2004). Timing of pubertal maturation in girls: An integrated life history approach. *Psychological Bulletin, 130,* 920–958.

Ellis, B. J., & Garber, J. (2000). Psychosocial antecedents of variation in girls' pubertal timing: Maternal depression, stepfather presence, and marital and family stress. *Child Development, 71,* 485–501.

Ellis, B. J., Bates, J. E., Dodge, K. A., Fergusson, D. M., Horwood, L. J., Pettit, G. S., et al. (2003). Does father absence place daughters at special risk for early sexual activity and teenage pregnancy? *Child Development, 74,* 801–821.

Ellis, B. J., McFadyen-Ketchum, S., Dodge, K. A., Pettit, G. S., & Bates, J. E. (1999). Quality of early family relationships and individual differences in the timing of pubertal maturation in girls: A longitudinal test of an evolutionary model. *Journal of Personality and Social Psychology, 77,* 387–401.

Ellis, N. B. (1991). An extension of the Steinberg accelerating hypothesis. *Journal of Early Adolescence, 11,* 221–235.

Ellison, P. T. (1990). Human ovarian function and reproductive ecology: New hypotheses. *American Anthropologist, 92,* 933–952.

Ellison, P. T. (1996). Developmental influences on adult ovarian hormonal function. *American Journal of Human Biology, 8,* 725–734.

Ellison, P. T. (2001). *On fertile ground: A natural history of human reproduction.* Cambridge, MA: Harvard University Press.

Farber, S. L. (1981). *Identical twins reared apart: A reanalysis.* New York: Basic Books.

Ferin, M. (1999). Clinical review 105: Stress and the reproductive cycle. *Journal of Clinical Endocrinology and Metabolism, 84,* 1768–1774.

Foster, A., Menken, J., Chowdhury, A., & Trussell, J. (1986). Female reproductive development: A hazards model analysis. *Social Biology, 33,* 183–198.

Ge, X., Conger, R. D., & Elder, G. H., Jr. (1996). Coming of age too early: Pubertal influences on girls' vulnerability to psychological distress. *Child Development, 67,* 3386–3400.

Geary, D. C. (2000). Evolution and proximate expression of human paternal investment. *Psychological Bulletin, 126,* 55–77.

Geary, D. C., & Flinn, M. V. (2001). Evolution of human parental behavior and the human family. *Parenting: Science and Practice, 1,* 5–61.

Golden, W. L. (1981). Reproductive histories in a Norwegian twin population: Evaluation of the maternal effect in early spontaneous abortion. *Acta Geneticae Medicae et Gemellologiae, 30,* 91–165.

Graber, J. A., Brooks-Gunn, J., & Warren, M. P. (1995). The antecedents of menarcheal age: Heredity, family environment, and stressful life events. *Child Development, 66,* 346–359.

Graber, J. A., Lewinsohn, P. M., Seeley, J. R., & Brooks-Gunn, J. (1997). Is psycho-pathology associated with the timing of pubertal development? *Journal of American Academy of Child and Adolescent Psychiatry, 36,* 1768–1776.

Grayson, D. A. (1989). Twins reared together: Minimizing shared environmental effects. *Behavior Genetics, 19,* 605–608.

Hoel, D. G., Wakabayashi, T., & Pike, M. C. (1983). Secular trends in the distributions of the breast cancer risk factors—menarche, first birth, menopause, and weight—in Hiroshima and Nagasaki, Japan. *American Journal of Epidemiology, 118,* 78–89.

Hughes, P. E., Philip, G., & Siswadi, R. (1997). The effects of contact frequency and transport on the efficacy of the boar effect. *Animal Reproduction Science, 46,* 159–165.

Hulanicka, B. (1999). Acceleration of menarcheal age of girls from dysfunctional families. *Journal of Reproductive and Infant Psychology, 17,* 119–132.

Hulanicka, B., Gronkiewicz, L., & Koniarek, J. (2001). Effect of familial distress on growth and maturation of girls: A longitudinal study. *American Journal of Human Biology, 13,* 771–776.

Jorm, A. F., Christensen, H., Rodgers, B., Jacomb, P. A., & Easteal, S. (2004). Association of adverse childhood experiences, age of menarche and adult reproductive behavior: Does the androgen receptor gene play a role? *American Journal of Medical Genetics Part B: Neuropsychiatric Genetics, 125,* 105–111.

Kadlubar, F. F., Berkowitz, G. S., Delongchamp, R. R., Wang, C., Green, B. L., Tang, G., et al. (2003). The CYP3A4*1B variant is related to the onset of puberty, a known risk factor for the development of breast cancer. *Cancer Epidemiology Biomarkers and Prevention, 12,* 327–331.

Kanazawa, S. (2001). Why father absence might precipitate early menarche: The role of polygyny. *Evolution and Human Behavior, 22,* 329–334.

Kantero, R. L., & Widholm, O. (1971). II. The age of menarche in Finnish girls in 1969. *Acta Obstetrica et Gynecologica Scandinavica, 14*(Suppl.), 7–18.

Kaplan, H. S., & Lancaster, J. B. (2003). An evolutionary and ecological analysis of human fertility, mating patterns, and parental investment. In K. W. Wachter & R. A. Bulatao (Eds.), *National Research Council (2003): Fertility behavior in biodemographic perspective* (pp. 170–223). Washington, DC: National Academy Press.

Kaprio, J., Rimpela, A., Winter, T., Viken, R. J., Rimpela, M., & Rose, R. J. (1995). Common genetic influences on BMI and age at menarche. *Human Biology, 67,* 739–753.

Kelsey, J. L., Gammon, M. D., & John, E. M. (1993). Reproductive factors and breast cancer. *Epidemiologic Reviews, 15,* 36–47.

Ketelaar, T., & Ellis, B. J. (2000). Are evolutionary explanations unfalsifiable? Evolutionary psychology and the Lakatosian philosophy of science. *Psychological Inquiry, 11,* 1–21.

Khan, A. D., Schroeder, D. G., Martorell, R., Haas, J. D., & Rivera, J. (1996). Early childhood determinants of age at menarche in rural Guatemala. *American Journal of Human Biology, 8,* 717–723.

Kim, K., & Smith, P. K. (1998). Childhood stress, behavioural symptoms and mother-daughter pubertal development. *Journal of Adolescence, 21,* 231–240.

Koziel, S., & Jankowska, E. A. (2002). Effect of low versus normal birthweight on menarche in 14-year-old Polish girls. *Journal of Paediatrics and Child Health, 38,* 268–271.

MacDonald, K. (1999). An evolutionary perspective on human fertility [Special issue: Perspectives on fertility and population size]. *Population and Environment: A Journal of Interdisciplinary Studies, 21,* 223–246.

Marcus, M. D., Loucks, T. L., & Berga, S. L. (2001). Psychological correlates of functional hypothalamic amenorrhea. *Fertility and Sterility, 76,* 310–316.

Marshall, L. M., Spiegelman, D., Goldman, M. B., Manson, J. E., Colditz, G. A., Barbieri, R. L., et al. (1998). A prospective study of reproductive factors and oral contraceptive use in relation to the risk of uterine leiomyomata. *Fertility and Sterility, 70,* 432–439.

McPherson, C. P., Sellers, T. A., Potter, J. D., Bostick, R. M., & Folsom, A. R. (1996). Reproductive factors and risk of endometrial cancer: The Iowa Women's Health Study. *American Journal of Epidemiology, 143,* 1195–1202.

Meyer, F., Moisan, J., Marcoux, D., & Bouchard, C. (1990). Dietary and physical determinants of menarche. *Epidemiology, 1,* 377–381.

Miller, E. M. (1994). Optimal adjustment of mating effort to environmental conditions: A critique of Chisholm's application of life history theory, with comments on race differences in male paternal investment strategies. *Mankind Quarterly, 34,* 297–316.

Moffitt, T. E., Caspi, A., Belsky, J., & Silva, P. A. (1992). Childhood experience and the onset of menarche: A test of a sociobiological model. *Child Development, 63,* 47–58.

Nappi, R. E., & Facchinetti, F. (2003). Psychoneuroendocrine correlates of secondary amenorrhea. *Archives of Women's Mental Health, 6,* 83–89.

Olivier, G., & Devigne, G. (1983). Biology and social structure. *Journal of Biosocial Science, 15,* 379–389.

Parent, A. S., Teilmann, G., Juul, A., Skakkebaek, N. E., Toppari, J., & Bourguignon, J. P. (2003). The timing of normal puberty and the age limits of sexual precocity: Variations around the world, secular trends, and changes after migration. *Endocrine Review, 24,* 668–693.

Qamra, S. R., Mehta, S., & Deodhar, S. D. (1991). A mixed-longitudinal study on the pattern of pubertal growth: Relationship to socioeconomic status and caloric-intake—IV. *Indian Pediatrics, 28,* 147–156.

Quinlan, R. J. (2003). Father absence, parental care, and female reproductive development. *Evolution and Human Behavior, 24,* 376–390.

Rivier, C., & Rivest, S. (1991). Effect of stress on the activity of the hypothalamic-pituitary-gonadal axis: Peripheral and central mechanisms. *Biology of Reproduction, 45,* 523–532.

Roff, D. (1992). *The evolution of life histories: Theory and analysis.* New York: Chapman & Hall.

Rowe, D. C. (2000a). Environmental and genetic influences on pubertal development: Evolutionary life history traits. In J. L. Rodgers, D. C. Rowe, & W. B. Miller (Eds.), *Genetic influences on human fertility and sexuality: Theoretical and empirical contributions from the biological and behavioral sciences* (pp. 147–168). Boston: Kluwer Academic.

Rowe, D. C. (2000b). Review of the book *Death, hope and sex: Steps to an evolutionary ecology of mind and morality. Evolution and Human Behavior, 21,* 347–364.

Rowe, D. C. (2002). On genetic variation in menarche and age at first sexual intercourse: A critique of the Belsky-Draper hypothesis. *Evolution and Human Behavior, 23,* 365–372.

Rowe, D. C., Jacobson, K. C., & Van den Oord, E. J. C. G. (1999). Genetic and environmental influences on vocabulary IQ: Parental education level as moderator. *Child Development, 70*, 1151–1162.

Sellers, T. A., Kushi, L. H., Potter, J. D., Kaye, S. A., Nelson, C. L., McGovern, P. G., et al. (1992). Effect of family history, body-fat distribution, and reproductive factors on the risk of postmenopausal breast cancer. *New England Journal of Medicine, 326*, 1323–1329.

Shonkoff, J., & Phillips, D. (2000). *From neurons to neighbourhoods: The science of early child development*. Washington, DC: National Academy Press.

Stavrou, I., Zois, C., Ioannidis, J. P., & Tsatsoulis, A. (2002). Association of polymorphisms of the oestrogen receptor alpha gene with the age of menarche. *Human Reproduction, 17*, 1101–1105.

Stearns, S. (1992). *The evolution of life histories*. Oxford, UK: Oxford University Press.

Stearns, S., & Koella, J. C. (1986). The evolution of phenotypic plasticity in life-history traits: Predictions of reaction norms for age and size at maturity. *Evolution, 40*, 893–913.

Steinberg, L. (1988). Reciprocal relation between parent–child distance and pubertal maturation. *Developmental Psychology, 24*, 122–128.

Surbey, M. K. (1990). Family composition, stress, and the timing of human menarche. In T. E. Ziegler & F. B. Bercovitch (Eds.), *Socioendocrinology of primate reproduction* [Monographs in Primatology, 13, pp. 11–32]. New York: Wiley-Liss.

Surbey, M. K. (1998). Parent and offspring strategies in the transition at adolescence. *Human Nature, 9*, 67–94.

Tanner, J. M. (1962). *Growth and adolescence* (2nd ed.). Oxford, UK: Blackwell Scientific.

Tanner, J. M. (1990). *Fetus into man* (2nd ed.). Cambridge, MA: Harvard University Press.

Thompson, L. H., & Savage, J. S. (1978). Age at puberty and ovulation rate in gilts in confinement as influenced by exposure to a boar. *Journal of Animal Science, 47*, 1141–1144.

Treloar, S. A., & Martin, N. G. (1990). Age at menarche as a fitness trait: Nonadditive genetic variance detected in a large twin sample. *American Journal of Human Genetics, 47*, 137–148.

Turkheimer, E., Haley, A., Waldron, M., D'Onofrio, B., & Gottesman, I. I. (2003). Socioeconomic status modifies heritability of IQ in young children. *Psychological Science, 14*, 623–628.

Udry, J. R. (1979). Age at menarche, at first intercourse, and at first pregnancy. *Journal of Biosocial Science, 11*, 433–441.

Udry, J. R., & Cliquet, R. L. (1982). A cross-cultural examination of the relationship between ages at menarche, marriage, and first birth. *Demography, 19*, 53–63.

van den Akker, O. B. A., Stein, G. S., Neale, M. C., & Murray, R. M. (1987). Genetic and environmental variation in menstrual cycle: Histories of two British twin samples. *Acta Geneticae Medicae et Gemellologiae (Roma), 36*, 541–548.

van Noord, P. A., & Kaaks, R. (1991). The effect of wartime conditions and the 1944–45 "Dutch famine" on recalled menarcheal age in participants of the DOM breast cancer screening project. *Annals of Human Biology, 18*, 57–70.

Veronesi, F. M., & Gueresi, P. (1994). Trend in menarcheal age and socioeconomic influence in Bologna (northern Italy). *Annals of Human Biology, 21*, 187–196.

Voland, E. (1998). Evolutionary ecology of human reproduction. *Annual Review of Anthropology, 27,* 347–374.

Wasser, S. K., & Barash, D. P. (1983). Reproductive suppression among female mammals: Implications for biomedicine and sexual selection theory. *Quarterly Review of Biology, 58,* 513–538.

Wellens, R., Malina, R., Beunen, G., & Lefevre, J. (1990). Age at menarche in Flemish girls: Current status and secular change in the 20th century. *Annals of Human Biology, 17,* 145–152.

Wellens, R., Malina, R., Roche, A., Chumlea, W., Guo, S., & Siervogel, R. (1992). Body size and fatness in young adults in relation to age at menarche. *American Journal of Human Biology, 4,* 913–924.

West-Eberhard, M. (2003). *Developmental plasticity and evolution.* Oxford, UK: Oxford University Press.

Wilson, M., & Daly, M. (1997). Life expectancy, economic inequality, homicide, and reproductive timing in Chicago neighbourhoods. *British Medical Journal, 314,* 1271–1274.

Worthman, C. M. (1999). Evolutionary perspectives on the onset of puberty. In W. Trevethan, E. O. Smith, & J. J. McKenna (Eds.), *Evolutionary medicine* (pp. 135–163). New York: Oxford University Press.

Wu, M. L., Whittemore, A. S., Paffenbarger, R. S., Jr., Sarles, D. L., Kampert, J. B., Grosser, S., et al. (1988). Personal and environmental characteristics related to epithelial ovarian cancer: I. Reproductive and menstrual events and oral contraceptive use. *American Journal of Epidemiology, 128,* 1216–1227.

8

SOME FUNCTIONAL ASPECTS OF HUMAN ADOLESCENCE

GLENN E. WEISFELD
HEATHER C. JANISSE

DEVELOPING A FUNCTIONAL THEORY OF HUMAN ADOLESCENCE

Aside from psychoanalytic theories, which have met with rather severe criticism from contemporary scholars, theories of specific stages of the lifespan have been notable for their rarity. Theories of adolescence have been especially lacking, so that research proceeds on particular topics but without much conceptual guidance. The closest thing to an accepted, general theory of adolescence is probably that of Piaget, but his is a specifically cognitive theory that largely neglects social and emotional behavior, among other limitations. Lacking a general theory of human adolescence, most textbooks mainly cover individual differences in, say, drug use or academic success. Statements are largely restricted to U.S. adolescents, and hence beg the question of whether or not they are also true of adolescents elsewhere, whether they are universal, and whether they are true of adolescents in other primate species as well. Thus, we need a framework, or context, for understanding human adolescence and its normal and pathological variants.

This chapter constitutes an essay into the still largely uncharted terrain of human adolescence. It addresses the following questions: What is true of most adolescents everywhere? What features distinguish adolescents from older and younger individuals? What are the phylogenetic origins of these universals of adolescence? What are the functions of these features of normal adolescence? We describe pubertal development, puberty rites, the adolescent's family context, peer competition, and mate choice from a comparative, functional perspective.

In order to identify these basic features of human adolescence, it is necessary to identify those adolescent traits with an evolved basis. It is sometimes stated that the nature–nurture distinction is chimerical, that all behaviors are compounded of inseparable genetic and environmental influences. The latter is certainly true, but there still remains the very real distinction between traits that are part of the evolved equipment of a species and traits that arise because of atypical experience. As evolutionists, we want to know whether, in the old parlance, a trait is innate or learned. This attention to evolutionary questions is what distinguishes us from other developmentalists, including those who acknowledge neural and hormonal factors in behavioral development.

In *The Expressions of the Emotions in Man and Animals*, Darwin (1872/1965) introduced his classic research strategies for identifying behaviors with evolved bases. These include testing for specieswide prevalence, for presence in phylogenetically related species, for stereotypy (an indicator of a specific, purpose-built genetic mechanism), and for early onset (or presence even with crucial deprivation experience). As research on physiology expanded, testing for a specific neural or hormonal mechanism was added to this research toolkit. For further discussion, see Archer (1992), Lorenz (1965), and Weisfeld (1999).

Once an evolved trait is identified, its function can be investigated. It is often claimed that many specieswide traits are not adaptive, and never were, that they arose by genetic drift, pleiotropy, or linkage to adaptive traits, and somehow remained in the genome. We would argue that a specieswide trait is adaptive until proven otherwise. Consider specieswide anatomical traits, whose functions are better known than those of behavioral traits. What superfluous anatomical structures do we humans possess? The candidate that is usually proposed is the vermiform appendix. This structure no longer serves its original function of aiding in digestion of raw meat. However, it is still functional; it is now part of the immune system and is filled with lymphatic tissue. Nature does not saddle us with purposeless anatomical, physiological, or behavioral traits that would waste valuable bodily energy. Even the tiny and nonnutritive male nipple may function to attract or reassure infants. The seemingly random convolutions of the outer ear actually serve to amplify sounds in the register of the human voice. Even if we are ignorant of the function of a given specieswide anatomical or behavioral trait, it is likely that there is one, or was one in prehistory. As we continue to discover the functions of various specieswide traits, such as fever, which kills pathogens, the notion that many of these features lack function will become ever less plausible. Some features may be side effects of adaptive alleles, but selection will tend to suppress these side effects even if some are inevitable; thus, the overall impact of a common allele will almost always be beneficial. Moreover, precisely neutral traits are improbable; any structure or behavior consumes calories and is therefore deleterious unless counteracted by some benefit, which is unlikely to exactly equal its cost.

Functional analysis is an empirical undertaking. A functional hypothesis is proposed, even guessed at, but then must be tested. This is usually done by first delineating the extent, or distribution, of the trait. The trait may be present in all vertebrates, or all female mammals, or all mature Old World primates. Whatever its distribution, the hypothesized function must account for that particular pattern, just as the source of an epidemic of food poisoning is traced systematically by determining what foods the victims ate that were not consumed by the nonvictims. If the proposed functional explanation does not account for some animals that lack the trait or for presence of the trait elsewhere, the explanation must be rejected or modified.

Functional explanations can also be tested by determining their ability to account for the precise features of the trait. Last, a functional explanation can be tested by seeing what happens to fitness if the trait is absent, as in Tinbergen's (1963) experiment of gluing eggshell fragments into the nest so the parent could not discard them, and observing an increase in predation on the hatchlings. These various functional methods are illustrated by analysis of morning sickness. Profet (1992) hypothesized that emesis during pregnancy protects the fetus against toxins. Since all fetuses are vulnerable to toxins, we would expect to find emesis commonly during pregnancy in other human cultures and mammals, which indeed is the case (Flaxman & Sherman, 2000). The fact that morning sickness occurs mainly in the first trimester, when the fetus is most vulnerable to toxins, parasites, and microorganisms, is also evidence in favor of this explanation, as is the particular aversion to foods commonly high in toxicity, such as spices, alcohol, meat, and fish. Last, the demonstration that women with more severe morning sickness are less likely to miscarry clinches the case.

Functional analysis can sometimes explain a pattern of cross-cultural diversity. For example, adult status is conferred on young men at different average ages in different societies, but a pattern exists. Adult status tends to be enhanced by eligibility to marry (van den Berghe, 1980). In societies in which men require many years to accumulate sufficient wealth or economic skills to afford marriage, adult status usually comes relatively late. Thus, cultural differences can best be explained in functional terms rather than as historical accidents, or the consequences of linguistic features or belief systems. Practices that enhance reproductive success under extant ecological conditions will tend to prevail in a population. Note that such a practice need not have any specific evolved basis; nevertheless, individuals or populations that embrace the practice will gain a selective advantage and it will spread.

An evolutionary theory of adolescence must use these research strategies to identify the general, specieswide features of adolescence and specify their functions. This means that research on adolescence in other cultures and species, and on the effects of pubertal hormones, is especially valuable. These sources of information reveal many examples of specieswide characteristics of human adolescents. General statements about adolescence, to the extent that they can be established, will provide a functional framework for viewing this stage of life.

PUBERTY, THE KEYSTONE OF ADOLESCENCE

Sex Differentiation during Puberty

Probably the most obvious universal of adolescence is puberty. The body undergoes a gradual but profound metamorphosis at puberty. Appetite increases in adolescent boys and girls concomitantly with their growth spurts. The ravenous appetite of the adolescent is an obvious fact, but it serves to illustrate the point that bodily and behavioral developmental changes act in concert; they are functionally compatible. This implies that knowledge of the bodily changes of puberty can inform us about the behavioral changes. Similarly, the sequence of pubertal developments in each sex is quite invariant, again demonstrating the adaptive importance of concerted ontogenetic sequences and not just arrival at the final adult form. The organism must survive at each step of the way, and not just reach adulthood. For this reason, the notion that adolescents pass through an "awkward stage" in which some bodily features are temporarily out of sync with others is unrealistic.

Likewise, sex differentiation of the body must generally be compatible with sex differentiation of behavior. For example, in many species, the males become more aggressive, as well as larger, at reproductive maturity. Their greater size would do them little good if it were not matched by an increase in aggressiveness, and vice versa. In humans, sex differentiation in body and behavior, although in evidence throughout ontogeny (Bjorklund & Pellegrini, 2002), becomes pronounced at puberty. Before puberty, the sexes are quite similar (Willner & Martin, 1985); after puberty, hardly anything can be said about adolescents that applies equally to boys and girls. In fact, the dearth of compelling theories about adolescence may stem partly from failure to fully appreciate behavioral sex differences and their hormonal roots.

Sex differences emerge or intensify at puberty in libido, spatial skills, verbal skills, strength, sensory acuities, nurturance, and aggression, among other behaviors (Hoyenga & Hoyenga, 1979, 1993). Gonadal hormones are known to contribute to most of these sex differences (Hampson, 2002; Kimura, 1999). This evidence, plus the fact that many of these sex differences are cross-cultural or present in other mammals too (Christiansen, 1998; Kimura, 1999; Mitchell, 1981), suggests that they are likely to have evolved bases. Hormones can affect adolescents' behavior directly, not just by altering their body and thus changing others' reactions to them (e.g., Nottelmann, Inoff-Germain, Susman, & Chrousos, 1990). Furthermore, others' reactions to an adolescent's observable transformation may themselves have evolved bases. For example, in many species, male maturity markers antagonize males and attract females. Evidence of similar effects of human bodily traits and pheromones is accumulating (see below).

Why is sex differentiation so marked at puberty? Puberty constitutes sexual maturation; it prepares males and females to fulfill their specialized reproductive roles. In old age, as fertility and gonadal hormone levels decline, sex differentiation is again reduced. The general function of adolescence, then, may be said to be reproductive maturation, successful transformation into a reproductively competent male or female (see Charlesworth, 1988; Schlegel, 1995). Primatologists define *adolescence* as the period from the onset of puberty to the attainment of fertility (Pereira & Altmann, 1985). Before maturity, the child depends heavily on parents and others for assistance. After maturity, adolescents themselves become, potentially, the parents of dependents. Given the great amount of parental care exhibited by our species, this constitutes a radical transformation that entails dramatic changes in body and behavior.

Patterns of Growth

The growth spurt is a uniquely primate feature (Janson & van Schaik, 1993; Jones, Martin, & Pilbeam, 1992; Worthman, 1993). Most other mammals follow a smooth growth trajectory, growing fast initially and then leveling off as maturity approaches. The growth spurt is more pronounced in the male in most primates, because males need to be larger than females (referred to as *sexual size dimorphism*) in order to fight for mates. There may not be much of a female growth spurt in most primates. However, the large size of the human fetus necessitates an appreciable growth spurt in girls in order to allow parturition (Harvey & Clutton-Brock, 1985). The primate growth spurt is thought to compensate for another uniquely primate trait, the juvenile growth plateau that precedes the growth spurt. So it is slow juvenile growth that is fundamental and requires explanation.

Monkeys and apes remain small as juveniles for several adaptive reasons (Pereira & Altmann, 1985). Their small size is advantageous for traveling on thin branches and for conserving calories. Primates can afford to remain small because they are protected from most predators by their arboreality or, in many terrestrial species, by their mother and adult males. Small size also reduces the need for food competition with older animals. Much of the metabolic energy that other, faster growing mammals devote to foraging and growth is devoted by primates to play. Primate behavior is extremely flexible, so monkeys and apes need to play extensively in order to learn how to develop this behavioral versatility. Play is particularly variegated in human children (Bjorklund & Pellegrini, 2002; Smith, Chapter 11, this volume).

A related aspect of the primate pattern of growth is delayed maturation. Juvenile primates not only grow slowly but also grow for a comparatively long time. Why this delay in reaching maturity and in beginning reproductive life? Delayed maturity is thought to allow time for learning. Juvenile primates learn how to select food, locomote through trees, identify predators, and care for their young (Janson & van Schaik, 1993). Enhanced survival and care of offspring compensate for the delay in beginning reproduction.

The juvenile growth plateau is especially protracted in humans, who reach puberty about 3 years later than chimpanzees (Goodall, 1986) and begin to reproduce about 6 years later (Bjorklund & Pellegrini, 2002). Our hominid ancestors evidently benefited from a very long period of learning before maturity. This long period of dependency both necessitated efficient parental behavior and permitted time for developing skills for provisioning and protecting the young, and of course, for survival (Bogin, 1999; see also Flinn & Ward, Chapter 2, this volume). In particular, the extraordinarily long period of immaturity and brain flexibility may have allowed hominids to learn to hunt and to forage for roots and tubers (Kaplan, Hill, Lancaster, & Hurtado, 2000). Tool-using humans have been calculated to extract about twice the calories from a savannah habitat as nonhuman primates (Bogin, 1988). Other skills may not require prolonged practice but are improved by increased size, strength, and walking speed (Bird & Bird, 2002a, 2002b; Blurton Jones & Marlowe, 2002). In addition, human social relationships are highly complex and presumably require time and cognitive sophistication to develop (e.g., Bjorklund & Pellegrini, 2002). Consistent with the technical and social complexity of hominid life, the human brain is two to three times as large as that of the chimpanzee (Jerison, 1973).

Puberty in Boys

Both sexes undergo a juvenile growth plateau and adolescent growth spurt; this pattern is one of the *monomorphic* changes of puberty. However, males take longer to reach adult size than do females, because their ancestors needed more time to grow and also to master fighting skills and hunting techniques. Play fighting is the main factor accounting for the greater playfulness of male primates than females, and their longer (earlier and later) juvenile play period (Walters, 1987). The period of play fighting is regulated by testosterone, much as the growth spurt is started and ended mainly by gonadal hormones; castrated male rhesus monkeys continued to play to an older age (Mitchell, 1981).

Puberty prepares boys to compete for mates and enter into married life and parenthood. Secondarily, large size and greater strength may have allowed hominid males to become better hunters and defenders of the family, and stronger laborers. Pubertal boys also become hairier. Why? Comparative analysis often reveals the function of this trait. Dark, thick, curly, conspicuous hair of the type that covers men's bodies generally functions in mammals to exaggerate body size and hence intimidate rivals (Guthrie, 1976). In primates, anatomical features that are important in fighting, such as the jaws, chest, and shoulders, are often especially hirsute. Similarly, men's deep voices, deep-set eyes, and large jaws constitute general primate threat or dominance features that attract females and intimidate males (Keating, 1985). These morphological changes are complemented by an increase in dominance aggression enhanced by testosterone (Ellis, 1986). Observational research indicates that adolescent boys become rougher in their competition (Boulton, 1992; Cairns, Cairns, Neckerman, Ferguson, & Gariepy, 1989; Loeber & Hay, 1997; Neill, 1985), just as aggressiveness and mate competition increase in the maturing males of many other species. In no culture studied are adolescent girls more competitive than boys (Schlegel, 1995). Another observational study revealed that adolescent boys were more inclined than girls to use force and threats of force against rivals (Savin-Williams, 1987).

Puberty in Girls

Puberty in girls likewise functions mainly to prepare them for reproduction. The reproductive "tasks" that females must perform include attracting and selecting a desirable mate, and bearing and caring for children effectively. Adolescent girls undergo widening of the pelvis for childbirth, accumulate subcutaneous fat to fuel pregnancy and lactation, become attractive to males and infants, and begin to evaluate males as possible mates (Tanner, 1990). Other clearly adaptive pubertal changes in girls have also been documented. Women surpass men in remembering the location of objects, a skill of value in gathering plant food, their ancestral livelihood (Silverman & Phillips, 1993). By contrast, males excel at finding their way and at hurling projectiles accurately, skills that would have aided them in hunting and warfare (Kimura, 1999). Women tend to surpass men in manual dexterity, which is useful for gathering plants and for delicate handiwork (Kimura, 1999). They also exceed men on verbal and nonverbal communication tasks; these skills would be especially advantageous in teaching and raising (preverbal) infants and children (Babchuk, Hames, & Thompson, 1985).

Cross-cultural evidence suggests that girls, like other female primates, also become more attracted to infants at puberty (Coe, 1990; Goldberg, Blumberg, & Kriger, 1982). However, throughout the lifespan, females perform more parental care than males in all cultures and all mammals (Daly & Wilson, 1983; Friedl, 1975; Schlegel & Barry, 1991). Various pubertal, pregnancy, and lactational hormones, including estrogens, progesterone, oxytocin, and prolactin, have been implicated in human maternal behavior (Altemus, Deuster, Galliven, Carter, & Gold, 1995; Uvnas-Moberg, 1997). But men, like a few other male mammals, typically aid their own offspring as well. Rising levels of prolactin and falling levels of testosterone during his mate's pregnancy seem to render a man more parental, as is the case in other paternal mammals (Storey, Walsh, Quinton, & Wynne-Edwards, 2000).

The male specialization in family defense may have allowed females to be smaller than they would have been otherwise (Willner & Martin, 1985). Similarly, the less threatening size and more pedomorphic (juvenile) appearance of females may help make them less frequent targets for aggression (McArthur & Berry, 1987). The generally greater sensory acuity and fearfulness of females can also be interpreted as adaptive for the less muscular and aggressive—but more parental—sex (Baker, 1987; Campbell, 1999). Another advantage of sexual size dimorphism is that food competition is reduced between females and males if they eat somewhat different foods; for example, men show a greater preference for protein-rich foods than do women, and women prefer carbohydrates more than do men. Females mature earlier than males (*sexual bimaturism*) partly because this allows them to embark on reproduction sooner. Because mammalian gestation is lengthy, females need to maximize their reproductive span; on the other hand, males can afford a delay in maturation if it results in greater success in competing for mates.

Other Pubertal Changes in Both Sexes

Some pubertal changes involve pheromones that affect courtship and male rivalry. Pair-bonding is enhanced by a steroid present on men's skin, androstadienone, which when introduced intranasally produces contentment and physiological relaxation in women (Monti-Bloch, 1999). Male axillary odors help to induce ovulation (Cutler et al., 1986) and to draw women to men (Cowley & Brooksbank, 1991). Women become more attracted to men's odors at ovulation, when they are fertile. In turn, pheromones that are present in vaginal secretions at ovulation raise men's testosterone levels, thereby aiding sperm production and libido (Grammer, 1996). Thus, pheromones coordinate and prime sexual behavior. The axillary odors of mature males also repel rivals, being literally offensive. This occurs in male chimpanzees too, and likewise under conditions of social tension (Guthrie, 1976). Sensitivity to male pheromones increases at puberty in boys and girls (Baker, 1987), and long, thin hairs of the form that disperse pheromones in mammals appear in the axillae and groins of boys and girls (Guthrie, 1976).

In addition, male and female adolescents develop the sex drive, whose intensity gradually increases with the rise in androgens. But they also become romantically motivated; they seek to establish pair-bonds. Development of libido and amorousness may stem from a rise in dihydroepiandrosterone (DHEA) from the adrenal cortex during late childhood (McClintock & Herdt, 1996). This hormone also seems to be involved in the rise in gonadal hormones that leads to most of the somatic changes of puberty. Oxytocin, a pituitary hormone, seems to consolidate social bonds; it is released at orgasm in both sexes, and during parturition and lactation.

The sequencing of pubertal changes is adaptive. The first stage of male puberty consists of development of the internal and external genitalia, including penile growth and sperm production. Why do boys begin sperm production before their bodies are fully grown? If bodies matured first, then boys would be using their mature bodies to fight for mates—without being fertile! By beginning sperm production first, a male may perchance succeed in fertilizing some females even before he can successfully fight with mature males. In the later stages of puberty, boys become larger, more muscular, and more intimidating to aid them in face-to-face competition with rivals. On the other hand, girls do not reach fertility until their bodies are almost fully grown and capable of childbearing. Fertility is one of the last changes of puberty in girls. A pregnancy before the pelvis is wide enough for parturition might be fatal.

A related example of analysis of sequences of development concerns initiation of sexual behavior. Although fertility in girls does not occur until late in puberty, and then increases only gradually until the early 20s, their external genitals become functional early in the sequence of pubertal events. Sexual lures such as pubic hair and the breasts also develop very early, as do the vaginal rugae, which stimulate the penis. Pubic hair and the mons veneris also presumably protect the skin during intercourse. This developmental pattern suggests that in prehistory, sexual experimentation by girls typically began early in puberty. Cross-cultural data confirm that adolescent sexual experimentation is normative in most traditional cultures (Broude & Greene, 1976; Murdock, 1949). Likewise, boys become capable of orgasm about a year before they produce semen, and fertility increases gradually thereafter. Early sexual experimentation may have provided practice in sex and courtship, and in assessing one's own and others' mate value. Girls in prehistory may also have received gifts in exchange for sex.

Individual and Cultural Differences

The interplay of hormonal and experiential factors in individual differences in behavior is illustrated by research on the development of sexual behavior in adolescents. Individual differences in testosterone level are associated with the strength of libido in adolescents of both sexes (Cashdan, 1995; Udry, 1988). The fact that males' testosterone levels eventually become about 10 times those of women partially accounts for the greater urgency of the male libido, although there is a ceiling effect beyond which further increases do not raise libido (Christiansen, 1998). But U.S. adolescent girls' sex drive is also affected appreciably by their attitudes toward sexual experimentation—which is not true for boys, whose libido was correlated mainly with testosterone level (Udry, 1988). On the other hand, the age of onset of sexual activity for boys depends considerably on their attractiveness to girls and not just their testosterone level (Udry & Billy, 1987). Girls' onset of sexual activity was associated mainly with attitudes. Udry's research is noteworthy for its measurement of the respective contributions of hormone levels and attitudes to behavior.

Hormones affect behavior, but various experiences can alter hormone levels too, thus resulting in individual differences in pubertal development. Most stressors raise corticosteroid levels and lower the levels of growth hormone and gonadotropins, thereby sometimes retarding growth and sexual maturation (see Ellis, Chapter 7, this volume). But hormone levels continue to respond to environmental factors after puberty is attained. Stressors can interfere with reproductive physiology in mature men and women. Also, in mammals generally, testosterone rises in competitive situations to mobilize the individual for aggression. Youth who lived in violent neighborhoods tended to have higher testosterone levels than those living in peaceful ones, controlling for various factors (Mazur & Booth, 1998). Similarly, when men marry, their testosterone levels tend to fall as they withdraw from mating competition—and to rise again if they divorce.

PUBERTY RITES

Just as body and behavior must be functionally compatible, the genetic and cultural programs need to mesh for the successful survival and reproduction of the organism. This notion is illustrated by puberty rites, which may be regarded as a cultural growth spurt analogous to the changes of puberty; both provide intensive preparation for adulthood. Therefore, functional analysis of the various features of puberty rites may reveal some general characteristics of adolescence. Although only 56% of preliterate cultures have a formal initiation ceremony (Schlegel & Barry, 1980), virtually all have an intensive training period before induction into adulthood (Schlegel & Barry, 1991; Weisfeld, 1997), and so puberty rites, broadly construed, are a constant of adolescence.

Puberty rites vary widely across cultures, because different environments demand the cultivation of different skills and behaviors, but some general patterns emerge in research on traditional cultures. Initiates are tutored in sex-specific adult economic, familial, and cultural skills. The same-sex parent is typically the main teacher of subsistence skills, but the initiate is tutored by some other same-sex adult in social and ceremonial matters (Schlegel & Barry, 1991). In addition, puberty rites usually entail some challenging or hazardous ordeal that boys, in particular, must endure. This is analogous to the more rigorous competition that males, as opposed to females, undergo to reproduce. Boys also have to refine their economic skills in order to compete for a wife, such as by paying a bride price or performing bride service. Consistent with this interpretation, the theme of boys' initiation rites is typically graduation, rebirth, or accomplishment (Hotvedt, 1990). The theme for girls' rites is usually fertility or beauty (Sommer, 1978). Thus, for both sexes, traits important for reproductive success are valued. Interestingly, for both sexes, initiation occurs shortly before the onset of fertility, thus underscoring the significance of this institution as a preparation for family responsibilities.

Several other features of puberty rites seem to be functionally analogous to various pubertal changes. The sexes are invariably segregated during the training period, just as primates, including children, spontaneously sex segregate before puberty and often are drawn to older, same-sex models (Goodall, 1986; Mackey, 1983). Sex segregation doubtlessly aids acquisition of sex roles in traditional cultures and other primate species, as do the bodily and behavioral changes of pubertal sex differentiation. Also, initiates usually have their bodies specially marked, much as primates take on adult bodily features that signal sexual maturity.

Initiates are separated from their parents as well, just as mature simians distance themselves from their mothers and increasingly spend time with peers. Emotional distance from parents also increases in human adolescents (Silverberg & Steinberg, 1987). Parent–adolescent distancing in humans may be promoted by pubertal hormones, as suggested by observational research on family conflict. As adolescents enter puberty, discussions with their parents (especially the mother) tend to increase in acrimony (Hill, Holmbeck, Marlow, Green, & Lynch, 1985; Holmbeck & Hill, 1991; Sagrestano, McCormick, Paikoff, & Holmbeck, 1999; Steinberg, 1987). Fewer explanations are offered, and more harsh words are exchanged. Contentiousness peaks and self-disclosure dips at the height of the adolescent growth spurt (Rivenbark, 1971), suggesting that these trends are driven either directly by hormonal effects on behavior or indirectly by the bodily changes of puberty triggering perceptual changes in the parents. Offering support for this view are studies by Molina and Chassin (1996) and Sagrestano et al. (1999). These researchers found the effects of puberty to be present after controlling for chronological age.

Parent–child conflict tends to be harshest between mother and son (Montemayor & Hanson, 1985; Paikoff & Brooks-Gunn, 1991; Silverberg, 1989). After the velocity of growth peaks, conflict usually subsides. However, at this point, adolescent sons tend to win most arguments with their mothers, whereas previously the mothers usually prevailed (Jacob, 1974; Steinberg, 1987). In effect, mother and adolescent son reverse their dominance relationship, just as happens in chimpanzees (Goodall, 1986). Dominance reversal between sons and mothers probably occurs universally, in that in all cultures, males are assigned higher status than females, and youth defers to age (Stephens, 1963). By contrast, human mothers remain dominant over daughters, and fathers over sons and daughters. Parent–adolescent distancing and renegotiation of dominance relations may be necessary for adolescents to gain appropriate independence from their parents. Given the ubiquity of this adaptive problem, a genetic basis for this separation probably evolved gradually. It is likely that some dependable, hormonally based mechanism provided a basis for parent–adolescent distancing, although cultural and individual factors probably modify it.

Adolescents may come into conflict with parents for other reasons, of course. Adolescents possess the independence of thought and critical thinking skills to challenge their parents, and are less dependent on them, and so can risk confrontations. Furthermore, being more independent, adolescents can better pursue their own genetically based impulses, to seek a personally congenial environment, perhaps leading to conflict with parents.

In addition, adolescents may exhibit little kin altruism, because they are preoccupied with their own reproductive interests. By contrast, grandparents tend to be quite devoted to their grandchildren and other kin. They are past their reproductive years and so can only increase the representation of their genes in subsequent generations by practicing kin altruism. For example, postmenopausal Hadza women in Tanzania worked even more than childbearing women, allowing their daughters to have more and healthier children

(Hawkes, O'Connell, & Blurton Jones, 1989). Adolescent Hadza boys, by contrast, shared some food with siblings but also engaged in gathering honey and in hunting, evidently in order to cultivate reputations that would make them desirable to girls (Blurton Jones, Hawkes, & O'Connell, 1997).

Other widespread features of puberty rites make functional sense too. Newly initiated youth often serve as warriors, just as young male monkeys are forced to the periphery of the group to act as sentinels and shock troops (Chance & Jolly, 1970). These youth have undergone the rigors of puberty rites together, and have developed solidarity that will serve them well in warfare. They are unmarried and have no dependents, and so are somewhat expendable. Girls, on the other hand, are invariably initiated singly, as soon as they reach menarche. This ensures that a girl will be initiated, and hence eligible for marriage, just as she approaches the onset of fertility, when her *reproductive value* peaks: her expected future number of offspring (Daly & Wilson, 1983). She will then be most in demand as a bride; her mate value will peak too. By marrying such a woman, who cannot be carrying another man's child but has all of her childbearing years ahead of her, a man maximizes his reproductive prospects.

THE ADOLESCENT'S FAMILY CONTEXT
IN TRADITIONAL CULTURES

A virtually universal feature of not only forager societies but also all preliterate human societies is the extended family, if we define it as three generations of family members typically dwelling together or nearby (Stephens, 1963). Almost all of ancestral adolescents' social contacts would have been with kin, including clan members of more remote consanguinity. Through the genetic benefit of kin altruism, this arrangement would have rewarded cooperation in essential endeavors such as hunting, gathering, warfare, and child care. In addition, because foraging communities tend to be small (hunting requires low population density), ancestral human settlements were probably limited to no more than about 60 individuals (van den Berghe, 1980). Therefore, adolescents would have had few agemates and so would have socialized extensively with older and younger kin. Contact with neighboring bands and their adolescents (i.e., members of the same tribe sharing a language) would have occurred on occasion.

This pattern of age integration would have fostered adolescents' assisting and teaching younger children. In turn, there would have been ample opportunity for observing and being instructed by adults. Cross-cultural research suggests that contact with adult men tempers adolescent boys' aggressiveness (Schlegel, 2004). In most traditional cultures, children and adolescents perform important work for their families, especially instructing and supervising younger children (Cicirelli, 1994). As they grow older and more competent, they undertake increasingly difficult and valuable tasks, and their prestige increases concomitantly. For example, contemporary Mayan children become net producers during adolescence (Kramer & Boone, 1999). In traditional cultures, adolescents usually begin full-time work at ages 10–12 and assume an adult workload at ages 14–16 (Neill, 1983). The labor contributions of children and adolescents, unique among the primates, are thought to have allowed women to wean their children sooner and hence bear more children (Zeller, 1987).

Labor is strongly sex-segregated everywhere, with males and females undertaking tasks congruent with their interests, aptitudes, and training, and with practicalities such as distance from the settlement (Friedl, 1975; Murdock & Provost, 1973). In all preliterate cultures, women perform most of the domestic tasks, including child care, cooking, and cleaning, and men specialize in work requiring strength, such as handling heavy and hard materials (van den Berghe, 1980). Vestiges of this arrangement can be seen in modern society; men predominate in occupations requiring heavy manual labor and in the military, and women gravitate toward the service sector, which demands interpersonal skills at which females excel (Hall, 1984).

What sort of labor do adolescents perform specifically, and how does it aid the family economy? Hadza adolescent girls often dig for roots while tending younger siblings. This is an inefficient foraging technique, but it frees the mothers to forage more efficiently (Blurton Jones et al., 1997). In many preliterate cultures, adolescents do not perform arduous labor. In the !Kung of southern Africa, for example, adolescents are discouraged from working hard until about age 15 (Blurton Jones, Hawkes, & Draper, 1993). Evidently, the optimal reproductive strategy in this forager society is extensive care of offspring, including prolonged breast-feeding. This line of research suggests that cultural and individual differences in adolescent industriousness and other traits can sometimes be explained by ecological factors and labor availability (Bock, 2002; Kramer, 2002). One adolescent may be "lazy" because cultural selection has favored an easy life under his ecological or family circumstances. Another adolescent may be industrious because she will maximize her fitness by acquiring a reputation for industry, or by aiding kin. Adolescents apply themselves to subsistence activities, honing of skills, supervision of children, and courtship in patterns that vary across cultures and individuals, but this variation seems to fall into functional patterns.

PEER COMPETITION

Intensity of Competition

Competition for mates begins at reproductive maturity. As noted earlier, competition is especially intense among males, since the variation in reproductive success among males tends to exceed that among females—the Bateman effect, demonstrated in many species. In the adolescent sexual arena, a few boys gain many sex partners, and quite a few boys have none (Forrest &

Singh, 1990; Laumann, Gagnon, Michael, & Michaels, 1994). Adolescent boys are at a disadvantage in that they are competing against older, more established males. But competition is intense among girls too. Most have little trouble finding a sex partner, but what they ideally want is an exclusive relationship with one of the few highly desirable, pubertally mature boys. Female competition over males has been documented cross-culturally (Burbank, 1987) and in modern societies (Campbell, 1986). Adolescent girls are also under intense competitive pressure to marry while still young. Furthermore, both sexes are under intense competitive pressure, because few of them can secure their claim to a mate through marriage. Adolescent society is in effect promiscuous, especially early in adolescence, when sexual relationships tend to be brief. The precarious state of young breeders may help explain why primate mothers often preferentially back up a pregnant adolescent daughter in dominance encounters, thereby raising the latter's dominance rank above those of her older sisters (Hrdy, 1981).

Criteria of Success

In many species, males compete among themselves, and the females mate with the successful, dominant competitors (Ellis, 1995). Similarly, adolescent boys who are socially successful among their male peers also tend to be popular with girls (Miller, 1990; Weisfeld, Omark, & Cronin, 1980). And the same criteria that determine success among same-sex peers generally determine success among opposite-sex peers (Weisfeld et al., 1980; Dong, Weisfeld, Boardway, & Shen, 1996).

What are these criteria? As in other species, physical traits figure strongly for adolescents and adults of both sexes in various cultures (Buss, 1994; Ford & Beach, 1951; Weisfeld, Muczenski, Weisfeld, & Omark, 1987). Even well before puberty, boys who are dominant, popular leaders tend to be strong, athletic, handsome, and "tough" (Rodkin, Farmer, Pearl, & Van Acker, 2000). In a study of Québécois boys, ages 6–13 years, body mass and testosterone level each predicted dominance (Tremblay et al., 1998). Physical traits may be especially salient in settings with a minimum of adult supervision, such as street gangs (Feldman & Weisfeld, 1973). On the other hand, even in intellectually oriented U.S. high schools, athletic ability and physical attractiveness are paramount attributes of popular boys (Weisfeld, Bloch, & Ivers, 1983; Weisfeld et al., 1980). Physical traits are salient for girls' popularity too. Popular girls tend to be pretty, well-dressed, and nonaggressive (Merten, 1997; Tulkin, Muller, & Conn, 1969; Weisfeld, Bloch, & Ivers, 1984). The ubiquity of physical traits as criteria of social success suggests that there was some evolved advantage to seeking these attributes in a mate or ally. Health, vigor, and attractiveness in oneself, a spouse, or ally would be advantageous in any economy. Data indicate further that attractive individuals are likely to be healthy and highly fertile (Manning, Scutt, & Lewis-Jones. 1998; Shackelford & Larsen, 1999).

However, nonphysical traits may be important as well in peer judgments of both sexes. Chinese male and female adolescents admired intelligence in both sexes above all other traits measured (Dong et al., 1996). For centuries in China, success on written examinations has opened the way to desirable civil service jobs. Similarly, intelligence has been found to be salient for gaining respect among British (Boardway & Weisfeld, 1994) and Canadian (Brown, 1990) adolescents. It makes adaptive sense for mate choice to be influenced by local ecological and economic factors.

Both sexes prefer their mates to be somewhat more sex differentiated than average, physically and psychologically (reviewed in Weisfeld, 1999). Young women tend to like somewhat masculine men, just as young men like feminine women. Why this affinity for a sex-differentiated mate? The degree of sex differentiation of an organism reflects a compromise between the demands of reproductive physiology and of survival. Immature males and females of a given species resemble each other, because natural selection has molded their bodies to maximize survival in their common ecological niche. Likewise, in old age, men and women increasingly resemble each other as gonadal hormone levels decline. But as the reproductive years approach, as in human adolescence, the sexes differentiate markedly in order to allow reproduction, even at some risk of death. Reproductive competition is, after all, risky to the competitive male and the gestating female. In choosing a mate, an organism does not care about the mate's long-term survival as much as about short-term reproductive efficiency. Mates may stay together only briefly, so each takes a shorter term view of the other than does the other of itself. In other words, we are going to be with ourselves for the rest of our lives, and are profoundly interested in our long-term fitness. But our mate is mainly invested in our reproductive success together over what may prove to be a very short term. Therefore, a relatively high degree of sex differentiation is sought in a mate, because this will maximize one's reproductive success. This notion is similar to the genomic imprinting phenomenon that paternally active genes (derived from the father) tend to enhance fetal growth and survival, whereas maternally active genes promote kin altruism by the offspring, that is, survival of all of the mother's offspring (Trivers, 1997).

Pubertal Timing

Reasoning similar to that discussed earlier on the preference for strongly sex-differentiated mates would lead to the prediction that early-maturing mates would be preferred to late maturers. Speed of maturation depends partly on favorable gene–environment interaction during development. Individuals that enjoy a propitious developmental course will require less time to mature. These individuals will be in demand as mates because of their genetic quality, current healthiness, and longer projected reproductive span (including later menopause). Of course, there is a lower limit to the age of reproductive maturation, because the adolescent needs a minimal amount of time to develop essential skills for adult functioning.

Are early-maturing adolescents more popular than late maturers? This is clearly the case for boys; early maturity is associated with boys' social success among male and female peers (Graber, Lewinsohn, Seeley, & Brooks-Gunn, 1997; Jones & Bayley, 1950; Udry, 1987). However, longitudinal research shows that boys' social success among peers is a highly stable trait; therefore, early pubertal maturity does not itself cause a rise in social rank even though they are correlated (Bronson, 1966; Kagan & Moss, 1962; Weisfeld et al., 1987). In other words, socially dominant adolescent boys were dominant as children too. Moreover, these dominant, early-maturing boys were more sociable and cooperative even at age 38 (Livson & Peskin, 1980). Even if reaching puberty early confers a temporary advantage in strength and hence in athletics, it does not affect social ranks very much.

We are left with the conclusion that socially successful boys are attractive, tough, athletic, muscular, masculine, and early maturers; these traits are highly intercorrelated (reviewed in Weisfeld, 1999). One might expect, then, that natural selection would result in runaway selection for high testosterone production, which mediates this complex of traits. However, high testosterone production and strong sex differentiation are in a sense a luxury available only to those fortunate individuals whose development has been relatively unperturbed. In other words, the heritability of testosterone production is limited. Moreover, stabilizing selection seems to have operated, in that high testosterone levels are associated with more criminality (reviewed by Christiansen, 1998), earlier mortality (Hamilton & Mestler, 1969), lower income, less likelihood of marrying, and more marital instability (Booth & Dabbs, 1993; Dabbs, 1992)—the revenge of the nerds. Evidence suggests that men with lower testosterone levels also spend more time with their wives, apparently pursuing a mate-guarding or paternal investment ("dad") strategy more than a promiscuous ("cad") one (Baker & Bellis, 1995). Thus, uxoriousness may have a hormonal basis.

Early-maturing girls tend to be desirable as brides and to be reproductively successful (e.g., Borgerhoff Mulder, 1989). However, the consequences of early maturity for girls seem to be complicated by some unusual factors in U.S. society. Early-maturing American girls may experience some temporary distress as they enter puberty ahead of their peers (Faust, 1960). This may be due to embarrassment as a result of being obese, as they often are (Hayward et al., 1997; Simmons, Blyth, & McKinney, 1983). In Scotland, too, early maturing girls often were low in self-esteem and were concerned with their weight (Williams & Currie, 2000). Another possible source of embarrassment is the sexual connotations of puberty; the United States is relatively puritanical in its sexual attitudes compared with other Western nations. In Germany, for example, early-maturing girls seem not to suffer from low self-esteem (Silbereisen, Petersen, Albrecht, & Kracke, 1989). But even in the United States, whatever social or self-esteem problems early-maturing girls suffer are usually temporary. After age 11, these girls tend to be relatively popular and to suffer few sequelae. Moreover, they are popular with boys and with adults right from the start, and come to be popular with girls later, after age 12 and in adulthood (Faust, 1960; Jones & Mussen, 1958; Peskin & Livson, 1972; Simmons et al., 1983).

On the other hand, early-maturing girls are at risk of neglecting their studies and, in the United States and Europe, even engaging in delinquent behaviors (Silbereisen et al., 1989). This may be due partly to involvement with boys, since it was not observed in an all-girl school in New Zealand (Caspi, Lynam, Moffitt, & Silva, 1993) or in early-maturing Swedish girls who did not socialize with older adolescents (Magnusson, Stattin, & Allen, 1985). The values of adolescent peer culture and those of adults differ somewhat, so an adolescent may be popular with her peers at the expense of acceptance by adults, who are liable to regard her behavior as delinquent. In a U.S. study, early maturing adolescents were prone to use drugs, but were not especially distressed emotionally (Tschann et al., 1994).

Overall, attractive early maturers of both sexes are relatively successful with their peers. They enjoy many social advantages—they tend to be respected, attended to, relaxed, given leadership experience, and treated favorably—and usually continue to exercise social privileges throughout life and to develop positive social attributes (Charlesworth & Hartup, 1967; Coie & Kupersmidt, 1983). Physical attractiveness is a strong predictor of various measures of social success throughout the lifespan (Jackson, 1992). It is sometimes maintained that entering puberty, especially before one's peers, is traumatic—but, to the contrary, delayed puberty and hypogonadism, and even normal but late pubertal onset, are more typically associated with peer rejection and other psychological problems (Graber et al., 1994; Higham, 1980; Williams & Currie, 2000).

MATE CHOICE

Awareness of our ancestral way of life can help make sense of the cross-cultural commonalities in the criteria of mate choice and the correlates of marital satisfaction (Weisfeld & Weisfeld, 2002). Both sexes seek kindness in a mate, which is understandable given the ubiquitous strains of marriage and child rearing (Buss, 1994). They also seek a mate that they are likely to be able to retain, that is, one of similar mate value. Likewise, they seek someone who appears to be committed to them emotionally. And of course, like other species (Andersson, 1994), people tend to prefer a sexually mature, physically attractive mate, one who is likely to be healthy and fertile, and to carry high-quality genes. Naturally, not everyone can attract someone who is above average in desirability, so people usually wind up with mates who lack some ideal features, but the preferences that most people express are often clear and specific, and generally hold even across racial lines (Cunningham, 1986).

Human mates, including dating adolescents, tend to be similar on all sorts of traits, a finding that is difficult to explain solely in terms of spousal social and ideological compatibility, because it also occurs in insects, birds, and simians (Thiessen & Gregg, 1980). Why would genetic similarity (or *homogamy*) be advantageous in mate choice? One possibility is that it conserves locally adaptive gene combinations that would be fragmented if the mates were genetically dissimilar. Consistent with this idea, homogamy reduces the likelihood of miscarriage (Thomas, Harger, Wagener, Rabin, & Gill, 1985) and low birthweight (Ober et al., 1987). In any case, people tend to choose similar mates, and similar mates tend to stay together longer (Hill, Rubin, & Peplau, 1976). Evidence suggests that men tend to select mates who resemble their mothers, which would effectively result in homogamy (Bereczkei, Gyuris, Koves, & Bernath, 2002; Wilson & Barrett, 1987); women too tend to select husbands who resemble their fathers (Bereczkei, Gyuris, & Weisfeld, 2004; Jedlicka, 1980). Similar imprinting effects on mate choice are common in male birds (reviewed by Bereczkei et al., 2002). In addition, homogamy could be accomplished by phenotypic matching.

Extreme consanguinity, of course, risks the deleterious effects of inbreeding depression. Given the advantages and disadvantages of homogamy, one would expect that a moderate degree of genetic similarity between mates is ideal, as indeed is indicated by avian and mammalian data (Andersson, 1994). Since sexually reproducing species must guard against inbreeding, they evolved countermeasures such as dispersion from the natal area before reproductive maturity. Genetic studies suggest that, like female great apes, hominid females tended mate outside their natal group (Owens & King, 1999; Pennisi, 2001; Seielstad, Minch, & Cavilli-Sforza, 1998). We are protected against the adverse genetic effects of incest partly by close social contact in childhood (Erickson, 1993; Silverman & Bevc, Chapter 12, this volume). Sexual aversion for first-degree relatives may be imprinted in part through olfaction (Weisfeld, Czilli, Phillips, Gall, & Lichtman, 2003). The only relationships between nuclear family members that exhibited mutual olfactory aversion were father–daughter and brother–sister, those with the greatest risk of incest. Similarly, men and women prefer the odors of mates who are moderately different from them genetically (Jacob, McClintock, Zelano, & Ober, 2002; Wedekind & Furi, 1997).

Cultural norms supplement these biological mechanisms. Foragers and other traditional societies often idealize marriage between cousins, whose relationship may approach the optimal degree of consanguinity (Coon, 1971). The incest taboo augments the biological mechanisms and adds refinements. The taboo applies to different kin relationships in different societies. This presumably allows for adjustment to local factors, such as overall level of genetic similarity in the population and cultural practices that would raise the genetic risks of inbreeding (van den Berghe, 1979).

In addition to seeking kindness, availability, commitment, and similarity in a mate, the sexes exhibit some differences in their respective mate-choice criteria. Men seek a youthful but fertile mate who would enhance their life-time reproductive success (Buss, 1994). Adolescent boys have been found to prefer a woman in her early 20s to an age peer (Kenrick, Keefe, Gabrielidis, & Cornelius, 1996). Males also seek a sexually faithful wife, in order not to be deceived into caring for the children of a rival.

Women likewise exhibit definite mate preferences. They tend to desire a man who is older than they—but not necessarily an old man. Because of menopause and other factors, a man retains his fertility longer than a woman, so youth is less advantageous in a groom than in a bride. Most women also prefer a man who is taller and who earns more money. Even women with high incomes prefer a man with an even higher income (Buss, 1994), suggesting that economic need is not as important as respect for the man. The husband's income and economic power strengthen a marriage in societies around the world (Friedl, 1975; Goode, 1993; Pearson & Hendrix, 1979), whereas the wife's may even weaken it (Cready, Fossett, & Kiecolt, 1997). These preferences suggest that many women seek a man who is somewhat dominant over them—taller, richer, stronger, older. In traditional societies, high-ranking men tend to have more children than low-ranking ones (Barkow, 1989). High-status men have more sexual partners, even in monogamous societies (Perusse, 1993). Additional data confirm that male dominance in nonverbal behavior, assertiveness, self-confidence, and bodily features attracts females in various cultures and is associated with marital stability (reviewed by Gray-Little & Burks, 1983; Weisfeld, 1999). The cloying bravado, exhibitionism, risk taking, aggressive humor (Apte, 1985), and insubordination of adolescent boys may seem foolish and even dangerous, but if it demonstrates dominance to girls, it probably was selected for.

Most of the criteria of marital satisfaction mirror those of mate choice. Marital satisfaction and stability are associated with moderate male dominance, moderate homogamy, sexual satisfaction, actual (as opposed to putative) fecundity, fidelity, and mutual respect (Betzig, 1989; Weisfeld & Weisfeld, 2002). Moderate male dominance in decision making—but not extreme dominance—has usually, but not always, been correlated with marital satisfaction in various countries (Corrales, 1975; Gray-Little & Burks, 1983; Kotlar, 1965; Lucas et al., 2004).

CONCLUSIONS

Obviously, a great deal of new research, as well as integration of past findings, will be necessary to develop an acceptable model of human adolescence. Research is especially needed on neural, hormonal, and pheromonal factors in adolescent behavioral development. Gross brain development continues through adolescence, particularly of the prefrontal cortex, thus accounting for the continued decline in impulsiveness and increase in planned behavioral sequences (Gross, Carstensen, Pasupathi, & Tsai, 1997). The brain attains the final 10% of its volume after age 10 (Bjorklund & Pellegrini, 2002). Improvements in memory doubtless contribute to enhancement of abstract reasoning, and the accumulation of experience allows the adolescent to deal with more and more situations. During adolescence, the cortex undergoes a period of pruning of neural connections (Restak, 2001), perhaps corresponding to increased specialization and individuation of behavior as adult tasks are practiced. The corpus callosum continues to grow as the sexes develop their hemispheric specializations. Just as the body reaches its apex in size and health in response to the challenge of initiating reproduction, the brain reaches its peak in cognitive power. The prefrontal cortex and the association areas become the last cortical regions to myelinate. Although most cognitive capacities improve during adolescence as brain volume and myelination increase (Kolb & Whishaw, 2003), some capacities decline, such as acquisition of foreign languages.

The neural bases of motivational changes during adolescence are even less well understood than the cognitive ones, although some connections between medial temporal lobe function and anxiety (Rosenzweig, Breedlove, & Leiman, 2002), and between prefrontal cortex volume and homicide (Raine, 1993), have been documented in adults. The cardinal emotional changes of adolescence, including those in amorousness, libido, competitiveness, and parental care, are mediated by subcortical and hormonal mechanisms that are still poorly understood. For example, men and women tend to undergo different hormonal changes when threatened: Whereas men undergo sympathetic arousal, women's oxytocin levels rise, prompting them to seek help and to protect their children (Taylor et al., 2000). Some have argued that the study of cognition has unduly eclipsed that of emotion, and that emotional development is often inappropriately explained in cognitive terms (Panksepp, Moskal, Panksepp, & Kroes, 2002). This sort of explanation is rather improbable given that motivation—feeding, mating, defense, and so on— phylogenetically preceded the evolution of higher cognitive processes and therefore is unlikely to depend on them (Weisfeld, 2002). The resurgence of interest in emotion (e.g., Panksepp, 1998) may help to counteract the traditional emphasis on cognition in U.S. psychology, including evolutionary psychology.

Some aspects of adolescent behavior have been particularly neglected from a comparative perspective, such as friendship, subsistence activity, female–male competition (cf. Weisfeld, 1986), sibling relations, leisure activities, and relations with nonparent adults. In addition, we need a better understanding of the evolution of adolescent behavior in the hominid line, cross-cultural and historical variation, and the role of nonshared environmental factors such as disease, attractiveness, peers, mentors, and parent–adolescent compatibility. In summary, more integration across social science and biological disciplines seems essential for the study of human development (Archer, 1992; Bjorklund & Pellegrini, 2002; Segal, Weisfeld, & Weisfeld, 1997).

REFERENCES

Altemus, M., Deuster, P. L. Galliven, E., Carter, C., & Gold, P. (1995). Suppression of hypothalamic–pituitary–adrenal axis responses to stress in lactating women. *Journal of Clinical Endocrinology and Metabolism, 80,* 2954–2959.

Andersson, M. (1994). *Sexual selection.* Princeton, NJ: Princeton University Press.

Apte, M. L. (1985). *Humor and laughter: An anthropological approach.* Ithaca, NY: Cornell University Press.

Archer, J. (1992). *Ethology and human development.* Hemel Hempstead, UK: Harvester Wheatsheaf.

Babchuk, W. A., Hames, R. B., & Thompson, R. A. (1985). Sex differences in the recognition of infant facial expressions of emotion: The primate caretaker hypothesis. *Ethology and Sociobiology, 6,* 89–101.

Baker, M. A. (1987). Sensory functioning. In M. A. Baker (Ed.), *Sex differences in human performance* (pp. 5–36). New York: Wiley.

Baker, R. R., & Bellis, M. A. (1995). *Human sperm competition: Copulation, masturbation and infidelity.* London: Chapman & Hall.

Barkow, J. H. (1989). *Darwin, sex, and status: Biological approaches to mind and culture.* Toronto: University of Toronto Press.

Bereczkei, T., Gyuris, P., Koves, P., & Bernath, L. (2002). Homogamy, genetic similarity, and imprinting: Parental influence on mate choice preferences. *Personality and Individual Differences, 33,* 667–690.

Bereczkei, T., Gyuris, P., & Weisfeld, G. (2004). Sexual imprinting in human mate choice. *Proceedings of the Royal Society of London, B, 271,* 1129–1134.

Betzig, L. (1989). Causes of conjugal dissolution. *Current Anthropology, 30,* 654–676.

Bird, D. W., & Bird, R. B. (2002a). Children on the reef: Slow learning or strategic foraging? *Human Nature, 13,* 269–297.

Bird, R. B., & Bird, D. W. (2002b). Constraints of knowing or constraints of growing?: Fishing and collecting by the children of Mer. *Human Nature, 13,* 239–267.

Bjorklund, D. F., & Pellegrini, A. D. (2002). *The origins of human nature: Evolutionary developmental psychology.* Washington, DC: American Psychological Association.

Blurton Jones, N. G., Hawkes, K., & Draper, P. (1993). Differences between Hadza and !Kung children's work: Original affluence or practical reason? In E. S. Burch (Ed.), *Key issues in hunter–gatherer research* (pp. 189–215). Oxford, UK: Berg.

Blurton Jones, N. G., Hawkes, K., & O'Connell, J. F. (1997). Why do Hadza children forage? In N. L. Segal, G. E. Weisfeld, & C. C. Weisfeld (Eds.), *Uniting psychology and biology: Integrative perspectives on human development* (pp. 279–313). Washington, DC: American Psychological Association.

Blurton Jones, N. G., & Marlowe, F., W. (2002). Selection for delayed maturity: Does it take 20 years to learn to hunt and gather? *Human Nature, 13,* 199–238.

Boardway, R. H., & Weisfeld, G. E. (1994, August). *Social dominance among English adolescents.* Poster presented at the International Society for Human Ethology congress, Toronto.

Bock, J. (2002). Learning, life history, and productivity: Children's lives in the Okavango Delta, Botswana. *Human Nature, 13,* 161–197.

Bogin, B. (1988). *Patterns of human growth.* Cambridge, UK: Cambridge University Press.

Bogin, B. (1999). *Patterns of human growth* (2nd ed.). Cambridge, UK: Cambridge University Press.

Booth, A., & Dabbs, J. (1993). Testosterone and men's marriages. *Social Forces, 72,* 463–477.

Borgerhoff Mulder, M. (1989). Early maturing Kipsigis women have higher reproductive success than late maturing women and cost more to marry. *Behavioral Ecology and Sociobiology, 24,* 145–153.

Boulton, M. J. (1992). Rough physical play in adolescents: Does it serve a dominance function? *Early Education and Development, 3,* 312–333.

Bronson, W. C. (1966). Central orientation: A study of behaviour organization from childhood to adolescence. *Child Development, 37,* 125–155.

Broude, G. J., & Greene, S. J. (1976). Cross-cultural codes on twenty sexual attitudes and practices. *Ethnology, 15,* 409–429.

Brown, B. (1990). Peer groups. In S. Feldman & G. Elliott (Eds.), *At the threshold: The developing adolescent.* Cambridge, MA: Harvard University Press.

Burbank, V. (1987). Female aggression in cross-cultural perspective. *Behavioral Science Research, 21,* 70–100.

Buss, D. M. (1994). *The evolution of desire.* New York: Basic Books.

Cairns, R. B., Cairns, B. D., Neckerman, H. J., Ferguson, L. L., & Gariepy, J. L. (1989). Growth and aggression: Childhood to early adolescence. *Developmental Psychology, 25,* 320–330.

Campbell, A. (1986). Self report of fighting by females. *British Journal of Criminology, 26,* 28–46.

Campbell, A. (1999, June). *Female aggression: Fear, form and frequency.* Paper presented at the convention of the Human Behavior and Evolution Society, Salt Lake City, UT.

Cashdan, E. (1995). Hormones, sex, and status in women. *Hormones and Behavior, 29,* 354–366.

Caspi, A., Lynam, D., Moffitt, T., & Silva, P. (1993). Unraveling girls: Delinquency: Biological, dispositional, and contextual contributions to adolescent misbehavior. *Developmental Psychology, 29,* 19–30.

Chance, M. R. A., & Jolly, C. J. (1970). *Social groups of monkey, apes and men.* New York: Dutton.

Charlesworth, W. R. (1988). Resources and resource acquisition during ontogeny. In K. B. MacDonald (Ed.), *Sociobiological perspectives on human development* (pp. 24–77). New York: Springer-Verlag.

Charlesworth, W. R., & Hartup, W. W. (1967). Positive social reinforcement in the nursery school peer group. *Child Development, 38,* 993–1002.

Christiansen, K. (1998). Behavioural correlates of testosterone. In E. Nieschlag & H. M. Behre (Eds.), *Testosterone: Action-deficiency–substitution* (pp. 107–141). New York: Springer.

Cicirelli, V. G. (1994). Sibling relationships in cross-cultural perspective. *Journal of Marriage and the Family, 56,* 7–20.

Coe, C. L. (1990). Psychobiology of maternal behavior in nonhuman primates. In N. A. Krasnegor & R. S. Bridges (Eds.), *Mammalian parenting: Biochemical, neurological, and behavioral determinants* (pp. 157–183). New York: Oxford University Press.

Coie, J. D., & Kupersmidt, J. B. (1983). A behavioral analysis of emerging social status in boys' peer groups. *Child Development, 54,* 1400–1416.

Coon, C. S. (1971). *The hunting peoples.* Boston: Little, Brown.

Corrales, R. G. (1975). Power and satisfaction in early marriage. In R. E. Cromwell & D. M. Olson (Eds.), *Power in families* (pp. 197–216). New York: Wiley.

Cowley, J. J., & Brooksbank, B. W. L. (1991). Human exposure to putative pheromones and changes in aspects of social behavior. *Journal of Steroid Biochemistry and Molecular Biology, 39,* 647–659.

Cready, D. M., Fossett, M. A., & Kiecolt, K. J. (1997). Mate availability and African American family structure in the U.S. nonmetropolitan South, 1960–1990. *Journal of Marriage and the Family, 59,* 192–203.

Cunningham, M. R. (1986). Measuring the physical in physical attractiveness: Quasiexperiments in the sociobiology of female facial beauty. *Journal of Personality and Social Psychology, 50,* 925–935.

Cutler, W. G., Preti, G., Krieger, A., Huggins, G. R., Garcia, C. R., & Lawley, H. J. (1986). Human axillary secretions influence women's menstrual cycles: The role of donor extract from men. *Hormones and Behavior, 20,* 463–473.

Dabbs, J. (1992). Testosterone and occupational achievement. *Social Forces, 70,* 813–824.

Daly, M., & Wilson, M. (1983). *Sex, evolution and behavior* (2nd ed.). Boston: Willard Grant.

Darwin, C. (1965). *The expression of the emotions in man and animals.* Chicago: University of Chicago Press. (Original published in 1872)

Dong, Q., Weisfeld, G., Boardway, R. H., & Shen, J. (1996). Correlates of social status among Chinese adolescents. *Journal of Cross-Cultural Psychology, 27,* 476–493.

Ellis, L. (1986). Evidence of neuroandrogenic etiology of sex roles form a combined analysis of human, nonhuman primate, and nonprimate mammalian studies. *Personality and Individual Differences, 7,* 519–551.

Ellis, L. (1995). Dominance and reproductive success among nonhuman animals: A cross-species comparison. *Ethology and Sociobiology, 16,* 257–333.

Erickson, M. T. (1993). Rethinking Oedipus: An evolutionary perspective of incest avoidance. *American Journal of Psychiatry, 150,* 411–416.

Faust, M. S. (1960). Developmental maturity as a determinant of prestige in adolescent girls. *Child Development, 31,* 173–184.

Feldman, R., & Weisfeld, G. (1973). An interdisciplinary study of crime. *Crime and Delinquency, 19,* 150–162.

Flaxman, S. M., & Sherman, P. W. (2000). Morning sickness: A mechanism for protecting mother and embryo. *Quarterly Review of Biology, 75,* 113–148.

Ford, C. S., & Beach, F. A. (1951). *Patterns of sexual behavior.* New York: Harper & Row.

Forrest, J. D., & Singh, S. (1990). Public-sector savings resulting from expenditures for contraceptive services. *Family Planning Perspectives, 22,* 6–15.

Friedl, E. (1975). *Women and men: An anthropologist's view.* New York: Holt, Rinehart & Winston.

Goldberg, S., Blumberg, S. L., & Kriger, A. (1982). Menarche and interest in infants: Biological and social influences. *Child Development, 53,* 1544–1550.

Goodall, J. (1986). *The chimpanzees of Gombe: Patterns of behavior.* Cambridge, MA: Harvard University Press.

Goode, W. J. (1993). *World changes in divorce patterns.* New Haven, CT: Yale University Press.

Graber, J., Lewinsohn, P., Seeley, J., & Brooks-Gunn, J. (1997). Is psychopathology associated with the timing of pubertal development? *Journal of the American Academy of Child and Adolescent Psychiatry, 36*, 1768–1776.

Grammer, K. (1996, June). *The human mating game: The battle of the sexes and the war of signals.* Paper presented at the Human Behavior and Evolution Society convention, Evanston, IL.

Gray-Little, B., & Burks, N. (1983). Power and satisfaction in marriage: A review and critique. *Psychological Bulletin, 93*, 513–538.

Gross, J. J., Carstensen, L. L., Pasupathi, M., & Tsai, J. (1997). Emotion and aging: experience, expression, and control. *Psychology and Aging, 12*, 590–599.

Guthrie, R. D. (1976). *Body hot spots: The anatomy of human social organs and behavior.* New York: Van Nostrand Reinhold.

Hall, J. (1984). *Nonverbal sex differences: Communication accuracy and expressive style.* Baltimore: Johns Hopkins University Press.

Hamilton, J. B., & Mestler, G. E. (1969). Mortality and survival: Comparison of eunuchs with intact men and women in a mentally retarded population. *Journal of Gerontology, 24*, 395–411.

Hampson, E. (2002). Sex differences in human brain and cognition: The influence of sex steroids in early and adult life. In J. B. Becker, S. M. Breedlove, D. Crews, & M. M. McCarthy (Eds.), *Behavioral endocrinology* (2nd ed., pp. 579–628). Cambridge, MA: MIT Press.

Harvey, P. H., & Clutton-Brock, T. H. (1985). Life history variations in primates. *Evolution, 39*, 559–581.

Hawkes, K., O'Connell, J., & Blurton Jones, N. (1989). Hardworking Hadza grandmothers. In V. Standen & R. Foley (Eds.), *Comparative socioecology: The behavioural ecology of mammals and man* (pp. 341–366). London: Blackwell Scientific.

Hayward, C., Killen, J. D., Wilson, D. M., Hammer, L. D., Litt, I. F., Kraemer, H. C., et al. (1997). Psychiatric risk associated with early puberty in adolescent girls. *Journal of the American Academy of Child and Adolescent Psychiatry, 36*, 255–262.

Higham, E. (1980). Variations in adolescent psychohormonal development. In J. Adelson (Ed.), *Handbook of adolescent psychology* (pp. 472–494). New York: Wiley.

Hill, C. T., Rubin, Z., & Peplau, L. (1976). Breakups before marriage: the end of 103 affairs. *Journal of Social Issues, 3*, 147–168.

Hill, J. P., Holmbeck, G. N., Marlow, L., Green, T. M., & Lynch, M. E. (1985). Pubertal status and parent–child relations in families of seventh-grade boys. *Journal of Early Adolescence, 5*, 31–44.

Holmbeck, G., & Hill, J. (1991). Conflictive engagement, positive affect, and menarche in families with seventh-grade girls. *Child Development, 62*, 1030–1048.

Hotvedt, M. E. (1990). Emerging and submerging adolescence sexuality: Culture and sexual orientation. In J. Bancroft & J. M. Reinisch (Eds.), *Adolescence and puberty* (pp. 157–172). New York: Oxford University Press.

Hoyenga, K. B., & Hoyenga, K. T. (1979). *The question of sex differences: Psychological, cultural, and biological issues.* Boston: Little, Brown.

Hoyenga, K. B., & Hoyenga, K. T. (1993). *Gender-related differences: Origins and outcomes.* Boston: Allyn & Bacon.

Hrdy, S. B. (1981). *The woman that never evolved.* Cambridge, MA: Harvard University Press.

Jackson, L. A. (1992). *Physical appearance and gender: Sociobiology and sociocultural perspectives.* Albany: State University of New York Press.

Jacob, S., McClintock, M. K., Zelano, B., & Ober, C. (2002). Paternally inherited HLA alleles are associated with women's choice of male odor. *Nature Genetics, 30,* 175–179.

Jacob, T. (1974). Patterns of family conflict and dominance as a function of age and social class. *Developmental Psychology, 10,* 21–24.

Janson, C. H., & van Schaik, C. P. (1993). Ecological risk aversion in juvenile primates: Slow and steady wins the race. In M. E. Pereira & L. A. Fairbanks (Eds.), *Juvenile primates: Life history, development, and behavior* (pp. 57–76). New York: Oxford University Press.

Jedlicka, D. (1980). A test of the psychoanalytic theory of mate selection. *Journal of Social Psychology, 122,* 295–299.

Jerison, H. J. (1973). *Evolution of brain and intelligence.* New York: Academic Press.

Jones, M. C., & Bayley, N. (1950). Physical maturing among boys as related to behavior. *Journal of Educational Psychology, 41,* 129–148.

Jones, M. C., & Mussen, P. H. (1958). Self-conceptions, motivations, and interpersonal attitudes of early- and late-maturing girls. *Child Development, 29,* 492–501.

Jones, S., Martin, R., & Pilbeam, D. (Eds.). (1992). *Cambridge encyclopedia of human evolution.* Cambridge, UK: Cambridge University Press.

Kagan, J., & Moss, H. A. (1962). *Birth to maturity: A study in psychological development.* New York: Wiley.

Kaplan, H., Hill, K., Lancaster, J., & Hurtado, A. M. (2000). A theory of human life history evolution: Diet, intelligence, and longevity. *Evolutionary Anthropology, 9,* 156–185.

Keating, C. F. (1985). Gender and the physiognomy of dominance and attractiveness. *Social Psychology Quarterly, 48,* 61–70.

Kenrick, D. T., Keefe, R. C., Gabrielidis, C., & Cornelius, J. S. (1996). Adolescents' age preferences for dating partners: Support for an evolutionary model of life-history strategies. *Child Development, 67,* 1499–1511.

Kimura, D. (1999). *Sex and cognition.* Cambridge, MA: MIT Press.

Kolb, B., & Whishaw, I. Q. (2003). *Fundamentals of human neuropsychology* (5th ed.). New York: Worth.

Kotlar, S. L. (1965). Middle-class marital role perceptions and marital adjustment. *Sociology and Social Research, 49,* 283–294.

Kramer, J. L. (2002). Variation in juvenile dependence: Helping behavior among Maya children. *Human Nature, 13,* 299–325.

Kramer, K. L., & Boone, J. (1999, June). *Does children's work increase household production? Production, consumption and family size among subsistence agriculturalists.* Paper presented at the convention of the Human Behavior and Evolution Society, Salt Lake City, UT.

Laumann, E. O., Gagnon, J. H., Michael, R. T., & Michaels, S. (1994). *The social organization of sexuality: Sexual practices in the United States.* Chicago: University of Chicago Press.

Livson, N., & Peskin, H. (1980). Perspectives on adolescence form longitudinal research. In J. Adelson (Ed.), *Handbook of adolescent psychology* (pp. 47–98). New York: Wiley.

Loeber, R., & Hay, D. (1997). Key issues in the development of aggression and violence from childhood to early adulthood. *Annual Review of Psychology, 48,* 371–410.

Lorenz, K. (1965). *Evolution and modification of behavior.* Chicago: University of Chicago Press.

Lucas, T. W., Weisfeld, G. E., Wendorf, C. A., Weisfeld, C. C., Imamoglu, E. O., & Shen, J. (2004). *Marital satisfaction in four cultures as a function of homogamy, male dominance, and female attractiveness.* Manuscript in preparation.

Mackey, W. C. (1983). A preliminary test for the validation of the adult male–child bond as a species-characteristic trait. *American Anthropologist, 85,* 391–402.

Magnusson, D., Stattin, H., & Allen, V. L. (1985). Biological maturation and social development: A longitudinal study of some adjustment processes from mid-adolescence to adulthood. *Journal of Youth and Adolescence, 14,* 267–284

Manning, J. T., Scutt, D., & Lewis-Jones, D. I. (1998). Developmental stability, ejaculate size, and sperm quality in men. *Evolution and Human Behavior, 19,* 273–282.

Mazur, A., & Booth, A. (1998). Testosterone and dominance in men. *Behavioral and Brain Sciences, 21,* 353–397.

McArthur, L. Z., & Berry, D. S. (1987). Cross-cultural agreement in perceptions of baby-faced adults. *Journal of Cross-Cultural Psychology, 18,* 165–192.

McClintock, M., & Herdt, G. (1996). Rethinking puberty: The development of sexual attraction. *Current Directions in Psychological Science, 5,* 178–183.

Merten, D. (1997). The meaning of meanness: Popularity, competition and conflict among junior high school girls. *Sociology of Education, 70,* 175–191.

Miller, K. E. (1990). Adolescents' same-sex and opposite-sex peer relations: Sex differences in popularity, perceived social competence, and social cognitive skills. *Journal of Adolescent Research, 5,* 222–241.

Mitchell, G. (1981). *Human sex differences: A primatologist's perspective.* New York: Van Nostrand Reinhold.

Molina, B. S. G., & Chassin, L. (1996). The parent–adolescent relationship at puberty: Hispanic ethnicity and parent alcoholism as moderators. *Developmental Psychology, 32,* 675–686.

Montemayor, R., & Hanson, E. (1985). A naturalistic view of conflict between adolescents and their parents and siblings. *Journal of Early Adolescence, 5,* 23–30.

Monti-Bloch, L., (1999, June). *Behavioral and physiological effects of androstadienone in human subjects.* Paper presented at the convention of the Human Behavior and Evolution Society, Salt Lake City, UT.

Murdock, G. P. (1949). *Social structure.* New York: Macmillan.

Murdock, G. P., & Provost, C. (1973). Factors in the division of labor by sex: A cross-cultural analysis. *Ethnology, 12,* 203–219.

Neill, S. R. St. J. (1983). Children's social relationships and education—An evolutionary effect? *Social Biology and Human Affairs, 47,* 48–55.

Neill, S. R. St. J. (1985). Rough-and-tumble and aggression in school children: Serious play? *Animal Behaviour, 33,* 1380–1382.

Nottelmann, E. D., Inoff-Germain, G., Susman, E. J., & Chrousos, G. P. (1990). Hormones and behavior at puberty. In J. Bancroft & J. M. Reinisch (Eds.), *Adolescence and puberty* (pp. 88–123). New York: Oxford University Press.

Ober, C., Simpson, J. L., Ward, M., Radvany, R. M., Andersen, R., Elias, S., et al. (1987). Prenatal effects of maternal–fetal HLA compatibility. *American Journal of Reproductive Immunology and Microbiology, 15,* 141–149.

Owens, K., & King, M. C. (1999). Genomic views of human history. *Science, 286,* 451–453.

Paikoff, R., & Brooks-Gunn, J. (1991). Do parent–child relationships change during puberty? *Psychological Bulletin, 110,* 47–66.

Panksepp, J. (1998). *Affective neuroscience: The foundations of human and animal emotions.* New York: Oxford University Press.

Panksepp, J., Moskal, J. R., Panksepp, J. B., & Kroes, R. A. (2002). Comparative approaches in evolutionary psychology: Molecular neuroscience meets the mind. *Neuorendocrinology Letters, 23*(Suppl. 4), 105–115.

Pearson, W., Jr., & Hendrix, L. (1979). Divorce and the status of women. *Journal of Marriage and the Family, 41,* 375–385.

Pennisi, E. (2001). Tracing the sexes by their genes. *Science, 291,* 1733–1734.

Pereira, M. E., & Altmann, J. (1985). Development of social behavior in free-living nonhuman primates. In E. S. Watts (Ed.), *Nonhuman primate models for human growth and development* (pp. 217–309). New York: Liss.

Perusse, D. (1993). Cultural and reproductive success in industrial societies: Testing the relationship at proximate and ultimate levels. *Behavioral and Brain Sciences, 16,* 239–242.

Peskin, H., & Livson, M. (1972). Pre- and postpubertal personality and adult psychological functioning. *Seminars in Psychiatry, 4,* 343–353.

Profet, M. (1992). Pregnancy sickness as adaptation: A deterrent to maternal ingestion of teratogens. In J. H. Barkow, L. Cosmides, & J. Tooby (Eds.), *The adapted mind: Evolutionary psychology and the generation of culture* (pp. 327–365). New York: Oxford University Press.

Raine, A. (1993). *The psychopathology of crime: Criminal behavior as a clinical disorder.* San Diego: Academic Press.

Restak, R. M. (2001). *The secret life of the brain.* Washington, DC: Dana Press.

Rivenbark, W. H. (1971). Self-disclosure patterns among adolescents. *Psychological Reports, 28,* 35–42.

Rodkin, P., Farmer, T., Pearl, R., & Van Acker, R. (2000). Heterogeneity of popular boys: Antisocial and prosocial configurations. *Developmental Psychology, 36,* 14–24.

Rosenzweig, M. R., Breedlove, S. M., & Leiman, A. L. (2002). *Biological psychology: An introduction to behavioral, cognitive, and clinical neuroscience* (3rd ed.). Sunderland, Ma: Sinauer.

Sagrestano, L. M., McCormick, S. H., Paikoff, R. L., & Holmbeck, G. N. (1999). Pubertal development and parent–child conflict in low-income, urban, African American adolescents. *Journal of Research on Adolescence, 9,* 85–107.

Savin-Williams, R. C. (1987). *Adolescence: An ethological perspective.* New York: Springer-Verlag.

Schlegel, A. (1995). A cross-cultural approach to adolescence. *Ethos, 23,* 15–32.

Schlegel, A. (2004, March). *A place of adolescents in human social structure.* Paper presented at the meeting of the Society for Research on Adolescence, Baltimore, MD.

Schlegel, A., & Barry, H., III. (1980). Adolescent initiation ceremonies: A cross-cultural code. In H. Barry, III. & A. Schlegel (Eds.), *Cross-cultural samples and codes* (pp. 277–288). Pittsburgh: University of Pittsburgh Press.

Schlegel, A., & Barry, H., III. (1991). *Adolescence: An anthropological inquiry.* New York: Free Press.

Segal, N. L., Weisfeld, G. E., & Weisfeld, C. C. (1997). *Uniting psychology and biology: Integrative perspectives on human development.* Washington, DC: American Psychological Association.

Seielstad, M. T., Minch, E., & Cavilli-Sforza, L. (1998). Genetic evidence for a higher female migration rate in humans. *Nature Genetics, 20,* 278–280.

Shackelford, T. K., & Larsen, R. J. (1999). Facial attractiveness and physical health. *Evolution and Human Behavior, 20,* 71–76.

Silbereisen, R., Petersen, A., Albrecht, H., & Kracke, B. (1989). Maturational timing and the development of problem behavior: Longitudinal studies in adolescence. *Journal of Early Adolescence, 3,* 247–268.

Silverberg, S., & Steinberg, L. (1987). Adolescent autonomy, parent–adolescent conflict, and parental well-being. *Journal of Youth and Adolescence, 16,* 293–312.

Silverberg, S. B. (1989, April). *Parents as developing adults: The impact of perceived distance in the parent–adolescent relationship.* Poster presented at the biennial meeting of the Society for Research in Child Development, Kansas City, MO.

Silverman, I., & Phillips, K. A. (1993). Effects of estrogen changes during the menstrual cycle on spatial performance. *Ethology and Sociobiology, 14,* 257–269.

Simmons, R. G., Blyth, D. A., & McKinney, K. L. (1983). The social and psychological effects of puberty on white females. In J. Brooks-Gunn & A.C. Petersen (Eds.), *Girls at puberty: Biological and psychosocial perspectives* (pp. 229–272). New York: Plenum Press.

Sommer, B. B. (1978). *Puberty and adolescence.* New York: Oxford University Press.

Steinberg, L. (1987). The impact of puberty on family relations: Effects of pubertal status and pubertal timing. *Developmental Psychology, 23,* 451–460.

Stephens, W. N. (1963). *The family in cross-cultural perspective.* New York: Holt, Rinehart & Winston.

Storey, A. E., Walsh, C. J., Quinton, R. L., & Wynne-Edwards, K. E. (2000). Hormonal correlates of paternal responsiveness in new and expectant fathers. *Evolution and Human Behavior, 21,* 79–95.

Tanner, J. M. (1990). *Foetus into man: Physical growth from conception to maturity.* Cambridge, MA: Harvard University Press.

Taylor, S. E., Klein, I. C., Lewis, B. P., Grunewald, T. L., Gurung, R. A. R., & Updegraff, J. A. (2000). Female responses to stress: Tend-and-befriend, not fight-or-flight. *Psychological Review, 107,* 411–429.

Thiessen, D., & Gregg, B. (1980). Human associative mating and genetic equilibrium: An evolutionary perspective. *Ethology and Sociobiology, 1,* 111–140.

Thomas, M. L., Harger, J. H., Wagener, D. K., Rabin, B. S., & Gill, T. J. (1985). HLA sharing and spontaneous abortion in humans. *American Journal of Obstetrics and Gynecology, 151,* 1053–1058.

Tinbergen, N. (1963). The eggshell menace. *Natural History, 72,* 28–35.

Tremblay, R., Schaal, B., Boulerice, B., Arseneault, L., Soussignan, R., Paquette, D., et al. (1998). Testosterone, physical aggression, dominance and physical development in early adolescence. *International Journal of Behavioral Development, 22,* 753–777.

Trivers, R. L. (1997). Genetic basis of intrapsychic conflict. In N. L. Segal, G. E. Weisfeld, & C. C. Weisfeld (Eds.), *Uniting psychology and biology: integrative perspectives on human development* (pp. 385–395). Washington, DC: American Psychological Association.

Tschann, J. M., Adler, N. E., Irwin, C. E., Jr., Millstein, S. G., Turner, R. A., & Kegeles, S. M. (1994). Initiation of substance abuse in early adolescence: The roles of pubertal timing and emotional distress. *Health Psychology, 13*, 326–333.

Tulkin, S. R., Muller, J. P., & Conn, L. K. (1969). Need for approval and popularity: Sex differences in elementary school children. *Journal of Consulting and Clinical Psychology, 33*, 35–39.

Udry, J. R. (1987). Hormonal and social determinants of adolescent sexual initiation. In J. Bancroft (Ed.), *Adolescence and puberty* (pp. 70–87). New York: Oxford University Press.

Udry, J. R. (1988). Biological predispositions and social control in adolescent sexual behavior. *American Sociological Review, 53*, 709–722.

Udry, J. R., & Billy, J. (1987). Initiation of coitus in early adolescence. *American Sociological Review, 52*, 841–855.

Uvnas-Moberg, K. (1997). Physiological and endocrine effects of social contact. In C. Carter, I. Lederhendler, & B. Kirkpatrick (Eds.), *The integrative neurobiology of affiliation* (pp. 146–163). New York: New York Academy of Sciences.

van den Berghe, P. (1979). *Human family systems: An evolutionary view.* New York: Elsevier.

van den Berghe, P. L. (1980). The human family: A sociobiological look. In J. S. Lockard (Ed.), *The evolution of human social behavior* (pp. 67–85). New York: Elsevier.

Walters, J. R. (1987). Transition to adulthood. In B. B. Smuts, D. L. Cheney, R. M. Seyfarth, R. W. Wragham, & T. T. Struhsaker (Eds.), *Primate societies* (pp. 358–369). Chicago: University of Chicago Press.

Wedekind, C., & Furi, S. (1997). Body odour preferences in men and women: Do they aim for specific MHC combinations or simply heterozygosity? *Proceedings of the Royal Society of London B, 264*, 1471–1479.

Weisfeld, C. C. (1986). Female behavior in mixed-sex competition: A review of the literature. *Developmental Review, 6*, 278–299.

Weisfeld, G. E. (1997). Puberty rites as clues to the nature of human adolescence. *Cross-Cultural Research, 31*, 27–54.

Weisfeld, G. E. (1999). *Evolutionary principles of human adolescence.* New York: Basic Books.

Weisfeld, G. E. (2002). Neural and functional aspects of pride and shame. In G. A. Cory & R. Gardner, Jr. (Eds.), *The neuroethology of Paul MacLean: Convergences and frontiers* (pp. 193–214). Westport, CT: Praeger.

Weisfeld, G. E., Bloch, S. A., & Ivers, J. W. (1983). A factor analytic study of peer-perceived dominance in adolescent boys. *Adolescence, 18*, 229–243.

Weisfeld, G. E., Bloch, S. A., & Ivers, J. W. (1984). Possible determinants of social dominance among adolescent girls. *Journal of Genetic Psychology, 144*, 115–129.

Weisfeld, G. E., Czilli, T., Phillips, K. A., Gall, J. A., & Lichtman, C. M. (2003). Possible olfaction-based mechanisms in human kin recognition and inbreeding avoidance. *Journal of Experimental Child Psychology, 85*, 279–295.

Weisfeld, G. E., Muczenski, D. M., Weisfeld, C. C., & Omark, D. R. (1987). Stability of boys' social success among peers over an eleven-year period. *Contributions to Human Development, 18*, 58–80.

Weisfeld, G. E., Omark, D. R., & Cronin, C. L. (1980). A longitudinal and cross-sectional study of dominance in boys. In D. R. Omark, F. F. Strayer, & D. G. Freedman (Eds.), *Dominance relations: An ethological view of human conflict and social interaction* (pp. 205–216). New York: Garland.

Weisfeld, G. E., & Weisfeld, C. C. (2002). Marriage: an evolutionary perspective. *Neuroendocrinology Letters, 23*(Suppl. 4), 47–54.

Williams, J. M., & Currie, C. (2000). Self-esteem and physical development in early adolescence: Pubertal timing and body image. *Journal of Early Adolescence, 20,* 129–149.

Willner, L. A., & Martin, R. D. (1985). Some basic principles of mammalian sexual dimorphism. In J. Ghesquiere, R. D. Martin, & F. Newcombe (Eds.), *Human sexual dimorphism* (pp. 1–42). London: Taylor & Francis.

Wilson, G. D., & Barrett, P. T. (1987). Parental characteristics and partner choice: Some evidence for Oedipal imprinting. *Journal of Biosocial Science, 19,* 157–161.

Worthman, C. M. (1993). Biocultural interactions in human development. In M. E. Pereira & L. A. Fairbanks (Eds.), *Juvenile primates: Life history, development, and behavior* (pp. 339–358). New York: Oxford University Press.

Zeller, A. C. (1987). A role for children in hominid evolution. *Man, 22,* 528–557.

9

SEX DIFFERENCES
IN COMPETITIVE
AND AGGRESSIVE BEHAVIOR

A View from Sexual Selection Theory

ANTHONY D. PELLEGRINI
JOHN ARCHER

Discussions of sex differences are basic to many fields, including developmental psychology and evolutionary biology. In the field of developmental psychology, chapters on sex differences have been included in the *Handbook of Child Psychology* since the first edition (Terman, 1946). Correspondingly, seminal contributions by Eleanor Maccoby and colleagues (Maccoby, 1998; Maccoby & Jacklin, 1974) have, correctly, stressed the centrality of sex and gender for developmental functioning. Sex differences are also basic to the field of evolutionary biology (Clutton-Brock, 1983; Trivers, 1985), and the allied fields of evolutionary psychology (e.g., Buss, 1989) and evolutionary developmental psychology (Bjorklund & Pellegrini, 2002). Darwin (1871) himself was aware of the importance of sex differences when he proposed the theory of sexual selection to complement his theory of evolution by natural selection.

We present an exploratory model for the development of sex differences in competitive and aggressive behavior that is rooted in both developmental psychology and evolutionary biology, particularly Darwin's sexual selection theory and its later elaboration, parental investment theory (Trivers, 1972). The complementary role of evolutionary biology in developmental–

psychological expositions of sex differences is needed, following Maccoby's (1998) acknowledgment of the limitations of socialization explanations for sex differences in social behaviors. In this chapter, we examine the dynamic relations between children's social experiences and evolutionary forces, and how they relate to sex differences in aggression, agonistic behavior, and competitive behavior.

Organizationally, we first, and briefly, outline basic tenets of sexual selection theory and parental investment theory, with a focus on competitive and aggressive behaviors, because the theory points specifically to differences in competition and aggression. It also points, more indirectly, to the importance of sex segregation, which provides the developmental context for contrasting patterns of aggression in the two sexes. Second, we specify the dynamic relations between evolutionary history and the context in which individuals develop. Third, we present evidence for a model of sex differences in both sex segregation and agonistic behavior during childhood. The model (Figure 9.1) posits that mating systems and resources (in the form of nutrition) influence each other. For example, in marginal ecologies, such as the high Arctic, there is a tendency toward monogamy. The confluence of meager nutrition and ecologically imposed monogamy attenuates sex differences in size. The degree of sexual dimorphism in size should, in turn, predict differences in physical activity, aggression, and sex segregation. In segregated groups, males exhibit high levels of physically vigorous, rough, and aggressive behavior, as they sort out dominance relationships and maximize their physical conditioning. Agonistic behavior in male groups is characterized by competitive, dominance-related encounters and by physical aggression.

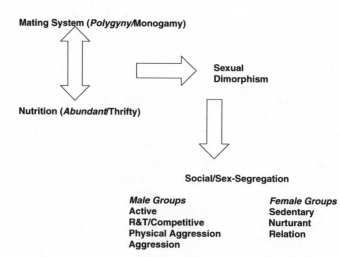

FIGURE 9.1. A model for sex differences in agonistic behavior.

SEXUAL SELECTION
AND PARENTAL INVESTMENT THEORY

Sexual Selection Theory

Darwin (1871) recognized explicitly that, in many species, males and females differed in terms of both size and "ornamentation," and he observed that such differences seemed to be related to differences in mating strategies: In polygynous species, relative to monogamous ones, males are larger than females and also are more ornamental. Males' ornamentation and body size is also associated with weaponry; for example, males' antlers and horns are both ornamental and related to combat.

The first component of sexual selection theory relates to intrasexual competition. Specifically, Darwin suggested that the differences in body size and weaponry were due to the fact that males are more competitive than females. Males, he observed, compete with one another for access to females. Competition is especially evident when there is a shortage of females and in polygynous mating systems. "Polygyny" is technically defined as greater male than female variance in reproductive success. To the extent that individual males monopolize sexual access to more than one female, male–male competition and variance in reproductive success is increased. Darwin could not, however, determine why males were more competitive and females more choosy, and not *vice versa*.

Males compete with each other, using resources associated with their body size, physical conditioning, and weaponry as one way in which they can gain access to mates. Relatively large size and natural weaponry are clearly advantageous in mating competition and have probably each been influenced by similar selection pressures (Clutton-Brock, 1983). From this viewpoint, males are selected to be more physically vigorous, competitive, and physically aggressive than females. These are also characteristics of all-male groups.

Wood and Eagly (2002) have recently questioned this view. Briefly, they have challenged the role of different mating systems and sexual dimorphism in determining sex differences in behavior. They suggest that sexual dimorphism in humans is not large and, indeed, not similar to that of other primates. While they acknowledge minimal sex differences in size, they suggest that these differences reflect a bias in humans for monogamy rather than polygyny. Furthermore, they minimize the role of size differences in psychological functioning

We are skeptical of these conclusions on the following grounds. First, though the differences in human's sexual dimorphism are not great, they are certainly consistent with sexual selection theory and in the range of those of the great apes. Specifically, in chimpanzees, bonobos, and human forager groups, males are approximately 15% larger than females (deWaal & Lanting, 1997; Pellegrini, in press; Zihlman, 1996). This difference in size masks much larger differences in upper body strength and grip strength. Humans often fight by utilizing upper body strength and weapons; thus, real differences exist between men's and women's aggressive abilities. Second, evidence, some of which was also cited by Wood and Eagly, from nonhuman (e.g., Plavcan & van Schaik, 1999) and human primate sources (Miller, 1998), suggests that the small but consistent difference in body size would have supported a tendency toward polygyny in our phylogenetic history. In support of this position, sexual dimorphism is clearly related to polygynous and monogamous tendencies. For example, in severe ecological niches, such as the high Arctic, monogamy is ecologically rather than culturally determined, because the efforts of both parents are required to successfully rear an offspring. In these cases, relative to less severe niches, there is lower sexual dimorphism (Alexander, Hoogland, Howard, Noonan, & Sherman, 1979). In short, and consistent with sexual selection theory, we suggest that differences in mating relate to sexual dimorphism, sexual segregation, and difference in aggression.

The second component of sexual selection theory relates to female choice (see Smuts, 1985). Darwin recognized that females do not passively wait to be chosen by the most dominant males. Female apes and monkeys often choose males that are healthy and dominant, as well as being a genetically appropriate partner. These preferences function to increase the probability that their offspring will have both a strong and healthy genetic makeup and that the female and her offspring will be protected by the chosen male. In humans, females also choose males on the basis of their willingness and ability to provision offspring. Finally, females choose genetically appropriate partners. In some cases, females shun healthy and dominant males in favor of low-status, new emigrants. This aspect of female choice functions to promote outbreeding vigor and prevent inbreeding depression.

Parental Investment Theory

The reasons why males are usually the larger and more competitive and aggressive sex, whereas females are usually the smaller and more choosy sex, remained unclear until the middle of the 20th century. The beginnings of the solution to this puzzle were presented by Bateman (1948, cited in Trivers, 1985) in a series of experiments with fruit flies (*Drosophilia melanogaster*). In these experiments he experimentally supported dimensions of sexual selection theory by finding that males, relative to females, were more variable in terms of reproductive success. Furthermore, he demonstrated that frequency of copulation had a positive effect on males' but not on females' reproductive success. There was no effect for number of copulations on female reproductive success, beyond the first copulation.

Bateman explained the sex differences in terms of corresponding differential physiological expense, or investment, by males and females in reproduction. Reproduction in fruit flies, as well as in many species, and especially in mammals, is more expensive for females than for males. For example, egg cells are more expensive to produce and keep than are sperm cells. For this reason there tends to be limited numbers of eggs produced in each female.

Variation in the number and quality of eggs within females is a result of their more general resource status, typically expressed in terms of food reserves.

Sperm, by contrast, is not expensive to produce, and males can fertilize dozens of females with relatively little expense; thus, males have a tendency toward promiscuity. The implication of this strategy is that a few males will mate more frequently than most males. Indeed, some males will not mate at all. This, in turn, leads to males competing with each other for access to a limited number of females. In evolutionary perspective, sexual dimorphism and differences in aggression result from this difference in parental investment.

An interesting test of hypotheses derived from parental investment theory is to examine cases where males' parental investment exceeds the parental investment of females; in these cases, where reproductive roles are reversed, males take on much care of offspring and females are more sexually aggressive. The best examples come from polyandrous shorebirds, such as the spotted sandpiper, *Actitis macularia* (Erckmann, 1983) and the American jacana, *Jacana spinosa* (Jenni, 1974): Females are larger than males, there is sexual segregation, mating is often polyandrous (females have multiple mates), and intrasexual competition is more intense among females than among males (Erckmann, 1983).

The optimal male strategy in most species is to mate as frequently as possible and to invest minimally in offspring. Lack of paternal certainty attenuates any male tendency to invest in offspring. Competition between members of the sex that invest less in offspring (usually males) for access to members of the sex that invest more in offspring (usually females) results in morphological, social, and behavioral differences between males and females.

Females generally invest highly in offspring. Expenses are not only costs associated with egg production but also with provisioning the fetus and the newborn, as well as protecting it from hostile forces. Females, unlike males, are certain that the offspring has about 50% of her genes, which means that investment is less risky. Males, on the other hand, are less certain of paternity (given the possibility of cuckoldry); thus, they are less likely to invest in the offspring; that is, there is always the possibility that the offspring is not theirs, and it is against their reproductive interests to invest their resources in another male's offspring.

Females seek "high-quality" mates, as indicated by their status and resources (e.g., dominance, wealth), health (e.g., symmetry, physical attractiveness), and genetic compatibility. This level of choice means that the offspring will benefit from outbreeding vigor and a strong and healthy genetic stock, as well as from the resources and protection that the female might accrue from a strong mate. Females also try to form alliances and coalitions that maximize their accessing mates and protecting their offspring (Smuts, 1985).

According to Trivers (1972, 1985), these differences in parental investment are responsible for a number of sex differences in morphology and behavior across species. The theory posits that the sex that invests more in offspring (usually females) will be more choosy in selecting mates and more concerned with maximizing investment in the offspring. From this view, females are less likely than males to put themselves at risk of harm or danger, because it would compromise their ability to provision and protect the offspring. As Campbell (1999) put it, females are concerned with "staying alive." This means that female behavior—mate-choice strategies, group formations, and allocation of time and resources more generally—heavily focuses on protecting and provisioning offspring. Furthermore, females' aggressive and agonistic strategies are less direct and confrontational than those of males (as discussed below).

Males are generally much less choosy in selecting a mate. To illustrate this point, Trivers (1985) gave examples of males from various species mating with members of other species and even mounting inanimate objects! This view is also supported for humans by Schmitt et al.'s (2003) findings that there are widespread sex differences in the desire for sexual variety (see also Symons, 1978). The strategy of frequent mating and lack of paternal investment results in intrasexual competition, sexual dimorphism, and sex differences in aggression.

THE MODEL: CONTEXTUAL MODERATION OF SEXUAL DIMORPHISM AND RELATIONS WITH ACTIVITY, SEXUAL SEGREGATION, AND AGGRESSION

We have argued that evolutionary history has an impact on human development. With this said, however, we must further clarify the role of evolutionary history and the moderating role of contextual effects in understanding human development. Indeed, evolutionary approaches to human development have been criticized on the grounds that they have not explicated the role of "context" in human psychology (e.g., Wood & Eagly, 2002). First, we do not take a deterministic view of phylogenetic history and genes on human behavior, even if continuity across common ancestry is found in dimensions of social behavior and organization. Our orientation leads to the position that genes, environment, and behavior dynamically influence each other (Archer & Lloyd, 2002; Bateson & Martin, 1999; Bjorklund & Pellegrini, 2002; Gottlieb, 1983; Stamps, 2003). Unlike Lorenz's (1950) classical ethological position (e.g., on instinct), we assume that environmental conditions and behavior modify the ways in which genes are expressed and development unfolds. Our view is more consistent with Tinbergen's (1951) view of ethology (and his correspondingly different views on instinct). He recognized that in order to understand the function of behavior, we need to study the ways in which distal factors (e.g., phylogenetic history) and proximal factors (e.g., socialization practices) affect behavioral development.

Bateson and Martin (1999) use a jukebox metaphor to describe this process. Individuals within each species have a genetic endowment that can be realized through a wide variety of options (similar to the collection of records in a jukebox) but the specific developmental pathway taken by an individual (similar to the specific record selected) is influenced by the perinatal (i.e., from conception through infancy) and childhood environments of the developing organism. Thus, a number of developmental pathways are possible, but which one is selected is influenced by the environment in which the organism develops (Archer, 1992; Caro & Bateson, 1986). This type of "gene × environment interaction" has been recently demonstrated in rhesus monkeys (Suomi, in press) and in humans (Moffitt, 2002). Specifically, a genetic predisposition toward aggression can be attenuated by supportive rearing conditions.

For the purposes of this chapter, perhaps the most relevant aspect of the environment is nutrition, because it affects the sexual dimorphism in size, which in turn affects activity, sex segregation, and agonistic behaviors, as specified in Figure 8.1. Specifically, the nutritional history of human mothers impacts the physical size of the offspring, and more particularly, that of males (Bateson & Martin, 1999). Furthermore, and more convincingly, ecological conditions and the availability of resources seem to affect human mating systems and sexual dimorphism.

Alexander et al. (1979) used the Human Relations Area File to partition human societies as ecologically imposed monogamy (e.g., Lapps of Norway, Cooper and Labrador Eskimo), polygynous (e.g., Bedouin Arabs and Khmer), and culturally monogamous (most Western societies). While it may have been an oversimplification for Alexander and colleagues to categorize mating systems into monogamous and polygynous, by doing so they underscored the importance of the dynamic relations between environment and mating. They found that the ecological-imposed groups were significantly less dimorphic than the other two, and there were no differences between the polygynous and culturally imposed monogamy groups. They argued that in ecologically imposed monogamous cultures, efforts of both parents are needed to protect and provision the offspring. Furthermore, monogamy is the result of ecological constraints, because individual men are unable to gain by attempting to provision for offspring of more than one wife. From this view, sexual dimorphism results from the confluence of ecological and mating systems. Dimorphism is in turn hypothesized to be an antecedent condition for different energetic demands of males and females, as well as an antecedent to both sex segregation and sex differences in agonistic behavior.

Differences in body size are associated with differences in physical activity and with competitiveness and aggressiveness, such that males and females view themselves differently very early in development and then segregate (see Pellegrini, 2004, for a fuller discussion). Later, these differences are translated into different levels of energetic behavior, social roles, and differences in agonistic behaviors associated with different energetic demands.

Difference in body size is also related to the reproductive patterns of humans and great apes, and possibly different social roles and uses of aggression associated with these mating systems (Pellegrini, 2004, in press).

Polygynous mating systems predict that males will be more competitive, active, and larger relative to females. Monogamous systems, on the other hand, result in less competition, less aggression, and less dimorphism. In the former case, there is likely to be more competition among males for females, resulting in more physical aggression and rough play among males in segregated groups of juveniles.

These patterns, however, vary according to predictable conditions in natural and experimental environments. Specifically, sex segregation and differences in agonistic behavior are related to sexual dimorphism. Differences in body size are due to genes and the nutritional status of pregnant mothers, as well as mating systems (Alexander et al., 1979; Bateson & Martin, 1999). Although physical stature is heritable within species, it is also affected by the perinatal environment; that is, our evolutionary history therefore provides a catalogue of options from which to choose. The option taken is related to the environment in which the individual develops. Given the vastly different environments into which individuals with comparable genetic histories are born, a single "genetic program" would not be equally effective across these different niches.

The human anthropological evidence used by Alexander and colleagues suggests that alternative strategies are used by human males and females, depending upon ecological constraints. When resources are scarce, both mothers and fathers are needed to rear and provision offspring; thus, monogamy is favored (Alexander et al., 1979). In such cases, sex differences in body size, sex segregation, and agonistic behavior should be attenuated. In polygamous cases with abundant resources, individual males compete with each other, using dominance-related roles and behaviors. Their status in these groups, in turn, relates to access to females. Males under these conditions should be bigger and physically more aggressive, and segregate themselves into juvenile groups where they can further develop associated physical conditioning and skills. Human cross-cultural studies support this claim. Specifically, male juveniles are socialized into more competitive and aggressive roles, especially in polygynous societies, where roles are not stratified (Low 1989).

Sex-Segregated Peer Groups

Sex-segregated peer groups are the contexts in which sex differences in aggressive behavior are socialized and develop. Like our closest genetic relatives, chimpanzees (*Pan troglodytes*) and bonobos (*Pan paniscus*), humans are sexually dimorphic, with males being around 15% larger than females (Alexander et al., 1979; deWaal & Lanting, 1997; Pellegrini, in press). Two interrelated hypotheses (the energetic hypothesis and the social roles hypothesis) have been presented to explain the existence of social group sex segregation among mammals more generally (Main, Weckerly, & Bleich, 1996; Ruckstuhl, 1998; Ruckstuhl & Neuhaus, 2002, in press) and humans in particular (Pellegrini, 2004).

First, the energetic hypothesis is based on the notion that differences in size have implication for energetic demands for males and females. Males, compared to females, are more physically active and require more exercise and space for physical conditioning. The second hypothesis suggests that adult social (reproductive) roles are responsible for segregation. For example, males segregate to learn and practice competitive and agonistic roles, such as rough-and-tumble (R&T) play. Both energetics and social roles, we suggest, are responsible for juvenile sex segregation. We suggest that males, more than females, are biased to high-energy models and behavior. With development, they are socialized to enact correspondingly energetic social roles that are associated with male and female reproductive roles.

The energetic hypothesis has two components, and each assumes that segregation is based on sexual dimorphism and corresponding differences in body size (Main et al., 1996). First, the *energetics* view posits that males and females choose different niches to maximize their physical growth and physical fitness. For example, typically larger-bodied male ungulates select areas that maximize body size and conditioning. This translates to larger males feeding on abundant, low-quality, high-fiber forage. Second, the *behavioral synchrony* aspect further clarifies this position by suggesting that male and female juveniles adjust their behavior in response to the behavior of the larger group (Ruckstuhl, 1998). Juvenile male ungulates (Ruckstuhl, 1998) and human juvenile males alike (Maccoby, 1998) exhibit less active behavior when in female groups, relative to being in a male groups. In short, participants may adjust their behavior to match that of the majority of their conspecifics.

The social factors hypothesis posits that the function of sex segregation is to learn the different male and female reproductive roles. Male groups, for example, are typified by R&T and physical aggression, because the male role is related to competing with others for access to mates. Female groups, on the other hand, are small and nurturant. When they become mothers and invest in their offspring, females spend time in dyadic units (with their offspring) caring for them and protecting them from infanticidal males.

The two hypotheses are developmentally complementary, however. Infant males and very young boys differentiate themselves from female peers, along lines associated with physically vigorous behaviors. During childhood, boys' and girls' groups differ in terms of energetics (Eaton & Enns, 1986). With development, and increases in social-cognitive competence, these energetic behaviors take the form of stereotypical social roles. During childhood, males' behavior, relative to females that of, is indeed more physically vigorous, but this vigor is typically expressed in behaviors related to social roles associated with dominance. Female behavior is more sedentary and embedded in the context of a small, often dyadic group, and this is associated with the nurturing role. In the following sections, we present evidence in support of the two hypotheses.

Energetic Hypothesis

Considering the energetic hypothesis, high levels of exercise can have both immediate *and* delayed benefits (Byers & Walker, 1995) for *both* males and females. That physical exercise may be *more* important for males, relative to females, is, however, at the heart of the energetic hypothesis for sex segregation. Exercise is more important for males, because it maximizes behavioral and morphological characteristics that are useful in competition with other males.

There is evidence for an early bias in males toward high-energetic behavior. In a meta-analysis of sex differences in activity level, Eaton and Enns (1986) found that male fetuses were more active than female ones. Differences in activity continue after birth. Furthermore, early sex differences have been found in males' and females' preference for action-based stimuli. For example, studies of infants suggest that boys and girls use body movement to discriminate between males and females (Kujawski & Bower, 1993).

More recently, Campbell, Shirley, Heywood, and Crook (2000) conducted a longitudinal experiment with infants at 3, 9, and 18 months of age. Using a visual preference paradigm, they showed video clips of children in male-typical activities (e.g., chasing, wrestling, climbing, jumping) and female typical activities (e.g., doll play, pat-a-cake, whispering, drawing). They found that male, compared to female, 9-month-olds looked longer at male activities, possibly reflecting an innate bias in males' preference for activity. At 18 months, both boys and girls preferred the male activities, possibly reflecting females' later attention and attraction to action-based stimuli. This bias continues into childhood, such that toddler males are more likely to imitate male models engaged in male-typical behavior than in female-typical behavior (Bauer, 1993). Gonadal hormones may bias males initially to high activity (Berenbaum & Hines, 1992; Hines & Kaufman, 1994). Consequently, males may express this bias by preferring to interact with others showing high activity—other males.

The finding from the meta-analysis cited earlier, that males are more active than females, and that these differences appear prenatally (Eaton & Enns, 1986), suggests that differences in activity were not due to socialization. Instead, exposure to androgens prenatally is probably the mechanism through which the selection pressure for more physically active males operates (Archer & Lloyd, 2002). These differences, in turn, may be responsible for male infants' preference for high-energy behaviors (Campbell et al., 2000). During preschool and later childhood, Eaton and Enns's (1986) meta-analysis found effect sizes (d) in sex differences in activity level for all studies reviewed of 0.44 and 0.66, respectively.

Although the degree of dimorphism in size is virtually nonexistent in childhood, there is still sex segregation. This may be because early experience in physical activity influences the development of systems that are relevant to later social roles and energetic demands. In lower mammals (e.g., rats and cats), Byers and Walker (1995) suggested that vigorous physical play during the juvenile period influences cerebellar synapse distribution and muscle fiber differentiation. These systems are important for subsequent development of skilled locomotive behavior and vigorous male reproductive social roles associated with hunting and predation, such as R&T. Thus, the juvenile period seems to be a sensitive period for the development of the neural and muscular basis of subsequent behaviors associated with sex segregation.

To further evaluate the energetic hypothesis of sex segregation, we can examine sex differences in physically vigorous play and caloric expenditure at different points in development. We would expect to find sex differences in caloric expenditure in physical activity during those periods when there is sex segregation, but little or no sex differences before that time: Sex segregation begins at around 3 years of age and peaks between 8 and 11 years (Maccoby, 1998).

Two experiments compared the caloric expenditure of the activity of boys and girls on the primary school playground during recess. The first experiment (Pellegrini, Horvat, & Huberty, 1998) examined two age groups (6.8 and 9.9 years), and found that the boys' play, relative to that of girls, became more costly (in terms of calories) with age, whereas girls' caloric expenditure remained constant. The second experiment reported in the study (Pellegrini et al., 1998) also involved two groups of children (ages 7.3 and 9.5 years), and found a sex-by-age interaction: Boys were more active than girls, and boys became more active with age, whereas girls remained at the same level. These findings show that sex differences in caloric expenditure in play do correspond to periods of peak sex segregation.

The second part of the energetic–behavioral synchrony hypothesis involves behavioral compatibility. Ruckstuhl (1998) proposed that this forms the basis of sex segregation in ungulates. To be a member of a group requires synchrony in individuals' behavior. For example, when young males are in all-male groups, their behavior is vigorous, but when they are in female groups, their behavior is more sedentary. Maccoby (1998) suggested that a similar process ("behavioral compatibility") underlies children's sex segregation. As noted earlier, Campbell et al. (2000) found that boys preferred looking at a sex-congruent activity at 9 months of age. This early bias may provide a basis upon which males differentiate themselves from females.

Studies examining the preference for playmates in relation to the child's sex and behavioral style provide more impressive evidence supporting the behavioral compatibility hypothesis. Alexander and Hines (1994) showed that boys (ages 4–8 years) expressed a preference for playing with girls who showed a masculine style, compared to a boy with a feminine play style. At 8, but not 4 years, girls also expressed a preference for playmates based on style rather than sex. Girls between 3 and 8 years of age who were exposed prenatally to high levels of male hormones (as a result of congenital adrenal hyperplasia [CAH]), were more likely than controls to choose males as playmates (Hines & Kaufman, 1994). Thus, behavioral style, rather than sex of the actor, seems to be an important dimension of sex segregation during child-hood. This evidence, in conjunction with that from the infancy preference studies, indicates that the bias toward compatible behaviors appears very early in development and is only minimally related to social learning.

The evidence in support of the behavioral compatibility hypothesis is sim-ilar during the period of early adolescence (Pellegrini, 1992). When youngsters in 6th and 7th grades (mean age of 13 years) were observed during free time at school, girls more often chose to remain indoors, and their activities were characterized by dyadic peer interaction and "passive social behavior" (in-cluding talking with peers and adults, comfort contact, and hugging). Males, in contrast, tended to be observed outdoors, and their groups were larger in number and characterized by rough play and dominance-oriented interac-tions. When males were observed with girls, however, their behavior was less rough and active.

Social Factors Hypothesis

With development, the social factors hypothesis posits that it is the need to learn sex-specific social skills that is responsible for segregation. In these groups, males and females learn and practice specific behaviors associated with the reproductive roles. The skills learned in segregated groups should be related to both immediate and delayed benefits. It is in these social roles that differences in energetics are realized in different types of agonistic behaviors for boys and girls. Males, for example, should segregate around dominance-related activities, such as R&T, competitive games, and physical aggression (Archer, 1992; Pellegrini & Smith, 1998). These behaviors are related to affili-ation with a variety of peers, and to physical conditioning during childhood. Females' segregation is in the service of forming close bonds and alliances with other females and, more distally, learning and practicing maternal skills, as well as avoiding physical aggression (Campbell, 1999). Females use safer, indirect aggression, to form these alliances and coalitions.

Studies of the choice of models for gender-appropriate roles and behavior provide a clear indication of this bias toward the activity level of roles chosen by boys and girls. Barkely, Ullman, Otto, and Brecht (1977) asked children to imitate a person carrying out gender-appropriate and -inappropriate activities. Boys imitated male activities and girls imitated female activities, regardless of the sex of the model. More recently, Alexander and Hines (1994) found in interviews that boys and girls, ages 4–8 years, generally preferred to play with other children on the basis of their play style (masculine or feminine) rather than on the basis of the sex of the actor (male or female).

The roles enacted by males tend to involve rough, competitive, and vigor-ous behaviors, which may have their ultimate origins in different levels of parental investment (Trivers, 1972), although the level of activity, and the social roles, may be, as we speculated earlier, moderated by environmental factors, such as availability of nutritional resources. Furthermore, males are socialized to express their physical activity in the form of rough play and aggression, often by their fathers. Indeed, fathers of young males spend significantly more time with sons, relative to their daughters (Parke & Suomi, 1981). During this time, fathers often engage in R&T and other forms of vigorous play with their sons (Carson, Burks, & Parke, 1993; MacDonald & Parke, 1986).

These physically rough and competitive behaviors have implications for male peer-group status. Male groups are hierarchically organized in terms of dominance, which is determined by a combination of agonistic and affiliative strategies used in the service of resources acquisition. Thus, in male groups, juveniles are using R&T, aggression, reconciliation, and facility in competitive games, as means of achieving status. Males tend to use aggressive strategies when their social groups are in the formative stages. After status is achieved, instances of physical aggression decrease, and dominant members use more affiliative strategies to reconcile former foes (Pellegrini, 2003; Pellegrini & Bartini, 2001).

After the second year of life, girls' interactions with their peers also reflect their roles in adult society. Specifically, the literature on children's pretend play is unequivocal in documenting sex differences in themes enacted in fantasy (Power, 2000). When fantasy play begins to emerge, at around 18 months of age (Fein, 1981), girls' play reflects domestic and nurturing themes (McLoyd, 1980; Saltz, Dixon, & Johnson, 1977). For example, Saltz et al. labeled the sorts of fantasy play that girls enacted as "social dramatic" and boys' play as "thematic fantasy." In social dramatic play, domestic and familial themes are enacted, with girls "mothering" or teaching younger children. Boys' thematic fantasy, on the other hand, is rooted in the world of superheroes and has themes associated with dominance, fighting, and competition.

With older, school-age children, boys' and girls' groups continue to differ. First, playgroups remained segregated, along rough/competitive and sedentary dimensions. Specifically, boys engage in competitive and physical games (Pellegrini, Kato, Blatchford, & Baines, 2002). Males' status in games, in turn, is related to their dominance status. Girls, on the other hand, spend significantly more time alone rather than in social interactions, exhibit more positive affect, and show more sedentary play than boys (Blatchford, Baines, & Pellegrini, 2003). The roles enacted in male and female groups tend to vary along energetic dimensions, and the roles tend to follow themes consistent with sexual selection theory: Males are competitive and aggressive, and females are sedentary and nurturant.

Females may avoid males because they represent threats, in the form of general aggression to themselves and, more distally, to their offspring. Consistent with the idea that females segregate for protection from males is the finding that adult presence increases the likelihood of girls interacting with boys (Maccoby, 1998). While male children seem to be more concerned with segregation than females, at least during childhood, females actively withdraw from interactions with males, often to seek the protection of their parents (Maccoby, 1998). In experimental studies of unacquainted toddlers, in which children were observed in mixed-sex dyads, girls often withdrew and stood next to their mothers (Maccoby, 1998). This sort of withdrawal was not observed in female dyads. Similar findings were reported for older children (5- and 6-year-olds). When quartets were observed in an experimental playroom, girls tended to stay near an adult when in mixed-sex, but not in all-girl groups (Greeno, 1991, cited in Maccoby, 1998).

In short, boys' and girls' peer groups are segregated in preschool, and males' and females' interaction is organized around different activities and toys by both adults and peers. The themes of the interactions, in turn, reflect males' bias toward competitive and dominance-oriented roles, and females' bias toward nurturing and domestic roles. It may be that the energetic dimensions of behaviors initially bias males and females to each other. Then, with subsequent social-cognitive development, children learn the behaviors associated with male and female roles in the wider society.

Sex Differences in Aggression

We have so far considered the developmental and broader social contexts of male and female groups, and the contrasting types of behavior that these involve. It is clear that in childhood, male groups involve more energetic play involving bodily contact (R&T) and concerns about dominance, largely based on physical prowess (e.g., Weisfeld, Block, & Ivers, 1983; Weisfeld, Omark, & Cronin, 1980). Female social groups are typically smaller and involve more disclosure of personal information and feelings, with closer social bonds. The evidence from studies of sex differences in aggression, in childhood and in adulthood, parallel these sex differences and can be understood in terms of fitting the different social contexts of male and female groups, as well as ultimately being the consequence of sexual selection. Broadly, these sex differences entail a higher frequency of direct aggression (physical and verbal) by males and a higher frequency of indirect or covert forms of aggression by females (Bjorkqvist, 1994).

These sex differences in indirect and direct aggression could be, following Campbell (1999), the result of different mating strategies. Following sexual selection theory, females, more than males, invest in the reproductive effort. They bear the fetus, protect it, and provision it. In the case of human infants, with their relatively long juvenile period, this investment is especially great. Females may use indirect, rather than direct, aggression to protect their offspring, because it is safer; that is, indirect aggression is less confrontational than direct aggression and, consequently, the perpetrators of indirect aggression are less likely to be the target of retaliation (relative to direct aggression). This indirectness, in turn, is more likely to result in the mother "staying alive" to care for her offspring (Campbell, 1999).

Physical Aggression

Sex differences in physical aggression are observed early in life, when children first interact with other children, between their second and third year. For example, two older observational studies (Sears, Rau, & Alpert, 1965; McGrew, 1972) yielded very large effect sizes for physical aggression at 4 years of age (d = 1.27 and 1.29, respectively: Archer, in press). Hay, Castle, and Davies (2000) reported observations from toddlers ages 18–30 months: Boys showed more frequent assaults on peers than did girls (d = 0.64 for sex differences in studies reviewed in Archer, in press). Campbell, Shirley, and Caygill (2002) observed children with a mean age of 27 months and found considerably greater numbers of negative interactions with peers for boys than girls. These included grabbing another child's toy (d = 1.42) and resisting another child's attempt to grab their toy (d = 0.86). Data from the Quebec longitudinal study (Baillargeon, 2002), in which children's behavior was rated by the child's primary caregiver (usually the mother), found sex differences at 17 months of age for kicking, biting, and hitting other children. Effect sizes were expressed in terms of odds ratios (1.53, 1.30, and 1.97, respectively), which is probably the statistic of choice for frequencies. Overall, these studies show that the sex difference in physical aggression occurs very early in postnatal life, in fact, as early as children engage in social interactions. The consensus from the few observational studies at young ages is that the magnitude of the sex difference is large. There is no indication of a progressive widening of the difference as boys and girls are exposed to different socialization influences (Tremblay et al., 1999).

In a large, representative-sample longitudinal study, Tremblay et al. (1999) showed that physical aggression (in the form of hitting, biting, and kicking) was most frequent at 24 and 27 months of age and progressively declined after these ages. Measures were taken at three monthly intervals from 24 months to 11 years of age, and involved maternal reports. At most ages, boys showed higher frequencies than girls.

Indirect Aggression

Physical (and its accompanying verbal) aggression are direct forms that have their counterparts in nonhumans. Individuals confront an opponent in a way that commands immediate attention and usually evokes a response. Fight or flight neatly sums up the main options, although aggressive intentions may lead to a number of other actions. First, aggression may be displaced to other targets that are unlikely to retaliate (Marcus-Newhall, Pedersen, Carlson, & Miller, 2000). Second, direct aggression may be inhibited and become the subject of revenge fantasies (e.g., Kenrick & Sheets, 1993). Third, aggression may take the form of actions designed to harm the opponent, without involving direct confrontation (Bjorkqvist, 1994). These three alternatives avoid the costs of violent retaliation associated with direct confrontation. They can be viewed as low-cost aggressive responses—the first two have no benefits, because they do not harm potential opponents, or make them comply. The third, "indirect aggression," has considerable effects on its victims, in terms of manipulating their behavior or excluding them from a social group.

Indirect aggression typically involves deliberate social exclusion and ostracism. Bjorkqvist and his colleagues (Lagerspetz, Bjorkqvist, & Peltonen, 1988; Bjorkqvist, Lagerspetz, & Kaukiainen, 1992) emphasized the indirect nature of these forms of aggression, whereas Crick and her colleagues (Crick, 1995; Crick & Grotpeter, 1995) emphasized their manipulation of social relations, referring to "relational" aggression. Some actions fall within one definition but not the other, and vice versa (Archer, 2001), but core items are consistent across the two categories.

The earliest studies of indirect aggression (Feshbach, 1969; Feshbach & Sones, 1971) involved introducing children into established dyads or small groups, and observing any acts of social exclusion or rejection that were directed toward them. Feshbach and Sones specifically viewed such actions as functionally comparable with direct aggression. Lagerspetz et al. (1988) used a peer-rating measure to study both direct and indirect forms of aggression among 11- and 12-year-old children. Children evaluated all others of the same sex in their class in response to the question, "What do they do when angry with another boy/girl in the class?" They did so by rating 18 possible responses along a 4-point scale. These involved items of both direct and indirect aggression and two more peaceful means of solving conflicts. Nearly all the responses loaded highly onto one of two factors, the first reflecting indirect and the second direct acts of aggression. For example, telling an untruth behind someone's back and suggesting to others that a child should be ignored both loaded heavily on the first (indirect) factor. Shoving, swearing at someone, and tripping him or her up, loaded heavily on the second (direct) factor. Two scales were formed from the factors, and these revealed a clear sex difference in the female direction for indirect aggression ($d = 0.80$), and in the male direction for direct aggression ($d = 1.15$). The researchers commented that the neglect of indirect aggression by most previous researchers had led to an incorrect characterization of girls as "nonaggressive." Girls are in fact aggressive, but they are more likely to express this by covert means than are boys.

A number of subsequent studies have confirmed this sex difference in indirect aggression among children (e.g., Bjorkqvist, Lagerspetz, & Kaukiainen, 1992; Crick & Grotpeter, 1995; Owens, 1996), although when all the available evidence is examined (Archer, in press), the overall difference is much smaller than that found in the better known studies. It does seem that there is a clear sex difference by 11 years of age and that this is maintained until around 18 years. During adulthood, it is likely that the sex difference is absent, at least in the sorts of educated, middle-class, Western samples that have been studied so far (Archer, in press).

In the original paper on indirect aggression (Lagerspetz et al., 1988), the authors commented on why indirect aggression is found more frequently in girls' than in boys' groups. As we have seen in earlier sections, girls' peer groups are characterized by a few emotionally important relationships. Such relationships make a person vulnerable to being psychologically harmed through tactics such as betraying confidences, threatening rejection, or actual rejection. Boys' social groups, on the other hand, involve less emotionally close relationships, but a recognized dominance order based on physical attributes and skills, and, particularly at older ages, social skills in areas such as storytelling, humor, and "banter" (Benson & Archer, 2002).

Kaukiainen et al. (1999) measured the association between social intelligence, empathy, and direct and indirect aggression in 10-, 12-, and 14-year-old children. Social intelligence involved being able to guess others' feelings, knowing how to make them to laugh, being able to persuade, and getting on with them. At all three ages, indirect aggression was positively associated with social intelligence, although the value at 12 years was low ($r = .18$). However, social intelligence showed no associations with direct forms of aggression at any of the ages studied. Green, Richardson, and Lago (1996) tested a suggestion from the original study of indirect aggression—that people with more dense social networks would use indirect forms of aggression more frequently. Consistent with this, they found that young men whose social networks were denser reported more indirect aggression (and less direct aggression) than men whose networks were less dense. In contrast, women reported similar levels of indirect aggression irrespective of their network density. Thus, when men's social networks are more like those of typical women, their pattern of aggression is also more like that of women. However, we should note that in this study, although women showed more indirect aggression than did men ($d = -0.38$), the difference was not large.

These two studies show that indirect aggression is linked both to a person's social intelligence and his or her social network. Thus, someone who has the social skills to manipulate others, operating within a social context in which social relationships and others' opinions are valued, will be more likely to use these forms of aggression. Girls' social groups, particularly at ages when their social skills become well developed, provide the ideal context for indirect aggression. Studies of the social groups of boys and girls confirm this pattern of more extensive and diffuse social relations among boys, and more intense relations with a best friend or small number of friends among girls (Griffin, 1986; Maccoby & Jacklin, 1987; Waldrop & Halverson, 1975).

The Development of Overt and Indirect Aggression

We have already indicated that direct aggression appears early in a child's development. Bjorkqvist, Osterman, and Kaukiainen (1992) proposed a developmental theory of changes in overt and indirect forms of aggression, based on their studies involving children at different ages. They viewed direct aggression as being replaced partly by more indirect forms as social intelligence develops. The extent to which this occurs depends on the individual (e.g., some children maintain a preference for physical aggression into middle childhood) and the context (direct aggression is more effective in certain circumstances). Although boys show more physical aggression than girls overall, and girls show more indirect aggression than boys, there is a decline in physical aggression with age for both sexes. According to the cross-sectional evidence presented by Bjorkqvist and his colleagues, verbal abuse increases from ages 8 to 11 years, and shows a slight decline from ages 15 to 18 years. Indirect aggression increases in both sexes from ages 8 to 11 years, and declines a little thereafter until age 18 years. The researchers suggest that men "catch up" with women by young adulthood, and that, as adults, both sexes engage in indirect aggression to similar extents.

Bjorkqvist, Osterman, and Lagerspetz (1994) qualified this view in a study of indirect aggression among Finnish university employees. They found two different types of indirect aggression, "rational-appearing aggression," aggression disguised as rational argument, and "social manipulation," involving backbiting and spreading false rumors. The first was more common among men and the second, more common among women, although these sex differences were relatively small. Campbell, Sapochnik, and Muncer (1997) also found a category involving social exclusion in a study of British undergraduates. This included telling stories, making others dislike the person, and seeking to exclude him or her. However, no sex differences were found in this study. But women did show more of a second category of indirect aggression, which involved actions such as cursing when the person had gone, and complaining to others about him or her. This seems to involve expressions of anger and annoyance when the person who had provoked these feelings had left, and may be related to displaced aggression (Marcus-Newhall et al., 2000). A further study (Archer, Monks, & Connors, 1997) did not find these two categories, or the sex differences, in another sample. Other research involving adults has usually found no sex differences in indirect aggression (Forrest, Etough, & Shevlin, 2002; Forrest & McGuckin, 2002; Green et al., 1996; Richardson & Green, 1999). Overall, these findings are consistent with the original suggestion by Bjorkqvist, Osterman, and Kaukiainen (1992) that men's indirect aggression increases in young adulthood, to reach levels similar to those found in women. We should qualify this conclusion by acknowledging that all the existing studies have involved educated samples from Western nations. In such social settings, the costs of more direct forms of aggression will be higher than in social environments that are less demanding in terms of required standards of public behavior.

In their original analysis of developmental trends in indirect aggression during childhood, Bjorkqvist, Osterman, and Kaukiainen (1992) used data from their peer-rating studies of indirect aggression at ages 8, 11, 15, and 18 years. Figure 9.2 shows the values for gossiping by age: An increase is appar-

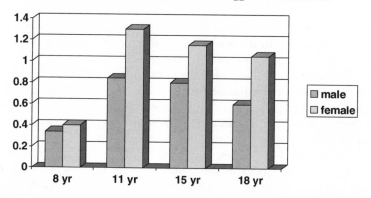

FIGURE 9.2. Age differences in indirect aggression (gossip): cross-sectional data. Based on Bjorkvist, Osterman, and Kaukiainen (1992).

ent in both sexes from 8 to 11 years of age, followed by a slight decline to 15 and 18 years. Sex differences are apparent at 11, 15, and 18 years of age. An Australian cross-sectional study (Owens, 1996), involving children ages 8, 12, 15, and 17 years, found greatly increased sex differences from 12 years ($d = 0.16$[1]), to 15 years ($d = 0.59$) to 17 ($d = 0.96$). These, and qualitative reports from the same sample (Owens, Shute, & Slee, 2000), suggest that covert aggression is particularly marked during teenage years among girls, and that it is used to manipulate social reputations and, ultimately, to manipulate other girls' prospects with boys.

In addition to this evidence from cross-sectional comparisons, there are two longitudinal studies of indirect aggression. In the Carolina Longitudinal Study (CLS; Cairns & Cairns, 1994), a multiple-cohort, multimethod study, begun in 1981–1982. There were large sex differences in self-reported indirect aggression at 8, 11, and 15 years of age ($d = 0.63, 0.96$, and 0.99[2]). Again, there was an increase from ages 8 to 11 years and older, but in this study, there was already a fairly large difference at 8 years of age.

A large (over 3,000) representative sample of Canadian children ages 4–11 years (Brendgen, Vaillancourt, Boivin & Tremblay, 2002) included measures of indirect aggression reported by the mother or the person most knowledgeable about the child. This study involved an accelerated longitudinal design using four cohorts. Factor analyses showed that the distinction between direct and indirect forms of aggression held across cohorts, time, and the sexes. From these data, longitudinal comparisons can be made across four age periods, using four different cohorts (ages 4, 6, and 8 years; ages 5, 7, and 9 years; ages 6, 8, and 10 years; and ages 7, 9, and 11 years).

There was an increase in indirect aggression from 4 to 6 years of age, which was more pronounced for girls than for boys: Sex differences were very small in magnitude at the two younger ages, and slightly larger at 8 years. In the next cohort, ages 5–9 years, indirect aggression increased with age for the girls, although, for the boys, it increased from ages 5 to 7 years and declined from ages 7 to 9 years. In this sample, sex differences were practically nonexistent at the younger ages and small (in the female direction) at 9 years of age. The third cohort showed that indirect aggression increased for both boys and girls from ages 6 to 8 years and declined by age 10. Sex differences were minimal at the youngest age and small (in the female direction) at the two oldest ages. In the fourth cohort, values were consistently high in the girls across ages 7, 9, and 11 years, yet they declined for boys from the youngest age. Sex differences were minimal at 7 years, and small (in the female direction) at ages 9 and 11 years. In these large Canadian samples, sex differences were small but consistently in the female direction from ages 8 to 11 years, based on mothers' reports. There was a broad trend for girls to show more indirect aggression than boys at these ages, but there were no large differences of the sort reported in the studies using peer ratings. It is indeed possible that mothers' reports underestimate the amount of indirect aggression, since it occurs in children's peer groups. This consideration alone should make peer reports the measure of choice for this type of aggression at these ages.

Overall, we can conclude that there is evidence from methodologically different studies that sex differences in indirect aggression are small in magnitude in middle childhood, and increase to age 11 years and older. The differences in middle childhood may have to do with sexually segregated groups, where girls' groups are smaller and more intimate, thus the importance of damaging social relations. The limited evidence from adults supports the view that the gap between the sexes closes by this time. The attenuation of sex differences in adulthood may be a result of males' learning to suppress direct confrontation in the modern world of commerce, business, and education.

CONCLUSIONS:
SEXUAL SELECTION AND AGGRESSION

Aggression was one of the main forms of behavior highlighted in the original formulation of sexual selection (Darwin, 1871). Higher male than female same-sex aggression follows from the principle of higher competition among members of the sex with the lesser parental investment, usually the male (Trivers, 1972). As we argued in the first part of this chapter, the extent to which this occurs depends on the characteristic mating system of the species, whether polygynous or monogamous. It also depends on environmental circumstances, in particular, nutrition. Nutritional stress will influence development in the direction of lesser sexual dimorphism and, possibly, lesser sex-segregation, leading to lower levels of aggression.

Examining the evidence from studies of human sex differences in direct forms of aggression, we were struck by the continuity with the pattern found in nonhumans. The developmental context of the greater male than female levels of direct aggression is that it occurs early in life, as part of the social relations characteristic of boys' groups. It forms part of a pattern that is probably initiated early in development by the action of testosterone on the preferred level of energetic play. From the perspective of sexual selection, it is interesting that this sex difference emerges in development though the interaction of early preferences with experiences in sex-segregated groups. Therefore, sex differences in direct aggression are found early in life and are closely connected with the social context in which they occur. They do not suddenly appear at puberty through the action of testosterone (Halpern, Udry, Campbell, & Suchindran, 1994). Evidence from studies of social development in nonhuman mammals suggests that here, too, males and females may have different developmental pathways leading to their respective adaptive end points.

The evidence from human studies of indirect aggression has fewer, if any, parallels in nonhuman animals. Campbell (1999) set out the reasons why a more cautious approach to direct confrontation would be expected from females as a consequence of sexual selection. These can be summarized as the greater fitness costs (in terms of offspring survival) of a female dying as a consequence of a risky activity, and the lower fitness benefits deriving from direct competition. The preference of girls for more covert methods of aggression can be viewed as an extension of this principle, and therefore as a further consequence of sexual selection. Again, these are patterns of behavior that develop in sex-segregated girls' groups rather than appearing at sexual maturity. Their occurrence in girls' groups during childhood shows the importance of considering the development of characteristics resulting from sexual selection, and the importance of the social context in which this development takes place.

NOTES

1. Effect sizes are taken from Archer (in press).
2. The values were calculated from the proportions of boys and girls showing different categories of aggression, using D-STAT software (Johnson, 1989).

REFERENCES

Alexander, G. M., & Hines, M. (1994). Gender labels and play styles: Their relative contributions to children's selection of playmates. *Child Development, 65*, 869–879.

Alexander, R. D., Hoogland, J. L., Howard, R. D., Noonan, K. M., & Sherman, P. W. (1979). Sexual dimorphisms and breeding systems in pinnipeds, ungulates, primates, and humans. In N. A. Chagnon & W. Irons (Eds.), *Evolutionary biology and human social behavior* (pp. 402–435). N. Scituate, MA: Duxbury Press.

Archer, J. (1992). *Ethology and human development.* Hemel Hemstead, UK: Harvester Wheatsheaf.

Archer, J. (2001). A strategic approach to aggression. *Social Development, 10,* 267–271.

Archer, J. (in press). Sex differences in aggression in real-world settings: A meta-analytic review. *Review of General Psychology.*

Archer, J., & Lloyd, B. (2002). *Sex and gender.* London: Cambridge University Press.

Archer, J., Monks, S., & Connors, L. (1997). Comments on SP0409: A. Campbell, M. Sapochnik and S. Muncer: Sex differences in aggression: Does social representation mediate forms? *British Journal of Social Psychology, 36,* 603–606.

Baillargeon, R. (2002). *Gender differences in physical aggression at 17 months of age.* Unpublished manuscript, Department of Psychology, University of Illinois at Urbana-Champaign.

Barkley, R. A., Ullman, D. G., Otto, L., & Brecht, J. M. (1977). The effects of sex-typing and sex-appropriateness of modeled behavior on children's imitation. *Child Development, 48,* 721–725.

Bateson, P. P. G., & Martin, P. (1999). *Design for life: How behaviour develops.* London: Jonathan Cape.

Bauer, P. J. (1993). Memory for gender-consistent and gender-inconsistent event sequences by twenty-five-month-old children. *Child Development, 64,* 285–297.

Benson, D. A., & Archer, J. (2002). An ethnographic study of sources of conflict between young men in the context of the night out. *Psychology, Evolution and Gender, 4,* 3–30.

Berenbaum, S. A., & Hines, M. (1992). Early androgens are related to childhood sex-typed toy preferences. *Psychological Science, 3,* 203–206.

Bjorklund, D. F., & Pellegrini, A. D. (2002). *Evolutionary developmental psychology.* Washington, DC: American Psychological Association Press.

Bjorkqvist, K. (1994). Sex differences in physical, verbal and indirect aggression: A review of recent research. *Sex Roles, 30,* 177–188.

Bjorkqvist, K., Lagerspetz, K. M. J., & Kaukiainen, A. (1992). Do girls manipulate and boys fight?: Developmental trends in regard to direct and indirect aggression. *Aggressive Behavior 18,* 117–127.

Bjorkqvist, K., Osterman, K., & Kaukiainen, A. (1992). The development of direct and indirect aggressive strategies in males and females. In K. Bjorkqvist & P. Niemela (Eds.), *Of mice and women: Aspects of female aggression* (pp. 51–64). San Diego: Academic Press.

Bjorkqvist, K., Osterman, K., & Lagerspetz, K.M.J. (1994). Sex differences in covert aggression among adults. *Aggressive Behavior, 20,* 27–33.

Blatchford, P., Baines, E., & Pellegrini, A. D. (2003). The social context of school playground games: Sex and ethnic differences, and changes over time after entry to junior school. *British Journal of Developmental Psychology, 21,* 481–505.

Brendgen, M., Vaillancourt, T., Boivin, M., & Tremblay, R. (2002, July). *A longitudinal analysis of indirect and physical aggression: Evidence for two factors over time?* In M. Brendgen (Chair), Developmental pathways of indirect aggression: Precursors and consequences. Symposium conducted at the XV World Meeting of the International Society for Research on Aggression, Montreal, Canada.

Buss, D. M. (1989). Sex differences in human mate preferences: Evolutionary hypotheses tested in 37 cultures. *Behavioral and Brain Sciences, 12,* 1–49 (including commentaries).

Byers, J. A., & Walker, C. (1995). Refining the motor training hypothesis for the evolution of play. *American Naturalist, 146,* 25–40.

Cairns, R. B., & Cairns, B. D. (1994). *Lifelines and risks: Pathways of youth in our time*. New York/London: Harvester Wheatsheaf.

Campbell, A. (1999). Staying alive: Evolution, culture and women's intra-sexual aggression. *Behavioral and Brain Sciences*, 22, 203–252 (including commentaries).

Campbell, A., Shirley, L., Heywood, C., & Crook, C. (2000). Infants' visual preference for sex-congruent babies, children, toys, and activities: A longitudinal study. *British Journal of Developmental Psychology*, 18, 479–498.

Campbell, A., Sapochnik, M., & Muncer, S. (1997). Sex differences in aggression: Does social representation mediate form of aggression? *British Journal of Social Psychology*, 36, 161–171.

Campbell, A., Shirley, L., & Caygill, L. (2002). Sex-typed preferences in three domains: Do two-year-olds need cognitive variables? *British Journal of Psychology*, 93, 203–217.

Caro, T. M., & Bateson, P. (1986). Ontogeny and organization of alternative tactics. *Animal Behaviour*, 34, 1483–1499.

Carson, J., Burks, V., & Parke, R. (1993). Parent–child physical play: Determination and consequences. In K. MacDonald (Ed.), *Parent–child play* (pp. 197–220). Albany: State University of New York Press.

Clutton-Brock, T. M. (1983). Selection in relation to sex. In D. S. Bendall (Ed.), *Evolution: From molecules to men* (pp. 457–481). London: Cambridge University Press.

Crick, N. R. (1995). Relational aggression: The role of intent attributions, feelings of distress, and provocation type. *Development and Psychopathology*, 7, 313–322.

Crick, N. R., & Grotpeter, J. K. (1995). Relational aggression, gender, and social, psychological adjustment. *Child Development*, 66, 710–722.

Darwin, C. (1871). *The descent of man and selection in relation to sex*. London: Murray.

deWaal, F., & Lanting, F. (1997). *Bonobo: The forgotten ape*. Berkeley: University of California Press.

Eaton, W., & Enns, L. (1986). Sex differences in human motor activity level. *Psychological Bulletin*, 100, 19–28.

Erckmann, W. W. (1983). The evolution of polyandry in shorebirds: An evaluation of hypotheses. In S. K. Wasser (Ed.), *Social behavior of female vertebrates* (pp. 113–168). New York: Academic Press.

Fein, G. (1981). Pretend play in childhood: An integrative review. *Child Development*, 52, 1095–1118.

Feshbach, N. (1969). Sex differences in children's modes of aggressive responses toward outsiders. *Merrill–Palmer Quarterly*, 15, 249–258.

Feshbach, N., & Sones, G. (1971). Sex differences in adolescents' reactions to newcomers. *Developmental Psychology*, 4, 381–386.

Forrest, S., Etough, V., & Shevlin, M. (March, 2002). *Developing a measure of adult indirect aggression*. Poster session presented at the Annual Conference of the British Psychological Society, Blackpool, UK.

Forrest, S., & McGuckin, C. (March, 2002). *Adult indirect aggression: Do men "catch up" with women in using indirect aggression?* Poster session presented at the Annual Conference of the British Psychological Society, Blackpool, UK.

Gottlieb, G. (1983). The psychobiological approach to developmental issues. In J. J. Campos & M. Haith (Eds.), *Handbook of child psychology: Infancy and developmental psychobiology* (Vol. II, pp. 1–26). New York: Wiley.

Green, L. R., Richardson, D. R., & Lago, T. (1996). How do friendship, indirect, and direct aggression relate? *Aggressive Behavior, 22*, 81–86.

Griffin, C. (1986). Qualitative methods and female experience: Young women from school to the job market. In S. Wilkinson (Ed.), *Feminist social psychology* (pp. 173–191). Milton Keynes, UK/Philadelphia: Open University Press.

Halpern, C. T., Udry, J. R., Campbell, B., & Suchindran, C. (1994). Relationships between aggression and pubertal increases in testosterone: A panel analysis of adolescent males. *Social Biology, 40*, 8–24.

Hay, D. F., Castle, J., & Davies, L. (2000). Toddlers' use of force against familiar peers: A precursor of serious aggression? *Child Development, 71*, 457–467.

Hines, M., & Kaufman, F. R. (1994). Androgen and the development of human sex-typical behavior: Rough-and-tumble play and sex of preferred playmates in children with congenital adrenal hyperplasia (CAH). *Child Development, 65*, 1042–1053.

Jenni, D. A. (1974). Evolution of polyandry in birds. *American Naturalist, 14*, 129–144.

Johnson, B. T. (1989). *Software for the meta-analytic review of research literatures.* Hillsdale, NJ: Erlbaum.

Kaukiainen, A., Bjorkqvist, K., Lagerspetz, K., Osterman, K., Salmivalli, C., Rothberg, S., et al. (1999). The relationship between social intelligence, empathy, and three types of aggression. *Aggressive Behavior, 25*, 81–89.

Kenrick, D. T., & Sheets, V. (1993). Homicidal fantasies. *Ethology and Sociobiology, 14*, 231–146.

Kujawski, J. H., & Bower, T. G. R. (1993). Same-sex preferential looking during infancy as a function of abstract representation. *British Journal of Developmental Psychology, 11*, 201–209.

Lagerspetz, K. M. J., Bjorkqvist, K., & Peltonen, T. (1988). Is indirect aggression typical of females?: Gender differences in 11- to 12-year old children. *Aggressive Behavior, 4*, 403–414.

Lorenz, K. (1950). The comparative method in studying innate behaviour patterns. *Symposia of the Society for Experimental Biology, 4*, 221–268.

Low, B. S. (1989). Cross-cultural patterns in the training of children: An evolutionary perspective. *Journal of Comparative Psychology, 103*, 311–319.

Maccoby, E. E. (1998). *The two sexes: Growing up apart, coming together.* Cambridge, MA: Harvard University Press.

Maccoby, E., & Jacklin, C. (1974). *The psychology of sex differences.* Stanford, CA: Stanford University Press.

Maccoby, E. E., & Jacklin, C. N. (1987). Gender segregation in childhood. In H. W. Reese (Ed.), *Advances in Child Development and Behavior, 20*, 239–287. New York/London: Academic Press.

MacDonald, K., & Parke, R. (1986). Parent–child physical play. *Sex Roles, 15*, 367–378.

McGrew, W. C. (1972). *An ethological study of children's behavior.* New York: Academic Press.

McLoyd, V. (1980). Verbally expressed modes of transformation in the fantasy and play of black preschool children. *Child Development, 51*, 1133–1139.

Main, M. B., Weckerly, F. W., & Bleich, V. C. (1996). Sexual segregation among ungulates: New directions for research. *Journal of Mammalogy, 77*, 449–461.

Marcus-Newhall, A., Pedersen, W. C., Carlson, M., & Miller, N. (2000). Displaced aggression is alive and well: A meta-analytic review. *Journal of Personality and Social Psychology, 78*, 670–689.

Miller, G. F. (1998). How mate choice shaped human nature: A review of sexual selection and human evolution. In C. Crawford & D. L. Krebs (Eds.), *Handbook of evolutionary psychology: Issues, ideas, and applications* (pp. 87–129). London: Heinemann.

Moffitt, T. (2002, August). *Behavioral genomics of antisocial behavior: How genetic research pushes environmental theory forward.* Invited address to the International Society for the Study of Behavioral Development, Ottawa, Canada.

Owens, L. D. (1996). Sticks and stones and sugar and spice: Girls' and boys' aggression in schools. *Australian Journal of Guidance and Counselling, 6*, 45–55.

Owens, L. D., Shute, R., & Slee, P. (2000). "Guess what I just heard!": Indirect aggression among teenage girls in Australia. *Aggressive Behavior, 26*, 67–83.

Parke, R. D., & Suomi, S. J. (1981). Adult male–infant relationships: Human and nonhuman primate evidence. In K. Immelman, G. W. Barlow, L. Petronovitch, & M. Main (Eds.), *Behavioral development* (pp. 700–725). New York: Cambridge University Press.

Pellegrini, A. D. (1992). Preference for outdoor play during early adolescence. *Journal of Adolescence, 15*, 241–254.

Pellegrini, A. D. (2003). Perceptions and function of playfighting in early adolescence. *Child Development, 74*, 1459–1470.

Pellegrini, A. D. (2004). Sexual segregation in childhood: A review of evidence for two hypotheses. *Animal Behaviour, 68*, 435–443.

Pellegrini, A. D. (in press). Sexual segregation in humans. In K. Ruckstuhl & P. Neuhaus (Eds.), *Sexual segregation in vertebrates.* Cambridge, UK: Cambridge University Press.

Pellegrini, A. D., & Bartini, M. (2001). Dominance in early adolescent boys: Affiliative and aggressive dimensions and possible functions. *Merrill–Palmer Quarterly, 47*, 142–163.

Pellegrini, A. D., Horvat, M., & Huberty, P. D. (1998). The relative cost of children's physical activity play. *Animal Behaviour, 55*, 1053–1061.

Pellegrini, A. D., Kato, K., Blatchford, P., & Baines, E. (2002). A short-term longitudinal study of children's playground games across the first year of school: Implications for social competence and adjustment to school. *American Educational Research Journal, 39*, 991–1015.

Plavcan, J. M., & van Schaik, C. P. (1999). Intrasexual competition and body weight dimorphism in anthropoid primates. *American Journal of Physical Anthropology, 103*, 37–68.

Power, T. G. (2000). *Play and exploration in children and animals.* Mahwah, NJ: Erlbaum.

Richardson, D. R., & Green, L. R. (1999). Social sanction and threat explanations of gender effects on direct and indirect aggression. *Aggressive Behavior, 25*, 425–434.

Ruckstuhl, K. E. (1998). Foraging behaviour and sexual segregation in bighorn sheep. *Animal Behaviour, 56*, 99–106.

Ruckstuhl, K. E., & Neuhaus, P. (2002). Sexual segregation in ungulates: A comparative test of three hypotheses. *Biological Review, 77*, 77–96.

Saltz, E., Dixon, D., & Johnson, J. (1977). Training disadvantaged preschoolers on various fantasy activities: Effects on cognitive functioning and impulse control. *Child Development, 48*, 367–380.

Schmitt, D. P., & the 118 Members of the International Sexuality Description Project. (2003). Universal sex differences in the desire for sexual variety: Tests from 52 nations, 6 continents, and 13 islands. *Journal of Personality and Social Psychology, 85*, 85–104.

Sears, R. R., Rau, L., & Alpert, R. (1965). *Identification and childrearing*. Stanford, CA: Stanford University Press.

Smuts, B. B. (1985). *Sex and friendship in baboons*. Hawthorne, NY: Aldine de Gruyter.

Stamps, J. (2003). Behavioural processes affecting development: Tinbergen's fourth question comes to age. *Animal Behaviour, 66*, 1–13.

Suomi, S. J. (in press). Genetic and environmental contributions influencing the expression of impulsive aggression and serotonergic functioning in rhesus monkeys. In R. E. Tremblay, W. W. Hartup, & J. Archer (Eds.), *Developmental origins of aggression*. New York: Guilford Press.

Symons, D. (1979). *Play and aggression: A study of rhesus monkeys*. New York: Columbia University Press.

Terman, L. M. (1946). Psychological sex differences. In L. Carmichael (Ed.), *Manual of child psychology* (pp. 954–1000). New York: Wiley.

Tinbergen, N. (1951). *The study of instinct*. London: Oxford University Press.

Tremblay, R. E., Japel, C., Perusse, D., Boivin, M., Zoccolillo, M., Montplaisir, J., et al. (1999). The search for the age of "onset" of physical aggression: Rousseau and Bandura revisted. *Criminal Behavior and Mental Health, 9*, 8–23.

Trivers, R. (1972). Parental investment and sexual selection. In B. B. Campbell (Ed.), *Sexual selection and the descent of man* (pp. 136–179). Chicago: Aldine.

Trivers, R. L. (1985). *Social evolution*. Menlo Park, CA: Benjamin/Cummings.

Waldrop, M. F., & Halverson, C. F., Jr. (1975). Intensive and extensive peer behavior: Longitudinal and cross-sectional analyses. *Child Development, 46*, 19–26.

Weisfeld, G. E., Bloch, S. A., & Ivers, J. W. (1983). A factor analytic study of peer-perceived dominance in adolescent boys. *Adolescence, 18*, 229–243.

Weisfeld, G. E., Omark, D. R., & Cronin, C. L. (1980). A longitudinal and cross-sectional study of dominance in boys. In D. R. Omark, F. F. Strayer, & D. G. Freedman (Eds.), *Dominance relations: An ethological view of human conflict and social interaction* (pp. 205–216). New York/London: Garland STPM Press.

Wood, W., & Eagly, A. H. (2002). A cross-cultural analysis of the behavior of women and men: Implications for the origins of sex differences. *Psychological Bulletin, 128*, 699–727.

Zihlman, A. E. (1996). Reconstructions reconsidered: Chimpanzee models and human evolution. In W. C. McGrew, L. F. Marchant, & N. Toshisada (Eds.), *Great ape societies* (pp. 293–304). Cambridge, UK: Cambridge University Press.

10

SOCIAL BEHAVIOR AND PERSONALITY DEVELOPMENT

The Role of Experiences with Siblings and with Peers

JUDITH RICH HARRIS

They lacked the fleetness of the deer, the teeth and claws of the lion, even the climbing ability of the chimpanzee; yet our ancestors managed to survive in a hazardous environment. The way they did it was by banding together. *Homo sapiens* is a highly social species. A basic tenet of evolutionary psychology is that "the human mind has been prepared by natural selection, operating over geological time, for life in a human group" (Bjorklund & Pellegrini, 2002, p. 4).

Survival in ancestral times hinged on becoming and remaining an acceptable member of a group. Through the trial and error of natural selection, evolution provided the members of our species with mental equipment designed to serve the evolutionarily important goals of winning the acceptance and esteem of their groupmates. In this chapter, I use evidence from several areas of psychology to draw conclusions about how these mental mechanisms operate during childhood and what environmental information they are tuned to receive.

THE CHALLENGE FACING THE CHILD

Since societies differ in the social behaviors their members deem appropriate, social behaviors cannot all be built in. But it is not simply a question of tailoring one's behavior to one's society because, within every society, social behav-

245

iors deemed appropriate differ for children versus adults and for males versus females. In large, complex societies, there may be other relevant social categories as well.

And the job is still more complicated than that, because within every social category there are individual differences in social behavior—differences that are not only tolerated but expected. The clearest example is the dominance hierarchy, found in nonhuman animal groups as well as in humans. The dominant members of groups behave differently from the lower downs. A small, puny member of a group would quickly find itself in trouble if it attempted to behave in an aggressive fashion. Other examples of within-category differences may be peculiar to our own species; for example, pretty girls behave differently from plain ones (Etcoff, 1999). Thus, individuals must adjust their social behavior not only to their group but also to their status or niche within the group.

Clearly, children have a lot to learn about social behavior. I argue in this chapter that this learning involves at least two different processes, each regulated by a specialized mental mechanism. The *socialization mechanism* makes the members of a given society—and, within a society, the members of a given social category—more alike in their social behavior. Since I have elsewhere discussed socialization in detail (Harris, 1995, 1998, 2000b), the lion's share of this chapter is devoted to the second process: one that maintains, increases, or produces individual differences in social behavior. This process is regulated by what I call the *behavioral strategy mechanism*.

When individual differences in social behavior are observed in adults and are maintained over long periods of time and in a variety of situations, we attribute them to differences in personality. *Personality development*, then, is the development during childhood of chronic patterns of behavior (along with their cognitive and emotional concomitants) that differ from one individual to another. Some individuals are chronically more outgoing, or more aggressive, or more rule-abiding than others.

Research in behavioral genetics (see Segal & Hill, Chapter 5, this volume) has shown that roughly half the variation in personality within a given population is genetic in origin; people differ in part because they have different genes. This chapter focuses on the other part of the variation—the part attributed to the environment. How do children respond to signals from the environment and to what signals do they respond? Which signals lead to short-term, context-dependent changes in behavior, and which are responsible for longer term shaping of the personality?

"If one knows what adaptive functions the human mind was designed to accomplish," observed Cosmides, Tooby, and Barkow, "one can make many educated guesses about what design features it should have" (1992, p. 10). One can then test these guesses either by using existing evidence or by designing new studies. The proposals I make here—that there are two separate mechanisms, both operating in the domain of social behavior but having different adaptive functions and different design features—are, as I will show, consistent with the preponderance of existing evidence. It is my hope that these proposals will point the way to new research designed specifically to test them.

SOCIALIZATION

On average, people in different societies differ somewhat in personality (McCrae, 2004). Are these differences entirely cultural or is there also a genetic component? The behavioral-genetic evidence is uninformative on this question, since the participants in these studies almost always come from the same broad culture. What the evidence does suggest, however, is that cultural effects on personality occur on a societywide level rather than on a family-by-family level. Siblings who grew up in the same family are not noticeably more alike in personality than those who grew up in separate families, which means that differences among families within the society have little or no effect on adult personality (Bouchard & Loehlin, 2001; Rowe, 1994).[1] If there are subcultural differences among the families of the people who participate in these studies, or if their homes differed from the norm in some way, these differences have negligible effects on the aspects of personality that have been measured.

The implication of these results is that children acquire culturally approved patterns of social behavior outside the home. Though this conclusion is at odds with the standard theory of socialization, it can explain things that the standard theory cannot: for example, why the children of immigrants, and the hearing children of Deaf parents, adopt the culture and language of the neighborhood in which they grow up, and abandon the culture and language of their parents (Harris, 1998); and why a child who obeys rules such as "Do not cheat" and "Do not lie" at home may nonetheless cheat on tests in the classroom or in games on the playground (Hartshorne & May, 1930/1971).

Although atypical families provide the clearest examples, the conclusion that socialization occurs outside the home is not restricted to such families. All children, no matter how "normal" their homelife, have to learn what behaviors are acceptable in public, and they cannot do this simply by imitating their parents. Adults do many things that children are not permitted to do, and children do many things they never see adults doing.

My conclusion about socialization also explains why girls and boys continue to behave differently in public despite the best efforts of many contemporary parents to raise them in an androgynous fashion (Serbin, Powlishta, & Gulko, 1993), and why boys reared in fatherless homes are no less masculine in their behavior than boys with fathers (Stevenson & Black, 1988). During middle childhood, children spontaneously divide into all-male and all-female groups wherever their numbers are sufficient to permit such a division (Edwards, 1992). Socialization of gender-specific behavior occurs within these groups (see Pellegrini & Archer, Chapter 9, this volume).

The job of learning how to behave appropriately can be broken down into several components. The child has to figure out which social categories exist in her society. She has to figure out which of these categories she belongs in. She has to observe and record how the members of each social category— especially her own—behave. Finally, she has to adjust her behavior, as best she can given her genetic makeup, to that of her own social category. It is a formidable cognitive challenge.

I propose that evolution has provided children with a specialized device— the socialization mechanism—that enables them to acquire acceptable social behavior and provides the motivation to do so. This mechanism makes use of information provided by a submodule that does the job of categorization (see Barrett, Chapter 17, this volume). A sizable body of research shows that people—adults and children—do categorize other people (e.g., Serbin et al., 1993). When we meet someone new, we automatically categorize him or her by age, gender, and race; the stereotypes associated with these social categories are activated, usually without conscious awareness (Macrae & Bodenhausen, 2000). A stereotype is a generalization about a category of people. The fact that we have stereotypes and that the stereotypes—at least those for familiar groups such as men and women—tend to be reasonably accurate (Swim, 1994) suggests that the human mind contains a device for computing averages or central tendencies. Atypical examples are given little weight in the formation of stereotypes.

This averaging process can explain why children reared in atypical homes nonetheless become acceptable members of their society—why the family makes so little difference, once genetic influences have been taken into account. The goal furnished by the socialization mechanism is to become a typical member of one's social category, based on the template provided by the submodule that calculates central tendencies. It is safer to base one's behavior on a calculated average than on a particular exemplar such as a parent or sibling, because there is always the risk that the particular exemplar might be atypical.

To succeed in adult life, children have to look beyond the nuclear family, to a world inhabited by people who are not their close relatives and who are not motivated by kinship to accept them. Behaviors acquired within the family will not necessarily serve them well in that larger world. For long-term adjustments in social behavior, it is to the child's advantage to use as much information about that larger world as the environment provides.

INDIVIDUAL DIFFERENCES IN PERSONALITY

The socialization mechanism cannot account for the fact that, within social categories in a given society, people differ chronically in behavior for reasons other than their different genes. Even identical twins reared in the same home differ in personality (Bouchard, Lykken, McGue, Segal, & Tellegen, 1990). It is the second mechanism, the behavioral strategy mechanism, that accounts for individual differences.

Consider dominance hierarchies. Within a group of chickens, wolves, chimpanzees, or humans, some individuals have higher status than others—hence, greater access to resources such as food and mates. In nonhuman animals and to some extent in human males (especially young ones), these hierarchies are based primarily on size and strength. An individual at or near the top of the hierarchy can get away with aggressive behavior that would be foolish, even suicidal, in one near the bottom. Individuals who lack the ability to dominate in an aggressive encounter have to learn to avoid evoking the anger of those bigger and stronger than themselves.

The prolonged human childhood provides individuals with the opportunity to try out behavioral strategies at a time when a mistake is less likely to have serious consequences. Equally important, it provides the opportunity to acquire the self-knowledge that is required for the selection of a workable strategy. Children have to learn, while they are growing up, what sort of people they are. Are they big or small, strong or weak, fast or slow, smart or dumb, pretty or plain? This information cannot be built in, because the genes that make individuals strong, smart, or pretty are scrambled by sexual recombination in each new generation (Tooby & Cosmides, 1990), and because such characteristics are affected by environment as well as by genes. Yet this information is essential. Without it, an individual has no basis for deciding whether to try to dominate others or give up without a fight, to make suggestions or follow the suggestions of others, to turn down potential mates in the hope of doing better or take whatever comes along.

In order to select an appropriate behavioral strategy that they can carry with them to adulthood, children have to learn from their experiences. I posit a mechanism honed by evolution to be sensitive to certain kinds of information gained through social interactions. Social interactions are not equally informative; some provide more useful information than others. What do children learn from their interactions with siblings and with peers? Because there is a rich trove of data on aggressive behavior and dominance, I use that as my primary example in figuring out how the behavioral strategy mechanism operates and what kind of information it uses.

Interactions with Siblings

Behavioral-genetic evidence has shown that people who grew up in the same family—whether they are twins, ordinary siblings, or adoptive siblings—are alike in personality only to the degree that they share genes by common descent. Adoptive siblings, who have no genes in common, are no more alike in adulthood than adoptees picked at random from the population. Summarizing these data in a groundbreaking article, Plomin and Daniels (1987) asked, "Why are children in the same family so different from one another?"

For many psychologists and nonpsychologists, the answer was obvious: because they differ in birth order. An explicit effort to use birth order to explain the personality differences between siblings, and to make the explanation consistent with Darwinian theory, was presented by Sulloway in his book *Born to Rebel* (1996).

According to Sulloway (1996), "Siblings become different for the same reason that species do over time: divergence minimizes competition for scarce resources" (p. xv). Because ordinary siblings share, on average, only 50% of their genes, their interests do not entirely coincide; each wants a larger share of family resources such as parental attention. This conflict of interests leads to competition—a competition in which the higher status sibling (in Sulloway's view, generally the firstborn) has the edge. Competition between individuals who differ in power or status leads, in turn, to divergence—an effort to fill different niches in the family in order to reduce competition. Typically, firstborns "employ their superior size and strength to defend their special status" (p. xiv), and consequently develop a personality that is dominant, jealous, and in favor of maintaining the status quo. Laterborns develop their own counterstrategies to the firstborn's attempt to dominate; they compete primarily "through good-natured sociability and cooperation" (p. 79). This is a good description of the behavioral consequences of a dominance hierarchy.

That dominance hierarchies exist among siblings is unquestionably true. But there are problems, both theoretical and empirical, with using this approach to account for the personality differences among adults. The first problem is the widely held premise that siblings become different as a result of growing up together. This premise is based on a misinterpretation of the behavioral genetic data.

As Plomin and Daniels (1987) explained, differences in genes account for no more than half the variance (the variation among all the subjects who participated in a given study) in personality. The environment shared by siblings accounts for little or none of it. Behavioral geneticists attribute the remainder of the variance—around 50% of the total—to what they call the *nonshared environment*. And the nonshared environment is commonly defined as the environment that "makes siblings differ from one another" (e.g., Dick & Rose, 2002, p. 70).

This definition has been interpreted to mean that something in the home environment, or in the sibling relationship itself, causes siblings to diverge in personality. But this is incorrect; growing up together does not cause siblings to diverge. Sharing a home does not increase the differences between siblings: It simply fails to make them more alike. The effects attributed to the nonshared environment are *uncorrelated* between siblings (Plomin & Daniels, 1987, p. 5), not negatively correlated. If growing up together caused siblings to diverge, there should be negative correlations between adoptive siblings reared together, and identical twins reared together should be more dissimilar than those reared apart. Research does not confirm these predictions. It is true that reared-together twins become less alike as they mature, but that is because the home environment produces some transient similarities in the early years, especially in IQ (McCartney, Harris, & Bernieri, 1990). Growing up together can temporarily make siblings a little more alike; it does not make them different.

The second problem for birth order theories in general, and Sulloway's (1996) theory in particular, is how to account for the differences between twins. The behavioral-genetic findings hold true for all kinds of sibling pairs, twins and nontwins alike. In a major study (Reiss, 2000), five different types of sibling pairs—identical twins, fraternal twins, ordinary siblings, half-siblings, and stepsiblings—were all assessed with the same exhaustive battery of tests, and the findings for shared and nonshared environment were essentially the same for all. The results led Reiss to conclude that "there are not important differences in shared or nonshared environment" (p. 142) among the various types of sibling pairs. In other words, once one deducts the similarities and differences that are due to genes, the remaining differences between sibling pairs are about the same. The implication is clear: Whatever environmental influences cause ordinary siblings to differ also cause identical twins to differ, and to differ just as much.

Twins do not differ in birth order, at least in the usual sense. However, even identical twins may differ in status or power within the family; Sulloway's (1996) theory attributes sibling differences to the competition produced by differences in status or power. The problem is that competition is not uniform across sibling types. According to kin selection theory, close relatives should compete less and cooperate more than distant relatives or nonrelatives. Support for this principle has been found in many species, including our own. Though the underlying mechanism is still unknown, even immature humans appear to have some way of assessing genetic relatedness. Identical twins compete with each other less and cooperate more than fraternal twins (Segal, 1999; Segal & Hershberger, 1999). In polygamous communities, children feel closer to their full siblings than to their half-siblings (Jankowiak & Diderich, 2000). If competition were the engine that produces nongenetic sibling differences, we should expect such differences to be sizable between adoptive or step-siblings, moderate between ordinary siblings, and small between identical twins. What we find instead is that the nongenetic differences are about the same for all these pairs.

The third problem is the assumption, implicit in Sulloway's (1996) theory, that diverging from each other will aid children in their attempt to gain a larger share of scarce family resources such as parental attention. To my knowledge, there are no data to support this assumption; nor does it follow from principles of evolutionary psychology. It is at least as plausible to assume that younger children would profit from acting more like their older siblings, or that older ones would do well to behave like their younger siblings, depending on whether parents favor older children or younger ones.

Oddly enough, there is no agreement among evolutionary psychologists regarding the effects of children's age on parental favoritism. Some (e.g., Daly & Wilson, 1988) believe that parents favor older children, because they are closer to the time when they can reproduce. If this is the case, then it would seem that a younger child's best strategy would be to act as mature as possible—sensible, responsible, not too clingy. Other evolutionary psychologists (e.g., Trivers, 1985) believe that parents favor younger offspring, because that is where a given amount of parental investment can produce the greatest benefit. Trivers used this reasoning to account for "regression" in older offspring—in particular, the infantile behavior displayed in human and nonhuman offspring around the time of weaning.

Although infants are at greater risk of being killed by their parents than are older children (Daly & Wilson, 1988), this may reflect the infant's vulnerability rather than the parents' preferences. Evidence from families functioning within the normal range supports the view that most parents actually favor younger, more dependent offspring. In two studies (Dunn & Plomin, 1990; McHale, Crouter, McGuire, & Updegraff, 1995), British and American parents of two preadolescent children were asked if they felt more affection for one child than the other. More than half admitted they did. The overwhelming majority of these parents—87% of the mothers and 85% of the fathers in the second study—said that they favored the younger child. Another study (Jenkins, Rasbash, & O'Connor, 2003) focused on the parents' behavior, rather than their feelings, in families with two or more children. The amount of "positive parenting," defined as warmth and involvement, declined steadily as the age of the child increased, over the age range of 4–11 years.

It would seem, then, that the best strategy for firstborns would be to act younger and more helpless than they really are. But, though there may be brief periods of regression, this is not a strategy they stick with. On the contrary, many of the terms often used by family members to describe firstborns— serious, responsible, bossy (Ernst & Angst, 1983)—are associated with greater maturity. Such behavior has been interpreted as an attempt to curry favor with parents (Sulloway, 1996), but other evidence supports a different explanation: The reason why firstborns are often seen by their parents as responsible, and by their younger siblings as bossy and aggressive, is that these behaviors are *evoked* by the presence of younger children.

In a cross-cultural survey, Edwards (1992) reported that two behaviors are seen consistently around the world in older children's interactions with younger ones: nurturance and dominance. Boys and girls of preschool age or older tend to be nurturant toward babies and toddlers, whether or not they are siblings. Once the younger child is past toddlerhood, nurturance may still be detectable in the older child's behavior, but it is likely to be accompanied, and eventually outweighed, by attempts to dominate. Dominance does not necessarily involve aggression, but it often does. As Edwards observed, "A pecking order of size and strength consistently emerges in multi-age [play] groups" (p. 303).

Goodall (1986) has described a similar pattern in chimpanzees. Like other group-living mammals, she explained, chimpanzees "tend to behave in varied and predictable ways to members of the several age-sex classes" (p.

173). Age and sex distinctions are made on the basis of physical appearance: "Thus small body size, pale skin, and white tail tuft indicate infancy" (p. 116). According to Goodall, juvenile male and female chimpanzees are attracted to infants of their species and are relatively gentle with them.

In our own species, studies have shown that children as young as age 4 "talk down" to still younger children: They use shorter, simpler sentences when conversing with toddlers than with children of their own age (Shatz & Gelman, 1973). They do this whether or not they have younger siblings and whether or not the younger children are related to them. These observations call into question the view that firstborns behave in a nurturant manner toward their younger siblings in an attempt to win parental approval. The same kind of behavior occurs in the absence of parents and when the younger child is not a sibling or even a close acquaintance.

Summary

Growing up together does not make siblings different. Nongenetic personality differences are about equal in magnitude for all kinds of sibling pairs, including identical twins. Both these findings present difficulties for a theory that attributes personality differences to competition between siblings. Other evidence suggests that firstborns are unlikely to increase parental investment by acting more mature. The nurturance and dominance shown by firstborns toward their younger siblings are typical of the way older children act toward younger ones; these behaviors appear to be evoked by the presence of a younger child.

Interactions with Peers

Although firstborns spend much of their time at home "talking down" to their younger siblings (Dunn, 1985), no one expects firstborns to use shorter, simpler sentences in conversing with adults or with their peers. It is taken for granted that children, like adults, adjust their style of speech to their interlocutor. Yet many psychologists make the assumption that other kinds of behaviors acquired within the family become a permanent part of the personality. This assumption is the fourth problem for birth order theorists.

According to Sulloway (1996), firstborns acquire bossy or aggressive patterns of behavior as a result of interacting with, and competing with, their younger siblings. These behaviors are assumed to transfer or generalize to other social interactions, involving people outside the family. It is not just that firstborns are more aggressive at home: Sulloway's theory predicts that they will be more aggressive wherever they go.

To produce such results, there would have to be an underlying mental mechanism that forms lifelong behavioral strategies on the basis of experiences within the family in the first 5 or 10 years of life. There are questions to be asked about such a hypothetical mechanism. Would it increase an individ-

ual's chances of surviving and reproducing, under the conditions that prevailed in ancestral times? If not, why would it have evolved? Why would a
mechanism that operated in this fashion have beaten out, in the competition
of Darwinian selection, one that operated in some other way?

The flaw in this hypothetical mechanism is that experiences within the
family in the first 5 or 10 years of life might be a poor indicator of the conditions one will have to face outside the family in adulthood, which means that
basing one's lifelong behavioral strategy on these experiences could be a serious mistake. As Tooby and Cosmides (1990) pointed out, there is a cost
involved in locking in a behavioral strategy too early: "The individual is subsequently committed to pursuing that strategy, even if it finds itself in situations where that strategy is radically inappropriate" (pp. 46–47). It makes
more sense to choose a behavioral strategy "as a response to what environment one finds oneself in; for example, be aggressive in those environments
where one is victimized for passiveness and peaceful in those environments
where one is penalized for aggressive behavior" (p. 46). In other words, retain
the ability to adjust one's behavior to a variety of social contexts, because a
behavioral strategy that worked in one context will not necessarily work in
others.

Aggression does not work in every context. A child can get away with
behaviors with family members that would not be tolerated by nonrelatives. A
firstborn who had grown accustomed to dominating his younger siblings
could put himself in jeopardy if he tried to act in a dominating manner with
his peers. What if he turned out to be the smallest and weakest child in his age
group? Being bigger and stronger than one's younger siblings is not a good
predictor—not a predictor at all—of one's ability to successfully employ an
aggressive strategy in life outside the family. I conclude that evolution would
be unlikely to produce a mechanism that caused long-term selection of behavioral strategies to be based on experiences within the family.[2] Only if children
lacked the mental capacity to store behavioral programs for more than one
context would it make sense for them to keep using the one they learned first,
and there are no signs that the child's mind is lacking in storage capacity.
Children can learn, for instance, to speak one language at home and a different language outside the home, and to switch back and forth between them
with ease. They show no preference for the language they learned first; on the
contrary, the children of immigrants show an increasingly strong preference,
as they mature, for the language they learned outside the home (Harris, 1998;
Pinker, 2002).

In considering the evidence on aggressive behavior, there is an important
caveat to keep in mind. Children do not inherit a predisposition to speak English, but they may inherit a predisposition to behave aggressively. If children
who behave aggressively at home also behave aggressively outside the home,
how can we tell whether they are transferring a pattern of behavior acquired
at home to other social contexts, or whether they have a genetic predisposition to behave aggressively wherever they go? The research design used in
most developmental studies provides no way of distinguishing these alterna-

tives. This is one case in which birth order studies, when done properly, can be useful. Because there are no systematic genetic differences (as far as we know) between firstborns and laterborns, birth order provides a built-in control for genetic influences. If firstborns are more aggressive than laterborns both at home and outside the home, then this would support the view that aggressive behavior generalizes across social contexts.

Relevant evidence is provided by two studies in which the behavior of the same children was assessed in two different contexts. The first, by Abramovitch, Corter, Pepler, and Stanhope (1986), showed that firstborns do tend to dominate their younger siblings, often by behaving aggressively. However, the researchers reported, "There was no evidence of individual differences in sibling interactions carrying over into peer interactions" (p. 228). Firstborns who dominated their siblings were not more likely to try to dominate their peers; laterborns were not more likely to allow their peers to dominate them. As the researchers put it, "Even the second-born child, who has experienced years in a subordinate role with an older sibling, can step into a dominant role when the situation permits" (p. 228).

The second study, by Deater-Deckard and Plomin (1999), used behavioral-genetic methods; about half the sibling pairs in this study were adoptive. The aggressiveness of both siblings was judged five times by their parents and judged independently by five different teachers, over a 6-year period. As the researchers explained, the parents' judgments must have been based primarily on "children's behavior at home and with other family members," whereas the teachers observed how the children behaved at school, in an "environment that provides opportunities for peer interaction" (p. 145). Again, the results showed that older siblings are more aggressive at home but not outside the home: Parents judged the older sibling to be more aggressive, teachers' judgments were about the same for the two siblings.

These findings are backed up by other evidence on the independence of children's sibling and peer relationships. Children who have hostile relationships with their siblings are not at greater risk of having hostile relationships with peers (Stocker & Dunn, 1990). Children who lack siblings are not handicapped in any way in their peer relationships (Falbo & Polit, 1986). Whatever is learned in the course of sibling interactions neither helps nor hinders children in learning to get along with their peers.

Birth order—the disparities in age, size, and strength between nontwin siblings—can account for differences in the way firstborns and laterborns behave within the family. Birth order cannot, however, account for the behavioral-genetic findings on personality that caused Plomin and Daniels (1987) to wonder why siblings are so different. The data they reviewed came chiefly from studies using standard personality tests—self-report questionnaires. As Sulloway himself has admitted (1999), significant birth order effects seldom turn up on such tests. If birth order cannot account for a detectable portion of the variance on standard personality tests, then it cannot explain the nongenetic differences between siblings that mystified Plomin and Daniels.

Sulloway (1996, 1999) has argued that self-report questionnaires produce inaccurate or misleading results, and that a better way to test for birth order effects is to make direct comparisons between siblings in the same family. He favors a method in which personality is judged by parents or siblings—a method that usually does produce significant results. The problem is that these people see each other only within the family context. My interpretation of the evidence I have surveyed (Harris, 1998, Appendix 1; 2000a) is that the difference in outcome does not depend on whether self-report questionnaires are used or whether direct comparisons are made between siblings: It depends on whether the method assesses behavior within the family or outside of it. Paulhus, Trapnell, and Chen (1999) used self-report questionnaires but asked subjects to compare themselves to their siblings and did find birth order effects; Deater-Deckard and Plomin (1999) used judgments by teachers to assess children's behavior outside the family and did not find birth order effects. Both studies made use of direct comparisons between siblings in the same family.

Earlier I mentioned the study by Reiss (2000), which included five different types of sibling pairs. The purpose of this ambitious, 12-year study was to find the source of the nonshared variance—the unexplained, nongenetic differences between siblings. The attempt was unsuccessful; the only interesting findings were negative ones. Reiss concluded that neither "differential parenting toward siblings" (the parents' tendency to give more affection or criticism to one child than the other) nor the "asymmetrical relationships the sibs construct with each other" (p. 407) could account for the measured sibling differences. Though Reiss did not specifically mention birth order (many of the participants in this study were twins), "asymmetrical relationships" would include any in which one sibling dominated the other.

Summary

Sibling and peer relationships are independent. Children who dominate or behave aggressively with siblings show no tendency to generalize these behaviors to peers; children without siblings suffer no social impediments. The evidence from birth order studies using a variety of methods suggests that firstborns and laterborns differ in their behavior within the family but not in other social contexts. The fact that significant birth order effects are seldom found in studies using standard personality tests means that birth order cannot explain why siblings score so differently on these tests.

When Does Learned Behavior Generalize?

The assumption that early experiences within the family are formative underlies not just birth order theories but most current theories of child development. The idea, seldom stated explicitly, is that patterns of behavior learned within the family become deeply ingrained and are generalized—carried along to other social contexts—without conscious volition. Individuals do not *choose* to reenact behaviors acquired in the course of interacting with parents or siblings, but they cannot help it and are usually not even aware they are doing it.

The evidence used to support this assumption consists of correlations found between a individual's behavior in different contexts. Children who are securely attached to their mothers are found, at least in some studies, to have a slightly better chance of having successful relationships with other social partners (Sroufe, Egeland, & Carlson, 1999). Children who behave in a "coercive" manner with their parents are slightly more likely to behave in a coercive manner with their peers (Dishion, Duncan, Eddy, Fagot, & Fetrow, 1994). Children who cheat or lie at home are slightly more likely to cheat or lie elsewhere (Hartshorne & May, 1930/1971). Though many children who are shy in one social context are not particularly shy in others, some are shy wherever they go (Rubin, Hastings, Stewart, Henderson, & Chen, 1997).

The problem with this evidence—and there is a lot more where that came from—is that it is correlational and there are no controls for genetic influences on behavior. Studies using a technique called *multivariate genetic analysis* have called into question the assumption about generalization. This technique enables researchers to assess the degree to which genetic and environmental influences each contribute to the correlations found between behavior in two different contexts. Researchers found that a genetic predisposition to be physically active or inactive accounts for the entire correlation between activity level in different contexts, and that a genetic predisposition to be shy or bold accounts for almost the entire correlation between shyness in different contexts (Saudino, 1997). This technique has not, to my knowledge, been used to assess cross-contextual genetic influences on coercive behavior, but the substantial heritability of such traits as aggressiveness and disagreeableness means that genetic influences could easily account for the slight tendency for some children to be coercive both at home and on the playground.[3]

Because children have a lot to learn, generalization would seem to make sense: If they did not generalize, they would presumably have to learn things all over again in every new context. On the other hand, generalization can be risky: What works in one context may be inappropriate or even dangerous in another. Whether generalizing or not generalizing makes more sense for an organism of a given species depends on how easily new behaviors are learned and on the storage capacity of the organism's brain. Learning different patterns of behavior for different contexts requires not only the ability to learn quickly but also a mental filing system that keeps track of which behaviors go with which contexts. For an organism possessing these attributes, not generalizing would appear to be the safer policy.

There is good evidence that human infants are indeed equipped with these attributes, and that they are born with a bias against generalizing (Harris, 2000a). Young babies taught to kick one foot in order to make a mobile jiggle will remember this trick a few days later and will kick the foot again, but only if nothing has been changed (Rovee-Collier, 1993). If the doodads dangling from the mobile are a different color, or the crib has been wheeled into another room, the infant will stare cluelessly at the mobile. Social behavior, too, is context-specific at an early age. Babies whose mothers are suffering from postpartum depression behave in a subdued manner with their depressed mothers, but they behave normally with caregivers who are not depressed (Pelaez-Nogueras, Field, Cigales, Gonzalez, & Clasky, 1994). The babies' subdued behavior, according to the researchers who studied them, is "specific to their interactions with their depressed mothers" (p. 358).

These results appear to conflict with other evidence that babies do indeed generalize. After all, the toddler who learned to speak English at home does not have to learn it all over again at the day care center! But Rovee-Collier's (1993) experiments with jiggling mobiles demonstrated not only that babies are born with a bias against generalizing, but also that this bias can be overcome. To teach a baby to generalize the foot-kicking trick, Rovee-Collier found, all it takes is to vary the training setup. A baby who has been trained with a variety of mobiles or in a variety of contexts learns that kicking the foot has wider applicability and will kick even with a brand new mobile. Similarly, a toddler who discovers that English works in a variety of social contexts will soon become confident enough to use that language even in unfamiliar settings. Experience can teach a child not only how to behave in a given context but also when it makes sense to generalize that behavior to other contexts.

The evidence on aggressive behavior cited in the previous section indicates that children do not make the mistake of generalizing aggressive or nonaggressive behavior from the family context to social contexts outside the family. The child who behaves in a dominating manner with a younger sibling, or in a submissive manner with an older one, does not automatically transfer these behaviors to the playground. Despite the fact that children inherit suites of genes that predispose them to behave in certain ways wherever they go, they nonetheless behave differently in different contexts. They do so because they have different experiences in different contexts.

The need to adapt, first to the immediate family, and later to the wider world outside the family, is a recurrent problem in human ontogeny. It would be surprising if evolution had not equipped the human mind with mechanisms for dealing with it.

Summary

The assumption that patterns of behavior acquired in the family are automatically generalized to other social contexts is based on correlational evidence from studies that failed to control for genetic influences on behavior. Research on infant learning suggests that humans are born with a bias against generalizing. Though this bias can be overcome (some behaviors are useful in a variety of settings), children do not make the mistake of transferring aggressive behaviors learned at home to other social contexts.

How Does the Behavioral Strategy Mechanism Work?

In his discussion of parent–offspring conflict, Trivers (1985) noted that the offspring has no choice but to comply with its parents' wishes, as long as it is dependent on its parents. But, he pointed out, the offspring should not allow itself to be *permanently* molded by parental rewards and punishments, because parents are looking out for their own interests, which do not necessarily coincide with those of the offspring. Were the offspring "to continue to act out parental wishes that were not in harmony with its own self-interest, it would continue to lower its own inclusive fitness" (p. 164).

Trivers' reasoning led him to speculate that children behave in accordance with their parents' wishes until they reach puberty, then abandon those behaviors and "reorganize their personalities" (1985, p. 164)—presumably by acquiring whole new patterns of behaviors. My proposal is less radical; it entails no major reorganization of the personality in adolescence. Children acquire patterns of behavior for getting along with their parents and siblings; they acquire other patterns of behavior tailored to their other social contexts. Because some behaviors work as well outside the family as within it, there will be some overlap; some of the things children learn at home will be retained. But in many cases—the boy who cries to evoke his mother's sympathy, the firstborn who dominates her siblings—the child will discover that behaviors that produced the desired effect within the family have undesirable effects outside it. In that case, the behavioral strategy mechanism is biased toward the outside-the-family behavior. Thus, the children of immigrants adopt the language and accent of their peers, men don't cry (boys who cry in the presence of their peers are teased or picked on), and firstborns are no more aggressive than laterborns in adulthood.

A mechanism that works this way is likely to win out, in Darwinian competition, over one that forms its long-term behavioral strategies on the basis of early experiences with parents and siblings. Under ancestral conditions, the short, slight young man whose belligerent personality was formed in childhood on the basis of his ability to beat up his younger brother was likely to lead a briefer life (and hence leave fewer descendants) than the equally short, slight young man who learned through encounters with peers that his best bet was to behave in a cooperative or conciliatory manner.

What about a young woman? For the sake of her descendants, she should choose the highest quality mate she is able to attract, and physically attractive women are able to attract higher status men (Buss, 1995). In order to work out an optimal mating strategy, a woman needs to have a reasonably accurate idea of how attractive she is, and she would be unwise to base her opinion of herself on what her parents think or what her brother says. If she underrates herself, she might be too ready to accept an inferior suitor; if she overrates herself, she might turn down opportunities that might not come again.

To make wise decisions about lifelong strategies, both the young man and the young woman have to consider information that neither their genes nor their mirror can provide—information that can be obtained only through social interactions with others. Their ability to dominate others and to win desirable mates depends not so much on whether they are objectively big and strong or pretty, but on how they compare with their rivals.

The behavioral strategy mechanism I am proposing gives individuals information about how they compare with their rivals on the basis of social cues—cues that tell them how they are regarded by others. The more informants contribute this information, the more valuable it is. A boy should not base his strategy on the fact that he once got beaten up by a bully, any more than he should base it on his ability to beat up his little brother. He needs more data than that. A recent article titled "Group Decision-Making in Animals" (Conradt & Roper, 2003) provides evidence for a submodule that the behavioral strategy mechanism might make use of: a device for counting votes. Groups of nonhuman animals make some of their group decisions, such as whether to move and which way to go, in a democratic fashion: The majority rules. African buffalo, for example, make decisions about which way to go on the basis of the direction of gaze of the majority of the adult females in the herd.

Humans, too, are responsive to the eye gaze of others (Baron-Cohen, 1995); in fact, there is evidence that they too count votes. A good predictor of whether an individual will speak out in a group situation is the number of eye gazes he or she receives from the others in the group (Vertegaal & Ding, 2002). It does not matter who does the gazing; nor does the timing of the gazes matter much. It is the sheer number of times eye contact occurs. The counter presumably does its work below the level of conscious awareness.

I am not suggesting that the number of eye gazes one gets during childhood determines one's personality in adulthood—only that this is one of the cues to which a behavioral strategy mechanism might be sensitive. It is a useful one, because how often individuals are looked at by the others in their group can serve as an indication of their social status. Those who rank high in the "attention structure" receive more gazes (Chance & Larsen, 1976).

Getting beaten up or pushed around repeatedly must matter too, at least for boys. Boys who are small for their age, either because they are maturing slowly or because they are destined to be small adults, are likely to be dominated or bullied by their peers (Weisfeld & Billings, 1988). Early maturers tend to have higher status in the peer group (Savin-Williams, 1979). In a classic longitudinal study, Jones (1957) found personality differences between slow-maturing and fast-maturing adolescent boys: The fast maturers—taller and stronger than most of their peers—were more socially poised and less anxious. Though the two groups ended up approximately equal in mean adult height, the fast maturers remained significantly more self-assured in adulthood; they scored higher on personality characteristics associated with dominance and were more likely to attain executive positions in their careers.

Jones's (1957) study is backed up by a newer, larger one. Persico, Postlewaite, and Silverman (in press) investigated the relationship, well known to evolutionary psychologists, between height and income in adult males. As Pinker (1997) noted, tall men earn more than short ones: about $600 per inch in annual income. Persico et al. used longitudinal data on more than 4,000 white males to show that what matters is not adult height but height during adolescence. It was the men who had been taller than most of their peers in adolescence—whether or not they remained the tallest in adulthood—who earned the highest salaries on average. The researchers ruled out some plausible explanations for this finding, such as differences in socioeconomic status, but declined to speculate on what attributes, acquired during adolescence, accounted for the higher salary in adulthood. Jones's study showed what these attributes are: Being taller than one's peers during adolescence gives males a more dominant and self-assured personality.

In contrast, being taller than one's siblings during childhood has no consistent long-term effects on personality. In one of the largest birth order studies of personality ever done, involving 7,582 participants, Ernst and Angst (1983) found no significant differences between firstborns and laterborns in dominance or aggressiveness.[4]

The Unexplained Variance in Personality

I have used height as my example because longitudinal data are available. However, these results cannot by themselves account for the variation in personality attributed to the nonshared environment—the unexplained differences between siblings—because height is largely genetic. Reared-together identical twins are usually similar in height, so the psychological consequences of being tall or short are also likely to be similar. Because behavioral-genetic analyses cannot distinguish between the direct effects of genes (being tall) and the indirect effects of genes (the social consequences of being tall), the effects of being tall or short will contribute mostly to the portion of the variance attributed to genes (heritability) rather than to environmental variance (see Harris, 1998).

However, the evidence on height can provide valuable insights into how the behavioral strategy mechanism works—the kind of input to which it responds and the output that results. The mechanism is designed to regulate social behavior, and the input it collects comes in the form of social cues, information provided by other people. No other kind of information could do the job required of it. But social cues can be ambiguous, and other people have their own agendas. A mechanism that works the way I propose could have some effects that are completely unrelated to genes.

Consider, for example, beauty. Physically attractive adults tend to have more assertive personalities than unattractive adults (Jackson & Huston, 1975). Physically attractive children and adolescents tend to have higher status among their peers (Kennedy, 1990). But other things besides beauty might give an adolescent girl high status among her peers. Her father might be wealthy. She might be a member of a large and powerful extended family.[5] She might have other assets, such as intelligence or charm. Or she might just be lucky. She once made a chance remark that was interpreted as a prediction, the prediction happened to come true, and people listened closely to her after that. If the social cues are similar, the behavioral strategy mechanism will respond to them in a similar way.

Nor is assertiveness the only personality characteristic that is likely to be affected by social cues. A short or puny boy who has learned through hard experience that he cannot dominate his peers could go in any number of directions. The outcome will depend in part on chance factors, such as which niche happens to be available in his group.

Buss (1995) has pointed out that "perceiving, attending to, and acting upon differences in others has been (and likely still is) crucial to solving adaptive problems" (p. 22). People not only collect information on social categories; they also collect data on individuals. They pass it along in the form of gossip. The information may not be correct; often it is not. On the basis of a chance event, a child or adolescent may get a reputation that persists for years. If the human mind is predisposed to perceive differences in others, as Buss suggested, then people will look for, and act upon, even the small differences between identical twins. The close associates of identical twins have no trouble telling them apart; someone who is sexually attracted to one is not necessarily attracted to the other (Segal, 1999; Lykken & Tellegen, 1993).

Though chance events may play a role in the way individuals are characterized by their associates, the long-term results of being characterized in a particular way are not random at all, if the behavioral strategy mechanism works the way I propose. To study these processes will not be easy; longitudinal data are required, and the method must provide adequate controls for the effects of genes. It is unrealistic, however, to expect that such studies will account for all of the unexplained variance in personality. Some of the variation is no doubt due to another kind of randomness: biological "noise," which makes neurophysiological development to some extent unpredictable (Pinker, 2002). The brains of identical twins differ slightly for the same reason their fingerprints do.

I have concentrated here on the mental mechanisms that lead to long-term changes in social behavior—the mechanisms involved in personality development. There are other mechanisms in charge of establishing and maintaining personal relationships; evidence reviewed elsewhere (Harris, 1995, 1998, 2000b) suggests that these mechanisms are context-dependent and do not produce long-term changes in behavior. As Bugental (2000) proposed, there may be several different relationship mechanisms, specializing in different types of relationships. These mechanisms could be activated and inactivated as needed during the lifespan; the relationships that matter most in childhood are not the ones that matter most in adolescence and adulthood.

FINDING OUT HOW THE CHILD'S MIND WORKS

I have proposed that there are two different innate mechanisms involved in personality development. The first adapts children to their society by enabling them to behave more like others of their age and sex. The second builds a workable lifetime behavioral strategy for the individual child, based on the feedback—the social cues—he or she receives from others. These social cues tell children how they compare with the rivals they will be competing against in adulthood and what might be the best way for them, given their own particular assets and liabilities, to compete successfully.

Innate mechanisms often provide their own motivation. Language acquisition, for example, proceeds without formal training and in the absence of extrinsic rewards or punishments. The two mechanisms I have described also provide their own motivations. Children *want* to behave, dress, and speak like others of their kind; they want to be seen as "normal." They also want to be better than others of their kind; they aspire to rise in the social hierarchy. The existence of these two separate and sometimes conflicting motives—the desire to conform and the desire to be best—is a clue that one mechanism is not adequate to do the job. As Pinker noted, "The mind has to be built out of specialized parts because it has to solve specialized problems" (1997, p. 30).

Leary (1999) has proposed that the mind contains a *sociometer* that keeps people informed about how they are doing socially—how others are reacting to them. Kirkpatrick and Ellis (2001) expanded on this idea by suggesting that the human mind is likely to contain a number of distinct psychological mechanisms for monitoring functioning in various areas of social endeavor. In other words, we may have several different sociometers, which "activate different psychological systems and processes" (p. 421). A study by Leary, Cottrell, and Phillips (2001) provides support for the multiple sociometer hypothesis by showing that different kinds of social feedback have independent effects on self-esteem. Feedback indicating acceptance by a group and feedback regarding one's status within the group have distinguishable effects, accounting for unique portions of the variance. I suggest that the sociometer that provides information about group acceptance is used by the socialization mechanism to monitor how well one is conforming to group norms, and that the sociometer that provides information about status within the group is used by the behavioral strategy mechanism.

These information-collecting devices are likely to differ in their degree of cognitive sophistication. The sociometer that serves the socialization mechanism can be very simple; the only signals it needs to transmit are social approval and disapproval. As pet owners know, even dogs are sensitive to signs of social disapproval.

The sociometer that serves the human behavioral strategy mechanism requires information of a more subtle kind. Working out a long-term strategy of behavior—figuring out which niche we can fill within the group—requires a more nuanced understanding of how we are regarded by others. We need to be able to look into other people's minds and guess what they are thinking about us. In short, we need a theory of mind (TOM) mechanism. Baron-Cohen (1995) presented evidence that three submodules, one of which is an eye-direction detector, provide information to the TOM mechanism. I am carrying his argument one step further (or one level higher) by proposing that the behavioral strategy mechanism makes use of information processed by the TOM mechanism.[6]

This proposal has a surprising implication: that nonhuman animals, including chimpanzees, may lack a mechanism that makes long-term modifications of "personality" on the basis of status in the juvenile group. In nonhuman primates, the behaviors associated with being an alpha male may be context-dependent; being at the top for a while may have no long-term consequences. If this sounds unlikely, consider that an animal's status in its dominance hierarchy changes drastically over the course of its lifetime, starting low, rising as maturation proceeds, then declining gradually due to aging or suddenly due to injury. Long-term modifications of behavioral strategy may have become useful only when the TOM mechanism was able to provide more subtle kinds of information, when the owner of the mechanism was able to make more subtle kinds of adjustments, and when longer preparation was required to fill specialized niches.

Another implication is that the behavioral strategy mechanism may do its work relatively late in the course of human development, since it depends on the prior development of the TOM mechanism. Though the desire to conform and the desire to be best are both apparent in children of preschool age, the socialization mechanism may complete its work sooner. Children's ability to acquire the accents of their peers generally ends around puberty (Pinker, 1994), but personality remains labile for a much longer time (Caspi & Roberts, 2001; McCrae, 2001). Persico et al. (in press) found that height in adolescence was a better predictor of adult salary than height in childhood.

Though the desire to conform and the desire for status often involve different kinds of behaviors and thus can coexist, these motives (as I mentioned) occasionally come into conflict. An illustration is provided by Asch's (1952/1987) famous experiment on group conformity, in which one subject made judgments of line lengths while others—actually the researcher's confederates—gave false judgments. Not all of Asch's subjects caved in and gave false judgments (only in children under the age of 10 did the majority succumb), but the subjects' comments afterwards made it clear that all experienced a struggle in which their desire not to be different vied with their desire to be the most accurate. Occasions in which two mental mechanisms issue conflicting commands—"the human heart in conflict with itself," as novelist William Faulkner put it—are a familiar part of human life.

Most of the time, however, the two mechanisms that I have proposed carry out their jobs unobtrusively, below the level of conscious awareness. The information they collect is stored in the form of implicit, rather than explicit, memories (see Bjorklund & Pellegrini, 2002, Chapter 5). People's explicit memories of childhood—their conscious thoughts about who or what influenced them—can therefore not be relied upon to confirm or disconfirm theories such as the one presented here.

Nor can we rely on parents' subjective feelings regarding their importance in their children's lives. These feelings may be an evolutionary adaptation, part of the package that motivates parents to take care of their children. Alternatively, they may be a peculiarity of our culture. Although close attention to the physical needs of infants and toddlers is almost (though not quite) universal, tender concern for the psychological well-being of older children is culturally unusual, perhaps unique. In hunter–gatherer and tribal societies, children past the age of weaning typically spend most of their time in the local play group and receive little parental attention or affection. In these traditional societies, according to Eibl-Eibesfeldt (1989), "it is in such play groups that children are truly raised" (p. 600).

The filling of niches goes on within families and in the world outside the family. Children are characterized or labeled by their parents, by their siblings, and by their peers; they have a certain status within their sibling group and a certain status—very likely a different one—within their peer group. The evidence reviewed in this chapter indicates that only the niche filling and status determining that go on outside the family have measurable long-term effects on personality. How you compare with your siblings mattered in childhood, but what matters in adulthood is how you compare with your peers.

SUMMARY

To account for findings on environmental influences on personality, I have proposed that the child's mind is equipped with two separate mental mechanisms for making long-term adjustments of social behavior on the basis of experience. These mechanisms provide different goals, are responsive to different environmental cues, and process the data in different ways. The socialization mechanism motivates children to behave like typical members of their age and gender category; it is responsive to social cues related to acceptance. The behavioral strategy mechanism collects information that tells children how they compare with others of their age and gender; it is responsive to social cues related to status. This second mechanism creates or maintains individual differences in social behavior and is the source of most of the nongenetic variation in personality. The goal of the behavioral strategy mechanism—to be best—sometimes conflicts with the goal of the socialization mechanism—to conform. The evidence suggests that these mechanisms make long-term adjustments of social behavior primarily on the basis of information collected outside the family. Information conveyed by experiences with peers is more useful in the long run than information conveyed by experiences with siblings.

ACKNOWLEDGMENTS

This chapter is dedicated to the memory of David C. Rowe (1949–2003), a good friend and stimulating colleague. Though his life was tragically cut short by cancer, his contributions to psychology remain remarkable in their quantity, quality, and lasting importance. I thank Gal Levin, Robert R. McCrae, and Irene Rebollo for their helpful suggestions on an earlier version of this chapter.

NOTES

1. Though shared environment effects on personality measures are generally close to zero, larger effects of shared environment have been found on certain specific behaviors, notably adolescent delinquency and alcohol use. These effects can be attributed to the influence of the environment siblings share outside the home: the neighborhood, school, or peer group (Harris, 2000b).
2. One might argue that evolution would be equally unlikely to cause long-term selection of behavioral strategies to be influenced by genes. Why is there heritable variation in personality? Tooby and Cosmides (1990) concluded that heritable psychological differences are "mostly evolutionary by-products, such as concomitants of parasite-driven selection for biochemical individuality" (p. 17). Another possibility is frequency-dependent selection: Genes for some personality traits might persist in a population because these traits are advantageous if they are relatively uncommon.
3. Genetic influences on behavior also account for continuities over time (Caspi & Roberts, 2001), such as the tendency for aggressive children to become aggressive adults.
4. Ernst and Angst (1983) measured 12 dimensions of personality, including dominance, aggressiveness, sociability, neuroticism, calmness, and openness. The only significant birth order effect they found was that lastborns in sibships of three or more were slightly lower in masculinity.
5. Being a member of a powerful family can have permanent effects on personality because it affects one's status—and hence one's experiences—outside the family, in the peer group or community.
6. According to Baron-Cohen (1995), children with autism lack a TOM mechanism; such a lack would severely impair the behavioral strategy mechanism. But these children appear to be deficient in every kind of sociometer; their socialization mechanism is impaired as well. Perhaps there are syndromes with less pervasive and less devastating effects that knock out one type of sociometer but not others.

REFERENCES

Abramovitch, R., Corter, C., Pepler, D. J., & Stanhope, L. (1986). Sibling and peer interaction: A final follow-up and a comparison. *Child Development, 57,* 217–229.

Asch, S. E. (1987). *Social psychology.* Oxford, UK: Oxford University Press. (Original work published 1952)

Baron-Cohen, S. (1995). *Mindblindness: An essay on autism and theory of mind*. Cambridge, MA: MIT Press.

Bjorklund, D. F., & Pellegrini, A. D. (2002). *The origins of human nature: Evolutionary developmental psychology*. Washington, DC: American Psychological Association.

Bouchard, T. J., Jr., & Loehlin, J. C. (2001). Genes, evolution, and personality. *Behavior Genetics, 31*, 243–273.

Bouchard, T. J., Jr., Lykken, D. T., McGue, M., Segal, N. L., & Tellegen, A. (1990). Sources of human psychological differences: The Minnesota study of twins reared apart. *Science, 250*, 223–228.

Bugental, D. B. (2000). Acquisition of the algorithms of social life: A domain-based approach. *Psychological Bulletin, 126*, 187–219.

Buss, D. M. (1995). Evolutionary psychology: A new paradigm for psychological science. *Psychological Inquiry, 6*, 1–30.

Caspi, A., & Roberts, B. W. (2001). Personality development across the life course: The argument for change and continuity. *Psychological Inquiry, 12*, 49–66.

Chance, M. R. A., & Larsen, R. R. (Eds.). (1976). *The social structure of attention*. London: Wiley.

Conradt, L., & Roper, T. J. (2003). Group decision-making in animals. *Nature, 421*, 155–158.

Cosmides, L., Tooby, J., & Barkow, J. H. (1992). Introduction: Evolutionary psychology and conceptual integration. In J. H. Barkow, L. Cosmides, & J. Tooby (Eds.), *The adapted mind: Evolutionary psychology and the generation of culture* (pp. 3–15). New York: Oxford University Press.

Daly, M., & Wilson, M. (1988). Evolutionary social psychology and family homicide. *Science, 242*, 519–524.

Deater-Deckard, K., & Plomin, R. (1999). An adoption study of the etiology of teacher and parent reports of externalizing behavior problems in middle childhood. *Child Development, 70*, 144–154.

Dick, D. M., & Rose, R. J. (2002). Behavior genetics: What's new? What's next? *Current Directions in Psychological Science, 11*, 70–74.

Dishion, T. J., Duncan, T. E., Eddy, J. M., Fagot, B. I., & Fetrow, R. (1994). The world of parents and peers: Coercive exchanges and children's social adaptation. *Social Development, 3*, 255–268.

Dunn, J. (1985). *Sisters and brothers*. Cambridge, MA: Harvard University Press.

Dunn, J., & Plomin, R. (1990). *Separate lives: Why siblings are so different*. New York: Basic Books.

Edwards, C. P. (1992). Cross-cultural perspectives on family-peer relations. In R. D. Parke & G. W. Ladd (Eds.), *Family-peer relationships: Modes of linkage* (pp. 285–316). Hillsdale, NJ: Erlbaum.

Eibl-Eibesfeldt, I. (1989). *Human ethology*. Hawthorne, NY: Aldine de Gruyter.

Ernst, C., & Angst, J. (1983). *Birth order: Its influence on personality*. Berlin: Springer-Verlag.

Etcoff, N. (1999). *Survival of the prettiest: The science of beauty*. New York: Doubleday.

Falbo, T., & Polit, D. F. (1986). Quantitative research of the only child literature: Research evidence and theory development. *Psychological Bulletin, 100*, 176–189.

Goodall, J. (1986). *The chimpanzees of Gombe: Patterns of behavior*. Cambridge, MA: Harvard University Press.

Harris, J. R. (1995). Where is the child's environment?: A group socialization theory of development. *Psychological Review, 102*, 458–489.

Harris, J. R. (1998). *The nurture assumption*. New York: Free Press.

Harris, J. R. (2000a). Context-specific learning, personality, and birth order. *Current Directions in Psychological Science, 9*, 174–177.

Harris, J. R. (2000b). Socialization, personality development, and the child's environments: Comment on Vandell (2000). *Developmental Psychology, 36*, 711–723.

Hartshorne, H., & May, M. A. (1971). Studies in the organization of character. In H. Munsinger (Ed.), *Readings in child development* (pp. 190–197). New York: Holt, Rinehart & Winston. (Original published in 1930)

Jackson, D. J., & Huston, T. L. (1975). Physical attractiveness and assertiveness. *Journal of Social Psychology, 96*, 79–84.

Jankowiak, W., & Diderich, M. (2000). Sibling solidarity in a polygamous community in the USA: Unpacking inclusive fitness. *Evolution and Human Behavior, 21*, 125–139.

Jenkins, J. J., Rasbash, J., & O'Connor, T. G. (2003). The role of the shared family context in differential parenting. *Developmental Psychology, 39*, 99–113.

Jones, M. C. (1957). The later careers of boys who were early or late maturing. *Child Development, 28*, 113–128.

Kennedy, J. H. (1990). Determinants of peer social status: Contributions of physical appearance, reputation, and behavior. *Journal of Youth and Adolescence, 19*, 233–244.

Kirkpatrick, L. A., & Ellis, B. J. (2001). An evolutionary–psychological approach to self-esteem: Multiple domains and multiple functions. In G. J. O. Fletcher & M. S. Clark (Eds.), *Blackwell handbook of social psychology: Interpersonal processes* (pp. 411–436). Malden, MA: Blackwell.

Leary, M. R. (1999). Making sense of self-esteem. *Current Directions in Psychological Science, 8*, 32–35.

Leary, M. R., Cottrell, C. A., & Phillips, M. (2001). Deconfounding the effects of dominance and social acceptance on self-esteem. *Journal of Personality and Social Psychology, 81*, 898–909.

Lykken, D. T., & Tellegen, A. (1993). Is human mating adventitious or the result of lawful choice?: A twin study of mate selection. *Journal of Personality and Social Psychology, 65*, 56–68.

Macrae, C. N., & Bodenhausen, G. V. (2000). Social cognition: Thinking categorically about others. *Annual Review of Psychology, 51*, 93–120.

McCartney, K., Harris, M. J., & Bernieri, F. (1990). Growing up and growing apart: A developmental meta-analysis of twin studies. *Psychological Bulletin, 107*, 226–237.

McCrae, R. R. (2001). Traits through time. *Psychological Inquiry, 12*, 85–87.

McCrae, R. R. (2004). Human nature and culture: A trait perspective. *Journal of Research in Personality, 38*, 3–14.

McHale, S. M., Crouter, A. C., McGuire, S. A., & Updegraff, K. A. (1995). Congruence between mothers' and fathers' differential treatment of siblings: Links with family relations and children's well-being. *Child Development, 66*, 116–128.

Paulhus, D. L., Trapnell, P. D., & Chen, D. (1999). Birth order effects on personality and achievement within families. *Psychological Science, 10*, 482–488.

Pelaez-Nogueras, M., Field, T., Cigales, M., Gonzalez, A., & Clasky, S. (1994). Infants of depressed mothers show less "depressed" behavior with their nursery teachers. *Infant Mental Health Journal, 15,* 358–367.

Persico, N., Postlewaite, A., & Silverman, D. (in press). The effect of adolescent experience on labor market outcomes: The case of height. *Journal of Political Economy.*

Pinker, S. (1994). *The language instinct.* New York: HarperCollins.

Pinker, S. (1997). *How the mind works.* New York: Norton.

Pinker, S. (2002). *The blank slate.* New York: Viking.

Plomin, R., & Daniels, D. (1987). Why are children in the same family so different from one another? *Behavioral and Brain Sciences, 10,* 1–16.

Reiss, D., with Neiderhiser, J. M., Hetherington, E. M., & Plomin, R. (2000). *The relationship code: Deciphering genetic and social influences on adolescent development.* Cambridge, MA: Harvard University Press.

Rovee-Collier, C. (1993). The capacity for long-term memory in infancy. *Current Directions in Psychological Science, 2,* 130–135.

Rowe, D. C. (1994). *The limits of family influence.* New York: Guilford Press.

Rowe, D. C. (2002). *Biology and crime.* Los Angeles: Roxbury.

Rubin, K. H., Hastings, P. D., Stewart, S. L., Henderson, H. A., & Chen, X. (1997). The consistency and concomitants of inhibition: Some of the children, all of the time. *Child Development, 68,* 467–483.

Saudino, K. J. (1997). Moving beyond the heritability question: New directions in behavioral genetic studies of personality. *Current Directions in Psychological Science, 6,* 86–90.

Savin-Williams, R. C. (1979). An ethological study of dominance formation and maintenance in a group of human adolescents. *Child Development, 49,* 534–536.

Segal, N. L. (1999). *Entwined lives: Twins and what they tell us about human behavior.* New York: Penguin.

Segal, N. L., & Hershberger, S. L. (1999). Cooperation and competition between twins: Findings from a prisoner's dilemma game. *Evolution and Human Behavior, 20,* 29–51.

Serbin, L. A., Powlishta, K. K., & Gulko, J. (1993). The development of sex typing in middle childhood. *Monographs of the Society for Research in Child Development, 58*(2, Serial No. 232).

Shatz, M., & Gelman, R. (1973). The development of communication skills: Modifications in the speech of young children as a function of listener. *Monographs of the Society for Research in Child Development, 38*(5, Serial No. 152).

Sroufe, L. A., Egeland, B., & Carlson, E. A. (1999). One social world: The integrated development of parent–child and peer relationships. In W. A. Collins & B. Laursen (Eds.), *Relationships as developmental contexts* (pp. 241–261). Mahwah, NJ: Erlbaum

Stevenson, M. R., & Black, K. N. (1988). Paternal absence and sex-role development: A meta-analysis. *Child Development, 59,* 793–814.

Stocker, C., & Dunn, J. (1990). Sibling relationships in childhood: Links with friendships and peer relationships. *British Journal of Developmental Psychology, 8,* 227–244.

Sulloway, F. J. (1996). *Born to rebel.* New York: Pantheon.

Sulloway, F. J. (1999). Birth order. In M. A. Runco & S. Pritzker (Eds.), *Encyclopedia of creativity* (Vol. 1, pp. 189–202). San Diego: Academic Press.

Swim, J. K. (1994). Perceived versus meta-analytic effect sizes: An assessment of the accuracy of gender stereotypes. *Journal of Personality and Social Psychology, 66,* 21–36.

Tooby, J., & Cosmides, L. (1990). On the universality of human nature and the uniqueness of the individual: The role of genetics and adaptation. *Journal of Personality, 58,* 17–67.

Trivers, R. (1985). *Social evolution.* Menlo Park, CA: Benjamin/Cummings.

Vertegaal, R., & Ding, Y. (2002). Explaining effects of eye gaze on mediated group conversations: Amount or synchronization? *Proceedings of CSCW 2002 Conference on Computer Supported Collaborative Work* (pp. 41–48). New Orleans: ACM Press.

Weisfeld, G. E., & Billings, R. L. (1988). Observations on adolescence. In K. B. MacDonald (Ed.), *Sociobiological perspectives on human development* (pp. 207–233). New York: Springer-Verlag.

11

PLAY

Types and Functions in Human Development

PETER K. SMITH

Play is often defined as activity that is both done for its own sake and is characterized by "means rather than ends"—the process of the play is more important than any end point or goal that is obvious to the participant or "naive" onlooker. These criteria contrast play with exploration (which may lead into play, as a child gets more familiar with a new toy or environment), and with work- or subsistence-related activities such as feeding (which have a definite, obvious goal) and fighting (different from play fighting, as discussed later). Additional common characteristics of human play are flexibility (objects being put in new combinations, roles acted out in new ways), positive affect (children often smile and laugh in play, and say they enjoy it) and pretense (use of objects and actions in nonliteral ways).

Although play may have no "obvious" goal, this does not mean that it has no positive benefits: Very many have been proposed! Also, it does not mean that play has no evolutionary function(s). In fact, the ubiquity of forms of play throughout most mammal species, and humans in all cultures studied to date, and the time, energy, and sometimes danger costs of engaging in them, strongly suggest that selective pressures have acted to favor play behaviors, and that they have some functional value for the player, even if he or she is not fully aware of it. However, the range of functions for play, and strength of evidence for them, is still a matter of considerable debate.

MAIN TYPES OF PLAY

Although play can be defined in broad terms, as mentioned earlier, it embraces a variety of behaviors that likely have different functions. The following main types of play are well recognized: physical activity play (rhythmic stereotypies, exercise play; rough-and-tumble play); object play; and pretend play (including sociodramatic play as a particularly complex form). Of these, physical activity play and object play are seen widely in other species of mammals. Pretend and sociodramatic play are only seen in humans, apart from some possibly very elementary forms of pretense in great apes. A related concept in developmental psychology is that of games. Games with rules describe more organized forms of play in which there is some clear and publicly expressed goal (such as winning the game in a manner accepted by other players); games with rules are not reviewed furthering this chapter. For a discussion of games from an evolutionary perspective, see Parker (1984).

UBIQUITY OF FORMS OF PLAY

All of the main forms of play—physical, object, pretense—have been described in a wide variety of human cultures, with no clear exceptions to date, although the detailed forms and relative frequencies do vary considerably according to cultural conditions (e.g., Bloch & Pellegrini, 1989; Bornstein, Haynes, Pascual, Painter, & Galperin, 1999; Haight, Wang, Fung, Williams, & Mintz, 1999; Lancy, 1996; Roopnarine, Johnson, & Hooper, 1994).

Observations of play in hunter–gatherer societies may be considered most relevant when examining evolutionary functions of play in postulated environments of evolutionary adaptedness. Konner (1972, 1976) describes play in the !Kung bush people of the Kalahari. Besides rough-and-tumble play (often in the context of chasing insects and small creatures) and object play, he describes pretend play such as play pounding, digging, cooking, and serving food. Children may use sticks and pebbles to represent village huts and herding cows. In the Hadza of Tanzania, children make dolls out of rags and play at being predators (Blurton Jones, 1993). Eibl-Eibesfeldt (1989) provides descriptions of all these forms of play in a range of societies.

Reviews of pretend play in non-Western societies by Schwartzman (1978) and Slaughter and Dombrowski (1989) mention over 40 articles describing pretend play. There are certainly variations in the amount and type of such play, and it can appear "impoverished" in some societies (Smilansky, 1968), but its presence appears ubiquitous. Gosso, Morais, and Otta (2004) compared play in native Indian (Parakana), rural (seashore), and three urban groups in Brazil. All forms of play were observed in all groups. Native Indian children were lower than other groups on overall play but nevertheless exhibited a lot of exercise play and pretend play, and some construction (object) and rough-and-tumble play.

INTEGRATIVE VIEWS OF PLAY

Although play can take a variety of forms, some authors have taken an integrative perspective. In *The Principles of Psychology* (1878/1898), Spencer proposed that play is carried out 'for the sake of the immediate gratifications involved, without reference to ulterior benefits'. He suggested that the higher animals are better able to deal with the immediate necessities of life, and that the nervous system, rather than remaining inactive for long periods, stimulates play. "Thus it happens that in the more evolved creatures, there often recurs an energy somewhat in excess of immediate needs. ... Hence play of all kinds—hence this tendency to superfluous and useless exercise of faculties that have been quiescent" (pp. 629–630). Spencer's approach embodies a modern definition of play, and a mechanism for its occurrence, but makes the assumption that play is "useless exercise." This has been labeled the "surplus energy" theory and has often been criticized, though skeptical views of the function of play have resurfaced later.

The work of Groos can be taken as a first major statement of a mainstream position in much developmental and educational thinking, namely, that play has a broad function as practice. In his two influential works, *The Play of Animals* (1898), and *The Play of Man* (1901), Groos criticized Spencer's theory on a number of grounds. He thought that surplus energy might provide 'a particularly favorable condition for play', but was not essential. He also thought play had a much more definite function than in Spencer's theory. Groos argued that a main reason for childhood was so that play could occur: "Perhaps the very existence of youth is largely for the sake of play" (p. 76). This was because play provided exercise and elaboration of skills needed for survival.

In his book *Adolescence* (1908) and elsewhere, Hall argued that Groos's practice theory was "very partial, superficial, and perverse" (p. 202). This was because Groos saw play as practice for contemporary activities. By contrast, Hall thought that play was a means for children to work through primitive atavisms, reflecting our evolutionary past, for example, "Play is not doing things to be useful later, but it is rehearsing social history" (p. 207). The function of play was thus cathartic in nature and allowed the "playing out" of those instincts that characterized earlier human history. This "recapitulation theory" of play has had little or no recent support, at least in the form proposed by Hall.

Although dated, these theories and speculations raised important issues that still concern us. Does play have real functions selected for in evolution, or is it just a by-product of selection for other processes? Would any functions selected for in evolutionary history still apply in contemporary environments? Does play function for future skills, or for present circumstances?

Evolutionary perspectives on play were neglected during the 1920s to 1970s. The writings of Vygotsky (1933/1966) and Piaget (1951) debate the immediate psychological mechanisms for playing, the relationships between play, thought, and language, and whether play is primarily assimilating new experiences to existing schemas (Piaget) or showing creativity through being liberated from immediate situation constraints (Vygotsky). Psychological theorists in this period concentrated on object and pretend play, probably because these more specifically human forms of play were perceived as educationally relevant (i.e., often approved of by teachers). Research on these forms of play became distorted by the "play ethos" (Smith, 1988), which assumed that (object and pretend) play was essential for normal development. Meanwhile, exercise play and rough-and-tumble play were ignored.

Ethologists were (sometimes) still studying animal play. The publication of Fagen's (1981) synthesis of animal and human play, and of Smith's (1982) review in *Behavior and Brain Sciences*, rekindled an interest in the evolutionary perspective on play. Fagen considered different classes of effects of animal play, which thus might be candidates for functional hypotheses. The one that he considered as the most supported by design, context, and sex differences was training of physical capabilities, and cognitive and social skills (for later use, although Fagen did not place much emphasis on the immediate or delayed benefits distinction in this context). He saw difficulties in applying a skills training hypothesis to certain kinds of play, such as adult play. A second effect was regulation of developmental rates. For example, rough play in kittens appears to accelerate the weaning process, as the mother is less willing to tolerate this. Fagen saw this as an effect (e.g., a signal to the mother) but not as a functional explanation for play (as the advantage to kittens of accelerating weaning, is unclear). Third, Fagen considered effects on cohesion, or social bonding. He saw the problem with this as a main functional hypothesis for play as being that other behaviors, such as grooming, could have the same result. Other effects Fagen considered were play as aggressive competition (related to "cheating" in play fighting, discussed later in this chapter), and behavioral flexibility, which he considered "suggestive at best" (p. 354).

Smith argued an integrative view that most forms of play were selected for practice functions, when a lot of direct practice might be difficult or dangerous (e.g., in fighting). Thus, rough-and-tumble play could have been selected for, such that young mammals gained relatively safe practice in fighting (and/or hunting) skills that would enhance their reproductive success as adolescents or adults, once conspecific competition for mates and resources (and/or hunting prey) became important for the individual; an animal that had not practiced in play could then be at a serious disadvantage. Such an analysis could also apply to, for example, play parenting, play courtship, or playful use of objects in relation to food acquisition skills. A few forms of play, such as adult play, could be explained either as by-products of mechanisms facilitating play in earlier periods or as play used for other purposes (e.g., to distract an older infant from suckling); alternatively, adult play too might still function for "tuning-up" skills, later in life (Bock, personal communication, 2004). These ultimate functions of play would be separate from the proximal mechanisms involved. Smith saw pretend play in humans as a mechanism for making play more complex and thus useful as practice than it would otherwise be (although this idea was left unelaborated). Alexander (1989) also saw play as primarily practice for later physical and intellectual competitive skills; in particular, he saw pretend play in humans as an efficient method for practice in "scenario-building," trying out social interaction possibilities in the mind.

A somewhat more skeptical view of the benefits of play was put forward by Martin and Caro (1985), who argued that the costs (time, energy, danger) of play were not very great, and that play had "low priority" when times were difficult; benefits of play might be correspondingly modest. Power (2000) has overviewed the animal and human literature, and sees the strongest case for an evolutionary function for play with rough-and-tumble play, but concludes generally that research on developmental functions of play needs more conclusive results and more studies of social as well as cognitive effects of play, before firm functional statements can be made. Bjorklund and Pellegrini (2002) however, reassert a functional significance for play. Documenting time and energy budgets, and other costs of play (such as injury) (also see Pellegrini & Bjorklund, 2004; Pellegrini, Horvat, & Huberty, 1998), they believe that physical, object, and pretend play would not be so prevalent if they had not been selected for in our evolutionary history.

HUMAN PLAY IN PHYLOGENY

Exercise play and rough-and-tumble play are very common in mammalian species. Forms of object play are also quite common, notably, in more intelligent species, including monkeys and apes (Fagen, 1981; Power, 2000). Pretend play is characteristically human, although very simple forms of what may be pretend play have been described in captive great apes. In chimpanzees, Morris (1962) recounted how, after a visit to a veterinarian for an injection, a chimpanzee gave itself pretend injections; and Hayes and Hayes (1952) gave a classic account of their chimpanzee Viki apparently having an imaginary pull toy. In bonobos, Savage-Rumbaugh (1986) described how Kanzi would hide and eat imaginary food. In gorillas, there are also examples of possible simple pretend episodes, including making loud sipping noises while "drinking" from an empty cup (Byrne, 1995). However there are no accounts of complex pretend play, role play, or sociodramatic play in nonhuman species.

Generally, play in mammals shows an inverted U curve, rising in infancy, peaking in the juvenile period, and falling off rapidly as sexual maturity is approached. This is especially true of peer–peer play, although in some species, including primates, there is appreciable parent–offspring play, which provides the main context for play in adulthood.

Human life history differs appreciably from that of other mammals and primates (Bogin, 1999; Kaplan, Lancaster, Hill & Hurtado, 2000). Human infants are immature and helpless; relative to brain size, the human gestation period is short when compared to other primates, probably because a longer pregnancy would have led to larger neonatal head size and severe birth complications (especially given bipedalism and concomitant constraints on the size of the birth canal; Trevathan, 1987). Besides a longer period of helpless infancy, there is a long period of childhood from around 3–7 years (when the child is weaned but still dependent on adults for food and protection), and of what has been described as a separate juvenile period from around age 7 years to adolescence, in which individuals are no longer dependent on parental care but are not yet sexually mature. In addition, there is a longer adolescent period before full adult stature and strength is reached (Bogin, 1999; Pereira, 1993). Growth is complete at around age 11 for chimpanzees and gorillas, and at around age 20 for humans.

Lancaster and Lancaster (1987) argued that the long period of immaturity in humans was adaptive for an environment in which extensive parental investment could pay off in terms of skill acquisition by offspring, in a situation in which immediate productive activity by children might be difficult due to hazards (e.g., hunting) or difficulty of extracting resources (e.g., foraging). "Skill acquisition" here could include both physical growth–related capabilities (strength, general coordination), and cognitive and social learning; in general, it has to do with acquiring useful competences for later life (but not necessarily very much later, bearing in mind that both subsistence responsibilities and reproductive opportunities would have started much earlier than is common in modern Western societies).

The parental (and also grandparental) investment envisaged by Lancaster and Lancaster (1987) and others (e.g., Hawkes, O'Connell, Blurton Jones, Alvarez, & Charnov, 1998; Kaplan et al., 2000) might take the form of allowing or encouraging play activities, a view consonant with Smith's (1982) hypothesis that play was broadly selected for when practice would be dangerous or ineffective. This view of play as an especially important characteristic of human childhood does not necessarily go so far as Groos's (1901) view that childhood largely existed so that play could occur; but it does see play as part of a package of adaptations involving prolonged immaturity, opportunities for learning (in a broad sense), and parental investment in such learning (Lovejoy, 1981).

HUMAN PLAY IN ONTOGENY

Play is primarily a phenomenon of the childhood period, and of the juvenile period for peer rough-and-tumble play. Starting with early physical activity play in infancy—rhythmic stereotypies (Pellegrini & Smith, 1998; Thelen, 1979) and sensorimotor object play (Piaget, 1951) in the first year or so—play becomes more fully differentiated in the age 3 to 6 year (childhood) range. Physical activity play (involving large muscle activity) now differentiates into exercise play (running, climbing, and other large body or muscle activity) and rough-and-tumble play (play fighting and play chasing). Exercise play increases in frequency from toddlers to preschoolers and peaks at early primary school (childhood) ages, then declines in frequency. Rough-and-tumble play increases from toddlers through preschoolers and primary school ages, to peak at late primary or middle school ages (juvenile period) and then decline.

Object (or construction) play is common in the preschool years; Pellegrini and Bjorklund (2004) cite conservative estimates of 10–15% of children's time being spent on object play. Pretend play emerges from about 15 months, in terms of simple nonliteral actions such as pretending to sleep, or to feed a doll. Much early pretend play can be with parents and older siblings. In Western societies, same-age peer pretend is common by ages 3 and 4 years; in traditional societies, mixed-age peer groups are more common (Konner, 1976). From around age 3 years, many children engage in sociodramatic play, with sustained role taking and a narrative line. Pretend play declines after about age 6 years (Humphreys & Smith, 1987; Piaget, 1951).

PHYSICAL ACTIVITY PLAY

Pellegrini and Smith (1998) argued that physical activity play has three main types following overlapping but sequential time courses: rhythmic stereotypies in the infancy period, exercise play in the childhood period, and rough-and-tumble play in (what is described here as) the juvenile period. Boys do more of all these kinds of play than girls. Rough-and-tumble play is considered separately in the next section.

Based on time courses of mammalian play and of neural maturation, Byers and Walker (1995; also Fairbanks, 2000) argued that physical play supports neural maturation and synaptic differentiation at important critical periods in development. Pellegrini and Smith (1998) argued that this applies to rhythmic stereotypies in infancy, such as body rocking and foot kicking. Exercise play in childhood is hypothesized to enhance physical training of muscles for strength and endurance, and skill and economy of movement. This is consistent with the design features of exercise play, and with the results of deprivation studies, which show that children engage in longer and more intense bouts of exercise play after being confined in smaller spaces and/or prevented from vigorous exercise (i.e., in classroom settings). Although proper cross-sectional studies are lacking, such rebound effects appear more important in the childhood and juvenile periods (i.e., children are more likely to get restless after long sedentary periods than are adults).

Another hypothesis relating to an adaptive function for exercise play is the "cognitive immaturity hypothesis" of Bjorklund and Green (1992), who argue that exercise play encourages younger children to take breaks from being overloaded on cognitive tasks, and that nonfocused play activities, such as those found at school break times, provide a release from more focused schoolwork. This is also consistent with the deprivation studies and results suggesting that exercise play in break time results in improved attention to school tasks (Pellegrini & Davis, 1993). However, its relevance to earlier human environments without schooling would need to be argued; this is conceivably an incidental benefit of exercise play rather than the main function for which it was selected.

ROUGH-AND-TUMBLE PLAY

Rough-and-tumble play (R&T) looks like real fighting but can be distinguished by several criteria (Pellegrini, 2002; Smith, 1997). These include the actual behaviors (e.g., presence of play face in R&T); antecedents and consequences (R&T does not commence with a threat and usually ends with continuing social activity between partners), choice of partners (R&T is often between friends), structure (R&T often involves self-handicapping and alternation of roles), and ecology (R&T frequency is strongly influenced by space and surface texture).

However, while both observational studies and interviews with children (Smith, Hunter, Carvalho, & Costabile, 1992) suggest that R&T and fighting are quite distinct behaviors in elementary and middle school years (i.e., childhood and juvenile periods), there is considerable evidence that this changes by adolescence. Humphreys and Smith (1987) found that at ages 7 and 9 years, children chose R&T partners in terms of friendship, not dominance, but that by age 11 years, dominance also became a factor (with children often initiating R&T with someone slightly below them in dominance). Pellegrini (1995) found partner choice related to dominance status in adolescent boys. Neill (1976) observed instances of "cheating" or manipulating R&T play conventions in adolescent boys, whereby one boy might encourage another into an R&T bout, and then inflict some actual hurt and/or display dominance, while justifying this as "just playing."

There are pronounced sex differences in R&T, which is much more frequent in males, especially contact forms such as fighting, kicking, wrestling (as compared to chasing). These sex differences are widely found cross-culturally (Gosso et al., 2004; Smith, 1997). In part, these sex differences are likely due to sex hormones, notably androgen, at a proximate level (while at an ultimate level being due to sexual selection favoring different reproductive strategies in males and females). Normal exposure to androgens during fetal developmental predisposes males, more than females, toward physical activity generally, and exercise play and R&T play more specifically. There is evidence that excessive amounts of these hormones during fetal development lead to masculinized play behavior in females (Collaer & Hines, 1995; Hines & Kaufman, 1994). Such sex-differentiated predispositions are often reinforced by parents, especially fathers, who engage in more R&T with sons than daughters (Parke & Suomi, 1981), and by boys coming to see R&T as a masculine behavior and choosing other boys as play partners (Maccoby, 1998).

Functional hypotheses for R&T need to take into account the form of the behavior (design features), age trends (with a peak frequency in middle childhood), and sex differences. Several have been proposed. Parke, Cassidy, Burks, Carson, and Boyum (1992) argued that parent–child R&T helps develop the child's ability to encode and decode social signals (e.g., facial expressions). However, this hypothesis does not explain the strong sex difference found, because ability to understand emotional expressions is equally important for females (Pellegrini, 2002). Pellegrini argues that this is only an incidental benefit of R&T, a position with which I agree. Skill in understanding emotional signals might also come from social contingency games in young children (with peers or parents), as well as other forms of social interaction.

Smith (1982) argued that R&T provides safe practice for developing fighting skills, as does Symons (1978) for rhesus monkey R&T. It is consistent with design features given that R&T is similar to play but safer due to self-handicapping and choice of friends as play partners. It is consistent with the sex difference, because physical fighting skills are more important for males. Pellegrini (2002) argues that it is less consistent with age trends, because safe practice of fighting skills would be especially important in adolescence, when R&T in fact declines. Against this, it could be argued that the development of fighting skills is especially important in the juvenile period of middle childhood to early adolescence (ages 7–11 years), in preparation for adolescence. In adolescence, real fighting and dominance become important for males in relation to desirability to females, as Pellegrini's own work demonstrates (Pellegrini & Long, 2003), and R&T may become less "safe" as practice as "cheating" in R&T becomes more common.

Related to the fighting skills hypothesis is the idea that R&T is (also) practice for hunting skills (i.e., physical aggression against prey animals rather than conspecifics) (Boulton & Smith, 1992). Konner (1972, p. 299) observed that "most of the components behaviours in rough-and-tumble play—chasing, fleeing, laughing, jumping, play-noise and play-face . . . along with completed 'object beats' (striking with an object) can be seen in Zhun/twa children annoying large animals . . . or trying to kill small ones'" and argued that "the basic primate pattern of rough and tumble play has become, in part, specialized in man to serve the acquisition of hunting behaviour" (p. 301). Again, this is consistent with sex differences (males primarily being the hunters in earlier human environments) and design features.

Pellegrini (2002) argued that the most important function for R&T is in relation to dominance, and that this takes two aspects: (1) in enabling an initiator to gauge the strength of another, and (2) in displaying dominance over others by pinning them down or intimidating them, through the "cheating" kinds of R&T, as described by Neill (1976). This latter function could be split into whether the intent is to establish dominance (in a challenge to a previously dominant partner) or to maintain dominance (already established).

This dominance function is certainly consistent with the sex difference in R&T, and with the new design features in adolescence, whereby cheating is more likely and partners are now chosen for more dominance-related reasons. Although Symons (1978) argued against a dominance function for R&T because of design features such as self-handicapping, Pellegrini (2002) countered this by pointing out that gauging strength can still occur despite self-handicapping, and that self-handicapping and similar features are less prominent in adolescence, when "cheating" becomes more common.

The fighting skills and dominance hypotheses are not incompatible and may form an ontogenetic and phylogenetic sequence. Ontogenetically, the high frequency of R&T in the juvenile period (middle childhood) approaching adolescence, and the design features of R&T in this period, appear very consistent with practicing fighting (and perhaps hunting) skills. Gauging strength of opponents (included by Pellegrini in the dominance hypothesis) could be considered a component of fighting skills. The specifically dominance-related aspect of the dominance hypothesis seems only consistent with the changed design features of R&T in adolescence, thus ontogenetically later, and possibly phylogenetically later too (as suggested by Pellegrini, 2002), if this was a function selected for as hominids became more socially intelligent.

OBJECT PLAY

In modern societies, play with objects typically involves toys purpose-made for children's play, often based on mass media prototypes. This was clearly not typical of earlier phases of human evolution. In traditional societies, play with objects is typically with surrounding materials, often involving pretend subsistence activities. Reanalyzing data on !Kung infants, Bakeman, Adamson, Konner, and Barr (1990) observed a lot of initiation of object play by infants. However, this was much more often ignored by caregivers than was the case in Western samples that they analyzed for comparison.

Argument from design would suggest that object play may help children develop proficiency in skills relevant to subsistence activities, and perhaps also foster creative problem-solving skills (Bruner, 1972). There is no pronounced sex difference in the frequency of object play between boys and girls, but object play in boys is typically more vigorous. Pellegrini and Bjorklund (2004) argue that object play develops skills useful in subsistence activities—such as hunting for boys, gathering for girls. Among the Parakana of Brazil, Gosso (personal communication, 2004) observed girls from age 4 to 6 playing making little baskets with palm leaves, like their mothers do. Their baskets could not be used, because they were very fragile. However, when they reach age 7 or 8, they stop engaging in playing with baskets and begin to make real baskets for use in helping their mothers or for their own use.

These causal relations between object play and subsistence skill acquisition are difficult to demonstrate. The best evidence comes from Bock's (1995, 2002) work with multiethnic, mixed-economy communities in the Okavango Delta, Botswana. Bock's (2002) most detailed analyses relate to "play pounding" of grain, an activity engaged in (in pretend context) by young girls. Parents may tolerate/encourage such play or require girls to take part in actual subsistence activities, such as actually pounding grain, sifting it, and so forth.

Pounding grain requires some combination of strength and skill that takes a few years to acquire near-adult proficiency. Bock's analyses show that play pounding frequency follows a characteristic inverted U curve, peaking at around ages 5–6 years and falling off steeply at around ages 8–9 years, when girls' productivity in actually pounding grain makes them useful for parents at this task (mothers then reallocate their time to mongongo nut processing, a more demanding skilled process). Another skill for girls to acquire is sifting grain. This is not something at which they play. It seems to be learned through instruction and by doing.

Parents tolerate children playing, even though they could be doing other productive tasks (e.g., food gathering or processing); indeed, they may encourage children to play when the benefits of skill acquisition with future payoff outweigh the benefits of immediate productivity. There is a developmental trade-off between the child doing actual productive work (albeit at low efficiency), and engaging in play that is not productive in immediate terms but can improve skills for later use. Bock's analyses certainly support the hypothesis that the play pounding helps develop related skills, and that these are indeed put to use as soon as it is productive to do so, in the sense that a reasonable level of skill has been reached and that further play brings "diminishing returns" in this respect. "Productive" here is most probably defined in terms of parental, maybe primarily maternal, interest. As Bock points out, there will be some conflict of interest between parents and children on time allocation to play or other activities; indeed, if children can reliably expect parents to provision them, it would be to their own advantage to spend much more time playing (with later payoffs to themselves) rather than contributing earlier on to productive activities for the family.

Bruner (1972), also taking an evolutionary perspective, emphasized more the flexible nature of play and its role in creative problem solving—findings solutions in new situations. This argument was apparently supported by experiments done on object play, usually using short sessions of about 10 minutes' duration (Dansky & Silverman, 1973, 1975; Smith & Dutton, 1978; Sylva, Bruner, & Genova, 1976). Children, usually of nursery school age, were given some play experience with objects; others were given an instructional session or an alternative materials condition (e.g., drawing), or put in a no-treatment control group. After the session was over, they were given an assessment of creativity (e.g., thinking of unusual uses for the objects they have played with), or problem solving (e.g., using the objects to make a long tool to retrieve a marble). A number of such studies claimed some form of superiority for the play experience, but subsequent work has not always borne these claims out (Smith & Whitney, 1987). In a review, Smith and Simon (1984) argued that these early studies were methodologically unsound due to the possibility of experimenter effects (see earlier discussion of "play ethos").

When the same experimenter administers the conditions and tests the children immediately after, some unconscious bias may come in. Some studies were criticized for inadequate control for familiarity with the experimenter. When these factors are properly taken into account, there is little evidence that the play experience helps, or indeed that such sessions have any real impact. Smith and Simon concluded that either the benefits of play in real life occur over a longer time period, or they are not substantial enough to measure by this sort of experimental procedure.

PRETEND PLAY, ROLE PLAY, AND SOCIODRAMATIC PLAY

The role of pretend play in development is perhaps one of the most debated areas in play research. It has been the form of play most described and discussed by play researchers such as Isaacs (1929) and Smilansky (1968; Smilansky & Shefatyah, 1990), and many developmental functions have been ascribed to it.

Studies of pretend play in hunter–gatherer and other traditional tribal societies point out how such play is imitative of adult activities and can be seen as practice for children in carrying them out (Bock, 1995; Konner, 1972). Martini (1994) observed children's play in the Marquesas Islands in Polynesia. Fantasy play constituted about 12% of all play episodes. Much of this was very simple behavior, such as making mud bananas. More complex role play involved subsistence activities such as hunting, fishing, and preparing feasts, but even these tended to be repetitive: "They follow the same fantasy script from one performance to the next" (Martini, 1994, p. 84). Such repetition is more consistent with a practice function than one related to creativity (see below).

Lancy (1996) observed play in Kpelle children in Liberia. He too believes that "make-believe play can provide opportunities for children to acquire adult work habits and to rehearse social scenes" (p. 89). For example, make-believe play at being a blacksmith involves the kinds of social roles (blacksmith, apprentice, client) and behavioral routines (fetching tools, lighting fire, hammering) that, obviously in more complex forms, are seen in the adult behavior.

One viable hypothesis, stemming from the writings of Piaget (1951), would be that pretend play is a reflection of a more general symbolic/representational ability. From this point of view, pretend play itself was not selected for but may be a symbolic expression of a more general playful tendency that is suited to one's ecological context. However, several researchers have postulated specific functions for pretend and/or sociodramatic play.

Smilansky (1968), working in Israel and with immigrant communities from other Arab countries, suggested that sociodramatic play was vital for language and cognitive development, creativity and role taking, and that pretend and sociodramatic play were less frequent and less complex in "disadvantaged" children. Such functions would be consistent with design features, in that complex language, imaginative thinking, and taking the role of others can occur in much complex pretend and sociodramatic play. Smilansky's ideas about the value of sociodramatic play were influential with Western psychologists in the 1970s and 1980s, and appeared to be supported by a number of experimental studies. However, critiques have been made of these studies due to selective interpretation of results, effects of experimental bias, and the use of inappropriate control groups (Christie & Johnsen, 1985; Smith, 1988). When proper precautions and controls are used, it appears that pretend and sociodramatic play do not assist these aspects of development any more than do instructional activities such as typify contemporary nursery schools.

Bretherton (1989) argued that pretend play helps the child explore and master emotional difficulties (e.g., fear of the dark, family conflicts). She pointed out that "securely attached" children show more elaborate, socially flexible play, with more benign resolution of pretend conflicts, whereas "insecure–avoidant" children have more aggressive and fewer nurturant themes and may become obsessive in their play. Paradoxically then, her proposed function of pretend play is "least open to those most in need of it" (p. 399). This disconfirming argument is also supported by Gordon's (1993) observation that children who have experienced emotional trauma show more nonresolution of negative affective experience through pretend activity, noncoordination and disorganization of play objects and activities, perseveration of activity and repetition of single schemes, and global inhibition of pretend play. These findings suggest that pretend play may be diagnostic of a child's emotional condition, but they actually argue against the hypothesis that a main function of pretend play is to help emotional mastery.

More recently, a new generation of researchers has proposed an important role for pretend play in theory of mind development. Perner, Ruffman, and Leekam (1994, p. 1236) stated that "pretend play is perhaps our best candidate for a cooperative activity which furthers the eventual understanding of false belief." Again, design features are consistent with this. Both pretend play and theory of mind are virtually unique to humans, with great apes showing elementary forms of both (Hare, Call, & Tomasello, 2001). The peak age for pretend play (childhood: 3–6 years) corresponds with the peak period for first-order theory of mind acquisition, as indexed by traditional false-belief tasks (Mitchell, 1997). Pretend play often involves talk about mental states (Brown, Donelan-McCall, & Dunn, 1996). Both pretend play and theory of mind appear delayed or lacking in people with autism and a few other clinical syndromes (Happé, 1995). Both probably have a genetic basis, as evidenced by twin studies (Hughes & Cutting, 1999). Both are influenced in similar ways by attachment quality to caregivers, with secure attachment apparently enhancing both (Meins, 1997). Pretend play from age 3 years onwards is often with older siblings or playmates (Konner, 1976), and experience with older siblings or playmates also accelerates theory of mind acquisition at this age period (Perner et al., 1994).

However the evidence base for pretend play having a causal influence on theory of mind abilities remains mixed (Lillard, 1993; Smith, 2002). Some studies have found correlations between aspects of pretend play and theory of mind abilities around ages 3 to 4 years, but results are not always consistent. As an example, Taylor and Carlson (1997) correlated various measures of pretend and fantasy (child and parent interviews, imaginary companions, impersonation, level of pretend play) with theory of mind tasks. There was no significant relationship for 3-year-olds but a significant relationship for 4-year-olds. The correlation for the whole sample was modest: $r = .16$ for the correlation of Principal Fantasy Component with theory of mind. Although statistically significant, this accounted for only 2.6% of the variance. Other findings are similarly mixed (Smith, 2002); if pretend play had a strong causal role in theory of mind, one might expect a stronger and more consistent pattern.

Training studies could give better evidence of a causal role, but their outcomes are similarly mixed. In two studies, Dias and Harris (1988, 1990) looked at effects of make-believe play (compared to nonplay conditions) on deductive reasoning at ages 5–6 years. Children in make-believe play conditions scored better on a syllogisms task. Dias and Harris argued that setting current reality aside and imagining a fictive alternative may be important in understanding false beliefs and theory of mind development. However their studies suffered some of the limitations of the earlier studies of the 1970s and 1980s, including testing not done blind to condition. Subsequently, Leevers and Harris (1999) carried out further studies within this paradigm, that led them to reinterpret the earlier work. Harris now argues that it is not the fantasy or pretend component, but simply any instruction which prompts an analytic, logical approach to the premises, which helps at these syllogistic tasks.

The only direct training study on pretend play and theory of mind to date is by Dockett (1998; personal communication, 2000). Children (mean age = 50 months) attended morning or afternoon sessions at the same preschool. One group of children received 3 weeks of sociodramatic play training; the control group experienced the normal curriculum. From an equal baseline, the play training group did increase significantly in frequency and complexity of group pretense relative to the control group, and, crucially, it did improve significantly more on the theory of mind tests, both at posttest and at follow-up 3 weeks later. This study provides the best evidence yet for a causal link from pretend play to theory of mind, but it has shortcomings (Dockett, personal communication, 2000; Smith, 2002); in particular, the testing was not done blind to condition, which is a serious reservation given previous findings about experimenter effects in studies of play and problem solving (Smith, 1988; Smith & Whitney, 1987).

The adaptive functions of pretend and sociodramatic play (if any) thus remain elusive. In traditional societies at least, such play is imitative of adult roles and subsistence activities. Thus, pretense might be a motivator for other forms of play (object play, R&T) that probably have their own practice functions. Bock (2002) observed how play pounding in Botswanan children was generally in a pretend context but probably assisted skill acquisition; the motivation to pretend may facilitate such play occurring. This would be consonant with Smith's (1982) argument that pretend makes play more complex and challenging than it would otherwise be. Alexander (1989) argues that social–intellectual play (or pretense) allows practice in "an expanding ability and tendency to elaborate and internalize social–intellectual–physical scenarios," using these to "anticipate and manipulate cause–effect relations in social cooperation and competition" (p. 480). Theory of mind skills would seem to be an important component of this.

In hypothesizing about pretend and sociodramatic play, we need to bear in mind that the forms of such play seen in contemporary Western, urban children are very different from those found in traditional societies. The kinds of "fantastic" themes often seen in Western children's play reflect influences of the mass media, and also—at least in higher socioeconomic groups—of a parental ethos valuing a prolonged play period in the childhood and juvenile periods, and of investment in this through the purchase of many toys (Kline, 1995), an absence of demands on children to help in subsistence activities, considerable parental involvement in initiating and sustaining play at home, and encouragement of play-based curricula in nursery and infant classes (which encourage object, pretend, and sociodramatic play, though not R&T).

Sociodramatic play, more than other kinds of play, appears sensitive to adult involvement and encouragement, and may reflect effects of increased parental investment (Haight & Miller, 1993; MacDonald, 1993). This investment can be seen in a positive light, as fostering the skills that sociodramatic play provides (whether as a main evolutionary function, which is debatable, or as incidental benefits, which are rather well documented). On the other hand, parents' interests are not identical with children's interests, and parents may be attempting to switch children from exercise and R&T play (which they may find noisy and irritating) to more "educational" forms of play; this may or may not be in the child's own interests. Parents themselves may be manipulated by media, commercial, and manufacturing interests to purchase and "consume" toys, backed up by a prevalent "play ethos" (Smith, 1994; Sutton-Smith, 1986).

SUMMARY

Given the near-universality of the various forms of play, its costs (time, energy) and the robust developmental mechanisms involved (e.g., hormonal influences on R&T play; peer and parental influences), we can expect there to be benefits to playing. These benefits may vary by species and by types of play. Some will be immediate benefits, as in adolescent R&T; others will be more delayed, as in object and pretend play, though not necessarily until adulthood. There may be a lot of "incidental" benefits to play: It keeps children active and more likely to encounter new situations.

Predictions can thus be made about the forms of play to be expected in an unknown tribal people, based on analogy with play in known tribal societies, and on assumptions about the developmental mechanisms underlying play and their adaptive functions. All major play forms should be observable, and the frequency of play should follow an inverted U curve, falling off in adolescence. In infancy, rhythmical stereotypies should be observed, followed by exercise play through the childhood years, and R&T in the childhood and juvenile years. Boys will exhibit more exercise and R&T play than females. These forms of play will be largely unsupervised by adults, and will occur in mixed-age peer groups (Konner, 1976). R&T is likely to be more frequent, and juvenile and adolescent R&T more aggressive, in an ecology involving high social competition with neighboring tribes (cf. Fry, 1990).

Object and pretend play will be based on subsistence activities, with cooking and caregiving more prominent in girls' play, and hunting and fighting more prominent in boys' play. Such play will be with naturally found or easily obtained materials, rather repetitive in nature, and imitative of adult roles in the tribe. The play will be tolerated by adults, but more rarely specifically encouraged. There will be expectations for, and pressure on, juveniles to help in subsistence activities—caretaking for younger siblings, simpler forms of food gathering and preparation. This pressure will be stronger on girls. If certain forms of object and pretend play develop such skills, these forms of play will be tolerated or mildly encouraged by parents, so long as the cost–benefit ratio to them does not yet favor requiring juveniles to actually help in subsistence activities.

With human children, and with object, pretend, and sociodramatic play, there is a balance between benefits of playing and of instruction; instruction can be more focused on a precise goal, but play is often more enjoyable for young children and, even if less efficient for a precise goal, may foster a more generally inquisitive and creative approach to problem solving. The "creative" benefits of play have been magnified in recent phases of human cultural evolution; it is not clear whether this was selected for in earlier evolutionary periods, but certainly the "play ethos" of modern Western societies, the toy industry, and the high investment of many parents in play activities and toys for their children have created a new spin-off for benefits of play. As always, "benefits" are a compromise between all actors concerned—children, their parents, and the wider society.

ACKNOWLEDGMENTS

I thank the editors and John Bock, Yumi Gosso, Tony Pellegrini, and Maria de Lima Salum e Morais for comments on an earlier draft of this chapter.

REFERENCES

Alexander, R. D. (1989). Evolution of the human psyche. In P. Mellars & C. Stringer (Eds.), *The human revolution* (pp. 455–513). Edinburgh: Edinburgh University Press.

Bakeman, R., Adamson, L. B., Konner, M., & Barr, R. G. (1990). !Kung infancy: The social context of object exploration. *Child Development, 61*, 794–809.

Bjorklund, D., & Green, B. (1992). The adaptive nature of cognitive immaturity. *American Psychologist, 47*, 46–54.

Bjorklund, D. F., & Pellegrini, A. D. (2002). *The origins of human nature: Evolutionary developmental psychology*. Washington, DC: American Psychological Association Press.

Bloch, M. N., & Pellegrini, A. D. (Eds.). (1989). *The ecological context of children's play*. Norwood, NJ: Ablex.

Blurton Jones, N. (1993). The lives of hunter–gatherer children: Effects of parental behavior and parental reproductive strategy. In M. E. Pereira & L. A. Fairbanks (Eds.), *Juvenile primates: Life history, development, and behaviors* (pp. 309–326). New York: Oxford University Press.

Bock, J. (1995). *The determinants of variation in children's activities in a southern African community*. Unpublished PhD thesis, Department of Anthropology, University of New Mexico, Albuquerque.

Bock, J. (2002). Learning, life history, and productivity: Children's lives in the Okavango Delta, Botswana. *Human Nature, 13*, 161–197.

Bogin, B. (1999). Evolutionary perspective on human growth. *Annual Review of Anthropology, 28*, 109–153.

Bornstein, M., Haynes, O. M., Pascual, L., Painter, K. M., & Galperin, C. (1999). Play in two societies. *Child Development, 70*, 317–331.

Boulton, M., & Smith, P. K. (1992). The social nature of play fighting and play chasing: Mechanisms and strategies underlying cooperation and compromise. In J. Barkow, L. Cosmides, & J. Tooby (Eds.), *The adapted mind* (pp. 429–444). Oxford, UK: Oxford University Press.

Bretherton, I. (1989). Pretense: The form and function of make-believe play. *Developmental Review, 9*, 383–401.

Brown, J. R., Donelan-McCall, N., & Dunn, J. (1996). Why talk about mental states?: The significance of children's conversation with friends, siblings and mothers. *Child Development, 67*, 836–849.

Bruner, J. S. (1972). The nature and uses of immaturity. *American Psychologist, 27*, 687–708.

Byers, J. A., & Walker, C. (1995). Refining the motor training hypothesis for the evolution of play. *American Naturalist, 146*, 25–40.

Byrne, R. (1995). *The thinking ape: Evolutionary origins of intelligence*. Oxford, UK: Oxford University Press.

Christie, J. F., & Johnsen, E. P. (1985). Questioning the results of play training research. *Educational Psychologist, 20*, 7–11.

Collaer, J. L., & Hines, M. (1995). Human behavioral sex differences: A role for gonadal hormones during early development. *Psychological Bulletin, 118*, 55–107.

Dansky, J., & Silverman, I. (1973). Effects of play on associative fluency of preschool-age children. *Developmental Psychology, 9*, 38–43.

Dansky, J., & Silverman, I. (1975). Play: A general facilitator of associative fluency. *Developmental Psychology, 11*, 104.

Dias, M., & Harris, P. L. (1988). The effect of make-believe play on deductive reasoning. *British Journal of Developmental Psychology, 6*, 207–221.

Dias, M., & Harris, P. L. (1990). The influence of the imagination on reasoning by young children. *British Journal of Developmental Psychology, 8*, 305–318.

Dockett, S. (1998). Constructing understandings through play in the early years. *International Journal of Early Years Education, 6*, 105–116.

Eibl-Eibesfeldt, I. (1989). *Human ethology.* New York: Aldine de Gruyter.

Fagen, R. (1981). *Animal play behavior.* New York: Oxford University Press.

Fairbanks, L. A. (2000). The developmental timing of primate play: A neural selection model. In S. T. Parker, J. Langer, & M. L. McKinney (Eds.), *Biology, brains and behavior: The evolution of human development* (pp. 131–158). Santa Fe, NM: SAR Press.

Fry, D. P. (1990). Play aggression among Zapotec children: Implications for the practice hypothesis. *Aggressive Behavior, 16*, 321–340.

Gordon, D. E. (1993). The inhibition of pretend play and its implications for development. *Human Development, 36*, 215–234.

Gosso, Y., Morais, M. L. S., & Otta, E. (2004). *Pretend play of Brazilian children: A window into different cultural worlds.* Manuscript submitted for review.

Groos, K. (1898). *The play of animals.* New York: Appleton.

Groos, K. (1901). *The play of man.* New York: Appleton.

Haight, W. L., & Miller, P. J. (1993). *Pretending at home: Early development in a sociocultural context.* Albany: State University of New York Press.

Haight, W. L., Wang, X.-L., Fung, H. H.-T., Williams, K., & Mintz, J. (1999). Universal, developmental, and variable aspects of young children's play: A cross-cultural comparison of pretending at home. *Child Development, 70*, 1477–1488.

Hall, G. S. (1908). *Adolescence.* New York: Appleton.

Happé, F. G. E. (1995). The role of age and verbal ability in the theory of mind task performance of subjects with autism. *Child Development, 66*, 843–855.

Hare, B., Call, J., & Tomasello, M. (2001). Do chimpanzees know what conspecifics know? *Animal Behaviour, 61*, 139–151.

Hawkes, K., O'Connell, J. F., Blurton Jones, N. G., Alvarez, H., & Charnov, E. L. (1998). Grandmothering, menopause, and the evolution of human life histories. *Proceedings of the National Academy of Sciences USA, 95*, 1336–1339.

Hayes, K. J., & Hayes, C. (1952). Imitation in a home-reared chimpanzee. *Journal of Comparative and Physiological Psychology, 45*, 450–459.

Hines, M., & Kaufman, F. R. (1994). Androgen and the development of human sex-typical behaviour: Rough-and-tumble play and sex of preferred playmates in children with congenital adrenal hyperplasia (CAH). *Child Development, 65*, 1042–1053.

Hughes, C., & Cutting, A. L. (1999). Nature, nurture and individual differences in early understanding of mind. *Psychological Science, 10*, 429–432.

Humphreys, A. P., & Smith, P. K. (1987). Rough-and-tumble play, friendship, and dominance in school children: Evidence for continuity and change with age. *Child Development, 58*, 201–212.

Isaacs, S. (1929). *The nursery years.* London: Routledge & Kegan Paul.

Kaplan, H. S., Lancaster, J. B., Hill, K., & Hurtado, A. M. (2000). A theory of human life history evolution: Diet, intelligence, and longevity. *Evolutionary Anthropology, 9,* 156–183.

Kline, S. (1995). The promotion and marketing of toys: Time to rethink the paradox? In A. D. Pellegrini (Ed.), *The future of play theory* (pp. 165–185). Albany: State University of New York Press.

Konner, M. (1972). Aspects of the developmental ethology of a foraging people. In N. Blurton Jones (Ed.), *Ethological studies of child behaviour* (pp. 285–304). Cambridge, UK: Cambridge University Press.

Konner, M. (1976). Relationships among infants and juveniles in comparative perspective. *Social Sciences Information, 13,* 371–402.

Lancaster, J. B., & Lancaster, C. S. (1987). The watershed: Change in parental-investment and family-formation strategies in the course of human evolution. In J. B. Lancaster, J. Altmann, A. S. Rossi, & L. R. Sherrod (Eds.), *Parenting across the lifespan: Biosocial dimensions* (pp. 187–205). New York: Aldine.

Lancy, D. F. (1996). *Playing on the mother-ground.* New York: Guilford Press.

Leevers, H. J., & Harris, P. L. (1999). Persisting effects of instruction on young children's syllogistic reasoning with incongruent and abstract premises. *Thinking and Reasoning, 5,* 145–173.

Lillard, A. S. (1993). Pretend play skills and the child's theory of mind. *Child Development, 64,* 348–371.

Lovejoy, C. O. (1981). The origin of man. *Science, 211,* 341–350.

Maccoby, E. E. (1998). *The two sexes.* Cambridge, MA: Belknap/Harvard University Press.

MacDonald, K. (1993). Parent–child play: An evolutionary perspective. In K. MacDonald (Ed.), *Parent–child play* (pp. 113–143). Albany: State University of New York Press.

Martin, P., & Caro, T. (1985). On the function of play and its role in behavioral development. In J. Rosenblatt, C. Beer, M. Bushnel, & P. Slater (Eds.), *Advances in the study of behaviour* (Vol. 15, pp. 59–103). Orlando, FL: Academic Press.

Martini, M. (1994). Peer interactions in Polynesia: A view from the Marquesas. In J. L. Roopnarine, J. E. Johnson, & F. H. Hooper (Eds.), *Children's play in diverse cultures* (pp. 73–103). Albany: State University of New York Press.

Meins, E. (1997). *Security of attachment and the social development of cognition.* Hove, UK: Psychology Press.

Mitchell, P. (1997). *Introduction to theory of mind.* London: Arnold.

Morris, D. (1962). *The biology of art.* London: Methuen.

Neill, S. R. St. J. (1976). Aggressive and non-aggressive fighting in twelve-to-thirteen year old pre-adolescent boys. *Journal of Child Psychology and Psychiatry, 17,* 213–220.

Parke, R. D., Cassidy, J., Burks, V. M., Carson, J. L., & Boyum, L. (1992). Familial contribution to peer competence among young children: The role of interactive and affective processes. In R. D. Parke & G. Ladd (Eds.), *Family–peer relationships* (pp. 107–134). Hillsdale, NJ: Erlbaum.

Parke, R. D., & Suomi, S. J. (1981). Adult male infant relationships: Human and non-human primate evidence. In K. Immelman, G. W. Barlow, L. Petronovitch, & M. Main (Eds.), *Behavioural development* (pp. 700–725). New York: Cambridge University Press.

Parker, S. T. (1984). Playing for keeps: An evolutionary perspective on human games.

In P. K. Smith (Ed.), *Play in animals and humans* (pp. 271–293). Oxford, UK: Blackwell.

Pellegrini, A. D. (1995). A longitudinal study of boys' rough-and-tumble play and dominance during early adolescence. *Journal of Applied Developmental Psychology, 16,* 77–93.

Pellegrini, A. D. (2002). Rough-and-tumble play from childhood through adolescence: Development and possible functions. In P. K. Smith & C. Hart (Eds.), *Blackwell handbook of social development* (pp. 438–453). Oxford, UK: Blackwell.

Pellegrini, A. D., & Bjorklund, D. F. (2004). The ontogeny and phylogeny of children's object and fantasy play. *Human Nature, 15,* 23–43.

Pellegrini, A. D., & Davis, P. D. (1993). Relations between children's playground and classroom behaviour. *British Journal of Educational Psychology, 63,* 88–95.

Pellegrini, A. D., Horvat, M., & Huberty, P. D. (1998). The relative costs of children's physical activity play. *Animal Behaviour, 55,* 1053–1061.

Pellegrini, A. D., & Long, J. D. (2003). A sexual selection theory longitudinal analysis of sexual segregation and integration in early adolescence. *Journal of Experimental Child Psychology, 85,* 257–278.

Pellegrini, A. D., & Smith, P. K. (1998). Physical activity play: The nature and function of a neglected aspect of play. *Child Development, 69,* 577–598.

Pereira, M. E. (1993). Evolution of the juvenile period in mammals. In M. E. Pereira & L. A. Fairbanks (Eds.), *Juvenile primates* (pp. 17–27). Oxford, UK: Oxford University Press.

Perner, J., Ruffman, T., & Leekam, S. R. (1994). Theory of mind is contagious: You catch it from your sibs. *Child Development, 65,* 1228–1238.

Piaget, J. (1951). *Play, dreams, and imitation in childhood.* London: Heinemann.

Power, T. G. (2000). *Play and exploration in children and animals.* Mahwah, NJ: Erlbaum.

Roopnarine, J. L., Johnson, J. E., & Hooper, F. H. (Eds.). (1994). *Children's play in diverse cultures.* Albany: State University of New York Press.

Savage-Rumbaugh, E. S. (1986). *Ape language: From conditioned response to symbol.* New York: Columbia University Press.

Schwartzman, H. (1978). *Transformations: The anthropology of children's play.* New York: Plenum Press.

Slaughter, D., & Dombrowski, J. (1989). Cultural continuities and discontinuities: Impact on social and pretend play. In M. N. Bloch & A. D. Pellegrini (Eds.), *The ecological content of children's play* (pp. 282–310). Norwood, NJ: Ablex.

Smilansky, S. (1968). *The effects of sociodramatic play on disadvantaged preschool children.* New York: Wiley.

Smilansky, S., & Shefatyah, L. (1990). *Facilitating play: A medium for cognitive, socio-emotional and academic development in young children.* Gaithersburg, MD: Psychosocial and Educational Publications.

Smith, P. K. (1982). Does play matter?: Functional and evolutionary aspects of animal and human play. *Behavioral and Brain Sciences, 5,* 139–184.

Smith, P. K. (1988). Children's play and its role in early development: A reevaluation of the "play ethos." In A. D. Pellegrini (Ed.), *Psychological bases of early education* (pp. 207–226). Chichester, UK: Wiley.

Smith, P. K. (1994). Play training: An overview. In J. Hellendoorn, R. van der Kooij, & B. Sutton-Smith (Eds.), *Play and intervention* (pp. 185–194). Albany: State University of New York Press.

Smith, P. K. (1997). Play fighting and real fighting: Perspectives on their relationship. In A. Schmitt, K. Atswanger, K. Grammar, & K. Schafer (Eds.), *New aspects of ethology* (pp. 47–64). New York: Plenum Press.

Smith, P. K. (2002). Pretend play, metarepresentation, and theory of mind. In R. Mitchell (Ed.), *Pretending in animals and humans* (pp. 129–141). Cambridge, UK: Cambridge University Press.

Smith, P. K., & Dutton, S. (1979). Play and training in direct and innovative problem solving. *Child Development, 50,* 830–836.

Smith, P. K., Hunter, T., Carvalho, A. M. A., & Costabile, A. (1992). Children's perceptions of playfighting, playchasing and real fighting: A cross-national interview study. *Social Development, 1,* 211–229.

Smith, P. K., & Simon, T. (1984). Object play, problem-solving and creativity in children. In P. K. Smith (Ed.), *Play in animals and humans* (pp. 199–216). Oxford, UK: Blackwell.

Smith, P. K., & Whitney, S. (1987). Play and associative fluency: Experimenter effects may be responsible for previous findings. *Developmental Psychology, 23,* 49–53.

Spencer, H. (1878, 1898). *The principles of psychology.* New York: Appleton.

Sutton-Smith, B. (1986). *Toys as culture.* New York: Gardner.

Sylva, K., Bruner, J. S., & Genova, P. (1976). The role of play in the problem-solving behaviour of children 3–5 years old. In J. S. Bruner, A. Jolly, & K. Sylva (Eds.), *Play: It's role in development and evolution* (pp. 244–261). New York: Basic Books.

Symons, D. (1978). *Play and aggression: A study of rhesus monkeys.* New York: Columbia University Press.

Taylor, M., & Carlson, S. M. (1997). The relation between individual differences in fantasy and theory of mind. *Child Development, 68,* 436–455.

Thelen, E. (1979). Rhythmical stereotypies in normal human infants. *Animal Behaviour, 27,* 699–715.

Trevathan, W. (1987). *Human birth: An evolutionary perspective.* New York: Aldine de Gruyter.

Vygotsky, L. S. (1966). Play and its role in the mental development of the child. *Voprosy Psikhologii, 12,* 62–76. (Original published in 1933)

1 2

EVOLUTIONARY ORIGINS AND ONTOGENETIC DEVELOPMENT OF INCEST AVOIDANCE

IRWIN SILVERMAN
IRENE BEVC

The question of how people develop dispositions not to engage in sexual relations with close relatives has been a focal point in the nature–nurture controversy for more than 100 years. In the pristine environmentalist perspective that pervaded the behavioral and social sciences for most of their existence, the contribution of genes to human behavior was generally conceptualized in terms of basic, undifferentiated drives. Thus, object preferences for the expression of sexual drives, including the avoidance of close kin, were regarded as exclusive products of culture. In the contemporary evolutionary view, however, genetic and environmental influences are considered to be largely interrelated in behavioral development.

In this chapter, we first examine the shortcomings of the pure environmental theories and present the case for the evolutionary model. In this context, we discuss the universality of incest avoidance across both human cultures and animal species, and its adaptive functions. We then review various mechanisms that have evolved in the service of incest avoidance and, where these have been discovered, the developmental processes underlying their expression.

THE PURE ENVIRONMENTAL VIEW

Two major theoretical positions emanated from the pure environmental view. The first, mainly associated with Freud (1950) and Malinowski (1927), holds that prohibitions against incest are socialized within family systems for the purpose of subverting natural sexual attractions between family members that may lead to violent confrontations driven by possessiveness and jealousy. The second, presented initially by Frazer (1910) and elaborated by Levi-Strauss (1969), maintains that the function of incest taboos is to facilitate, by the exchange of spouses, ties of reciprocity and alliances between kin groups. As such, incest taboos are assumed to mark the origins of human culture.

Van den Berghe (1983) described some of the shortcomings of both views. Regarding the family harmony model, he noted that possessiveness and jealousy may pertain to parent–offspring incest but not necessarily to sibling incest, particularly when there is just one of each sex in a family having reached the age of sexual maturity. He argued further that some societies permit or even prefer arrangements, such as sororal polygyny and stepdaughter marriage, which increase jealousy and competition among family members while avoiding incest.

In regard to the kin-group affiliations theory, he pointed out the fallacy of the premise that exogamy is an extension of the incest taboo. Fox (1967) had previously maintained that incest taboos have to do with sexual relations, while the rules of exogamy pertain to the more complex institution of marriage. Van den Berghe made the further point that while incest taboos prohibit sex between close kin, the rules of exogamy often discourage marriage outside the larger kin group, and thus could hardly function to increase ties between them.

The validity of van den Berghe's critiques notwithstanding, there is a broader basis on which one might question the value of the pure environmental viewpoint. The eschewal of evolution by the traditional behavioral and social science theories has rendered them highly teleological in their concepts of causation, which tend to rest on simplistic assumptions mirroring apparent consequences (Silverman & Fisher, 2001). As illustration, the implicit premise underlying the conditioning theories is that because learning often results in immediate rewards, the rationale for learning must be the attainment of immediate rewards. Similarly, because warfare entails physical aggression, social science explanations tacitly presume that a need for aggression is at cause, attributed to the effects of frustration or displaced death instincts, or the like.

The culture-bound theories of incest avoidance show the same trend. The model postulated by Freud and Malinowski maintains, in effect, that because incest taboos result in more harmonious households, their cause must reside in the need for familial harmony. The Frazer and Levi-Strauss theories hold that because resistance to incest serves to increase the scope of social affiliations beyond the family, such taboos must have originated in the need for wider social ties. Circular reasoning of this kind by pure environmentalists is somewhat of a paradox, inasmuch as it is the evolutionary-oriented behavioral theories that are frequently criticized as being teleological, "just-so-stories" (e.g., Gould & Lewontin, 1979).

Evolutionary theory provides the only explanation of the root causes of incest avoidance that does not suffer from circularity of this type. Moreover, the facts of incest avoidance are compatible with the two primary criteria for the presumption of evolutionary origins: universality across societies and a viable concept of adaptive function. Finally, the case for evolution is further supported by observations of analogous incest avoidance mechanisms in infrahuman species.

THE CASE FOR EVOLUTION

Universality of Incest Taboos and Avoidance

Incest taboos, defined as prohibitions against sexual relations between kin more closely related than cousins, are ubiquitous across human populations. There have been reports of a few societies throughout history that sanctioned incestuous matings (Bixler, 1982a, 1982b; Van den Berghe & Mesher, 1980), but in all but one, this was restricted to rulers and/or nobility. Bixler (1982b) has shown further that these cases generally involved institutionalized marriages of political convenience that often remained unconsummated.

There are a number of studies documenting the very low incidence levels of incest among contemporary human groups. Most of these studies suffer in that they do not separate the data according to specific kin relationships, sexual activities, or ages of the parties involved. Extrapolating from the few that did attend to these factors (e.g., Baker & Duncan, 1985; Bevc & Silverman, 1993; Russell, 1983), it appears that attempted or completed genital intercourse between relatives closer than cousins comprise about .5% of postpubertal relationships. Of these, the great majority are between siblings, and mother–son encounters are extremely rare.

Given that incest avoidance is universal, or as close to universal as one finds for any molar social behavior, it seems implausible to posit a pure cultural view of this phenomenon. The concept of culture, by definition, deals with diversity among human groups. When we find behavioral universals, we generally presume these are primarily based in human *nature* rather than culture.

One frequently cited demurrer to this conclusion maintains that if incest avoidance is an aspect of human nature, there would not be a need for social taboos. The rejoinder to this argument (e.g., Bixler, 1981; Van den Berghe, 1990) asserts that the role of taboos is to bolster innately based, implicit incest avoidance mechanisms. In support of this notion, Lieberman, Tooby, and Cosmides (2003) found that adults who had been raised in the same household as an opposite-sex sibling, and hence grew up in an environment where sibling incest was possible, expressed stronger moral sentiments against it.

This illustrates a basic tenet of evolutionary psychology, that consciously mediated processes in humans, such as social rules, are as much products of evolution as autonomous behaviors. The functions of the human brain evolved by the same principles of natural selection as did the functions of other human organs and the brains of other animal species. The human phenotype is unique in that it includes the ability for communication by symbol, but there is no reason to presuppose that this capacity did not evolve, as did other neural capacities, in the service of fitness. There are, for example, universal social and legal rules for the care of dependent children, but this does not vitiate the evolutionary and genetic roots of parental motives and behaviors.

Adaptive Functions

The major adaptive function of incest avoidance is intrinsically related to the major adaptive function of sexual reproduction, which is to increase diversity in the genotype. Such diversity is accomplished both by the fusion of gametes from each parent and, particularly, by the phenomenon of *crossover*, whereby pairs of chromosomes exchange material during meiosis.

One way by which diversity increases fitness is by providing a hedge against ecological change. Sexual, compared to asexual reproduction, results in the loss of 50% of the organism's genotype in the progeny, which will usually entail a loss of some degree of adaptation to the present niche. In exchange, however, the diversity accruing to the progeny will likely provide greater adaptability to a novel niche. As evidence, animals with potential for both asexual and sexual reproduction use the former when inhabiting a resource-rich environment, thus maintaining the same, successful genotype. They revert to the latter, however, when resources begin to abate, dispersal is imminent, and adaptability to a novel niche bears a greater benefit (Williams, 1975).

This proposed function of diversity as a hedge against change is also supported by neo-Darwinian theories and data suggesting that most directional selection, that is, change leading to new subspecies and species, has been episodic rather than gradual, a reaction to sudden, dramatic alterations in environmental circumstances (Mayr, 1954; Eldridge & Gould, 1972). Greater diversity in the genotype will tend to favor adaptation to sudden environmental change.

A relatively recent variant of the hedge theory maintains that a principal function of sexual reproduction is to create physiological defense systems capable of coping with a range of potentially harmful parasites and, also, able to adjust to rapidly evolving changes across generations in the parasite population (Hamilton & Zuk, 1982). One of the means by which this is accomplished is by disassortative mating for genes that control for specific immune responses, termed the major histocompatibility complex (MHC). Potts, Manning, and Wakeland (1991) discovered that the female mouse selects mating partners that display MHCs that are both different from her own and from other males with whom she has copulated, thus bestowing the widest possible range of immunities among her offspring. Recent studies suggest that the human female tends also to be more sexually attracted to a prospective mate featuring an MHC dissimilar to her own. As in the case of mice, this attraction also appears to be mediated by pheromones (Geary, 1998).

The relevance of all of this to incest avoidance is simple and straightforward; the magnitude of the diversity inherent in sexual reproduction, and the advantages to fitness thereof, would be sorely compromised by inbreeding between close relatives.

A second adaptive advantage of incest avoidance is the prevention of inbreeding depression. This pertains to a decline in the mean level of fitness in a population, based on a higher rate of deficiency symptoms (e.g., retarded growth, lowered immunity, shorter life expectancy, reduced fertility) under conditions of extreme inbreeding. The reason for the decline is that all individuals carry at least a few deleterious, recessive genes, which are more likely to be expressed when parents share a greater number of genes in common, and are thereby more likely to possess the same recessives.

Human inbred populations are rare, but there have been several studies of these, and most show increased mortality and morbidity. Considering the data of the two studies in which noninbred control groups were used (Adams & Neel, 1967; Seemanova, 1971), the rate of mortality and morbidity was about twice as high in the inbred groups. Inbreeding depression has also been reported in a wide range of animals raised in captivity (Ralls & Ballou, 1983)

Incest Avoidance in Animals

Incestuous matings and consequent inbreeding depressions are, however, rarely found where animals are left untrammeled in their natural habitats. In this setting, behaviors that promote incest avoidance have been reported in virtually every form of animal life in which they have been studied, including marine invertebrates, fishes, amphibians, reptiles, spiders, small mammals, lions, and primates (Thornhill, 1993). In a review of field studies of avarian and mammalian species, Harvey and Ralls (1986) concluded that father–daughter, mother–son, and brother–sister unions usually comprised fewer than 2% of total matings.

EVOLUTIONARY-BASED MECHANISMS
FOR INCEST AVOIDANCE

The ultimate question for an evolutionary-based approach to behavior is: What is inherited? A more precise way to phrase this question is: What is the nature of our evolved adaptations? (See Bock & Cardew, 1998.) In contemporary evolutionary psychology, evolved adaptations are generally conceptualized in terms of domain-specific, psychological mechanisms. These mechanisms remain broadly defined at this early stage of theoretical development, and may be described at the neurological, cognitive, or behavioral levels, as well as in terms of developmental processes. The essential feature of a domain-specific mechanism is that it is presumed to have evolved in response to a specific problem of survival or reproduction (Cosmides & Tooby, 1992).

Mechanisms for incest avoidance are quite diverse, often with more than one operating in the same species. Given, as previously described, the crucial adaptive functions of incest avoidance in maintaining diversity in the gene pool and preventing inbreeding depression, it is reasonable that virtually any heritable mechanism that could decrease the likelihood of intrafamilial mating was a prime candidate for natural selection. Furthermore, one mechanism often serves as a fail-safe for another.

One very simple mechanism is earlier maturity of the female, which increases the likelihood that she will have found extrafamilial mates before the males in her clutch or litter, or brothers of about the same age, are sexually mature (Bischof, 1972, 1975). Another concise mechanism, found in marsupials, is the death of fathers before their offspring are born (Cochburn, Scott, & Scotts, 1985).

The most common mechanisms, however, are *dispersal* and *behavioral avoidance*. Dispersal refers to voluntary or forced emigration of one or both sexes prior to sexual maturity (Clutton-Brock, 1989; Bischof, 1972; 1975). Behavioral avoidance pertains to an apparent lack of postpubertal sexual interest toward those who are likely to be close family members, usually expressed by active avoidant responses (Pusey, 1987, 1990). This mechanism undergoes a prolonged developmental process in early childhood, which we discuss in later sections.

Nonhuman Primates

Both dispersal and behavioral avoidance are evident in chimpanzees Most adolescent females voluntarily transfer out of their natal troops during their ovulatory periods. Some eventually return in response to aggression by the resident females of prospective new troops, but usually after completing their ovulatory cycles or becoming pregnant in the new troop. Some do not leave the natal troop, but these show avoidant behaviors toward male kin, regardless of the close associations they may have had as juveniles (Pusey, 1979, 1980; Van Lawick-Goodall, 1967, 1971, 1986). Temerlin (1975) reported anecdotally that a female chimpanzee, reared in his home and affectionate toward all family members, began to show hostility at puberty toward his son and himself, but not his wife. At the same time, the chimp began sexually presenting to visiting human males.

Male chimpanzees do not customarily transfer out of their natal troops, but researchers report a virtual complete absence of mating between mothers and their mature sons, despite the fact that affectionate attachments often continue through adulthood (Pusey, 1980, Sugiyama & Koman, 1979; Van Lawick-Goodall, 1967, 1971). Clark (1977) reported several instances of mounting of mothers by immature sons, with occasional intromissions, but these ceased before they reached maturity.

Both dispersal and behavioral avoidance, often working in concert, are also widely reported among baboons (Dunbar & Dunbar, 1975; Smuts, 1985). In olive baboons, most males transfer voluntarily from their natal troops within 1–2 years of reaching full size. Transfer was found not to be a function either of the number of available mates in the natal troop or the male's position in the dominance hierarchy. Mature males who had not yet transferred out of the troop made no effort to compete for ovulatory females with males who had transferred in. When they did attempt to mate, it was only with immature females, where conception was unlikely. Ovulatory females exhibited a marked preference for immigrant males as sexual partners, though prior to maturity, they had preferred to associate with familiar, related males (Packer, 1975, 1979, 1985).

Dispersal is sometimes accomplished by "bride capture." For example, young female hamadryas baboons are abducted by adolescent males from outside their troops, without apparent resistance from the normally protective alpha males. The abductors feed, groom, and defend their captives who, at maturity, become their mates (Kummer, 1968). This phenomenon has also been observed in mountain gorillas (Stewart & Harcourt, 1987).

Among Japanese macaques, mature males are encouraged to leave the natal group, although not all comply. Within the troop, two types of social bonds develop: affinitive bonds between close family members, characterized by frequent grooming, and consort bonds. The latter occur only during the mating season and mostly between nonrelated individuals. When consorts are related, they are generally distant kin (Baxter & Fedigan 1979; Chapais & Mignault, 1991; Wolfe, 1986).

Incest avoidance is also common among rhesus macaques (Drickamer & Vessey, 1973; Sade, 1968, 1972). Grooming behavior between mother and son is frequent and intense, and often extends past puberty, but copulations between them are extremely rare (Sade, 1968). Missakian (1973) observed mounting of mothers with some intromissions by immature males, but this did not appear to have a reproductive function and was generally a reaction to a disturbance of some kind. The sons did not exhibit typical consort behavior and, in almost all cases, the mother was anestrous at the time. Opportunities for inbreeding are further reduced by voluntary emigration of most mature males from their natal group during the mating season (Sade, 1972).

Gibbons live in pair-bonds, and incest is prevented by one or the other parent, who drives the same-sex offspring from the home range at maturity (Carpenter, 1964; Ellefson, 1968). Forced transfer was also noted by Carpenter (1964) in howler monkeys and, occasionally, in rhesus macaques.

Indian common langur troops are composed of several females, an adult male protector, and their offspring. The male protector customarily changes every 3–5 years, either through death, accident, or a challenge from a stronger male from outside the troop. Since sexual maturity is reached in 4 years, the possibility of father–daughter incest is thereby greatly reduced. The likelihood of brother–sister or mother–son incest is also diminished, inasmuch as the new alpha male drives off the immature male offspring and kills the infants of his predecessor. Similar patterns have been reported for hanuman langurs (Hrdy, 1974, 1977; Mohnot, 1971; Sugiyama, 1965, 1966, 1967; Yoshiba, 1968).

Other Mammals and Birds

Other social mammals show the same diversity of mechanisms as primates. Female dispersal is the primary mechanism in wild dogs (Packer, 1979); behavioral avoidance in prairie dogs (Hoogland, 1982). In lions, all males and about one-third of females emigrate from the natal pride. Although males frequently remain for a time after puberty, they do not mate until they enter a new pride (Pusey & Packer, 1987; Schaller, 1972). Incest avoidance is achieved in zebras by the abduction of young females from their harems by bachelor males (Joubert, 1972; Klingel, 1972; Grubb, 1981).

Rodents feature behavioral avoidance as their primary mechanism. Rodent incest avoidance also illustrates the particular mode of interaction between heredity and environment underlying the ontogenetic development of the behavioral avoidance mechanism; that is, the animal is genetically programmed to respond with sexual avoidance toward another with which it has been in continuous contact during an early critical period. Prairie voles, for example, rarely mate incestuously under their natural living conditions of close proximity to kin. When siblings were separated and fostered out at birth, however, they avoided mating as adults with the unrelated foster siblings with whom they were raised, but readily mated with their unfamiliar biological siblings (Gavish, Hofmann, & Getz, 1984). Similarly, opposite-sex prairie deer mice that were experimentally paired before puberty experienced a delay in reproduction and reproduced at a significantly lower rate than those paired after puberty, with the same effects holding for both sibling and nonsibling pairs (Hill, 1974).

For birds, dispersal is the most common mechanism of incest avoidance (Greenwood, 1980), though behavioral avoidance has been observed in a number of species (Bischof, 1972, 1975; Koenig & Pitelka, 1979; Kortmulder, 1968; Lorenz, 1970; Woolfenden & Fitzpatrick, 1978).

Similar to rodents, Canada geese have also been shown to develop behavioral avoidance through early association. Sexually mature geese seek mates only outside of their natal group but will mate with siblings from their clutch if the experimenter separated the eggs before hatching (Aberle et al., 1963).

Japanese quail, as well, will not mate with siblings when reared together, but will if reared apart. These birds also prefer first cousins as mates over any other category, including siblings reared apart, third cousins, and unrelated conspecifics. This is presumed to function in the service of maintaining an optimal balance between inbreeding and outbreeding (Bateson, 1982). These findings may bear particular significance for the human case, in which first-cousin relationships seem to represent the point in kin relatedness at which incest avoidance ceases to be universal (Van den Berghe, 1983).

Extrapolations to Humans

The propensity of our species for colonization suggests that genotypic diversity, and consequent adaptability to ecological change, was a critical aspect of our evolutionary heritage; hence, we would be expected to exhibit a wide range of incest avoidance mechanisms. The earlier maturation of females may be regarded as one such mechanism given that in early human societies, the female's eligibility for mating probably began much earlier than in contemporary life. Although humans do not produce litters, earlier maturation of the female serves to reduce the number of brothers close in age and sexually mature in the family group, during the interval between menarche and mating.

Contemporary tribal societies also show evidence of female dispersal, usually by bride exchange or capture, and bridal exchange exists in many modern cultures (Van den Berghe, 1990, Koenig, 1989). The social and psychological separation from family in favor of same-sex peer groups in early adolescence, ubiquitous in human societies (Geary, 1998), may represent another form of dispersal. Harlow (1962), in fact, noted the parallels between this phenomenon in humans and nonhuman primates.

The primary mechanism for humans, however, appears to be behavioral avoidance toward those with whom the individual has shared continuous early association, analogous to the various nonhuman species described earlier.

THE WESTERMARCK THEORY

Customarily, evolutionary-oriented theories of human behavior begin with extrapolations from animal life. In the case of the relationship of continuous early association to later sexual avoidance, however, it was the reverse. The existence of this mechanism in humans was first described in 1889 by Westermarck, who claimed that cohabitation throughout early childhood was the causative factor in later feelings of sexual aversion between siblings.

Aside from critical commentary by Freud (1950) and others, directed mainly at Westermarck's assumption of an innate basis for incest avoidance, the theory was generally ignored until the 1960s. Then there appeared a spate of supporting studies, focusing on societies in which unrelated individuals were reared together from a very early age.

The Israel Studies

Kibbutzim is the term for communes established in Israel shortly after the founding of that country. In the early kibbutzim, children of similar ages from different families were reared in small, stable, heterosexual peer groups from early infancy through high school. The children lived in communal houses separate from their parents' residences and were supervised by trained nurses and educators. They visited their parents and siblings from 1 to 4 hours each day, depending on their ages, and spent the balance of their time in each other's company. Boys and girls slept in the same rooms and used the same shower and toilet facilities, and adult attitudes toward nudity and sex play were generally permissive.

The implications for the Westermarck theory began with the observations of several investigators of kibbutz life, who reported on the rarity of marriages and even postpubertal sexual interest between those who grew up together in the same peer group (Bettelheim, 1969; Fox, 1962; Rabin, 1965; Spiro, 1958; Talmon, 1964).

Shepher (1971a, 1971b, 1983) subsequently reported more extensive studies of this phenomenon. Initially, he analyzed marriage statistics for 2,769 adults who were raised in kibbutzim, comprising 98% of the total married population of their generation of kibbutz members. He found not a single marriage between individuals who had been raised continuously in the same peer group for the first 6 years of their lives. There were five marriages between individuals who had been in the same peer group for 2 years or less during their first 6 years, and eight marriages in which one of the partners joined the peer group after age 6. Given that 1,443 of the 2,769 subjects (53%) married a resident of the same kibbutz, Shepher calculated that under conditions of random mating, the most conservative estimate for the probable frequency of marriages between peer-group members would be 4%, or 110.

Shepher also directly observed one kibbutz over several years, interviewing members and their teachers, parents, caretakers, and peers. Among 65 members, he did not find a single case of postpubertal heterosexual activity between any pair who had belonged to the same peer group during their first 6 years. For the one case of heterosexual activity within a peer group that he did find, the male had joined at age 10.

In regard to the alternative possibility that peer-group members simply became bored with each other through overexposure, Shepher (1971b) followed up on the adult associations between some of the subjects in the kibbutz that he had directly observed. Although no statistical documentation was provided, he provided several examples of the "warm, friendly relationships" that he regarded as typical (pp. 296–297).

The China Studies

Wolf (1966, 1968, 1970, 1995) studied arranged marriages in China, comparing the *sim pua*, or minor form, to the major form. In contrast to the major form, in which the bride and groom usually do not meet each other until the day of the wedding, *sim pua* couples are betrothed in early childhood by parental arrangement and become married in early adulthood. The bride is brought to her future husband's home as an infant or young child, usually no more than 3 years old and often less than 1, and the couple is raised by the groom's family as if they were siblings. Pair members are typically close in age.

Parents customarily arrange *sim pua* marriages for economic reasons, because they cannot afford the payment of a dowry. The prospective mates, however, tend to show resistance to the arrangement from the time they are made aware of it, and often need to be pressured to live together as spouses. According to Wolf:

> One old man told me he had to stand outside the door of their room with a stick to keep the newlyweds from running away; another man's adopted daughter did run away to her natal family and refused to return until her father beat her; a third informant who had arranged minor marriages for both of his sons described their reactions this way: "I had to threaten them with a cane to make them go in there, and then I had to stand there with my cane to make them stay." (1970, p. 508)

Wolf initially assumed that *sim pua* marriages were unfulfilling, because they were less prestigious than the major form marriage. Based on his informants' reports, however, he began to consider that *sim pua* couples were simply not sexually attracted to each other. Thus, he examined the household registration records of two districts of northern Taiwan, comparing the outcomes of 132 *sim pua* and 171 major form marriages contracted during 1900–1925. He found that for *sim pua* compared to major form marriages, rates of divorce or permanent separation were 24.2% to 1.2%, and rates of reported adultery on the part of wives were 33.1% to 11.3%. Furthermore, *sim pua* unions produced 30% fewer children. Wolf also reported anecdotal evidence suggesting that at least 12 of the 132 *sim pua* couples had never engaged in sexual relations with each other, even after years of marriage.

In a wider demographic study, Wolf and Huang (1980) examined the household registration records of a large section of the population of northern Taiwan for 1845–1945, confirming that *sim pua* marriages had a significantly higher divorce rate and fewer children than major form marriages. There was also a significant negative relationship within the *sim pua* sample between the husband's age when the wife joined the family and the likelihood of divorce, suggesting that the earlier in childhood that intimate association begins, the stronger the marital problems that later develop. Divorce occurred in 16.4% of cases when the husband was under 5 years of age, 12% when the husband was between 5 and 9 years of age, and 5.4% when he was 10 years of age or older.

The Lebanon Studies

McCabe (1983) investigated a similar situation to Wolf's, involving marriages between first cousins in a southern Lebanese village. In this society, brothers tended to live in close proximity to each other, relying on each other for emotional and economic support. Their children were raised like siblings, constantly in each other's company from birth and often sleeping, eating, playing, and attending school together. In fact, the males became the physical and moral guardians of their female cousins, as was the customary role of brothers.

Arranged marriages between first cousins were fairly common in Lebanon. McCabe, however, found that marriages between cousins raised together were more than four times more likely to end in divorce and produced 23% fewer children than marriages in a control condition that comprised cousins raised apart and unrelated individuals. There were no apparent differences between the two groups comprising the control condition. In her interviews, McCabe found also that arranged marriages between familiar first cousins frequently required intense pressure on the part of their parents.

WESTERMARCK EXTENDED AND REVISED

Proximate Processes

There have been a number of theories, building on Westermarck, that attempted to explain the proximate processes by which early association leads to sibling incest avoidance.

Demarest (1977) took a physiological perspective, postulating that neural habituation in the amygdala, which mediates sexual arousal, is at the core of the Westermarck effect. He pointed out that these neurons increase their firing rates in the face of a novel stimulus but return to their baseline rates if the stimulus is continued, as would occur in the case of individuals raised together.

Both Fox (1962) and Wolf (1968) explained the process in terms of negative reinforcement for sexual contact incurred as a function of being co-socialized as children. For Fox, the negative reinforcer is, directly, the constant frustration of incomplete sexual encounters in childhood. For Wolf, it is punishment, in general, experienced during socialization, which becomes associated through classical conditioning to the presence of the sibling and thereby discourages sexual activity.

Shepher (1971a, 1971b) labeled the process *negative imprinting*, based on its similarity to classic imprinting as defined by Thorpe (1956); that is, fairly constant environmental circumstances occurring within a critical period and eliciting specific, stable, species-characteristic behaviors later in life. Though in the classic definition of social imprinting the individual is drawn closer to the imprinted object, Shepher argued that it is feasible to postulate an innately based negative imprinting process, operating in the opposite direction.

Bateson (1979) theorized that animals, including humans, have an innate, evolutionarily based process for mate selection that reflects a balance between inbreeding and outbreeding. During early socialization, the individual acquires, by means of social imprinting, a standard representing the characteristics of its close family members. Then it chooses a mate that is somewhat, but not entirely, different. In the case of Japanese quail and some other birds, the standard is color of plumage. In humans, Bateson asserts, the standard likely comprises a variety of physical and psychological characteristics.

Erickson (1989, 1993) proposed that there are two distinct and antithetical types of social attraction: *familial attraction*, which develops through close proximity to immediate kin during a *sensitive period* comprising the first 6 years of life, and *sexual attraction*, which may develop later between distantly related or unrelated individuals. Erickson maintained that if familial attraction is not well established because of inadequate familial bonding (Bowlby, 1969), altruism toward family members may be impaired, and the individual may form ambivalent incestuous feelings for parents, siblings, and offspring. In support, he cited clinical data suggesting that rejection and emotional deprivation during childhood tend to increase the probability of incestuous relations (Meiselman, 1978; Herman, 1981). He speculated further that family members who are separated in early life and thus unable to engage in familial bonding would likely, if reunited, find a very strong sexual attachment between them.

Thus, theories of the processes underlying the Westermarck effect have been numerous and diverse, and although no studies have been reported that attempt to test between theories, some recent data bear on several of the issues that have been raised.

Postadoption Incest

Postadoption incest and *genetic sexual attraction* are two terms invoked to describe a unique, highly intense sexual attraction, often leading to incestuous relations, experienced by close kin who have been separated at or soon after birth and reunited as adults. The data on this phenomenon are mostly anecdotal, though Greenberg and Littlewood's (1995) survey of postadoption counselors in London indicated that about 50% of clients who had been reunited with kin as adults experienced, "strong, sexual feelings" (p. 35). A recent media report ("Love at First Sight . . . ," 2003) described several support groups in Britain and America that deal specifically with this phenomenon, which may also suggest that it is more prominent than generally considered. All of these observations are on self-selected samples, however, limited to those seeking counseling for adoption-related problems; thus, a comprehensive, systematic study is required to establish the actual frequency of postadoption incest.

If postadoption incest proves to be more than an occasional event, it may have much theoretical importance. Neither the original Westermarck nor the rival Freudian theory would predict that separation would *enhance* the sexual attraction of close family members toward each other. On the other hand, both Bateson's and Erikson's theories of the processes underlying the Westermarck effect seem to relate in some respects to this phenomenon; that is, both emphasize the salience of early familial attachments to later, appropriate sexual attraction to exogamous others.

Neither Bateson nor Erikson, however, explain why the lack of opportunity to develop early familial attachments results in intense sexual attractions toward family members. Erikson speculates that this will happen but does not provide a rationale other than the implicit assumption that if familial attachment toward kin is not allowed to develop, sexual attraction will take its place. By the same token, Bateson's theory presumes that if familial objects have not been imprinted to serve as referents from which sexual attraction develops toward optimally dissimilar objects, the attraction will somehow turn inward to the family members themselves.

Another implication of the postadoption incest data pertains to the generality of the Westermarck effect to parent–child incest. Westermarck believed early association was specific to sibling incest, but several investigators (Parker & Parker, 1986; Williams & Finkelhor, 1995) have concluded that early separation of fathers also relates to later incestuous behavior. The relative frequency with which parent–child incest cases are noted in the both the Greenwood and Little (1995) paper and the media report may support this claim.

The Westermarck Effect in the Nuclear Human Family

Inasmuch as prior data in support of the Westermarck theory were mainly limited to studies of nonrelated siblings raised together, Bevc and Silverman (1993) assessed the generality of the phenomenon to the nuclear family. Based on a survey administered to approximately 500 university undergraduates, they compared those reporting postchildhood sibling sexual encounters with those reporting no such encounters. Comparisons were made in regard to whether or not the sibling pair had been separated for a year or more during their early years and on various aspects of early intimacy and proximity between them during early childhood.

Intimacy and proximity during childhood were included as antecedent variables to test the notion that has been occasionally inferred from the Westermarck theory, that these will be inversely related to later incestuous behavior. For example, Daly and Wilson suggest that "sexual prudery in child rearing may have an effect precisely opposite to that intended" (1983, p. 307), and Beckstrom advises that "to discourage sexual relations between youngsters after puberty, take whatever steps are practical to keep the youngsters in close proximity to one another in their prepubertal years" (1993, p. 34). The Bevc and Silverman study, however, failed to find any relationships between early proximity and intimacy variables (e.g., sleeping arrangements, physical play, practices with regard to nudity) and postpubertal sexual behavior of any kind.

The most compelling finding was a dichotomy in the relationship of early separation to postchildhood sexual activities. Early separation was significantly, positively related to the more mature sexual behaviors, labeled "consummatory" acts by the authors, and comprising completed or attempted genital, oral, or anal intercourse. (Given that the total sample size across these categories was 18, there were insufficient cases to enable more precise delineation.) Separation was not, however, characteristic of sibling pairs who engaged solely in immature or nonconsummatory sexual behavior, that is, exhibitionism, touching, fondling, or kissing.

A replication was subsequently undertaken with a larger sample of incest cases, in order to differentiate among the categories of mature sexual acts (Bevc & Silverman, 2000). Persons with sibling incest in their histories were mainly solicited by newspaper ads, and the control group was drawn from adult education courses. All answered the survey either by phone or mail. Respondents were sorted into three groups in terms of postpubertal sexual activity: completed or attempted genital intercourse ($N = 54$), sexual activities other than genital intercourse ($N = 35$), and no sexual activities ($N = 81$).

As in the first study, there was no evidence for a Westermarck effect in response to early intimacy and proximity. In fact, there were significantly higher levels of reported nudity and physical contact during childhood for both the genital intercourse group and the group reporting other sexual activities, compared to the no sexual activity group.

Regarding separation effects, however, 32% of sibling pairs in the genital intercourse group were separated for more than 1 year during childhood, compared to 3% in the group reporting other sexual activities, and 4% in the no sexual activities group. Within the total sample of 54 in the genital intercourse group, the subgroup of 19 respondents who reported attempted or incomplete intercourse (without ejaculation) was largely similar in percentage that had been separated to the subgroup of 35 reporting intercourse with ejaculation (36% vs. 29%).

Additionally, 13 of the 17 separated sibling pairs in the genital intercourse group had not lived together for the entire period when both were under 3 years of age, and two other pairs had been apart for at least 1 year during this interval. In contrast, none of the four separated pairs in the groups reporting other or no sexual activities had lived apart at any time when both siblings were younger than age 3. These findings would appear to bear out Wolf's (1995) contention that the critical period reaches a peak at age 3, based on his analysis of the effects of age at which the bride entered the groom's family on *sim pua* marital outcomes. Wolf also concluded from his analysis that the critical period wanes at about age 5, which is roughly equivalent to estimates of age 6 given by both Westermarck and Shepher.

Bevc and Silverman considered that the limitation of the Westermarck effect to genital intercourse was consistent with the evolutionary paradigm, inasmuch as the adaptive function of incest avoidance is presumed to reside in the restriction of reproductive attempts. Furthermore, continuous association in early childhood did not appear to cause sexual disinterest between siblings, as stated or implied by Westermarck and most followers of the theory. The frequency of early separation was approximately the same for sibling pairs reporting postpubertal sex play without genital intercourse as for those reporting no sexual contact. Early separation seemed to affect reproductive behavior in a more direct manner, by creating a specific barrier against copulation.

The Possible Role of Olfaction in the Westermarck Effect

What would be the nature of this barrier? One possibility is that it is olfactory. There are much data on the functions of pheromones in animals and humans for both kin recognition and sexual attraction (see Hepper, 1991; Kohl, Atzmuller, Fink, & Krammer, 2001). There is also evidence of a genetic basis for individual odors in humans. Parents can distinguish between the odors of their biological children, except in the case of identical twins (Wallace, 1977).

Although it is often presumed from these data that olfaction plays a role in incest avoidance, Weisfeld, Czilli, Phillips, Galli, and Lichtman (2003), studying human families, were the first to present direct evidence. They found that immediate family members exhibited particular patterns of aversions to each other's odors. Fathers showed aversions to their daughters' but not to their sons' odors. Opposite-sex, but not same-sex sibling pairs, showed aversions to each other's odors. These patterns occurred whether or not the source of the odor was recognized, and whether or not the individuals involved were biologically related.

Weisfeld et al.'s (2003) data present a compelling case for the notion that the effects of early continuous association in inhibiting incestuous behavior are mediated by the development of olfactory aversions. This may render more credible the various findings that separation of any significant duration can undermine the sexually inhibiting effects of early association, based on the presumption that the physiological process of developing an olfactory aversion to another person is gradual and progressive. The concept of a gradual, progressive process also appears adaptive from an evolutionary standpoint in that, under normal life circumstances, it would limit the aversive response to family members. Finally, it seems consistent with Bevc and Silverman's (1993, 2000) data showing that the Westermarck effect is limited to consummatory sexual activity, given that pheromonal secretions become stronger as sexual encounters become more physically intimate.

CONCLUSIONS AND FUTURE DIRECTIONS

Based on the adaptive functions of incest avoidance and its universality across human societies and animal species, it seems evident that evolutionary factors must be considered in any meaningful theory of its origins and development. This is further supported by the parallel mechanisms for the development of incest avoidance exhibited in humans and infrahuman animals.

The evolutionary approach has also generated productive research questions and data over the past four decades in what was previously a rather dormant area of inquiry. These have focused mainly on the Westermarck effect, and have convincingly demonstrated that continuous association between opposite-sex individuals during an early critical period functions to deter later sexual activity. Critical questions remain, however, which may contribute to the further refinement of this mechanism.

For one, the question is open as to whether the mechanism extends to parent–child incest. Further survey-type research along the lines of Williams and Finkelhor (1995) might be instructive, particularly if greater attention was given to possible latent variables confounding cause and effect. For example, we would want to know whether the effects for parents separated from young children by reasons of estrangement within the pair-bond were the same as those for parents separated by other reasons, such as illness or occupation or military service. If only separation by estrangement was predictive of incestuous behavior, the effect might readily be based on paternal uncertainty or emotional instability associated with familial dissolution.

The question also remains as to whether early proximity deters sexual interest in general or operates specifically as a barrier to genital intercourse, as suggested by Bevc and Silverman (1993, 2000). Here, also, more tightly controlled survey studies would be useful. Studies with rodents or fowl, which also show deterrent effects on sexual interest of continuous early association, would enable more precise experimental methods and may thereby provide a useful complement.

Finally, there is the question of the proposed role of olfaction in mediating early proximity effects. Animal experiments may also be undertaken on this question, and human studies might focus on differences in olfactory preferences between related individuals raised together or apart.

REFERENCES

Aberle, D., Bronfenbrenner, U., Hess, E., Miller, D., Schneider, D., & Spuhler, J. (1963). The incest taboo and the mating pattern of animals. *American Antropologist, 65,* 253–265.

Adams, M. S., & Neel, J. V. (1967). Children of incest. *Pediatrics, 40,* 55–62.

Baker, A. W., & Duncan, S. P. (1985). Child sexual abuse: A study of prevalence in Great Britain. *Child Abuse and Neglect, 9,* 457–467.

Bateson, P. (1979). How do sensitive periods arise and what are they for? *Animal Behaviour, 27,* 470–486.

Bateson, P. (1982). Preferences for cousins in Japanese quail. *Nature, 295,* 236–237.

Baxter, M. J., & Fedigan, L. M. (1979). Grooming and consort partner selection in a troop of Japanese monkeys (*Macaca fuscata*). *Archives of Sexual Behavior, 8,* 445–458.

Beckstrom, J. H. (1993). *Darwinism applied: Evolutionary paths to social goals.* Westport, CT: Praeger.

Bettelheim, B. (1969). *Children of the dream.* New York: Macmillan.

Bevc, I., & Silverman, I. (1993). Early proximity and intimacy between siblings and incestuous behavior: A test of the Westermarck hypothesis. *Ethology and Sociobiology, 14,* 171–181.

Bevc, I., & Silverman, I. (2000). Early separation and sibling incest: A test of the revised Westermarck theory. *Evolution and Human Behavior, 21,* 151–161.

Bischof, N. (1972). The biological functions of the incest taboo. *Social Science Information, 11,* 7–36.

Bischof, N. (1975). Comparative ethology of incest avoidance. In R. Fox (Ed.), *Biosocial anthropology* (pp. 37–67). London: Malaby Press.

Bixler, R. H. (1981). Incest avoidance as a function of environment and heredity. *Current Anthropology, 22,* 639–654.

Bixler, R. H. (1982a). Comment on the incidence and purpose of royal sibling incest. *American Ethnologist, 9,* 580–582.

Bixler, R. H. (1982b). On genes, environment, and behaviour. *Current Anthropology, 23,* 581–582.

Bock, G. R., & Cardew, G. (Eds.). (1998). *Characterizing human psychological adaptations: CIBA Foundation Symposium 208.* New York: Wiley.

Bowlby, J. (1969). *Attachment.* London: Hogarth Press.

Carpenter, C. R. (Ed.). (1964). *Naturalistic behavior of nonhuman primates.* University Park: Pennsylvania State University Press.

Chapais, B., & Mignault, C. (1991). Homosexual incest avoidance among females in captive Japanese macaques. *American Journal of Primatology, 23,* 171–183.

Clark, C. B. (1977). A preliminary report on weaning among chimpanzees of the Gombe National Park, Tanzania. In S. Chevalier-Skolnikoff & F. E. Poirier (Eds.), *Primate biosocial development: Biological, social, and ecological determinants* (pp. 235–260). New York: Garland.

Clutton-Brock, T. H. (1989). Female transfer and inbreeding avoidance in social mammals. *Nature, 337,* 70–72.

Cochburn, A., Scott, M. P., & Scotts, D. J. (1985). Inbreeding avoidance and male-biased natal dispersal in *Antechinus* spp. (*Marsupialia: Dasyuridae*). *Animal Behaviour, 33,* 908–915.

Cosmides, L., & Tooby, J. (1992). Cognitive adaptations for social change. In J. H. Barkow, L. Cosmides, & L. Tooby (Eds.), *The adapted mind: Evolutionary psychology and the generation of culture* (pp. 163–228). New York: Oxford University Press.

Daly, M., & Wilson, M. (1983). Sex, evolution, and behavior (2nd ed.). Boston: Willard Grant.

Demarest, W. J. (1977). Incest avoidance among human and nonhuman primates. In S. Chevalier-Skolnikoff & F. E. Poirier (Eds.), *Primate biosocial development* (pp. 323–342). New York: Garland.

Drickamer, L. C., & Vessey, S. H. (1973). Group changing in free-ranging male rhesus monkeys. *Primates, 14,* 359–368.

Dunbar, R. I., & Dunbar, P. (1975). *Social dynamics of gelada baboons* [*Contributions to primatology* series, Vol. 6]. Basel: Karger.

Eldridge, N., & Gould, S. J. (1972). Punctuated equilibria: An alternative to phyletic gradualism. In T. J. M. Schopf (Ed.), *Models in paleobiology* (pp. 82–115). San Francisco: Freeman, Cooper.

Ellefson, J. O. (1968). Territorial behavior in the common white-handed gibbon, *Hylobates lar* Linn. In P. Jay (Ed.), *Primates: Studies in adaptation and variability* (pp. 180–200). New York: Holt, Rinehart & Winston.

Erickson, M. (1989). Incest avoidance and familial bonding. *Journal of Anthropological Research*, 45, 267–291.

Erickson, M. (1993). Rethinking Oedipus: An evolutionary perspective of incest avoidance. *American Journal of Psychiatry*, 150, 411–416.

Fox, R. (1962). Sibling incest. *British Journal of Sociology*, 13, 128–150.

Fox, R. (1967). *Kinship and marriage*. Hammondsworth, UK: Penguin.

Frazer, J. G. (1910). *Totemism and exogamy* (Vols. 1–4). London: Macmillan.

Freud, S. (1950, translated from 1913 edition). *Totem and taboo*. New York: Random House.

Gavish, L., Hofmann, J., & Getz, L. (1984). Sibling recognition in the prairie vole, *Microtus ochrogaster*. *Animal Behaviour*, 32, 362–366.

Geary, D. C. (1998) *Male, female: The evolution of human sex differences*. Washington, DC: American Psychological Association.

Gould, S. J., & Lewontin, R. C. (1979). The spandrels of San Marco and the Panglossian paradigm: A critique of the adaptionist programme. *Proceedings of the Royal Society London B*, 205, 581–598.

Greenberg, M., & Littlewood, R. (1995). Post-adoption incest and phenotypic matching: Experience, personal meanings and biosocial implications. *British Journal of Medical Psychology*, 68, 29–44.

Greenwood, P. J. (1980). Mating systems, philopatry, and dispersal in birds and mammals. *Animal Behaviour*, 28, 1140–1162.

Grubb, P. (1981). *Equus burchelli*. *Mammalian Species*, 157, 1–9.

Hamilton, W. D., & Zuk, M. (1982). Heritable true fitness and bright birds: A role for parasites? *Science*, 218, 384–387.

Harlow, H. F. (1962). The heterosexual affectional system in monkeys. *American Psychologist*, 17, 1–9.

Harvey, P. H., & Ralls, K. (1986). Do animals avoid incest? *Nature*, 320, 575–576.

Hepper, P. G. (Ed.). (1991). *Kin recognition*. Cambridge, UK: Cambridge University Press.

Herman, J. (1981). *Father–daughter incest*. Cambridge, MA: Harvard University Press.

Hill, J. L. (1974). *Peromyscus*: Effect of early pairing on reproduction. *Science*, 186, 1042–1044.

Hoogland, J. L. (1982). Prairie dogs avoid extreme inbreeding. *Science*, 215, 1639–1641.

Hrdy, S. B. (1974). Male–male competition and infanticide among langurs (*Presbytis entellus*) of Abu Rajastan. *Folia Primatologica*, 22, 19–58.

Hrdy, S. B. (1977). *The langurs of Abu*. Cambridge, MA: Harvard University Press.

Joubert, E. (1972). The social organization and associated behaviour in the Hartmann zebra, *Equus zebra Hartmannae*. *Madoqua*, 1, 17–56.

Klingel, H. (1972). Social behaviour of African Equidae. *Zoologica Africana*, 7, 175–186.

Koenig, W. D. (1989). Sex based dispersal in the contemporary United States. *Ethology and Sociobiology*, 10, 263–278.

Koenig, W. D., & Pitelka, F. (1979). Relatedness and inbreeding avoidance: Counterploys in the communally nesting acorn woodpecker. *Science*, 206, 1103–1105.

Kohl, J. V., Atzmueller, M., Fink, B., & Krammer, K. (2001). Human pheromones: Integrating neuroendocrinology and ethology. *Neuroendocrinology Letters*, 22, 309–321.

Kortmulder, K. (1968). An ethological theory of the incest taboo and exogamy. *Current Antrhopology, 9*, 437–449.

Kummer, H. (1968). *Social organization of hamadryas baboons.* Chicago: University of Chicago Press.

Levi-Strauss, C. (1969). *The elementary structures of kinship.* Boston: Beacon Press.

Lieberman, D., Tooby, J., & Consmides, L. (2003). Does morality have a biological basis?: An empirical test of the factors governing moral sentiments related to incest. *Proceedings of the Royal Society of London B, 270*, 819–826.

Lorenz, K. (1970). *Studies in animal and human behavior.* Cambridge, MA: Harvard University Press.

Love at first sight—for my brother. (2003, May 4). *The Observer/UK News.* Available online at: *http://www.observer.co.uk*

Malinowski, B. (1927). *Sex and repression in savage society.* London: Kegan Paul.

Mayr, E. (1954). Change of genetic environment and evolution. In J. S. Huxley, A. C. Hardy, & E. B. Ford (Eds.), *Evolution as a process* (pp. 157–180). London: Allen & Unwin.

McCabe, J. (1983). FBD marriage—further support for the Westermarck hypothesis of the incest taboo. *American Anthropologist, 85*, 50–69.

Mieselman, K. C. (1978). *Incest.* San Francisco: Jossey-Bass.

Missakian, E. A. (1973). Geneological mating activity in free-ranging groups of rhesus monkeys (*Macaca mulata*). *Primates, 12*, 1–31.

Mohnot, S. M. (1971). Some aspects of social changes and infant-killing in the hanuman langur, *Presbytis entellus*, in western India. *Mammalia, 35*, 175–198.

Packer, C. (1975). Male transfer in olive baboons. *Nature, 255*, 219–223.

Packer, C. (1979). Inter-troop transfer and inbreeding avoidance in *Papio anubis*. *Animal Behaviour, 27*, 1–36.

Packer, C. (1985). Dispersal and inbreeding avoidance. *Animal Behaviour, 33*, 676–678.

Parker, H., & Parker, S. (1986). Father–daughter sexual abuse: An emerging perspective. *American Journal of Orthopsychiatry, 56*(4), 531–549.

Potts, W. K., Manning, C. J., & Wakeland, E. K. (1991). Mating patterns in seminatural populations of mice influenced by MHC genotype. *Nature, 352*, 619–621.

Pusey, A. E. (1979). Intercommunity transfer of chimpanzees in Gombe National Park. In D. Hamburg & E. McCown (Eds.), *The great apes* (pp. 465–479). Menlo Park, CA: Benjamin/Cummings.

Pusey, A. E. (1980). Inbreeding avoidance in chimpanzees. *Animal Behaviour, 28*, 543–552.

Pusey, A. E. (1987). Sex-biased dispersal and inbreeding avoidance in birds and mammals. *Trends in Ecology and Evolution, 2*, 295–299.

Pusey, A. E. (1990). Mechanisms of inbreeding avoidance in nonhuman primates. In J. Feierman (Ed.), *Pedophilia: Biosocial dimensions* (pp. 201–220). New York: Springer-Verlag.

Pusey, A. E., & Packer, C. (1987). The evolution of sex-biased dispersal in lions. *Behaviour, 101*, 275–310.

Rabin, I. A. (1965). *Growing up in a kibbutz.* New York: Springer.

Ralls, K., & Ballou, J. (1983). Extinction: Lessons from zoos. In C. M. Shonewald, S. M. Chambers, B. MacBryde, & W. L. Thomas (Eds.), *Genetics and conservation:*

A reference for managing wild animal and plant populations (pp. 164–184). Menlo Park, CA: Benjamin/Cummings.

Russell, D. E. (1983). The incidence and prevalence of intrafamilial and extrafamilial sexual abuse of female children. *Child Abuse and Neglect, 7,* 113–146.

Sade, D. S. (1968). Inhibition of son–mother mating among free-ranging rhesus monkeys. *Science and Psychoanalysis, 12,* 18–38.

Sade, D. S. (1972). A longitudinal study of social behavior in rhesus monkeys. In R. Tuttle (Ed.), *The functional and evolutionary biology of primates* (pp. 378–398). Chicago: Aldine.

Schaller, G. B. (1972). *The Serengeti lion.* Chicago: University of Chicago Press.

Seemanova, E. (1971). A study of children of incestuous matings. *Human Heredity, 21,* 108–128.

Shepher, J. (1971a). Mate selection among second generation kibbutz adolescents and adults: Incest avoidance and negative imprinting. *Archives of Sexual Behavior, 1,* 293–307.

Shepher, J. (1971b). *Self-imposed incest avoidance and exogamy in second generation kibbutz adults.* Unpublished doctoral thesis, Rutgers University, New Brunswick, NJ.

Shepher, J. (1983). *Incest: A biosocial view.* New York: Academic Press.

Silverman, I., & Fisher, M. L. (2001). Is psychology undergoing a paradigm shift?: Past, present and future roles of evolutionary theory. In A. Somit & S. A. Peterson (Eds.), *Evolutionary approaches in the behavioral sciences: Toward a better understanding of human nature* (pp. 203–216). New York: Elsevier.

Smuts, B. (1985). *Sex and friendship in baboons.* New York: Aldine.

Spiro, M. E. (1958). *Children of the kibbutz.* Cambridge, MA: Harvard University Press.

Stewart, K. J., & Harcourt, A. H. (1987). Gorillas. In B. Smuts, D. Cheney, R. Seyfarth, T. Truhsaker, & R. Wrangham (Eds.), *Primate societies* (pp. 155–164). Chicago: University of Chicago Press.

Sugiyama, Y. (1965). On the social change of hanuman langurs (*Presbytis entellus*) in their natural conditions. *Primates, 6,* 381–418.

Sugiyama, Y. (1966). An artificial social change in a hanuman langur troop (*Presbytis entellu*) in their natural conditions. *Primates, 7,* 41–42.

Sugiyama, Y. (1967). Social organization in langurs. In S. A. Altman (Ed.), *Social communication among primates* (pp. 221–236). Chicago: University of Chicago Press.

Sugiyama, Y., & Koman, J. (1979). Social structure and dynamics of wild chimpanzees at Bosou, Guinea. *Primates, 20,* 323–339.

Talmon, Y. (1964). Mate selection on collective settlements. *American Sociological Review, 29,* 491–508.

Temerlin, M. K. (1975). My daughter Lucy: Puberty of a chimpanzee. *Psychology Today, 9,* 59–62.

Thornhill, N. (Ed.). (1993). *The natural history of inbreeding and outbreeding.* Chicago: University of Chicago Press.

Thorpe, W. H. (1956). *Learning and instinct in animals.* London: Methuen.

Van den Berghe, P. L. (1983). Human inbreeding avoidance: Culture in nature. *Behavioral and Brain Sciences, 6,* 91–123.

Van den Berghe, P. L. (1990). *Human family systems: An evolutionary view* (2nd ed.) Prospect Heights, IL: Waveland Press.

Van den Berghe, P. L., & Mesher, G. M. (1980). Royal incest and inclusive fitness. *American Ethnologist, 7,* 399–317.

Van Lawick-Goodall, J. (1967). Mother–offspring relationship in free-ranging chimpanzees. In D. Morris (Ed.), *Primate ethology* (pp. 287–346). London: Weidenfeld & Nicholson.

Van Lawick-Goodall, J. (1971). *In the shadow of man.* London: Collins.

Van Lawick-Goodall, J. (1986). *The chimpanzees of Gombe.* Cambridge, MA: Harvard University Press.

Wallace, P. (1977). Individual discrimination of humans by odor. *Physiology and Behavior, 19,* 577–579.

Weisfeld, G. E., Czilli, T., Phillips, K. A., Galli, J. A., & Lichtman, C. M. (2003). Possible olfaction-based mechanisms in human kin recognition and inbreeding avoidance. *Journal of Experimental Child Psychology, 85,* 279–295.

Westermarck, E. (1889). *The history of human marriage.* New York: Allerton Press.

Williams, G. C. (1975). *Sex and evolution.* Princeton, NJ: Princeton University Press

Williams, L. M., & Finkelhor, D. (1995). Paternal caregiving and incest: Test of a biosocial model. *American Journal of Orthopsychiatry, 65,* 101–113.

Wolf, A. P. (1966). Childhood association, sexual attraction and the incest taboo: A Chinese case. *American Anthropologist, 68,* 883–898.

Wolf, A. P. (1968). Adopt a daughter-in-law, marry a sister: A Chinese solution to the problem of the incest taboo. *American Anthropologist, 70,* 864–874.

Wolf, A. P. (1970). Childhood association and sexual attraction: A further test of the Westermarck hypothesis. *American Anthropologist, 72,* 503–515.

Wolf, A. P. (1995). *Sexual attraction and early association: A Chinese brief for Edward Westermarck.* Stanford, CA: Stanford University Press.

Wolf, A. P. & Huang, C. (1980). *Marriage and adoption in China, 1845–1945.* Stanford, CA: Stanford University Press.

Wolfe, L. (1986). Sexual strategies of female Japanese macaques (*macaca fuscata*). *Human Evolution, 1,* 267–275.

Woolfenden, G. E., & Fitzpatrick, J. W. (1978). The inheritance of territory in group-breeding birds. *Bioscience, 28,* 104–108.

Yoshiba, K. (1968). Local and intertroop variability in ecology and social behavior in common Indian langurs. In P. Jay (Ed.), *Primates: Studies in adaptation and variability* (pp. 217–242). New York: Holt, Rinehart & Winston.

III

COGNITIVE DEVELOPMENT

13

INFANT PERCEPTION AND COGNITION

An Evolutionary Perspective on Early Learning

DAVID H. RAKISON

The young infant faces a seemingly daunting task in making sense of the world. The environment consists of a huge array of objects, entities, and events that possess and exhibit both considerable regularity and variability. For example, all things in the world tend to possess shape and size constancy, move as bounded wholes, follow the laws of physics, and possess clusters of correlated features. Yet some things move and act on their own volition, cause other things to move, and have goals and intentions, whereas others are caused to move and do not possess psychological states. Similarly, some things are potential threats, namely, certain animals, heights, and other humans, whereas others are benign or fundamental for the infant's survival.

The adaptive problems facing the human infant's perceptual and cognitive systems, and presumably that of the young of other species, are therefore to make sense of this multitude of information rapidly and in a veridical manner. Not only must the young of the species parse the array into individual objects, entities, and events, but they must sort these things into appropriate, sometimes context-dependent groups, recognize them when they are present, and learn which properties (e.g., agency, goal-directed, dangerous) are typical of which ontological kinds. Failure to accomplish this task efficiently, rapidly, and accurately would have dire consequences for the infant's probability of survival not only in the first years of life but beyond, into later childhood and adulthood.

317

Somewhat surprisingly, a scan of the developmental literature reveals that very few researchers consider an evolutionary approach in the study of early perceptual and cognitive development. A keyword search on PsychINFO—one of the most extensive databases available to psychologists—for infancy research on "perception" or "cognition" shows that over 3,000 articles or chapters have been published on each topic. However, the same database reveals that fewer than 100 articles or chapters have been published on infant perception and cognition as they relate to evolution, despite the fact that there are over 20,000 hits for the term "evolution" alone. What can explain this lack of focus on the evolutionary basis of perception and cognition?

There are a number of plausible answers to this question, but I propose just two here. First, many developmental psychologists, like psychologists in other fields, are unaware about evolutionary theory and have little exposure to it during their training. Second, developmental researchers are generally concerned with aspects of ontogenetic development rather than phylogenetic development; that is, the focus for those who study infant perception and cognition has usually been on what develops and when. For example, recent research on early categorization has shown that infants as young as 3 months of age can categorize cats as different from dogs and do so on the basis of surface properties such as facial features (Quinn, Eimas, & Rosenkrantz, 1993; Quinn & Eimas, 1996). However, few researchers discuss such important findings in light of the "how" and "why" questions: How do infants form category representations for diverse objects or, in other words, which mechanisms underlie such abilities? Why did these mechanisms, and not others, evolve? What adaptive problem is solved by the early onset of categorization? (Note that Quinn and colleagues do in fact consider such issues.) These kinds of questions are common to those who adopt an evolutionary approach to the study of the mind and behavior, but they are far from common in the developmental literature that addresses early perceptual and cognitive development. One of my goals in this chapter is to show that such an approach is necessary if researchers are to gain a complete understanding of development in these, and other, areas. Without it, researchers can appreciate only one part of the puzzle—what perceptual and cognitive abilities develop and when do they emerge—and they cannot hope to answer crucial questions relating to how these abilities develop and why they exist at all.

Although only a few researchers have explicitly adopted an evolutionary approach to perceptual and cognitive development, a number of theoretical views could be described as falling within the tenets of such an approach. These views, recently labeled as *core knowledge theories* (Siegler, DeLoache, & Eisenberg, 2003), have in common the view that the adaptive solution for rapid and efficient perceptual and cognitive development is to outfit infants with innate knowledge or specialized learning mechanisms in certain domains (e.g., Baillargeon, 1995; Carey & Spelke, 1994; Gelman & Williams, 1998; Mandler, 1992). (The term "innate" is used throughout the chapter to refer to mechanisms or content that "arise as a result of interactions that occur within the organism itself during ontogeny" [Elman et al., 1996, p. 22]). The core knowledge position is summarized succinctly by Gelman and Williams (1998, p. 600):

> The brain is no less a product of natural selection than the rest of the body's structure and functions. . . . Hearts evolved to support the process of blood circulation, livers evolved to carry out the process of toxin extraction, and mental structures evolved to enable the learning of certain types of information necessary for adaptive behavior.

In line with evolutionary psychologists who focus on aspects of adult behavior (e.g., Cosmides & Tooby, 1994; Buss, 2004), supporters of this view therefore stress that dedicated psychological mechanisms have evolved to solve adaptive problems faced by infants throughout human history. These perceptual and cognitive mechanisms have evolved, it is argued, because aspects or domains of the environment have been stable over time, and it is ontologically advantageous for the developing mind to be "prepared" to process inputs from such domains. Examples of environmental stability include the properties of objects, such as object boundedness or size constancy; the laws of physics, such as gravity and support; and aspects of mathematics, such as addition and subtraction. Because input in these domains has remained consistent over time, for instance, the force of gravity has been in effect on earth as long as life has existed on it, it is adaptive for organisms to come into the world expecting such consistencies to exist. According to this view, then, the most evolutionarily viable solution for making sense of the vast array of information in the world is for the brain to possess different mechanisms or modules that process different kinds of information.

In contrast to this view, a number of researchers have suggested that cognitive, and to some extent, perceptual development is grounded in a number of domain-general mechanisms that process a broad array of information (Cohen & Cashon, 2003; Johnson, in press; Quinn & Eimas, 1996; Rakison, 2003; Roberts, 1998; Smith & Heise, 1992). The term "domain-general mechanisms" is used here to refer to learning processes that can operate on a wide variety of inputs—for example, auditory, visual, and tactile stimuli—and that are not context- or information-specific. These mechanisms include, but are not limited to, associative learning, classical and operant conditioning, habituation, and imitation. Thus, the claim is that infants learn about varied aspects of the environment such as gravity, addition, and the properties of objects through the same basic learning mechanisms that are sensitive to, and are able to encode, regularities in the environment. How can such relatively simple and unrefined processes underpin the acquisition of a wide variety of complex information? Turning the evolutionary approach on its head somewhat, this view implicitly assumes that the presence over phylogenetic time of regularities in the environment means mechanisms that are sensitive statistical learners can be used to learn about those regularities. In other words, there is sufficient structure and regularity in the world across a wide range of domains that domain-general mechanisms can account for a good deal of early perceptual and cognitive development.

Although few theorists discuss this approach from an evolutionary viewpoint, I believe that it is important to note that such general learning mechanisms would have emerged to solve the adaptive problem of making perceptual and cognitive sense of the world; that is, domain-general processes, just like domain-specific ones, can be viewed as evolution's solution to learning. This argument goes against a number of intrinsic views within evolutionary psychology, most notably that an evolved psychological mechanism implies modularity and domain specificity. However, I suggest that it need not be the case that an evolved mechanism is a specialized one. The position I adopt in this chapter is that it is viable for humans, as well as animals, to possess both domain-general and domain-specific mechanisms for learning. Domain-general mechanisms, I suggest, operate for information that is highly structured in the environment and that has remained consistent over phylogenetic time. For example, such mechanisms are sufficient for infants to learn about the physical laws that govern objects in the world, develop object concepts for animals, and perceive speech components of one's native tongue. If domain-general mechanisms were the earliest to evolve and were sufficiently robust for rapid and veridical learning in these areas, there would be little selection advantage for the emergence of other specialized processes. Domain-specific mechanisms, in contrast, operate for information that is not as highly structured in the environment and/or that is relevant for survival and reproduction. For instance, heights, strangers, and snakes do not in and of themselves emit information that informs infants that they are to be avoided, yet failure to steer clear of them could result in injury or death. Some basic representational content could be prewired for such stimuli, what has been called minimal information-specific predispositions (Elman et al., 1996), as well as other areas of perception such as Gestalt principles and orientation to faces.

A similar view has recently been proposed by Geary and Huffman (2002), who provide an evolutionary framework for understanding brain and cognitive plasticity. In this context, they suggest that different kinds of plasticity have evolved as a result of different kinds of variability in the input. Thus, they argue that "information patterns that covary with survival and reproductive outcomes and that are invariant across generations favor the evolution of inherent, gene-driven constraints on brain organization and cognitive functions. Variable information patterns, in contrast, favor the evolution of brain and cognitive systems that are open to experience-driven modifications in these domains" (p. 677). Geary and Huffman call this approach *soft modularity* and suggest that domain-specific modules may have evolved to deal with the faces of conspecifics, the detection of favorably colored foods, and perhaps the acoustical patterns of conspecifics' vocalizations.

Although the framework presented in this chapter and that presented by Geary and Huffman (2002) have in common the notion that domain-general and domain-specific mechanisms can operate in tandem, it is important to note one key difference. Geary and Huffman suggest that regularity in the environment led to the evolution of mechanisms or modules to process this regularity. For example, they argue that humans may possess a module for understanding the physical world. In contrast, the view I suggest here is that domain-specific modules were unnecessary for many aspects of the environment that remained unchanged over phylogenetic time and that were not crucial to early survival. Infants do not, for example, need to have a naive understanding of physics to survive the first months of life, and the structure in physical events would allow more general learning mechanisms to process this information. One could argue that selection cannot, by definition, operate on environments that have no consequences for fitness, so selection for domain-general mechanisms for information irrelevant to fitness cannot occur. However, I suggest, albeit speculatively, that domain-general mechanisms were among the first phylogentically to evolve, because they represented a flexible solution to a multitude of adaptive problems. Over time, more specialized mechanisms have evolved to solve domain-specific problems; yet domain-general mechanisms remain the primary foundation for learning.

With this framework in mind, in the following sections I examine the evidence from the perceptual and cognitive development literature that learning in different domains is underpinned by domain-specific or domain-general mechanisms. Practically speaking, it is extremely difficult to determine whether one kind of mechanism or another is at work. How could one show, for example, whether specialized mechanisms or associative learning account for how infants learn about the motion properties of objects and entities in the world? Or that the expectation that things fall until they make contact with a horizontal surface is innately specified rather than learned through domain-general processes? In a few rare cases, evidence with newborns can speak directly to this issue (e.g., Slater, 1989; Morton & Johnson, 1991) by showing the presence of a behavior at birth (the absence of a behavior at birth is not evidence that it is not innately specified). Also, converging data suggest that specific behaviors develop with universality and with very little direct experience (e.g., Ainsworth, Blehar, Waters, & Wall, 1978; Gibson & Walk, 1960). One could also argue that development that occurs in a precise, regular, and predictable fashion despite considerable individual differences in childhood experiences is indicative of evolved, domain-specific mechanisms. But in the majority of areas covered in this chapter, no evidence exists that falls under these headings. For example, there is only limited evidence with newborns, and individual differences in experience are rarely recorded. To address this problem, I apply a relatively simple rule wherever appropriate: If domain-general mechanisms are sufficient to explain infants' behavior, this will be taken as suggestive, at least, that such mechanisms are present. Not surprisingly, this approach is far from perfect. Applying parsimony as a criterion is a good rule of thumb, but it can lead to both Type 1 and Type 2 errors. Nevertheless, it is the approach adopted here, and I endeavor to apply it with care.

PERCEPTUAL DEVELOPMENT IN INFANCY

Given the space limitations on a chapter of this sort, I confine my discussion in this section to fundamental aspects of perceptual development, and in particular I focus on early visual development. This may seem like a strange choice, because vision is perhaps the least well developed of the senses at birth, due most likely to the lack of visual input in the womb. And clearly, perceptual development of the other sensory modalities is crucial to early survival, and research on taste, smell, touch, and hearing are rife with evidence of phylogentically evolved adaptations. Newborns prefer the taste and smell of sweet nourishment over savory nourishment (and can discriminate a number of tastes), most likely because of the need for the energy given by sugar. Newborns—specifically those that are breast-fed—identify and prefer the smell of their mother's scent over that of a stranger (Porter, Bologh, & Makin, 1988). Newborns possess touch-based reflexes that facilitate eating, avoidance of stimuli (e.g., coughing, sneezing, blinking), and even clinging to a caretaker. And newborns can recognize and prefer the sound of their mother's voice to that of a stranger, though quite possibly this is the result of more general learning processes in operation while *in utero* (DeCasper & Fifer, 1980).

If there is such clear evidence for evolved mechanisms for survival in these areas of perception, why, one might ask, would this section focus on visual perception? The most compelling, and obvious, reason is that the visual array is the primary channel of information input for humans. To survive and reproduce, we must, among other things, identify caregivers, find and attract potential mates, and avoid predators. We must find food and shelter, and we must use tools and objects appropriately. Although the other sense modalities are involved in all of these actions, I suggest that it is visual information that is crucial for their success; that is, human and nonhuman primates are fundamentally visual creatures: Members of the opposite sex, caretakers, predators, food, shelters, and tools are easily identified by their visual appearance. A second reason, and one that stems from the importance of visual perception throughout the lifespan, is that research on this area is more extensive and in-depth than that on the other sensory modalities. Consequently, in the following section I focus on depth perception, shape, size, and form perception, face perception, movement and object perception, and causal perception.

Depth Perception

A seminal study by Gibson and Walk (1960) with the visual cliff, which was one of the first specifically to examine perceptual development, is often cited as evidence for an evolved perceptual mechanism. In the study, 6- to 14-month-old infants rarely crawled across an apparent "deep" illusory drop when called by their mothers. At the very least, this suggests that by 6 months of age infants perceive depth. However, the authors suggested a more controversial conclusion:

> Common sense might suggest that the child learns to recognize falling-off places by experience—that is, by falling and hurting himself. But is experience really the teacher? Or is the ability to perceive and avoid a brink part of the child's original endowment? (Gibson & Walk, 1960, p. 64)

Evidence on depth perception with infants considerably younger than 6 months of age could be taken as evidence to support this position. Infants as young as 1 month of age blink at objects that appear to approach them (Yonas, 1981), and at 2 months show a decrease in heart rate when placed on the deep side of the drop (revealing interest and processing) but not the shallow side (Bertenthal & Campos, 1990). Infants at 2 months of age also show binocular convergence, and at 5 months reveal sensitivity to kinetic information such as texture accretion and deletion that occurs as objects move closer or farther away (Kellman & Banks, 1998).

Though infants may perceive depth in the first months of life, this does not necessarily mean that this ability and the fear that accompanies refusal to cross the visual cliff are part of a domain-specific "original endowment." For example, the 2-month-olds in the study by Berthental and Campos (1990) perceived the depth of the illusory drop in the visual cliff but showed little or no fear of it. Furthermore, it has been suggested that "experience is the teacher," but not infants' personal experience of falling. Sorce, Emde, Campos, and Klinnert (1985) found that 12-month-olds crossed the deep side of the cliff when their parent smiled and encouraged them to do so; but infants of the same age seldom crossed the same drop when their parent's face showed intense fear. Perhaps, then, infants perceive depth early in life but fear of falling appears considerably later when they become sensitive to and learn about the emotional cues of others or, alternatively, when the relevant adaptive problem is faced.

Shape and Size Perception

Although objects' shape and size remain constant over time, it would be easy for a naive observer to come to a quite different conclusion. As objects move, they often change in orientation or angle, and as they move toward or away from an observer, the retinal image they cast changes. A naive observer could interpret such changes as relating to changes in the shape and size of the objects themselves, and to interpret these changes correctly, an infant (and adult) must perceive shape and size as constant. Seminal work by Bower (1966) suggested that infants as young as 2 months of age possess both shape and size constancy. Bower conditioned infants to turn their head to one stimulus and then presented a number of novel stimuli that varied from that stimulus in orientation, distance, and retinal and real size. Infants responded (with head turns) to objects that were the same shape and size as the original stimulus regardless of their orientation and distance, which suggests that they perceive shape and size as constant.

It is quite possible, however, that 2 months spent observing objects as they move provides plenty of experience for a domain-general learning mechanism to acquire shape and size constancy. Slater and Morrison (1985; see also Slater, Mattock, & Brown, 1990) addressed this issue by testing whether 2-day-old infants also exhibit shape and size constancy in a preferential looking procedure. In one study, newborns' preference for a square (relative to preference for a trapezium presented in a frontoparallel plane) diminished as the orientation of the square moved away from the frontal plane. In a second study, infants were familiarized to changes in slant (thus desensitizing them) for a square or a trapezium. In the test trials, infants were then shown the familiar shape in a novel slant paired with the other, novel shape. All of the infants looked longer at the novel shape, which suggests that the familiar shape was perceived as familiar despite its appearance in a different slant. Similar studies with three-dimensional objects by Slater et al. (1990) provided converging evidence to support these findings, as does research on scanning preferences that showed neonates possess a bias to scan along the horizontal (Haith, 1991). Taken together, then, these studies suggest that even newborns perceive the shape and size of objects as constant.

Why should these aspects of perception be present at birth when depth perception, for example, is not? One possibility is that depth perception is indeed present at birth, but no studies have been sensitive enough to test for it. The finding that infants possess size constancy could be interpreted as meaning they can perceive depth; yet all that is needed for size constancy is to base responses on retinal image size. Another possibility is that shape and size constancy are crucial to survival, even for newborns and very young infants. Why be interested in a human face, or food, if they are perceived to be relatively small? A small morsel of food across the room is unlikely to be as enticing as a large morsel of food that is perceived to be smaller because of its distance from an observer. Alternatively, it is plausible that there is simply insufficient information in the array to specify that objects remain constant in shape and size irrespective of distance and slant. How could a baby learn, for example, that it is an object's retinal image that becomes smaller as that object moves away rather than that the object shrinks in size as it moves away? Regardless, the available data provide compelling evidence that human infants possess an evolved perceptual mechanism that interprets shape and size as constant.

Form Perception

Given that infants are sensitive to shape and size, an important next questions concerns when and how they show sensitivity to the pattern, or form, of objects. Objects are generally composed of a number of features, or parts, and a naive perceiver could interpret these features as unconnected or as bounded together. In fact, it has been suggested that for infants and adults to perceive objects as bound wholes, they must first decompose those objects into a number of parts and then recombine the parts into wholes (Rakison, 2003; Triesman, 1985). This issue has a long history in psychology, going back to the Gestalt theorists who suggested that infants innately perceive whole forms (Koffka, 1935), as well as theorists with a constructivist viewpoint, who suggested that such perception is learned through experience (Hebb, 1949; Piaget, 1952).

To examine this issue, Slater, Mattock, Brown, Burnham, and Young (1991) conducted an ingenious experiment in which newborns were familiarized simultaneously to stimulus compounds such as a green vertical stripe and a red diagonal stripe. In the test trials, the infants were shown a novel combination of the two elements—for example, a red vertical stripe alongside one of the familiar stimuli. All of the newborns showed a preference to look at the new combination of elements, which suggests that they had processed the color and slant of the line together rather than independently. Again, converging evidence to support this result was found using a similar design that showed that newborns processed two connected lines as a compound—that is, in terms of the angle formed by those lines—rather than independently (Slater et al., 1991; cf. Cohen & Younger, 1984). In conjunction, these studies suggest that infants are born with an evolved predisposition to parse wholes into their component parts, and to recombine them together into a unified whole.

Another important aspect of form perception relates to the ability to categorize objects by forming prototypes. A "prototype" is an average or ideal of a category that can be a specific class (e.g., an average dog is a Labrador) or a more abstract notion (e.g., a square has four equal sides with internal angles of 90 degrees). There is now considerable evidence that infants are able to form perceptual prototypes within the first months of life and do so for a variety of stimuli. In one classic study, Bomba and Siqueland (1983) familiarized 3- and 4-month-olds with distorted shapes (either squares, diamonds, or triangles) and then presented the infants one of the same distorted shapes, as well as the prototypical shape (that was not shown during familiarization). Somewhat counterintuitively, infants looked longer at the distorted shape than at the prototypical shape, which the authors interpreted to mean that they treated the previously unseen prototype as familiar; that is, the prototype did not hold infants' visual attention because it was closer to their representation for the shape than the distorted image. Infants in the first months of life have also been shown to form prototypes for a variety of stimuli, including human faces (Langlois, Roggman, & Musselman, 1994; Rubenstein, Kalakanis, & Langlois, 1999) and schematic animals (Younger, 1985), which could be interpreted as evidence that a prototype formation mechanism is not specific to any particular input and is domain-general. However, as shown in the next section, there is reason to question whether the same perceptual mechanism operates for one class of particularly important stimuli; namely, faces.

Face Perception

If we are experts in nothing else, all adults are experts in the field of face recognition. We can recognize thousands if not tens of thousands of faces; we remember those that were last seen over 30 years ago, and we can identify sex and age from facial information alone. Does this expertise mean that faces are "special" in some sense and that their perception is driven by an evolved mechanism dedicated to faces? According to one view, this is exactly the correct characterization. Our ancestors needed to recognize specific faces to determine who were enemies, who were friends, and who were family members. They also used facial information in mating to determine health and vitality. And infants who quickly learned the faces of those who protected them and provided for their physical and emotional needs would have been more likely to survive than those who did not. Face expertise, it is therefore argued, is a consequence of the importance of faces in our evolutionary past and is grounded in an innate psychological mechanism that facilitates early orientation to, and learning about, faces (Johnson & Morton, 1991). According to another perspective, however, expertise in face recognition is a product of experience with many faces, and the same domain-general mechanism can be applied, and is applied, to other stimuli. For example, adults with relevant experience are able to make exceptionally fine discriminations between dogs of the same subordinate category (Diamond & Carey, 1986) and are able to sex-type chickens with over 99% accuracy (Gibson, 1969). Clearly, in contrast to the other aspects of perceptual development discussed thus far, the case for or against an evolved face-processing mechanism is far from unequivocal.

Impressive evidence to support the first view was presented in a prominent series of studies by Johnson, Dziurawiec, Ellis, and Morton (1991; see also Goren, Sarty, & Wu, 1975). Newborn infants were presented with stimuli that moved laterally back and forth at about 5 degrees per second, and the experimenters coded the amount of looking and orienting to the stimuli. The stimuli were head-sized paddles that depicted a schematic face (with eyes, eyebrows, a nose, and a mouth), a scrambled face (the same features rearranged in a symmetrical configuration), or a blank face (without any features). Impressively, the newborns looked at and tracked the schematic face more than the scrambled face and the blank face, and they looked at and tracked the scrambled face more than the blank face.

Based on these and related findings (for a review, see Johnson & Morton, 1991), it was proposed that infants are born with two separate but related mechanisms that are specific to information given by faces. The first, labeled CONSPEC, is a subcortical mechanism that causes infants to orient to faces or, at the very least, to face-like structures with eye and mouth elements (Simion, Valenza, & Umiltà, 1998). The second, labeled CONLERN, is cortically driven and allows infants to detect and learn about similarities and differences in faces. There are reasons to doubt at least part of this formulation, however. The study by Johnson et al. (1991) provides compelling evidence that newborns track human-like faces, which suggests the existence of something like a CONSPEC mechanism. There is little evidence, though, that infants possess a dedicated face-learning mechanism such as CONLERN over and above a more all-purpose learning mechanism. Furthermore, the claim that any such mechanism is cortically driven is undermined by evidence that infants discriminate between their mother and a stranger with the first days of life (Walton, Bower, & Bower, 1992). Indeed, Johnson and Morton (1993) acknowledge that CONLERN may be just a domain-general mechanism that "becomes specialized for faces as a result of massive experience of them provided by the species-typical environment" (p. 249). This view is supported by recent studies that examined processing of upright and inverted faces by infants and adults. For example, Pascalis, de Haan, and Nelson (2002; Johnson & de Haan, 2001) found that adults and 9-month-olds fixate visually longer to novel human faces than to familiar human faces but fixate equally long novel and familiar monkey faces. Infants at 6 months of age, however, visually fixate longer to novel than to familiar faces for humans as well as monkeys. The authors suggested that this narrowing of the ability to perceive faces is indicative of cortical specialization, a view that fits well with the idea that infants possess an initial bias for face orientation and, perhaps, recognition that is adapted following experience (Johnson, 2000; Nelson, 2001).

Another line of research provides further support, however, for the claim that newborns possess a dedicated face perception mechanism. In a classic body of work, Meltzoff and Moore (1977, 1994) showed that newborn infants will imitate facial gestures made by an adult, such as tongue protrusion and mouth opening, and by 6 weeks will repeat such gestures 24 hours after seeing them modeled. The basic imitation findings have since been replicated and extended in a number of laboratory conditions, most notably with emotional expressions such as happiness and sadness (Field, Woodson, Greenberg, & Cohen, 1982), and in non-Western cultures such as Nepal (Vinter, 1986). According to Meltzoff and Gopnik (1993), this imitation is possible because of an evolved "like me" mechanism. This mechanism, in combination with cross-modal matching of the visual input (e.g., a tongue protrusion) and the proprioceptive properties of his or her own mouth, leads an infant to draw a comparison between faces he or she observes and the infant's own face. Despite the appeal of such a view, the "like me" hypothesis currently remains controversial, and there is little in the way of direct evidence to support it; indeed, it is unclear how such a theory could empirically be tested. Nonetheless, the findings on imitation by newborns (Meltzoff & Moore, 1977, 1994) provide substantial evidence that infants are born with a predisposition to imitate human facial movements. In all likelihood, such contingent behaviors help to form an emotional bond between caretaker and infant, provide the foundation for communication between them, and may also constitute the first volitional motor activity of the newborn.

A final line of research that is worth noting concerns infants' preference for attractive faces. When infants at 2, 3, and 6 months of age are presented with attractive and unattractive faces (as rated by adults) in a paired-preference procedure, they look longer at the attractive faces than at the unattractive ones and do so for males and females (Langlois et al., 1987). This bias was not, however, a simple preference for symmetry, because infants have been shown to look at vertically symmetrical faces and asymmetrical faces equally long (Samuels, Butterworth, Roberts, Graupner, & Hole, 1994). Because infants have no experience of what is held by a culture as the standard for attractiveness, these findings could be interpreted as evidence for an evolved preference for attractiveness. According to one view, however, this early preference results from a more general information-processing capacity, namely, prototype formation (Langlois et al., 1987). The reasoning behind this argument is that average, or prototypical (e.g., the distance between facial features is average) faces tend to be highly attractive because humans possess a central tendency preference for prototypical exemplars over nonprototypical exemplars (Halberstadt & Rhodes, 2000). Indeed, adults find a composite face (made by averaging features across multiple faces) more attractive than nearly all of the individual faces from which it was formed (Langlois & Roggman, 1990), and infants as young as 6 months of age show a similar preference, as well as the ability to extract the central tendency from a set of faces (Rubenstein et al., 1999).

To summarize, three lines of research speak to whether infants possess one or more evolved mechanisms designed to facilitate learning of faces. The research on face tracking suggests that newborns orient to faces more than to other stimuli; the research on imitation suggests that newborns repeat facial movements by human faces, and the research on attractiveness suggests that a preference for attractiveness results from prototype formation. Taken together, these findings point to the existence of a bare-boned evolved mechanism for face perception that encourages infants to look at faces and repeat their movements. The findings also suggest, however, that beyond these initial predispositions, face recognition and perception—including the acquisition of information relating to age, gender, and specific exemplars, such as parents—result from more all-purpose, general learning mechanisms.

Movement and Object Perception

The world is primarily a static perceptual field interspersed with movement. Some of this movement has little relevance to the infant, such as the tree moving in the wind or the clouds drifting across the sky. Yet a good deal of movement carries with it important information. Moving entities may be dangerous, potential prey, or they may provide nourishment or protection. And understanding that different object kinds, namely, animates and inanimates, move in different ways is fundamental to reliable prediction about their behaviors. There is considerable evidence that sensitivity to motion is ubiquitous among animal species, and according to one view, this sensitivity has evolved as part of a predator avoidance mechanism: Young vervets, for instance, rely solely on motion cues to categorize potential predators, and will initially make false "eagle" alarm calls for a whole host of birds and even rapidly falling leaves (Evans & Marler, 1995; Seyfarth & Cheney, 1986). An important question is whether young infants are similarly sensitive to motion, how this sensitivity emerges, and how it relates to other aspects of object perception.

A good starting point is the study by Johnson et al. (1991) providing clear evidence that newborns respond to motion and track a moving object. More impressive, perhaps, newborns show a visual preference for moving stimuli over static ones, and they can extract shape information from such stimuli (Slater, 1989). These findings alone suggest that infants possess an evolved predisposition to find movement salient and orient to moving objects. Between 2 and 5 months of age, infants orient to a small moving object in a visual field of static objects (Dannemiller, 2000), and by 3 months of age, infants prefer a human moving point-light display to an unstructured point-light display (Bertenthal, 1993). This sensitivity to movement allows infants to extract information not only about shape but also spatial location. For example, Haith and colleagues (Haith, 1991; Haith, Wentworth, & Canfield, 1993) found that 3-month-olds develop an expectation, or anticipation, about the spatial location of stimuli when shown a repeating left–right pattern.

It might be predicted that it is more difficult for infants to extract information about an object's form when that object is moving, because the array is continuously changing. Similarly, it might be predicted that because objects are often partly occluded by other objects, infants initially perceive the world as made up of many fragments. However, classic research by Kellman and Spelke (1983) on infants' perception of partly occluded objects showed that quite the opposite is true. Infants at 4 months of age were habituated to a static central occluder behind which a rod moved back and forth. Importantly, only the top and bottom of the rod were visible. During the test trials, infants were shown a moving complete rod or two moving separate pieces of rod identical to those seen during habituation. Infants' looking behavior revealed that they interpreted the rod behind the occluder as complete; that is, they visually fixated longer to the incomplete rod than to the complete one. In subsequent studies with a similar design (Slater et al., 1990; Slater, Johnson, Kellman, & Spelke, 1994), newborn infants were found to show the opposite pattern of looking, such that they looked longer at the complete rod than at the incomplete rod. This was the case even if there was a considerable gap between the rod and the occluder (which means that one is definitely behind the other). However, 2-month-olds looked longer at the incomplete rod if the width of the occluder was reduced, so that more of the rod was visible (Johnson & Aslin, 1995; for a review, see Johnson, in press).

According to Kellman (1993; Kellman & Spelke, 1983) these data suggest that common motion, which he refers to as an innate, or maturational "primitive process," is a strong cue that indicates object unity, as does edge alignment. Yet at 4 months of age, neither cue is sufficient, on its own, to specify object unity. Although newborns are sensitive to common motion, it is possible that the fact that two separate pieces of rod (and not one) are seen overrides this dynamic information. However, that young infants require the two rods—or the variety of shapes used in the different experiments on object unity—to be similar suggests that their perception is guided by Gestaltist principles such as *common movement, good continuation* (edges that are unconnected are perceived as connected if the edges are relatable), *proximity,* and *similarity* (Kellman & Banks, 1998). These Gestalt principles are presumably an evolved perceptual predisposition that allow even very young infants to perceive the world as consisting of complete objects rather than unconnected fragments. Yet, at the same time, it is evident that experience is required before such principles supersede other available perceptual information.

Causal Perception

To make sense of the world, it is imperative that infants come to understand that actions have causal consequences. This is the case for their own actions, as suggested by Piaget (1952), as well as the actions of others around them. It is now well established that within the first year of life, infants are sensitive to various aspects of causality. Leslie and Keeble (1987), in perhaps the first series of studies to examine systematically this issue, showed 7-month-old infants a series of simple launching events based on those developed by Michotte (1963). Infants were habituated to a green, brick-shaped object that moved from left to right across a screen and contacted a second brick-shaped object (of a different color) that then moved in the same direction until off the screen. In a control condition, they were habituated to similar events, except that there was a short delay between contact and response. In the test phase, infants were shown the same events presented during habituation reversed. In other words, the brick shapes moved from the right side of the screen toward the left side of the screen. The rationale was that the reversal of the launching event changed the relationship between agent and recipient (the agent became the recipient and vice versa), whereas the reversal of the nonlaunching delay event did not. Impressively, 7-month-olds recovered visual attention to the reversal of the launching event more than did infants presented with the reversal of the nonlaunching event.

To explain these and other empirical data, Leslie (1984, 1994, 1995) proposed a nativist and modular view of early causal knowledge whereby infants are born with a three-part theory of agency. (The term "agency" refers to the stable and continuing aspect of objects as agents rather than a single display of agency.) According to Leslie, separate modules in the brain process the mechanical, intentional, and cognitive properties of agents, and it is these modules that direct infants to attend to, and interpret, diverse events in different ways. The perception of spatiotemporal patterns alone does not, according to Leslie, lead infants to interpret an animate as a causal agent; instead, one (or a number) of the causality modules construes spatial and temporal information as an abstract causal code. This is clearly an evolutionary-grounded perspective. The early perception of physical and psychological causality is of fundamental importance to human survival—we must determine which things engage in actions with causal consequences—and domain-specific causal processing mechanisms are an evolved solution to this adaptive problem.

This modular view has been challenged at both a theoretical and an empirical level. Rakison and Poulin-Dubois (2001), for example, pointed out that it is not clear how different causality modules are "triggered" by the same input, and questioned why infants must possess specific mental structures that draw attention to different kinds of causal information. Take, for instance, a seemingly simple causal event, such as when a human hand reaches for a ball; according to Leslie, such an event involves mechanical and intentional causation. Yet it remains to be seen how information-encapsulated modules work in concert to process such an event. The available empirical evidence has also suggested that causal perception may be learned during ontogeny, and that this learning is grounded in all-purpose information-processing mechanisms. Oakes and Cohen (1990) habituated 6- and 10-month-olds either to direct launching, delayed launching, or noncontact events. The direct launching and delayed launching events were identical to those in the study by Leslie and Keeble (1987). In the noncontact event, infants were habituated to a similar launching sequence except that there was a small gap between the final position of the first object and the starting position of the second object. In the test phase, infants in each condition were presented with the direct, delayed, and noncontact events. The results showed that 6-month-old infants looked equally long at all three test events, which was taken to mean that they did not discriminate causal from noncausal events. In contrast, 10-month-old infants who were habituated to the direct launching event looked longer at the two noncausal events, and those habituated to one of the noncausal events looked longer at the causal launching event but not at the other noncausal event. The authors interpreted these findings to mean that the ability to perceive causality is not automatic within the first year of life but rather emerges between 6 and 7 months of age.

Supporting evidence for this finding was generated in a follow-up study by Cohen and Oakes (1993) using a similar design in which 10- to 12-month-olds failed to discriminate causal launching events from noncausal events when different objects were used in each habituation trial. This finding can be explained within an information-processing perspective. Infants' processing of the different objects in each event meant that they failed to process the causal nature of the events themselves. Such an explanation is highly plausible and suggests that causal perception is not an automatic process that is controlled by evolved specialized modules. Thus, although causal perception is a viable candidate for an evolved psychological mechanism, there is little evidence to support such a possibility. Proponents of an information-processing approach argue that the available evidence points the other way: Causal perception is learned, appearing after 6 months of life, presumably through experience of spatial and temporal contiguities.

Summary of the Evidence for Evolved Mechanisms for Perceptual Development

In this section, I have examined evidence for evolved psychological mechanisms in early perceptual development by evaluating research on depth perception, shape, size, and form perception, face perception, movement and object perception, and causal perception. Overall, the available evidence indicates that infants may possess a number of evolved mechanisms that facilitate early perceptual development; however, in many cases, they are relatively simple mechanisms that simply help to get the baby's visual perception off the ground. For example, the reviewed data suggests that infants do not need to learn that objects have shape and size constancy, that objects can be closer or farther away, or that relatable edges imply that an occluded object is connected. They are also endowed with a number of *attention biases* (Rakison, 2003) that elevate the salience of particular aspects of the array. Specifically, young infants and newborns attend to motion and to simple face-like stimuli, prefer relatively complex over relatively simple stimuli, and parse simple forms into their component parts and then recombine them into wholes.

There is very little evidence, however, that other aspects of visual perception are underpinned by processes designed by evolution for specific inputs. Infants perceive depth within the first months but do not show fear of a drop until later in life. Infants learn about the specific shapes of objects, circles and squares, for example, as well as about the various faces they encounter through prototype formation and other general learning mechanisms. And infants may learn about physical causal perception—whereby one thing acts on another through contact—via experience with temporal and spatial contiguities. In these, and presumably other aspects of perceptual development not outlined here (e.g., speech perception), there is no need to posit specialized evolved mechanisms to explain how infants come to make sense of the world. In many cases, domain-general processes such as associative learning, prototype formation, conditioning, and imitation, coupled with simple attention biases and other basic perceptual principles—for example, those forwarded by the Gestaltists—can account convincingly for the available data.

COGNITIVE DEVELOPMENT IN INFANCY

The line between cognitive and perceptual development in infancy is often fuzzy. It is frequently hard to delineate where perceptual processes cease and cognitive ones begin. For example, it would be just as feasible to include the coverage of infants' understanding of causality in this section as in the section on perceptual development. As is the case for perceptual development, few researchers have explicitly set out to examine cognitive development from an evolutionary perspective—that is, in terms of adaptations designed to solve a particular problem that faced our ancestors—and, indeed, there are only a handful of studies on adult cognition that have adopted such a stance (cf. Cosmides & Tooby, 1994). Nonetheless, it is indisputable that humans' cognitive abilities distinguish us from other living things. Adult humans are able to remember a huge amount of relatively arbitrary information, solve complicated and multilevel, real-world abstract and mathematical problems, learn and use one or more languages, and form context-dependent categories online on the basis of surface and deep properties (Barsalou, 1983; Gelman, 2003). Are these abilities evolved specialized processes or modules? Or do they develop out of more general processes and simply reflect the multifaceted and complex world in which we live? To address these questions, at least in part, I examine a moderately small number of domains to assess the role of selection pressures on cognitive development, namely, an understanding of physics, math, and categorization and concept formation for objects.

Infants' Understanding of Simple Physics

To a naive reader, it may seem somewhat outlandish to consider whether infants understand or are sensitive to principles of physics. High school students find it difficult to understand such principles (as do I), so what, one might ask, could infants know about gravity, momentum, and inertia? As far as we know, the laws of physics have remained constant throughout human evolution. According to one view, therefore, it is adaptive for human infants and the young of other species to possess innate knowledge or specialized learning mechanisms that facilitate the ability to learn about such laws early in life. Evidence to support this view is drawn from a number of sources.

Classic work by Spelke, Breinlinger, Macomber, and Jacobson (1992) suggested that young infants appreciate that objects are solid. Two-month-old infants were shown a stage with a ball on one side and a box on the other side, after which a screen was lowered to occlude the box. Infants were then habituated to an event in which a ball rolled behind the screen, after which the screen was raised to show the ball resting against the box. In the test phase, infants were shown two similar events that included a second box placed nearer the ball and separated slightly from the first one. In the "impossible" event, after the screen was raised the ball was shown resting against the farthest box, having seemingly passed through the nearer box. In the "possible" event, the ball was shown resting against the nearest box. Infants visually fixated to the impossible event longer than to the possible event, which the authors interpreted to mean that they understood that one solid object cannot pass through another. A similar conclusion was drawn by Baillargeon and collaborators (Baillargeon, 1987, 1998; Baillargeon, Spelke, & Wasserman, 1985), who found that infants between 3 and 4 months of age looked longer at an event in which a rotating screen appeared to move through the space occupied by a box than at one in which the screen stopped at rest on the box.

Work examining infants' understanding of gravity has shown perhaps even more astounding results. Kim and Spelke (1992), for example, showed that 7-month-olds but not 5-month-olds looked longer at an event in which a ball rolls upward along a slope than at an event in which a ball rolls downward on a slope. The same authors also found that infants at 7 months looked longer at an event in which a ball decreased in speed as it moved down a slope relative to an event in which a ball accelerated in speed as it moved down a slope. Taken together, these findings suggest that toward the middle of the first year of life, infants start to appreciate that objects are affected by the laws of gravity and momentum. The findings on infants' early understanding of gravity were indirectly extended in a set of studies by Baillargeon and colleagues on the circumstances under which one object was supported by another (Baillargeon, 1998; Baillargeon, Needham, & DeVos, 1992; Needham & Baillargeon, 1993). Infants as young as 3 months of age looked longer at a box that was suspended in midair than at one that fell to the ground. However, it is not until 6 months of age that infants find anomalous a box that is only supported slightly by another box—even if only a small portion of the upper box is in contact with the lower one.

Although both Spelke and Baillargeon have been labeled core-knowledge theorists (Siegler et al., 2003), they have somewhat different views on how knowledge of the physical world is acquired by infants. Spelke suggests that infants are born with a set of innate domain-specific systems of knowledge such as, for example, that two objects cannot be located in the same physical space. Learning, according to this view, is guided by specialized processes that enrich this initial knowledge. Spelke claims that support for this view is the fact that there appears to be some overlap in core knowledge domains in humans and nonhuman animals; that is, "infants' core systems appear to be very similar to those of many nonhuman animals, suggesting that they have a long evolutionary history" (Spelke, 2000, p. 1233). Baillargeon (1995, 1998) similarly argues that infants possess specialized learning mechanisms that facilitate rapid learning in specific domains but does not claim that infants possess innate core knowledge that acts as the foundation for learning.

Once again, however, it is important to examine whether it is necessary to posit that infants are born with evolved domain-specific mechanisms for learning about physics or that they begin life with simple representations about how objects move through space. It certainly seems reasonable to assume that infants in the first 2–3 months of life would observe plenty of unsupported objects fall downward until they contact a horizontal surface. Given the regularity of such events—that objects invariably fall downward— could domain-general processes such as associative learning and habituation account for how infants develop expectations about the way in which objects move according to physical principles? That is, just as Haith et al. (1993) found that 3-month-olds develop an expectation about the spatial location of stimuli that follow a pattern of appearance, so it could be that infants develop an expectation about the motion of unsupported objects following repeated exposure to such events in the real world. A single mechanism that encodes regularities in the world and that operates across multiple modalities and inputs could, at least in principle, account for both sets of findings, as well as numerous others that putatively examine infants' understanding of physics. What of the claim that nonhuman animals possess core knowledge because they share many of the abilities observed in human infants? This too seems like a considerable assumption: It is well known that nonhuman animals learn about their environment in part through habituation, conditioning, associative learning, and imitation, and it is possible that these mechanisms can account for the similarity in behaviors of human infants and nonhuman animals.

Researchers have recently investigated the findings of Baillargeon with this more domain-general information-processing perspective in mind. These researchers do not directly examine whether domain-specific mechanisms or domain-general mechanisms underpin infants' behavior in tasks on physical principles. Instead, they address whether infants in such tasks are "reasoning" about physical events or responding to simpler aspects of the display. In a series of clever studies by Cashon and Cohen (2000; see also Bogartz, Shinskey, & Schilling, 2000) 8-month-olds' perception of object solidity and object permanence was tested in an extension of the rotating-screen studies discussed earlier (e.g., Baillargeon, 1987). Infants were habituated to one of four events on a computer screen and then tested with all four events. Some of the events were identical to those used by Baillargeon (e.g., a screen that rotated through either 180 degrees or 120 degrees without a block), and others were different (e.g., a screen that rotated through either 180 degrees or 120 degrees with a block sitting in its path). Infants' looking times suggested that they responded on the basis of perceptual novelty—that is, their visual fixation was affected by what changed between habitation and test—rather than on the basis of the possibility or impossibility of the events. Similarly, Rivera, Wakely, and Langer (1999) found that infants have a preference for the 180 degree rotation of the screen over the 120 degree rotation, which suggests that they were not reasoning about physically impossible object permanence events in the studies by Baillargeon and colleagues. The interpretation of the studies by Spelke et al. (1992) have also been questioned by Cohen, Gilbert, and Brown (1996), who found that, until 10 months of age, infants showed no understanding that one object cannot pass through another.

These studies suggest that it is not necessary to impute infants with an evolved specialized mechanism that facilitates early and rapid learning about physical principles. They bring into question whether infants are "little scientists" who reason about physical events by applying innate knowledge, or who possess innate mechanisms that allow them to learn about such events early in life. In contrast, they suggest that infants' behavior can be explained by their response to the introduction or deletion of aspects of the visual display. It is important to note, however, that, without exception, these studies rely on computer-presented animated events rather than real ones, and proponents of the core-knowledge view have suggested that infants process real events and animated computer-presented events differently. At the same time, the theoretical challenge that infants develop expectations about regularities in the world via domain-general processes suggests the possibility that they do not learn about physical events through specialized cognitive mechanisms. Unfortunately, it is unclear whether this issue can be resolved, because newborns and very young infants do not have the requisite perceptual abilities to view relatively complex events such as those in the studies by Spelke and

Baillargeon. Research continues at a brisk pace in this area, and the ever-growing database on infants' physical understanding promises to provide at least some answers to these issues.

Infants' Understanding of Mathematics

The study of infants' interpretation of physical events led researchers to consider other aspects of early science-like reasoning. Most notable among these areas was research on simple aspects of mathematics, such as addition and subtraction. Since the pioneering work of Piaget (1952) on conservation, developmentalists have generally assumed that young children, never mind infants, lack simple, as well as abstract, numerical abilities because, among other things, they do not possess the requisite representational structures. There is, however, considerable evidence that animals are capable of counting as high as 24 and perhaps considerably higher. For instance, rats will press a lever a specific number of times for numbers between 4 and 24 to obtain food (Platt & Johnson, 1971), and parrots and chimpanzees are able to combine numerical symbols in mathematically appropriate ways (Boysen & Berntson, 1989; Pepperberg, 1987). Indeed, perhaps spurred on in part by such work with nonhuman animals, researchers have come to believe that "more and more it appears that infants are capable of reasoning about the effects of the arithmetic operations of addition and subtraction" (Gelman & Williams, 1998, p. 588).

In one already classic study, Wynn (1992) habituated 5-month-olds to a single toy animal on a stage, which was then occluded by a screen. A human hand then placed a second, identical toy behind the screen. The screen was then removed to reveal either one or two toys (on alternating trials). The rationale for this design was that if infants did not represent the two objects over occlusion, they would be expected to fixate visually at the display of two toys longer than at the display of one toy, because only one toy was visible at a time. In contrast, if infants represented each object separately behind the occluder, that is, $1 + 1 = 2$, they would be expected to fixate visually longer at the display containing one toy than at the one containing two toys. In fact, Wynn found that infants showed the latter looking preference. Using a similar procedure, Wynn (1992) habituated infants to events in which two objects were shown and then occluded, after which one was removed from behind the screen. Infants in this study looked longer at the test event with two toys than at the event with one toy. This was interpreted to mean that they had represented the two toys behind the occluder and successfully computed the subtraction of two minus one.

In ensuing studies, moreover, infants who were presented with the task of adding one object to another looked longer at three objects than at two objects (Wynn, 1992). These basic findings have since been replicated and extended in a number of ways. Koechlin, Dehaene, and Mehler (1998) showed that infants responded appropriately to the number of objects even when the occluded objects moved on a turntable, which suggests that they responded to object number and not simply location. More impressive, perhaps, Simon, Hespos, and Rochat (1995) found that infants responded in a similar fashion even when the identity of the object changed while it was behind the screen, which could be taken to mean that they represented the number of occluded objects and not properties the objects had in common, such as their color or shape.

According to Wynn (1992, 1995), these findings suggest that infants possess an evolved innate system of numerical knowledge. Although such results are impressive, it is important to ask what adaptive problems simple numerical abilities such as addition and subtraction help infants to overcome. One can imagine that adults in our evolutionary past must have had to keep track of the number predators or prey, food, and even children in their environment. However, it is not so obvious why it is important or necessary for infants to keep track of such things. One possible answer concerns food; infants who discriminate one morsel of food from two morsels of food might opt to obtain the latter rather than the former and thus obtain more nourishment. Indeed, recent work by Feigenson, Carey, and Hauser (2000) showed that 8- to 12-month-old infants are more likely to crawl toward three cookies than toward two cookies. There is a difference, though, between discrimination of one from two—which can be guided by simple perceptual processes—and a numerical competence that supports addition and subtraction. Furthermore, infants' understanding of the effects of addition and subtraction are limited to small numbers, such that their competence is displayed only when the total number of objects is three or fewer.

These lines of reasoning have ignited a considerable body of research and theory that brings into doubt the findings by Wynn (1992). Most notably, Haith and Benson (1998; see also Clearfield & Mix, 1999) suggested that infants' behavior in the studies by Wynn and others is guided by a perceptual process called *subitizing* rather than numerical reasoning. Subitizing, they suggest, allows infants, children, and adults who observe a small number of items—namely, three or fewer—to immediately encode how many are present. A representation of the number of items is formed, along with any other items that are added or subtracted, and infants will therefore look longer at an image that contains more or fewer items than is stored in their representation. A corollary of this view is that infants will find it difficult to "add" or "subtract" in circumstances when it is more difficult to form a mental representation of the items, and research with 5-month-olds suggests that this is indeed the case (Uller, Carey, Huntley-Fenner, & Klatt, 1999). Although this argument is premised on the idea that infants are not calculating when they add or subtract, because the processes involved are inherently perceptual, it is important to bear in mind that subitizing is very much a specialized, and presumably evolved, mechanism for dealing with numbers.

Other researchers have evaluated the findings of Wynn (1992) and others from more of an empirical perspective. Cohen and Marks (2002) hypothesized that instead of reasoning about addition and subtraction, infants looked longer at events in the Wynn (1992) procedure because of a preference for familiarity in conjunction with a tendency to look longer when more items were presented. To test this idea, Cohen and Marks (2002) first replicated the basic Wynn (1992) study. In subsequent experiments, one group of 5-month-old infants was presented with the test events without exposure to the addition or subtraction habituation events, and another group was familiarized to either one or two items before each test trial, again without showing any addition or subtraction events.

The pattern of looking across the experiments supported the authors' explanation of the infants' behavior in studies on numerical competence; that is, infants tended to look longer at familiar arrays—having seen one object prior to the test phase, infants preferred to look at one object during the test phase—and they showed a general preference to look longer at more items than at fewer items (e.g., two rather than one). As one might expect given the contentious nature of claims about numerical competence in infants, the design and interpretation of the Cohen and Marks (2002) experiments have drawn criticism from a number of researchers on both sides of the fence (Carey, 2002; Mix, 2002; Wynn, 2002). Nevertheless, such studies do suggest that, as has been stressed throughout this chapter, it is necessary to be wary of a rich interpretation of infants' behavior in tasks that claim to show precocious cognitive abilities. In light of the issues under consideration, and in combination with the subitizing theory forwarded by Haith and Benson (1998), they also suggest that it is premature to conclude that infants possess an evolved specialized system that is dedicated to numerical reasoning. Indeed, as I suggested earlier in this section, it is unclear how and why such a system would have evolved in infants. That work in this area began relatively recently suggests that the answers to these concerns may yet be forthcoming; however, as things stand, it seems prudent to conclude that there is little evidence to support the view that humans possess an innate numerical competence system.

Categorization of Objects and Entities in Infancy

The ability to categorize, or group together things as the same, is perhaps the most fundamental of all the cognitive processes. It acts as the foundation for, among other things, language, problem solving, induction, and memory, and without it, the world would seem a chaotic and overwhelming place. Categorization, more specifically, is the process whereby discriminable properties, objects, or events are grouped into classes by means of some principle or rule. To categorize would be to treat, for example, various animals as equivalent and at the same time as different from various plants. The mental representation that encapsulates the qualities and features among items within categories, as well as the structure that exists across categories (e.g., dogs belong to the category of animals) is commonly referred to as a *concept*. Categories, then, tend to be sets of things in the world, whereas concepts are the internal mental representation of those sets (Margolis, 1994; Smith, 1995).

Clearly, it is crucial for young infants' survival to categorize the world appropriately. They must determine, for example, which objects can be acted upon and which things cause other things to act, which things are dangerous, and which things offer nourishment. Early categories must also constitute the foundation for those used in later life. Among other things, adults categorize people on the basis of their sex and abilities, animals on the basis of whether they are predators, prey, or companions, and objects on the basis of their function. Veridical categories and concepts of the world are therefore necessary not only to survive but also to reproduce. There is little debate that categorization in early infancy is fundamentally perceptual; that is, infants group together a variety of things on the basis of their surface appearance by attending to individual features, correlations among features, and by encoding the form of individual exemplars from which are produced prototypes (Bomba & Siqueland, 1983; Rubenstein et al., 1999). At the same time, however, theorists differ considerably in their view of the mechanisms for learning that allow infants to go beyond information given in the perceptual input. It is not enough for infants, and older children, to learn about only the surface features or shapes of objects: At some point in time, it is necessary to acquire knowledge about the motion properties of objects and entities (e.g., whether they act as agents or are self-propelled), their psychological properties (e.g., whether they are goal-directed or are potentially dangerous), and ultimately their internal biological or mechanical properties (e.g., whether they have a heart or an engine).

According to one group of theories, the acquisition of knowledge about such *nonobvious* properties is underpinned by evolved innate processes or structures (e.g., Leslie, 1995; Mandler, 1992; Gelman, 1990; Premack, 1990). The details of these theories vary somewhat, yet they share the view that infants, particularly those in the first year of life, quickly acquire knowledge about the nonobvious properties of objects and entities, and rely on this knowledge in their category membership decision. Leslie's (1984, 1995) theory of early concept development, which was outlined earlier in the chapter, is perhaps one of the most modular of these views. A similar, though less modular, perspective was proposed by Rochel Gelman (1990; Gelman, Durgin, & Kaufman, 1995). Gelman posited that infants are rapidly able to form concepts of animate entities and inanimate objects that include information about their nonobvious properties because of innate *skeletal causal principles*. These skeletal principles guide infants' attention to aspects of the type of motion and composition—that is, their energy source and materials—of objects and entities, and allow such properties to act as the basis for categorization. A related and equally nativist view was offered by Premack (1990), who suggested that specialized modules cause the perception of self-propelled objects that display goal-directed behaviors to be interpreted as intentional and to be assigned to the psychological domain.

Mandler (1992, 2003) presented one of the most prominent theories of category and concept development that is centered on the notion of an evolved and innate specialized process. According to Mandler, the earliest categories are perceptually based and are represented in terms of a prototype. She also suggests, however, that by 12 months of age or even earlier, an innate specialized process called *perceptual analysis* allows infants to form image schemas that summarize crucial characteristics of objects' spatial structure and movement. These image schemas are posited to recode the perceptual display into a more abstract but at the same more accessible format (Mandler, 1992). Once such information is abstracted, infants will no longer categorize objects on the basis of their appearance but instead group objects together because of a shared *meaning*. Thus, at 3 months of age, infants categorize cats as the same due to a perceptual prototype that specifies which feature values belong to that class (Quinn, et al., 1993), but at 12 months, infants categorize cats as the same because they are self-propelled entities that move nonlinearly.

Evidence to support this theory is drawn from three distinct, infant-related experimental procedures. In particular, Mandler (Mandler & McDonough, 1993, 1996, 1998; Mandler, Bauer, & McDonough, 1991) has used the object manipulation paradigm, in which infants touch sequentially the objects they consider to be the same; the object-examining paradigm, which is an object-based habituation task; and the inductive generalization paradigm, in which infants observe an action and imitate it with one of two test objects. Results from the first two procedures revealed that infants from 12 months of age form categories even when stimuli possess little within-class perceptual similarity—for example, animals, vehicles, or furniture (Mandler et al., 1991)—and by 9 months of age, they categorize as different perceptually similar items such as planes and birds (Mandler & McDonough, 1993). The results of the induction procedure are perhaps more surprising: Infants as young as 9–11 months extend behaviors such as drinking and sleeping to animals and behaviors such as "starting with a key" and "giving a ride" to vehicles.

The views just described have a common perspective: Infant category and concept development requires some kind of innate representational structure or mechanism that has evolved over phylogeny. Once again, however, before accepting this claim it is necessary to consider the nature of the input and whether the available data provide acceptable evidence. Regarding the nature of the input, a number of researchers have suggested that categories in the world are tightly structured not only in terms of their surface appearance but also their deeper, nonobvious properties. For example, dogs tend to look alike, both in terms of overall shape and the specific features they possess, move in similar ways, exhibit similar behaviors (e.g., wag their tails when happy, bark), and have similar internal properties (e.g., brains, dog DNA). Thus, it is argued, domain-general processes—such as associative learning—that are sensitive to regularities in a richly structured input will be sufficient to acquire concepts about surface properties, as well as deeper, nonobvious ones

(Jones & Smith, 1993; Rakison, 2003; Rakison & Hahn, in press; Smith, Colunga, & Yoshida, 2003). In support of this idea, there is substantial evidence that infants in the first and second year of life are sensitive to statistical regularities in the visual, as well as auditory, domains (e.g., Rakison & Poulin-Dubois, 2002; Saffran, Aslin, & Newport, 1996). Indeed, even preschoolers attend to such information in category membership decisions involving surface and nonobvious features (e.g., lives in trees, has a round heart) (Rakison & Hahn, in press).

On a related theme, a number of researchers have questioned the need to invoke abstract conceptual knowledge about objects' meaning in order to explain the available data (Quinn & Eimas, 2000; Quinn, Johnson, Mareschal, Rakison, & Younger, 2000; Rakison, 2003). I focus here on the evidence put forward by Mandler and colleagues (Mandler et al., 1991; Mandler & McDonough, 1993, 1996, 1998), because it constitutes the most substantial and influential body of work to date that is used to support the notion of a specialized mechanism for category and concept formation. One challenge to these data revealed that infants' category formation is grounded in surface features rather than in an understanding of the meaning of objects. Rakison and Butterworth (1998; Rakison & Cohen, 1999) found that object parts, such as legs and wheels, act as the basis for 14- to 18-month-old infants' superordinate category formation (e.g., animals, vehicles, and furniture). For example, infants categorize animals and furniture with legs as equivalent but as different from vehicles with wheels, but they do not categorize animals as different from vehicles when animals possess no legs and vehicles possess no wheels. Similarly, research with the inductive generalization procedure showed that infants' early knowledge of object motion is closely linked to object features. For example, if an experimenter models a cat walking, an infant will imitate this action with a dog and a table—which both have legs—but not with another animal without legs (e.g., a dolphin) (Rakison, in press).

These findings cast doubt over the presence of evolved psychological mechanisms for category and concept development. They suggest that all-purpose learning mechanisms and a sensitive perceptual system are adequate to account for a wide range of empirical data. Domain-general processes are sufficiently robust and sensitive for infants to acquire knowledge from the complex but richly structured input. There are some domains for categorization, however, in which the input is not so richly structured, and in which the cost of relatively slow concept formation may be high. One such domain that is probably more crucial to early survival than those described earlier (e.g., concept formation for animates and inanimates) is that of predator avoidance. The evolutionary psychology perspective suggests that it is more adaptive for predator detection processes, at least, to be innate, because it is not efficacious to learn which animals are dangerous through an encounter in a potentially life-threatening situation. Evidence to support this view is widespread in the animal behavior literature. For example, it has been suggested that the rabbit retina has a "hawk" detector (Marr, 1982), and salamanders bred from larvae show a predator response—by moving to shelter—in the presence of chemical cues of predatory fish (Kats, Petranka, & Sih, 1988). Perhaps more impressive, toad tadpoles show an antipredator response to three species that prey upon them—backswimmers, waterbugs, and garter snakes—but not to two potential predators that find them unpalatable (trout and newts) (Kiesecker, Chivers, & Blaustein, 1996).

With respect to the relevance of predator detection and avoidance mechanisms in humans, it is notable that the most common object-related phobias in adults are of snakes and spiders. Although the traditional view of phobic anxiety has generally relied on the concepts of fear conditioning (e.g., the pairing of a neutral stimulus with a negative event), more recent conceptualizations of phobias have taken evolutionary psychology into consideration. Work with adults, for instance, revealed that conditioned fear is more resistant to extinction with fear-relevant than with fear-irrelevant stimuli (Öhman & Mineka, 2001). Moreover, in one study by Mineka, Davidson, Cook, and Keir (1984), humans and nonhuman primates were conditioned to conspecifics exhibiting fear to dangerous items with evolutionary relevance (e.g., snakes) and nondangerous items (e.g., flowers). Impressively, both the humans and nonhuman primates acquired fear more rapidly and readily for the dangerous items than for the nondangerous items. This is not to say, however, that fears emerge in the absence of experience. Presumably, humans and nonhumans need to experience the fear exhibited by conspecifics in the presence of particular stimuli; however, there appears to be a bias to learn fears for some stimuli over others.

Based on this evidence, there is reason to suppose that infants, too, may be born with some kind of minimal, information-specific predisposition for things that were dangerous throughout human evolutionary history (for a review, see Barrett, in press). One indirect example of such a disposition is the classic work by Ainsworth et al. (1978) showing that when an unfamiliar adult, and in particular a male adult, approaches an infant, that infant is likely to show fear. Notably, this response is rarely shown toward small children, which indicates that infants' anxiety around strangers may result from a form of "predator" avoidance, whereby adults who are not familiar are treated as potentially dangerous. To examine this issue more directly, I recently gathered preliminary data that suggest that the basic perceptual structure of snakes and spiders may be specified early in life (Rakison, 2001). Infants at 10 months of age were familiarized with five different snakes or five different spiders. During the test phase, infants were shown a familiar predator (e.g., a snake, if familiarized to snakes), a novel predator (e.g., a spider, if familiarized to snakes), and a nonpredator (a frog or rabbit). Infants' looking times revealed that they recovered attention to the nondangerous animal but not to the novel or familiar dangerous animals; that is, infants looked equally long at the novel snake and novel spider, and they looked significantly longer at the frog or rabbit. It is important to stress that these results are tentative, and studies with younger infants and with moving images are currently under way. Note also that infants showed no external fear response—measured by affective behavior—to the stimuli, and that parents stated that their infants had little or no exposure to the various stimuli. The implication of this finding is that infants may have an innate representational construct that allows them to recognize predators, but the appropriate external fear response does not emerge until later.

In summary, although a number of theorists have suggested that innate specialized mechanisms are required for infants to learn about the complex categories of the world, the available evidence does not provide support for this view. Indeed, there is considerable reason to believe that domain-general processes are sufficient for infants to learn about the objects and entities around them. At the same time, there is good reason to believe that human infants, as with the young of other species, may have some specific predisposition for certain animals that have posed a threat to survival in the course of evolution. Initial evidence suggests that snakes, spiders, and adult humans may fall under this heading, though further research is needed to establish firmly whether indeed this is the case.

Summary of the Evidence for Evolved Mechanisms for Cognitive Development

In this section, I have examined evidence for evolved psychological mechanisms in early cognitive development for a naive understanding of physics, numerical reasoning, and object concept and category formation for animate entities and inanimate objects. In contrast to the review of the perceptual development literature, there is little incontrovertible evidence and considerably more debate over the existence of specialized cognitive mechanism in early development. Coverage of the literature on all three areas of early cognition revealed that there are both theoretical and empirical challenges to the idea that infants possess such mechanisms. At a theoretical level, I propose that domain-general processes are sufficient to encode the rich and consistent structure of the input in the domains of physics, mathematics, and categorization. It is unclear why specialized psychological mechanisms would have evolved for domains in which there are structured regularities that have existed over evolutionary time and that could be readily encoded by more general, all-purpose learning mechanisms. For example, all-purpose mechanisms such as habituation, conditioning, and associative learning can account for learning that unsupported objects fall until contacting a horizontal surface, that 1 + 1 is always 2, and that things with wings tend to fly; that is, given the (albeit brief) review of the literature presented here, it is far from clear that infants possesses (or need to possess) domain-specific mechanisms that prepare them more rapidly to learn about information in these areas.

At an empirical level, a number of researchers have presented data that directly contradict the interpretation that infants are precocious cognizers. For example, studies by Baillargeon and colleagues (Baillargeon, 1987, 1998;

Baillargeon et al., 1985) revealed putatively that infants understand that one object cannot pass through another object, yet several researchers have shown that perceptual preferences can account for such findings (Bogartz et al., 2000; Cashon & Cohen, 2000; Rivera et al., 1999). Similarly, Wynn's (1992) work suggested that in the first year of life, infants are capable of addition and subtraction for small numbers; yet Cohen and Mark's (2002; see also Haith & Benson, 1998) research implied that infants' behavior in numerical tasks is driven by perceptual and attention biases. Finally, Mandler's (Mandler et al., 1991; Mandler & McDonough, 1993, 1996, 1998) work suggested that infants rely on abstracted knowledge in categorization and induction decisions, but research by Rakison and collaborators (Rakison, in press; Rakison & Butterworth, 1998; Rakison & Cohen, 1999) indicated that the initial basis for such behavior is surface features.

There is, therefore, little unequivocal evidence that infants possess evolved cognitive mechanisms for learning about physics and simple mathematics, or for category and concept formation. Perhaps, this is not surprising given the later development of cognitive abilities relative to perceptual ones; that is, it is difficult to gather such data for abilities that emerge considerably after birth. At the same time, however, I have suggested that one domain in which one is more likely to find evidence for such mechanisms is that in which there is a high cost for failure to acquire the relevant information quickly and the input is not too richly structured. One such domain relates to predator detection and recognition, but conceivably research on other important areas relating to food and protection may impart similar findings.

CONCLUSIONS

In this chapter, I have reviewed a broad literature on early perceptual and cognitive development. The evaluated literature focused on perceptual and cognitive development in the visual modality but at the same time spanned a broad range of areas, including depth perception, shape, size, and form perception, face perception, movement and object perception, causal perception, naive physics and mathematics, and object category and concept formation. The overarching aim of the review was to determine whether there is evidence in these domains of inquiry for evolved, specialized psychological mechanisms or more general, all-purpose ones. Those who adopt an evolutionary perspective (e.g., Buss, 2004; Cosmides & Tooby, 1994) typically highlight the former as the adaptive solution to the problems faced by our hominid ancestors, while at the same time rejecting the idea that there exists any "general adaptive problem" (Symons, 1992). Thus, evidence that specialized, presumably modular mechanisms are present early in life and facilitate perceptual or cognitive development in particular domains could be interpreted as support for this view.

The review of the infant perceptual development literature revealed that infants may indeed possess evolved mechanisms that allow them to perceive shape and size as constant, depth, and occluded objects as connected. It was also suggested that infants are born with perceptual *attention biases* that cause them to attend to specific facets of the array. Included in these attention biases are a preference for dynamic over static cues, simple face-like stimuli, and complex rather than simple stimuli. There is also evidence that, across a range of stimuli, newborns and young infants process whole forms by breaking them down into their component features or dimensions. The review of the infant cognitive development literature was not as forthcoming in providing tangible evidence of evolved, specialized mechanisms that allow infants to learn about the world around them. Although a number of researchers claim that data on early physical understanding, mathematical reasoning, and category and concept development support, directly or indirectly, the evolutionary perspective (e.g., Baillargeon, 1987; Mandler & McDonough, 1993, 1998; Spelke et al., 1992; Wynn, 1992), in many cases, there is counterevidence suggesting that the data can be explained by more all-purpose mechanisms or perceptual preferences. Indeed, the review demonstrated that although a small number of evolved processes play an important role in the earliest aspects of perceptual and, perhaps, cognitive development, the brunt of the work in these domains is performed by more general mechanisms that operate across a range of domains.

As outlined earlier, I suggest that there is a clear pattern in these findings. Infants are endowed with a number of basic perceptual abilities, such as size constancy, as well as some perceptual preferences. These abilities and preferences, in conjunction with all-purpose mechanisms for learning, are sufficient for those domains in which there is a rich structure in the input and little survival cost in a relatively slow developmental time table. Attention to motion, coupled with size and shape constancy, and associative learning can explain, for example, how infants learn that unsupported objects will fall until they contact a horizontal surface. Similarly, associative learning, coupled with a perceptual bias to attend to specific object features and the motion characteristics of objects, can account for how infants learn about the way that animates and inanimates move in the world.

At the same time, the same underlying mechanisms are not adaptive for domains in which there is comparatively little structure in the input and/or those domains in which there is a high survival cost in a slow developmental timetable. For example, infants' ability to survive is contingent on recognizing the faces of caretakers, forming emotional bonds with them, and avoiding strangers. An evolved face-orienting mechanism and an innate wariness of unknown adults provides an important foundation for these behaviors. Likewise, infants must avoid dangerous predators and steep drops, and they cannot learn about the threat these things pose through experience. Infants may therefore have a minimal information-specific predisposition for snakes and spiders, as well as drops over a certain height. In both cases, however, experience is necessary to trigger the emotion or response that is appropriate for these contexts. Information-specific predispositions do not automatically come online at some point in development; rather, a small number of experiences with those events, and perhaps of conspecifics' reaction to them, is required.

Despite the fact that the review supports the idea that domain-general processes underlie a considerable amount of perceptual and cognitive development, it is important to note that these all-purpose mechanisms are adaptive solutions to the problems that infants have faced throughout human evolutionary history. This is not a popular view among evolutionary psychologists and will most likely be berated by those who adopt a more hardline evolutionary perspective. Yet it is impossible to dismiss the existence of such all-purpose mechanisms in humans and nonhuman animals, and the issue has been, and will remain, to what extent these mechanisms are responsible for our representation of the perceptual and cognitive world. I suggest that it is entirely feasible for domain-specific and domain-general mechanisms to have evolved alongside each other (for similar proposals, see Bjorklund & Pellegrini, 2002; Geary & Huffman, 2002). In light of the ubiquity of domain-general mechanisms in the animal kingdom, it is likely that they were the earliest learning apparatus to evolve. Subsequent species-general adaptive problems would cause the emergence of species-general mechanisms such as depth perception, and species-specific adaptive problems would cause the emergence of species-specific mechanisms such as face orienting in humans.

Finally, it is worth noting that it is assumed that the mechanisms involved in early perceptual and cognitive development continue to play a fundamental role in perception and cognition throughout the lifespan. However, although some of the early cognitive-developmental mechanisms remain (e.g., associative learning), many are usurped by a more "advanced" level of cognitive processing that emerges through more explicit learning (e.g., mathematical reasoning). Thus, although infants across many cultures may start with the same evolved, domain-specific and domain-general mechanisms, it is entirely probable that as infants reach preschool age, there will be an observed developmental divergence in their cognitive and, less so, their perceptual abilities. The role of language and formal tuition will account for a good deal of this divergence (see e.g., Smith et al., 2003), but are unlikely to affect the basic learning mechanism that evolution has endowed upon the child.

ACKNOWLEDGMENTS

David Bjorklund, Bruce Ellis, and David Buss made extremely helpful comments on and contributions to this chapter.

REFERENCES

Ainsworth, M. D. S., Blehar, M., Waters, E., & Wall, S. (1978). *Patterns of attachment.* Hillsdale, NJ: Erlbaum.

Baillargeon, R. (1987). Object permanence in 3.5- and 4.5-month-old infants. *Developmental Psychology, 23,* 655–664.

Baillargeon, R. (1995). Physical reasoning in infancy. In M. S. Gazzaniga (Ed.), *The cognitive neurosciences* (pp. 181–204). Cambridge, MA: MIT Press.

Baillargeon, R. (1998). Infants' understanding of the physical world. In M. Sabourin, F. Craik, & M. Robert (Eds.), *Advances in psychological science: Vol. 2. Biological and cognitive aspects* (pp. 503–529). East Sussex, UK: Psychology Press.

Baillargeon, R., Needham, A., & DeVos, J. (1992). The development of young infants' intuitions about support. *Early Development and Parenting, 1,* 69–78.

Baillargeon, R., Spelke, E. S., & Wasserman, S. (1985). Object permanence in 5-month-old infants. *Cognition, 20,* 191–208.

Barrett, C. H. (in press). Adaptations to predators and prey. In D. M. Buss (Ed.), *The evolutionary psychology handbook.* New York: Wiley.

Barsalou, L. W. (1983). Ad hoc categories. *Memory and Cognition, 11,* 211–227.

Bertenthal, B. I. (1993). Infants' perception of biochemical motions: Intrinsic image and knowledge-based constraints. In C. Granrud (Ed.), *Visual perception and cognition in infancy: Carnegie-Mellon symposia on cognition.* (pp. 175–214). Hillsdale, NJ: Erlbaum.

Bertenthal, B. I., & Campos, J. J. (1990). A systems approach to the organizing effects of self-produced locomotion during infancy. In C. Rovee-Collier & L. P. Lipsitt (Eds.), *Advances in infancy research* (Vol. 6, pp. 1–60). Norwood, NJ: Ablex.

Bjorklund, D. F., & Pellegrini, A. D. (2002). *The origins of human nature: Evolutionary developmental psychology.* Washington, DC: American Psychological Association Press.

Bogartz, R. S., Shinskey, J. L., & Schilling, T. H. (2000). Object permanence in 5.5-month-old infants. *Infancy, 1,* 403–428.

Bomba, P. C., & Siqueland, E. R. (1984). The nature and structure of infant form categories. *Journal of Experimental Child Psychology, 35,* 294–328.

Bower, T. G. R. (1966). The visual world of infants. *Scientific American, 215,* 80–92.

Boysen, S. T., & Berntson, G. G. (1989). Numerical competence in a chimpanzee (*Pan troglodytes*). *Journal of Comparative Psychology, 103,* 23–31.

Buss, D. M. (2004). *Evolutionary psychology: The new science of the mind.* New York: Allyn & Bacon.

Carey, S. (2002). Evidence for numerical abilities in young infants: A fatal flaw? *Developmental Science, 5,* 202–204.

Carey, S., & Spelke, E. (1994). Domain-specific knowledge ad conceptual change. In L. A. Hirschfeld & S. A. Gelman (Eds.), *Mapping the mind: Domain specificity in cognition and culture* (pp. 169–200). New York: Cambridge University Press.

Cashon, C. H., & Cohen, L. B. (2000). Eight-month-old infants' perception of possible and impossible events. *Infancy, 1,* 429–446.

Clearfield, M. W., & Mix, K. S. (1999). Number versus contour length in infants' discrimination of small visual sets. *Psychological Science, 10,* 408–411.

Cohen, L. B., & Cashon, C. H. (2003). Infant perception and cognition. In R. M.

Lerner, A. Easterbrooks, & J. Mistry (Eds.), *Handbook of psychology: Developmental psychology* (Vol. 6, pp. 65–89). New York: Wiley.

Cohen, L. B., Gilbert, K. M., & Brown, P. S. (1996, April). *Infants' understanding of solidity: Replicating a failure to replicate.* Poster session presented at the International Conference on Infant Studies, Providence, RI.

Cohen, L. B., & Marks, K. L. (2002). How infants process addition and subtraction events. *Developmental Science, 5,* 186–201.

Cohen, L. B., & Oakes, L. M. (1993). How infants perceive a simple causal event. *Developmental Psychology, 29,* 421–433.

Cohen, L. B., & Younger, B. A. (1984). Infant perception of angular relations. *Infant Behavior and Development, 7,* 34–47.

Cosmides, L., & Tooby, J. (1994). Origins of domain specificity: The evolution of functional organization. In L. A. Hirschfeld & S. A. Gelman (Eds.), *Mapping the mind: Domain specificity in cognition and culture* (pp. 85–116). New York: Cambridge University Press.

Dannemiller, J. L. (2000). Competition in early exogenous orienting between 7 and 21 weeks. *Journal of Experimental Child Psychology, 76,* 253–274.

DeCasper, A. J., & Fifer, W. P. (1980). Of human bonding: Newborns prefer their mothers' voices. *Science, 208,* 1174–1176.

Diamond, R., & Carey, S. (1986). Why faces are and are not special: An effect of expertise. *Journal of Experimental Psychology: General, 115,* 107–117.

Elman, J. L., Bates, E. A., Johnson, M. H., Karmiloff-Smith, A., Parisi, D., & Plunkett, K. (1996). *Rethinking innateness: A connectionist perspective on development.* Cambridge, MA: MIT Press.

Evans, C. S., & Marler, P. (1995). Language and animal communication: Parallels and contrasts. In H. L. Roiblat, & J. A., Meyer (Eds.), *Comparative approaches to cognitive science* (pp. 341–382). Cambridge, MA: Mit Press.

Feigenson, L., Carey, S., & Hauser, M. (2002). The representations underlying infants' choice of more: Object files versus analog magnitudes. *Psychological Science, 13,* 150–156.

Field, T. M., Woodson, R. W., Greenberg, R., & Cohen, C. (1982). Discrimination and imitation of facial expression by neonates. *Science, 218,* 179–181.

Geary, D. C., & Huffman, K. J. (2002). Brain and cognitive evolution: Forms of modularity and functions of mind. *Psychological Bulletin, 128,* 667–698

Gelman, R. (1990). First principles organize attention to and learning about relevant data: Number and the animate–inanimate distinction as examples. *Cognitive Science, 14,* 79–106.

Gelman, R., Durgin, F., & Kaufman, K. (1995). Distinguishing between animates and inanimates: Not by motion alone. In D. Sperber & D. Premack (Eds.), *Causal cognition: A multidisciplinary debate* (pp. 150–184). Oxford, UK: Clarendon Press.

Gelman, R., & Williams, E. M. (1998). Enabling constraints for cognitive development and learning: Domain specificity and epigenesis. In W. Damon (Series Ed.) & D. Kuhn & R. S. Siegler (Vol. Eds.), *Handbook of child psychology: Vol. 2. Cognition, perception, and language* (5th ed., pp. 575—628). New York: Wiley.

Gelman, S. A. (2003). *The essential child: Origins of essentialism in everyday thought.* New York: Oxford University Press.

Gibson, E. J. (1969). *Principles of perceptual learning and adaptation.* New York: Appleton-Century-Crofts.

Gibson, E. J., & Walk. R. D. (1960). The "visual cliff." *Scientific American, 202,* 64–71.

Goren, C. C., Sarty, M., & Wu, P. Y. K. (1975). Visual following and pattern discrimination of face-like stimuli by newborn infants. *Pediatrics, 56,* 544–549.

Halberstadt, J., & Rhodes, G. (2000). The attractiveness of nonface averages: Implications for an evolutionary explanation of the attractiveness of average faces. *Psychological Science, 11,* 285–289.

Haith, M. M. (1991). Gratuity, perception–action integration and future orientation in infant vision. In F. Kessel, A. Sameroff, & M. Bornstein (Eds.), *Contemporary construction of the child: Essays in honor of William Kessen* (pp. 23–43). Hillsdale, NJ: Erlbaum.

Haith, M. M., & Benson, J. B. (1998). Infant cognition. In W. Damon (Series Ed.) & D. Kuhn & R. S. Siegler (Vol. Eds.), *Handbook of child psychology: Vol. 2. Cognition, perception, and language* (5th ed., pp. 199–254). New York: Wiley.

Haith, M. M., Wentworth, N., & Canfield, R. (1993). The formation of expectations in early infancy. In C. Rovee-Collier, & L. P. Lipsitt (Eds.), *Advances in infancy research* (Vol. 8, pp. 217–249). Norwood, NJ: Ablex.

Hebb, D. O. (1949). *The organization of behavior.* New York: Wiley.

Johnson, M. H. (2000). Functional brain development in infants: Elements of an interactive specialization framework. *Child Development, 71,* 75–81.

Johnson, M. H., Dziurawiec, S., Ellis, H. D., & Morton, J. (1991). Newborns' preferential tracking of face-like stimuli and its subsequent decline. *Cognition, 40,* 1–19.

Johnson, M. H., & de Haan, M. (2001). Developing cortical specialization for visual-cognitive function: The case of face recognition. In J. L. McClelland & R. S. Siegler (Eds.), *Mechanisms of cognitive development: Behavioral and neural perspectives* (pp. 253–270). Mahwah, NJ: Erlbaum.

Johnson, M. H., & Morton, J. (1991). *Biology and cognitive development: The case for face recognition.* Oxford, UK: Blackwell.

Johnson, M. H., & Morton, J. (1993). Authors' response. *Early Development and Parenting, 2,* 248–249.

Johnson, S. P. (in press). Building knowledge from perception in infancy. In L. Gershkoff-Stowe & D. H. Rakison (Eds.), *Building object categories in developmental time.* Hillsdale, NJ: Erlbaum.

Johnson, S. P., & Aslin, R. (1995). Perception of object unity in 2-month-old infants. *Developmental Psychology, 31,* 739–745.

Jones, S. S., & Smith, L. B. (1993). The place of perception in children's concepts. *Cognitive Development, 8,* 113–139.

Kats, L. B., Petranka, J. W., & Sih, A. (1988). Antipredator defenses and the persistence of amphibian larvae with fishes. *Ecology, 69,* 1865–1870.

Kellman, P. J. (1993). Kinematic foundations of infant visual perception. In C. Granrud (Ed.), *Visual perception and cognition in infancy: Carnegie–Mellon symposia on cognition* (pp. 121–173). Hillsdale, NJ: Erlbaum.

Kellman, P. J., & Banks, M. S. (1998). Infant visual perception. In W. Damon (Series Ed.) & D. Kuhn & R. S. Siegler (Vol. Eds.), *Handbook of child psychology: Vol. 2. Cognition, perception, and language* (5th ed., pp. 103– 146). New York: Wiley.

Kellman, P. J., & Spelke, E. S. (1983). Perception of partly occluded objects in infancy. *Cognitive Psychology, 15,* 483–524.

Kiesecker, J. M., Chivers, D. P., & Blaustein, A. R. (1996). The use of chemical cues in predator recognition by western toad tadpoles. *Animal Behavior*, *52*, 1237–1245.

Kim, K., & Spelke, E. S. (1992). Infants: Sensitivity to effects of gravity on visible object motion. *Journal of Experimental Psychology: Human Perception and Performance*, *18*, 385–393.

Koechlin E., Dehaene S., & Mehler J. (1998). Numerical transformations in five-month-old human infants. *Mathematical Cognition*, *3*, 89–104.

Koffka, K. (1935). *Principles of Gestalt psychology*. New York: Harcourt Brace.

Langlois, J. H., & Roggman, L. A. (1990). Attractive faces are only average. *Psychological Science*, *1*, 115–121.

Langlois, J. H., Roggman, L. A., Casey, R. J., Ritter, J. M., Rieser-Danner, L. A., & Jenkins, V. Y. (1987). Infant preferences for attractive faces: Rudiments of a stereotype? *Developmental Psychology*, *23*, 263–369.

Langlois, J. H., Roggman, L. A., & Musselman, L. (1994). What is average and what is not average about attractive faces? *Psychological Science*, *5*, 214–220.

Leslie, A. (1994). ToMM, ToBy, and agency: Core architecture and domain specificity. In L. Hirschfeld & S. Gelman (Eds.), *Mapping the mind: Domain specificity in cognition and culture* (pp. 119–148). New York: Cambridge University Press.

Leslie, A. (1995). A theory of agency. In D. Sperber, D. Premack, & A.J. Premack (Eds.), *Causal cognition* (pp. 121–141). Oxford, UK: Clarendon.

Leslie, A. M. (1984). Infant perception of a manual pick-up event. *British Journal of Developmental Psychology*, *2*, 19–32.

Leslie, A. M., & Keeble, S. (1987). Do six-month-old infants perceive causality? *Cognition*, *25*, 265–288.

Mandler, J. M. (1992). How to build a baby: II. Conceptual primitives. *Psychological Review*, *99*, 587–604.

Mandler, J. M. (2003). Conceptual categorization. In D. H. Rakison & L. M. Oakes (Eds.), *Early category and concept development: Making sense of the blooming, buzzing confusion* (pp. 103–131). New York: Oxford University Press.

Mandler, J. M., Bauer, P. J., & McDonough, L. (1991). Separating the sheep from the goats: Differentiating global categories. *Cognitive Psychology*, *23*, 263–298.

Mandler, J. M., & McDonough, L. (1993). Concept formation in infancy. *Cognitive Development*, *8*, 291–318.

Mandler, J. M., & McDonough, L. (1996). Drinking and driving don't mix: Inductive generalization in infancy. *Cognition*, *59*, 307–335.

Mandler, J. M., & McDonough, L. (1998). Studies in inductive inference in infancy. *Cognitive Psychology*, *37*, 60–96.

Margolis, E. (1994). A reassessment of the shift from classical theory of concepts to prototype theory. *Cognition*, *51*, 73–89.

Marr, D. (1982). *Vision: A computational investigation into the human representation and processing of visual information*. San Francisco: Freeman.

Meltzoff, A. N., & Gopnik, A. (1993). The role of imitation in understanding persons and developing a theory of mind. In S. Baron-Cohen, H. Tager-Flusberg, & D. Cohen (Eds.), *Understanding other minds: Perspectives from autism* (pp. 335–365). Oxford, UK: Oxford University Press.

Meltzoff, A. N., & Moore, M. K. (1977). Imitation of facial and manual gestures by human neonates. *Science*, *198*, 75–78.

Meltzoff, A. N., & Moore, M. K. (1994). Imitation, memory, and the representation of persons. *Infant Behavior and Development*, *17*, 83–99.

Michotte, A. (1963). *The perception of causality.* London: Methuen.

Mineka, S., Davidson, M., Cook, M., & Keir, R. (1984). Observational conditioning of snake fear in rhesus monkeys. *Journal of Abnormal Psychology, 93,* 355–372.

Mix, K. (2002). Trying to build on shifting sand: Commentary on Cohen and Marks. *Developmental Science, 5,* 205–206.

Morton, J., & Johnson, M. H. (1991). CONSPEC and CONLERN: A two-process theory of infant recognition. *Psychological Review, 98,* 164–181.

Needham, A., & Baillargeon, R. (1993). Intuitions about support in 4.5-month-old infants. *Cognition, 47,* 121–148.

Nelson, C. A. (2001). Neural plasticity and human development: The role of experience in sculpting memory systems. *Developmental Science, 3,* 115–130.

Oakes, L. M., & Cohen, L. B. (1990). Infant perception of a causal event. *Cognitive Development, 5,* 193–207.

Öhman, A., & Mineka, S. (2001). Fear, phobias and preparedness: Toward an evolved module of fear and fear learning. *Psychological Review, 108,* 483–522.

Pascalis, O., de Haan, M., & Nelson, C. A. (2002). Is face processing species-specific during the first year of life? *Science, 296,* 1321–1323.

Porter, R. H., Bologh, R. D., & Makin, J. W. (1988). Olfactory influences on mother–infant interactions. In C. Rovee-Collier & L. P. Lipsitt (Eds.), *Advances in infancy research* (Vol. 5, pp. 39–69). Norwood, NJ: Ablex.

Piaget, J. (1952). *The origins of intelligence in children.* New York: Norton.

Pepperberg, I. (1987). Evidence for conceptual quantitative abilities in the African grey parrot: Labeling of cardinal sets. *Ethology, 75,* 37–61.

Platt, J. R., & Johnson, D. M. (1971). Localization of position within a homogeneous behavior chain: Effects of error contingencies. *Learning and Motivation, 2,* 386–414.

Premack, D. (1990). The infants' theory of self-propelled objects. *Cognition, 36,* 1–16.

Quinn, P. C., & Eimas, P. D. (1996). Perceptual organization and categorization. In C. Rovee-Collier & L. Lipsitt (Eds.), *Advances in infancy research* (Vol. 10, pp.1–36). Norwood, NJ: Ablex.

Quinn, P. C., & Eimas, P. D. (2000). The emergence of category representations during infancy: Are separate perceptual and conceptual processes required? *Journal of Cognition and Development, 1,* 55–61.

Quinn, P. C., Eimas, P. D., & Rosenkrantz, S. L. (1993). Evidence for representations of perceptually similar natural categories by 3-month-old and 4-month-old infants. *Perception, 22,* 463–475.

Quinn, P. C., Johnson, M., Mareschal, D., Rakison, D., & Younger, B. (2000). Response to Mandler and Smith: A dual process framework for understanding early categorization? *Infancy, 1,* 111–122.

Rakison, D. H. (2001). *A snake in the grass?: Infants' categorization of dangerous animals.* Poster presented at the Cognitive Development Society Meeting, Virginia Beach, VA.

Rakison, D. H. (2003). Parts, motion, and the development of the animate–inanimate distinction in infancy. In D. H. Rakison & L. M. Oakes (Eds.), *Early category and concept development: Making sense of the blooming, buzzing confusion* (pp. 159–192). New York: Oxford University Press.

Rakison, D. H. (in press). Developing knowledge of objects' motion properties in infancy. *Cognition.*

Rakison, D. H., & Butterworth, G. (1998). Infants' use of parts in early categorization. *Developmental Psychology, 34*, 49–62.

Rakison, D. H., & Cohen, L. B. (1999). Infants' use of functional parts in basic-like categorization. *Developmental Science, 2*, 423–432.

Rakison, D. H., & Hahn, E. (in press). The mechanisms of early categorization and induction: Smart or dumb Infants? In R. Kail (Ed.), *Advances in child development and behavior* (Vol. 32). New York: Academic Press.

Rakison, D. H., & Poulin-Dubois, D. (2001). Developmental origin of the animate–inanimate distinction. *Psychological Bulletin, 127*, 209–228.

Rakison, D. H., & Poulin-Dubois, D. (2002). You go this way and I'll go that way: Developmental changes in infants' attention to correlations among dynamic features in motion events. *Child Development, 73*, 682–699.

Rivera, S. M., Wakely, A., & Langer, J. (1999). The drawbridge phenomenon: Representational reasoning or perceptual preference? *Developmental Psychology, 35*, 427–435.

Roberts, K. (1998). Linguistic and nonlinguistic factors influencing infant categorization: Studies of the relationship between cognition and language. In. C. Rovee-Collier, & L. P. Lipsitt (Eds.), *Advances in infancy research* (Vol. 11, pp. 45–107). London: Ablex.

Rubenstein, A. J., Kalakanis, L., & Langlois, J. H. (1999). Infant preferences for attractive faces: A cognitive explanation. *Developmental Psychology, 35*, 848–855.

Saffran, J. R., Aslin, R. N., & Newport, E. L. (1996). Statistical learning by 8-month-old infants. *Science, 274*, 1926–1928.

Samuels, C. J., Butterworth, G., Roberts, A., Graupner, L., & Hole, G. (1994). Facial aesthetics: Infants prefer attractiveness to symmetry. *Perception, 23*, 823–831.

Seyfarth, R. M., & Cheney, D. L. (1986). Vocal development in vervet monkeys. *Animal Behavior, 34*, 1640–1658.

Siegler, R., DeLoache, J., & Eisenberg, N. (2003). How children develop. New York: Worth.

Slater, A. (1989). Visual memory and perception in early infancy. In A. Slater & G. Bremner (Eds.), *Infant development* (pp. 43–72). Hove, UK: Erlbaum.

Simion, F., Valenza, E., & Umilta, C. (1998). Mechanisms underlying face preference at birth. In F. Simion & G. Butterworth (Eds.), *The development of sensory, motor, and cognitive capacities in early infancy: From perception to cognition* (pp. 87–101). Hove, UK: Psychology Press.

Simon, T. J., Hespos, S. J., & Rochat, P. (1995). Do infants understand simple arithmetic?: A replication of Wynn (1992). *Cognitive Development, 10*, 253–269.

Slater, A. M., Johnson, S. P., Kellman, P. J., & Spelke, E. S. (1994). The role of three-dimensional depth cues in infants' perception of partly occluded object. *Early Development and Parenting, 3*, 187–191.

Slater, A. M., Mattock, A., & Brown, E. (1990). Size constancy at birth: Newborn infants' responses to retinal and real size. *Journal of Experimental Child Psychology, 49*, 314–322.

Slater, A. M., Mattock, A., Brown, E., Burnham, D., & Young, A. W. (1991). Visual processing of stimulus compounds in newborn babies. *Perception, 20*, 29–33.

Slater, A. M., & Morrison, V. (1985). Shape constancy and slant perception at birth. *Perception, 14*, 337–344.

Smith, E. E. (1995). Concepts and categorization. In E. E. Smith & D. N. Osherson

(Eds.), *Thinking: An invitation to cognitive science* (pp. 3–33). Cambridge, MA: MIT Press.

Smith, L. B., Colunga, E., & Yoshida, H. (2003). Making an ontology: Cross-linguistic evidence. In D. H. Rakison & L. M. Oakes (Eds.), *Early category and concept development: Making sense of the blooming, buzzing confusion* (pp. 275–302). New York: Oxford University Press.

Smith, L. B., & Heise, D. (1992). Perceptual similarity and conceptual structure. In B. Burns (Ed.), *Percepts, concepts, and categories* (pp. 233–272). Amsterdam: Elsevier.

Sorce, J. F., Emde, R. N., Campos, J. J., & Klinnert, M. D. (1985). Maternal emotional signaling: Its effect on the visual cliff behavior of 1-year-olds. *Developmental Psychology, 21,* 195–200.

Spelke, E. S. (2000). Core knowledge. *American Psychologist, 55,* 1233–1243.

Spelke, E. S., Breinlinger, K., Macomber, J., & Jacobson, K. (1992). Origins of knowledge. *Psychological Review, 99,* 605–632.

Symons, D. (1992). On the use and misuse of Darwinism in the study of human behavior. In J. Barkow, L. Cosmides, & J. Tooby (Eds.), *The adapted mind* (pp. 137–159). New York: Oxford University Press.

Triesman, A. (1985). Preattentive processing in vision. *Computer Vision, Graphics, and Image Processing, 31,* 156–177.

Uller, C., Carey, S., Huntley-Fenner, G., & Klatt, L. (1999). What representations might underlie infant numerical knowledge? *Cognitive Development, 14,* 1–36.

Vinter, A. (1986). The role of movement in eliciting early imitation. *Child Development, 57,* 66–71.

Wakely, A., Rivera, S., & Langer, J. Can young infants add and subtract? *Child Development, 71,* 1525–1534.

Walton, G. E., Bower, N. J. A., & Bower, T. G. R. (1992). Recognition of familiar faces by newborns. *Infant Behavior and Development, 15,* 265–269.

Wynn, K. (1992). Addition and subtraction by human infants. *Nature, 358,* 749–750.

Wynn, K. (1995). Infants possess a system of numerical knowledge. *Current Directions in Psychological Science, 4,* 172–177.

Wynn, K. (2002). Do infants have numerical expectations or just perceptual preferences? *Developmental Science, 5,* 207–209.

Yonas, A. (1981). Infants' responses to optical information for collision. In R. N. Aslin, J. Alberts, & M. Petersen (Eds.), *Development of perception: Psychobiological perspectives: The visual system* (Vol. 2, pp. 313–334). New York: Academic Press.

Younger, B. A. (1985). The segregation of items into categories by ten-month-old infants. *Child Development, 56,* 1574–1583.

14

EVOLUTION AND DEVELOPMENT OF HUMAN MEMORY SYSTEMS

Katherine Nelson

Memory is a general cognitive function for preserving information gained from interactions in the environment that are relevant to the organism's behavioral repertoire and continued successful functioning in that environment. In this sense, memory is a general process appearing early in the evolution of complex organisms and applicable across many domains. Memory systems have presumably been selected in the evolution of species to fulfill needs for the retention of information relevant to survival and reproduction under life conditions in natural environments. The questions relevant to the present inquiry then are the following: What forms of memory are needed for human life? Are there particular forms of memory that are unique to humans, in contrast to other animals, especially in comparison with other primates? If so, when do these appear in development, and what are the circumstances of their emergence? With regard to the latter question, are particular forms of memory needed during particular developmental periods, while others enter the repertoire at later points? That is, is there evidence of ontogenetic adaptation (Bjorklund, 1997)? Are some forms of human memory specifically dependent upon cultural evolution and processes rather than biological evolution and processes? Can cross-cultural comparative studies provide answers to this and other issues?

Although memory is a general cognitive function, both comparative and developmental psychologists have identified particular domain-specific memory systems that may call on specialized learning mechanisms. For example, squirrels appear to have specialized memory abilities for identifying the location of previously stored nuts. Likewise, human infants appear to have specific memory systems tuned to speech (Kuhl, 1991) and to human faces (Johnson

& Morton, 1991). This evidence suggests to many theorists that the cognitive system of humans, as well as that of other animals, is organized in terms of cognitive modules for domain-specific knowledge with specific learning processes and dedicated memory systems (e.g., Gallistel, 1989). Domain-specific memory usually implies a specific genetic adaptation in human evolution.

An alternative developmental approach proposed by Karmiloff-Smith (1992, p. 17) is "reiterative representational redescription," whereby similar cognitive processes operate within different areas or domains to convert implicit procedures to representations that are progressively more explicit and more accessible to conscious manipulation. Through these processes, different domains of knowledge emerge over developmental time (e.g., physical understanding of weight and size, or procedures for drawing). This model is generally consistent with the view of memory development in Nelson (1996; see also Campbell & Bickhard, 1986) and with that described in this chapter, based on levels of representation within and across domains.

Memory and representation are equally functional capacities that preserve learning or experience over time, and the terms are often used interchangeably. Representation on the individual cognitive level may be either very general (i.e., object permanence) or very specific (e.g., a snake image), and may be innately specified in the nervous system (e.g., arguably the fear of snakes) or be built up through memory for individual experience, or a combination of the two. Memory and representation may then be seen as two sides of the same nervous system; here, I do not consistently distinguish between them except for the caveat that memory is a product of experience and not of an inherited template or a novel generation of the cognitive system. Memory systems are products of biological evolution as discussed here; however, their particular characteristics, forms, and functions may be subject to cultural evolution and individual experience, and the sum of memory contents is unique to each individual.

Plotkin (1988) proposed a theory of "evolutionary epistemology" based on levels of learning and memory, pointing out that the retention component of experience is essential to animals living in free environments where decisions about action must be made. When environmental conditions affecting survival and reproduction vary within a single generation, and therefore cannot be adapted to through genetic change, evolution will select individual learning as an adaptive mechanism. Such conditions are common among freely moving animals subject to predators and variable sources of food. Plotkin postulated general levels of individual learning, with levels of social learning arising among species in more complex and variable environments. Tomasello, Kruger, and Ratner (1993) proposed levels of cultural learning that can be considered an extension of this idea. On the other hand, Oakley's (1983) discussion of evolutionary levels emphasized the domain-specific memory systems particular to many different species, for example, memory for food locations in squirrels, and memory for birdsong. As already noted, human infants appear to have a limited number of such domain-specific memory systems. For reasons that will become clear in the discussion to follow, it is not assumed here that specific genes are associated with domain-specific memory systems. Rather, the discussion focuses on general memory systems at different developmental levels.

In this chapter, a functional developmental systems framework forms the context for the discussion, in which I argue that adaptive specialized attentional mechanisms for particular aspects of perceptual learning at the beginning of life are superceded in development by generalized event memory and social learning processes, and that these are in turn supplemented by cultural learning and memory systems during an extended developmental period. I do not attempt to relate the discussion to all of the distinctions that have been made in the psychology of memory between different systems, nor do I attempt to relate these to the neurocognitive psychological basis of memory. Both of these topics are important but beyond the scope of this chapter. However, I do address here two different claims about the unique status of human memory. The first is Tulving's (1983, p. 1) statement: "Remembering past events is a universally familiar experience. It is also a uniquely human one . . . To experience again now . . . happenings from the past, and know that the experience refers to an event that occurred in another time and in another place. . . . [Only humans can] travel back into the past in their own minds." Tulving calls this kind of memory *episodic* memory, and it is very much tied up with the idea of the self; he thus proposes that episodic memory is *autonoetic* (or self-knowing).

The other claim for the uniqueness of some forms of human memory is Donald's (1991) theory of the origin of the "hybrid mind" of modern humans, which proposes changes in the characteristics of memory and representation over three major transitions. In this theory, memory is embedded in transformations of cognitive and cultural functions, including the emergence of language, the organization of domain knowledge, levels of consciousness, and so on. For both Tulving and Donald, as for cognitive science generally, memory is a function that serves broad and complex cognitive goals and processes. By that token, it is inevitably connected with broad transformations in human cognition and culture.

In considering how the development of memory relates to its evolution, I rely on the idea of a dynamic developing system. This framework may differ from that of many chapters in this volume, and I therefore consider next some of its basic principles as they apply to the issues under discussion here.

THE DYNAMIC DEVELOPMENTAL SYSTEMS APPROACH

Developmental systems theory (DST; Oyama, 1985, 2000) is ideal for the purpose of understanding development in the context of evolution because, as Griffiths and Gray (2001, p. 206) state: "Fundamentally, the unit of both development and evolution is the developmental system, the entire matrix of interactants involved in the life cycle." These interactants may be resources of the organism (e.g., genes, intracellular processes) or of the environment (internal and external to the organism). Then evolution is understood as "change in the nature of populations of developmental systems," in which the developmental systems contain "all those features which reliably recur in each generation and which help to reconstruct the normal life cycle of the evolving lineage" (p. 207). On the individual developmental level, these features vary in ways that may lead to differential reproduction in either a positive or a negative direction. For example, a difference in the system of developmental resources may enable some individuals to cope more effectively when environmental conditions change. The difference within the system might lie in a genetic mutation or in some noxious component of the parental prenatal diet, for example, or in other intracellular components of the developing system. In this conception, adaptation is defined in terms of "change over time in the developmental system of a lineage," which in turn can be understood as the differential ability of developmental systems to "reconstruct" themselves (p. 209). (See Oyama, Griffiths, & Gray, 2001, for extensive discussion; see also Thelen & Smith, 1994.)

Evolutionary psychology and other variations on neo-Darwinism assume that an overall genetic program causally and predictably influences the biological course of development. By contrast, developmental biologists studying the epigenetic processes involving coaction at different levels of organization find that orderly development is a product of complex interactions, of which DNA is but one component (Keller, 2000; Gottlieb, 1997). Genes are, of course, critical to development, as well as to evolution, but as one element in its organization; other elements are equally critical (Keller, 2000). The systems perspective differs from traditional neo-Darwinism in its emphasis on developmental processes. Evolutionary psychologists assume that what evolves are structured relationships between genes and environments, as exemplified by the concept of *conditional adaptation*: "evolved mechanisms that detect and respond to specific features of childhood environments." Such features are assumed to reliably predict "the nature of the social and physical world into which children will mature" (Boyce & Ellis, in press). For example, Ellis (Chapter 7, this volume) employs the concept of conditional adaptations to explain variations in the onset of puberty: Low caloric intake is presumed to produce changes in gene expression that delay onset of pubertal development, whereas high caloric intake is presumed to produce changes in gene expression that hasten onset of puberty, in either case assumed to have enhanced reproductive success under variable conditions in human evolutionary history. Ellis notes that allelic variation identified in molecular genetic studies also influences the timing of onset of puberty (e.g., Kadlubar et al., 2003), presumably by establishing different reaction norms.

Developmental systems theorists argue that this is a narrow and nondynamic, as well as nonsystemic, conception of the process. The DST formulation recognizes the variability associated with differences in body mass; however, it assumes a much more variable relation between this resource and age of menarche (now varying in developed countries from as low as 8 years to as late as 16 years), reflecting the complexity of the self-organizing system, which cannot foresee reproductive success or failure, but follows and adjusts as needed a reliable developmental course. Developmental systems theorists view the widely variable outcomes of puberty onset as the emergence of a different organized state from the convergence of a field of contributory elements, of which the different alleles are but one component.

Related to this argument is the fact that only the most general characteristics of the human physical and social environmental resources can be predicted by genetic changes through natural selection. Since the emergence of *Homo sapiens* 150,000 or so years ago, humans have experienced, often within one generation, radically varying geographical, climatic, and social and cultural conditions of development. Following the logic of Plotkin's argument for evolutionary epistemology, a simple dichotomous genetic variation for conditional adaptation would not suffice for the adjustment of a complex socially and culturally dependent system such as human reproduction. Instead, a flexible self-organizing developmental system incorporating genes, as well as other developing structures and processes, provides a more adequate solution to such problems. Because human development is dependent upon a social and cultural environment that is essential to survival and a long postbirth developmental period, this point is critical to all aspects of human reproduction (Hrdy, 1999; see also Bjorklund & Pellegrini, 2002).

Organismic development as a systems process has an inherent temporal dimension, relying on mechanisms of self-organization that depend upon timing, as well as location of process (Gottlieb, 1997; Oyama, 1985; Turkewitz, 1993). The concept of *emergence* is critical to this perspective, whether in biological, cognitive, or cultural context. In the epigenetic biological sequence, organs emerge from undifferentiated cell clusters, neural organization emerges in the developing brain, arms and legs emerge from protolimbs, and so on. The concept of emergence is also important in the behavioral and cognitive development of the individual, as the later discussion makes clear.

Implications of DST for the Evolution and Development of Human Cognition

In the DST view, the organism and environment form an interlocked system. In human development, the social and cultural environment provides the critical interactive space for the development of the child and adult. These environments, physical and social, are highly variable across and within generations, sometimes requiring radical behavioral and cognitive change, and at all times considerable adaptive skills, as well as social guidance and cultural learning (Tomasello, 1999; Tomasello, Kruger, & Ratner, 1993). This was true in the evolution of *H. sapiens* as well as at the present time, and must be accounted for in our models of cognitive evolution.

The major critical evolutionary difference between the organism–environment systems of other primates and humans is arguably that of the complex and variable cultural setting of development. Complex culture is itself a biological adaptation of humans; survival of the young and thus of the species is utterly dependent upon cultural arrangements (Hrdy, 1999). But it may be argued that because evolution could not predict the provisions of the human cultural environment in any detail, human infants are more dependent upon learning and memory processes than any other species. For example, in contrast to the broad environmental "niche" of humans, our close relatives, the gorillas, are born into a restricted natural niche in the rain forests of Africa, wherein their preferred diet of plants is readily available. The complexity of learning and memory required in that environment is relatively slight compared with that of almost any human environment. It is quite conceivable that apes have the same basic capacity for memory as humans, but that cultural modes of memory have emerged in humans to facilitate the successful achievement of adult skills in their more complex human environments. There are relatively few comparative data on memory abilities of other primates compared to humans; comparisons are difficult to make because of the reliance on verbal memory by humans.

Complex culture involving wide use of symbols, including representational language, decorative and pictorial art, architectural dwellings, and narrative mythologies, did not arise until well after the emergence of *H. sapiens* in modern anatomical form, now thought to be around 150,000 years B.P. We have little knowledge about the cognitive capacities of the species at that point in time, or about cognition in the preceding hominid line, although we can trace the evolution of increasing brain size over these millions of years. Humans initially lived in very simple societies and cultures, although symbolic culture emerged in terms of paintings, emblems, and decorative objects, as well as language as early in human prehistory as 40,000 B.P. Gamble (1994) makes the point that humans were able to survive the many drastic changes in climate during the period from 300,000 to 15,000 years B.P., as well as to colonize the many varying geological and climatic settings in the world, through a "suite" of adaptations. These included bipedality, big brains, omnivorous diets, large size, and cultural innovations; Gamble emphasizes the advantages of a generalist strategy of diet, social arrangements, and cultural inventions. This observation is similar to the claim here that infants must be prepared rather generally to gain knowledge of their environments, because the details of the physical and social environments cannot be predicted in advance through innate knowledge. Although these claims are not necessarily in contradiction to the argument for narrow, domain-specific knowledge preparation (for object knowledge, face recognition, speech, etc.), they imply that in addition to whatever specific domains there may be, much of human cognition from birth must rely on generalized knowledge acquisition processes.

As the following discussion indicates, there are almost certainly memory systems unique to humans, and at least some of these are culturally rather than biologically specified. What we do not know, and cannot know, is whether the earliest humans shared the same developmental sequence as contemporary humans in terms of the emergence of different memory systems. But because of the embedding of culture in the organism–environment systems complex, these different memory kinds are no less relevant from an evolutionary perspective. I am not making the claim here that culture is solely a product of individual cognition, but rather that the transaction between the individual and the culture is two-way. The important point is that the developmental systems view extends to the system embracing cognition and culture in childhood, and that this view supports the expectation of the emergence of novel human memory systems in cultural context.

Insofar as certain kinds of human memory are cultural products, it remains possible that these were not available to the earliest humans (and may not be to some humans living in simple societies today), although they are virtual human universals at the present time. The point here is that some cognitive abilities (mathematics is one prime example) are in fact cultural inventions, although presently carried out by biological nervous systems (usually with prosthetics such as written numbers or computers). Some forms of memory are of this kind.

LEVELS AND KINDS OF MEMORY
IN HUMANS AND OTHER PRIMATES

Humans rely on learning and memory to a high degree, whether implicit (involving perceptual pattern learning) or explicit, including social learning, for the purpose of future recall and use in problem solving and other cognitive processes. One basic division in human memory made by Schacter (1993), Squire (1995), and others is that between declarative memory, which is accessible to deliberate recall, and nondeclarative memory (see Table 14.1). Procedural, perceptual, and priming memory are usually characterized as nondeclarative (or implicit). These are the kinds of memory that Tomasello and Call (1997), in their review of primate cognition, referred to as the products of perceptual and motor learning; they are evident in early human infancy (Schacter & Moscovitch, 1984).

The hypothesis here is that basic human memory and cognition, beginning in the later stages of infancy, are organized around the experience of events, where events may be characterized as whole scenes unfolding over time that involve people (and/or other animates) acting over time in a particular place and with particular objects (Donald, 1991; Nelson, 1986). Events may be very small capsules of time, for example, examining an object; or they may be long sequences of episodes, as in a movie or novel. Event organization of frequent experiences enables individuals to predict what will happen next and how to carry out action and interaction within the event. Evidence for the reliance on event memory by young children was reported from research on memory, lan-

TABLE 14.1. Types of Memory Proposed by Cognitive Scientists

Introduced/ described	Memory type	Unique to humans?	In human development
Schacter and Moscovitch (1984)	Implicit Explicit		From birth 1 year[a]
Squire (1992)	Nondeclarative Declarative		From birth 1–2 years[b]
Tulving (1983)	Semantic Episodic	Yes	? Late preschool[c]
Schacter, Wagner, and Buckner (2000)	Procedural Priming Perceptual representation Semantic Episodic	Yes	Infancy Infancy Infancy Toddlers Late preschool[d]
Schank and Abelson (1977)	Scripts		Infancy[e]
Rubin (1986)	Autobiographical	Yes	3–5 years[f]

[a] Rovee-Collier (1997) early infancy.
[b] McDonough and Mandler (1994).
[c] Perner (2001); but see text for different views.
[d] Wheeler (2000).
[e] Nelson (1993).
[f] Pillemer and White (1989).

guage, play, and story recall in Nelson (1986). More recent support for this proposal has emerged from research using delayed imitation of event sequences with infants as young as 9 months by Bauer and colleagues (Bauer & Mandler, 1989; Bauer, Hertsgaard, & Dow, 1994; Carver & Bauer, 2001).

Event organization also provides a frame for interpreting and organizing new experiences. This insight lay behind the proposal of script knowledge by Schank and Abelson (1977). Schank's (1982) later proposal of dynamic memory suggested that bits and pieces from initial scripts might be redistributed to different event organizations or reorganized into different frames. One such reorganization was proposed in Nelson (1983) in terms of "slot-filler" categories that emerge from children's familiar event scripts, for example, the category of food based on the filling of the "eat _____" slot in different meals. Mandler and McDonough (2000) have extended this idea to infant categories, arguing that the category distinctions made by 1-year-olds are based on observations of the kinds of events in which animals as opposed to nonanimates are involved in real-world experience.

The event memory proposal represents an alternative to the idea that domain-specific theories are constructed from basic-domain principles beginning in early infancy, for example in the domains of number, objects, space, causality and intentionality (or "theory of mind"). The latter idea assumes that somehow the initial infant systems begin parsing the world into bits and pieces in order to distribute knowledge into appropriate "bins" for abstract theory and category construction of the kind that will be used in human cognition—especially problem solving—at a later stage of development. Specific modules are proposed to get the system started on the job of building theories for different domains of cognitive entities. The event memory proposal assumes instead that human cognition continuously evolved with the cognition of other primates, particularly the great apes, with whom we shared an ancestor some 5 or 6 million years ago. Thus, memory and cognition in early human infancy are assumed to be similar to that of infants of closely related species, for example, chimpanzees, adapted to setting up basic parameters of perception and action. Indeed, the major difference between human and chimpanzee infant cognitive development appears to result from the greater immaturity in the human neonate of motor and neurological systems.

Cognition in nonhuman animals, including other primates, is quintessentially pragmatic, with capacities relevant to survival and reproduction of organisms in environments via developmental systems. Memory is demonstrably about the environment, including other members of a group, food sources, available mates, infant needs, and so on. In their detailed review of primate cognition, Tomasello and Call (1997) emphasize the different cognitive specialties of different primate species, but they refrain from positing domain-specific memory or processes. Rather, they conclude that primates appear to use both ecological and social-cognitive skills across different functional domains, supporting the idea that the cognitive capacities derived from the human phylogenetic inheritance are of a general rather than domain-specific nature. The main difference between apes and humans at the level of action, according to Tomasello and Call's analysis, is that nonhuman primates do not have the capacity to analyze causal or intentional relations as humans do, although they do understand one-to-one antecedent–consequent sequences. The relevant conclusion is that there is little evidence from the study of cognition in other primates for the domain-specific organization of early memory in humans. Domain specificity might, however, emerge as knowledge specialization differentiates between sources and domains and their causal relations over the course of development.

Evolution and Development of Different Kinds of Human Memory

Tulving (1983) proposed that declarative memory may be divided into semantic memory, essentially atemporal memory for facts, and episodic memory, temporally organized memory for specific episodes from the past, which he characterizes as "autonoetic" or "self-knowing." The latter type of memory, he claims, is unique to humans; it is the only memory that is "about" the past;

other kinds of memory are functional for action in the present and future. That episodic memory may be unique to humans, as Tulving claims, suggests that it arose during human evolution and implies that it might serve a uniquely human function. What that function is and when in development it becomes important are relevant questions that I address subsequently.

A different account of memory and representation was laid out by Donald (1991; see also Donald, 2001). Donald's comprehensive theory of the evolution of human language and cognition proposed three major transitions in the passage from general primate to modern human minds. In doing so, he considered the extensive fossil evidence from the *Australopithecines*—the earliest branch now known as departing from the common ancestor of chimpanzee and human—through the emerging hominid line over the succeeding 4–6 million years, eventuating in *Homo erectus* about 2 million years before the present followed by *H. sapiens* within the last 150,000 years. Of course, a great amount of evolutionary change took place over this span, including upright posture, omnivorous diet, extended infancy, and enlarged brain with special expansion of the cerebral cortex, among others.

Donald's focus is on representational modes and the emergence of symbolic language. Consistent with the argument in this chapter, he postulated that the general ape model of cognition is based on episodic or event memory not accessible to specific, self-initiated recall. There is some confusion in his use of "episodic" in that it is not meant in the same specific way as Tulving's definition of "episodic memory." Rather, Donald conceived of the general primate model as more equivalent to semantic memory, albeit perhaps of a specific happening from the past, but without temporal marking, similar to the event representation proposal (Nelson, 1986). Moreover, the distinctive characteristic of ape memory was conceived to be the lack of a self-cuing function. In this conception, some current episode might activate an episode from the past that was relevant to present action, but the ape would not be able to search deliberately for or activate that memory in the absence of a current external cue.

That the chimpanzee (or the common ancestor) was capable only of implicit memory (i.e., perceptual, procedural, or priming—see Table 14.1) is a possibility, but these types tend to retain for recognition recurrent patterns rather than specific events. It seems more likely from what we know of adult chimpanzee learning, whether social learning in the wild or in the laboratory, that they are capable of learning and remembering in context-specific relations among things, conspecifics, people, and spatial relations, and to use that information in cognitive operations (see Tomasello & Call, 1997; Byrne & Whiten, 1988; Parker & McKinney, 1999). Thus, we could grant the capacity for both general and specific memory accessible in context to the nonhuman primate, with declarative use of that memory for cognitive purposes. I believe that this fits Donald's conception of the limitations on primate event memory; what he claims to be absent in the ape is its accessibility to voluntary recall out of context.

Donald's more specific claim is that the kind of social learning made possible by true imitation, more generally what he calls *mimesis*, was and is unavailable to the common ancestor of apes and humans, and to present-day nonhuman primates. In confining imitative learning to the human line, Donald is in general agreement with Tomasello (1999), who argues that chimpanzees have only primitive imitative learning capabilities that he calls "emulation." In particular, Tomasello argues that the chimpanzee may see the relation between an action and a goal but not understand the causal mechanism behind it. Thus, for example, a young chimp might attempt to undertake an action like one he has seen performed in order to get at food, waving a stick at a termite mound, but not realize that a specific action is causally involved, and thus fail to imitate the details required to succeed.

Donald focused on a somewhat different aspect of the imitative learning mechanism, namely, the feasibility of replay of what has been previously observed, or delayed recall out of context. In Donald's view, imitation is a part of the general cognitive function of *mimesis*, which formed the basis for the first major transition from ape to human cognition, placed during the epoch occupied by *H. erectus* (or *ergaster*).[1] Mimesis has both external and internal components. It enables learning skills such as complex tool making from observation of others and the engagement with others in shared activities involving different roles, including ritual. It also enables individual practice of skills based on the accessibility of a representation of the actions involved and internalized through imitation or perceptual attention. Thus, mimesis opened up a wide scope for social learning of a specific kind that enabled the refinement of tool making, as well as the generation of social and cultural rituals and routines, and the initiation of symbol use by gesture. This complex of capabilities Donald saw as a necessary move toward the complexities of a fully grammatical and representational language, an achievement only of *H. sapiens*.

The second major cognitive transition in the hominid line then was to the linguistic level of functioning, principally exhibited in narratives. Donald theorizes that language is a cultural invention (based on the biological potential of symbols derived from mimesis), and that narrative composes a specific mode of representation in addition to the self-aware generative mimetic mode. Narrative encompasses the complexities of temporal relations, mental states, goals, problem solving, and the other cultural realities of human life. This level of complex language enabled the construction of communal myths and other linguistic forms (e.g., arguments) that promoted the cohesiveness of group mentalities. Memory is involved in narrative from two directions. First, it is necessary to have an adequate short-term memory to retain the representation of even a short narrative. In addition, narrative structure, based on event representations, supports the extension of memory through holistic framing. (These aspects are discussed later in terms of their developmental implications.)

From the perspective of both individual thought and group cohesion and cognition, complex language, narrative, and myth seem to serve important social and cognitive functions such that selective pressures might establish the genetic basis of language (see Pinker & Bloom, 1992, for such an account). However, from a developmental systems perspective, the account incorporated into Tomasello's theory of cultural origins seems to provide a more plausible basis for this move to language-based cognition and memory. Tomasello (1999) posits shared attention between infant and caretaker as the key to the onset of specific human cognition. It is the social sharing that begins in infancy that provides the foundation for shared understanding of symbols in this theory and then, eventually, for the shared understanding of goals, minds, and motives articulated in language. But shared attention itself is not something that is simply endowed in the human infant, but rather builds on a months-long history of infant helpless dependence on adult caretaking (see Hrdy, 1999, for similar accounts).

It is obvious from what has been said that the topics of memory and representation are not independent of what is being represented and of the state of the cultural environment that is being experienced. In particular, it is critical that language is a symbolic system, not a direct representation of objects or events. It is then a metarepresentation system, and memory and cognition *in* language must exist on a different level or in a different mode than memory and cognition of events in themselves. The point here is that however events in themselves are represented, that representation cannot be the same as the way events are represented in language; there must then be a dual system (Sun, 2002). To the extent that mimesis involves a prior move to a less direct system of representing perceptions and actions, that is, a reflected self-aware system, it may be seen as the first move to a new level of memory/representation. At this point the argument is that it is only after language emerged as a representational mode (i.e., with narrative) that complex events could be articulated and communicated in terms of their temporal, spatial, causal, and psychological relations. This level of complexity implies a new level of individual memory, usually termed "autobiographical memory." This memory system, typically organized as narratives of the social self, emerges later in childhood and is assumed to be unique to humans, dependent upon symbolic language.

Donald's third transition in cognitive evolution is posited to have taken place in the course of human history itself, in terms of the secondary distancing of written texts designed to represent spoken language. This transition is only 4 or 5 millennia old, but it has had enormous impact in terms of enabling the movement of individual memory storage to external means (libraries, universities, museums, etc.) and transferring vast quantities of knowledge systems across time and space over many generations. It has also enabled a new level of cognitive processing during which external means serve as memory stores, while the individual mind carries out operations on the information. One cannot understand the evolution of human memory without taking into account these products of cultural evolution, which have vastly transformed our cognitive processing capabilities. It might be noted, however, that the tradition of memory studies in psychological laboratories rarely incorporates these kind of combined cultural external memory aids with individual processing. These studies are thus not a good fit to the typical memory operations of contemporary adults. Moreover, because memory studies of adults are almost always carried out on verbal materials, comparisons with nonverbal creatures (including human infants) are not feasible.

A FUNCTIONAL SYSTEMS ANALYSIS OF HUMAN MEMORY DEVELOPMENT

The general argument in this section is that the sequential development of memory within and across cognitive domains from infancy through the preschool period is a reflection of those functions useful in these particular life periods, namely, infancy and early childhood. This argument is similar to Bjorklund's (1997) ontogenetic adaptation proposal and is viewed within the framework of developmental systems and the assumption that memory serves functional needs within the overall system, retaining information relevant to that system during that period. This perspective does not deny that earlier memory types, organization, or contents may be useful to or extend to later periods and developing systems, but it brings into question the idea that earlier functions are developed to *prepare* for later developing cognitive structures. The idea here is analogous to the evolutionary argument that, for example, stone tool making did not flourish for millions of years in preparation for more complex tools and artifacts of the Iron Age. No doubt, experience in tool making was a prerequisite for the later technological advances, but during the Stone Age, it served purposes and flourished for goals central to the needs of that era.

This fairly subtle distinction between preparation and prerequisite is nonetheless important in understanding and theorizing about the nature of memory and other cognitive characteristics of the infancy and childhood periods. For example, Spelke and her colleagues are inclined to view the infant's understanding of objects and physical relations as "building blocks" that anticipate theoretical structures of adult conceptual knowledge, in this way preparing the infant for later cognitive developments (Spelke, Breinlinger, Macomber, & Jacobson, 1992). But, as viewed here, the infants' perceptual and cognitive capacities evolved to meet the needs of primate infants for the intelligent discrimination of objects in space. Later understanding of objects may require the same perceptual organization, but the former does not, except in some metaphorical sense, prepare for the latter.

Much has been learned from research on the infant's perception and representation of objects in early infancy, supporting the claim that some such capacities are innate (Spelke et al., 1992). However, there is no evidence that these initial capacities are unique to humans rather than general in primate systems. Such capacities would be particularly adaptive for other primates that are more precocial in motor development than humans and thus more dependent on the discriminative abilities of their own perceptual systems. The point here is that evolution may have provided the conditions that direct the perceptual systems toward functional discriminations of the phenomenal world in early infancy, without the implication of an incipient "theory" of domain-specific knowledge of objects to guide acquisition. Moreover, the *meaning* of the phenomenal object world begins to be significant only toward the end of the first year within the social interactions of caretaking and play, as well as in the observation of other actors in the child's purview. It is the structure of events that provides the meaning for the objects of engagement. The perceptual organization of early infancy is functional for that period of life and need not be viewed as preparation for the later development of meaning, even though it is also necessary for that function.

Consideration of the issues of the functional basis of the levels of memory and representation in infancy and childhood supplements this argument. What function does memory serve in the early months of life? Given that the infant is primarily engaged at this point in developing and using perceptual systems (vision, audition, touch), building pattern recognition memory of the scenes, people, and things in the immediately experienced ecology would seem to be of utmost importance. Indeed, infant cognitive research is primarily built on this assumption, through the use of the habituation and novelty choice paradigms, in investigations of recognition of faces, phonemes, and categories. The first two of these areas may involve domain-specific memory systems, the last a domain-general system, but all draw on the capacity for pattern recognition and analysis, as does the recognition of prosodic patterns of speech that have been recently uncovered (Jusczyk, 2000). Only minor differences in memory development in these early systems among different primate species should be expected (although there might be variations in what aspects are critical to recognition).

Among the unique characteristics of the human infant in comparison with other primate infants is the protracted period of extreme immaturity; months after birth, human babies are still developing neural and physical structure systems that in other primate species are completed in the fetal period. Human infants are extraordinarily immobile and helpless for many months, during the time that their perceptual systems are already functional and are completing development in the extrauterine environment. Thus, human infants are totally dependent on the social care of adults for months, even to the extent of changes in posture, and to a somewhat lesser extent for many years. This enforced dependent sociality is both the foundation for the social mind of humans and for the particular course of social-cognitive development found in the human child (see Bjorklund & Bering, 2003, for an excellent review of these developments).

As Tomasello (1999) traced it, the infant moves from being the helpless member of the duality formed of total care toward becoming the more active, alert, and sharing member of an interactive social pairing. In this case, the former state provides the necessary conditions for the latter, while the latter state develops the social activities of imitation and play that in turn foster the move toward communicative speech, carried on within the boundaries of the previously established social circle. Within that circle, moves—of caretaking, play, or other active engagements—can be anticipated by the infant. Thus, the social development of the human infant has an inherent, temporally organized logic, culminating in the acquisition of the species-specific communication system, symbolic language. What has been termed the 9-month "revolution" in social engagement is characterized by the onset of triadic intersubjectivity involving the sharing of attention to objects *with* another, which, according to Tomasello, is a uniquely human development. Tomasello reports that other primates do not exhibit the human infant's fascination with objects; thus, human infants' attention to objects is as critical to developing human cognition as is its social basis.

The sum of these considerations is that it is functional for helpless human infants to build basic knowledge of the recurring particulars of the specific cultural world within which they find themselves. This activity requires considerable time and attention, because cultural variation in very basic conditions of life over both time and space imply that these particulars are not otherwise predictable on the basis of inbuilt patterns of parent–infant interactions, mobility, and feeding. There is significant perceptual, memorial, cognitive, and communicative work for the human infant to do in collaboration with social partners to master the pragmatics of everyday life. This contrasts with the simpler task of other primate infants, born with greater skills of mobility into worlds of less complexity and greater predictability.

An essential foundation of this claim is that there is no basis in the evolutionary history of *H. sapiens* for human infants to adopt the goal of constructing a general theory of reality. Human knowledge systems admittedly go beyond those that are pragmatically necessary for survival (although survival may depend on skills not generally recognized as such), but there is no reason to believe that such knowledge systems have their basis in the learning and memory systems developing in infancy. Reasons based on the economy of cognitive effort suggest that such knowledge systems would likely interfere with optimal development rather than promote it.

Perceptual pattern recognition processes and procedural (motor) memory that adequately serve behavioral and cognitive functions of early infancy are forms of implicit memory, that is, not accessible to deliberate cognitive manipulation and self-awareness. Some researchers of infant cognition, however, claim otherwise. For example, Rovee-Collier (1997; Rovee-Collier, Hayne, & Columbo, 2001) who developed the conjugate reinforcement technique of investigating infant memory, asserts that the infant's memory for a particular context, in which an association between kicking a foot and moving a mobile attached by a ribbon was learned, represents an explicit memory equivalent to the explicit declarative memory of adults. From a functional perspective, these claims are difficult to defend. The immature biological state of young infants suggests that implicit pattern recognition and procedural memory adequately serve their functional needs. From the perspective of ontogenetic adaptation (Bjorklund, 1997) building in complex cognitive goals, and mechanisms such as explicit or declarative memory for achieving them, appears burdensome and likely to interfere with the primary requirements of this period of life.

As for retaining explicit memories, given the enormous distance between the structure of the life space in infancy and that of early or later childhood or adulthood, the rapid absorption of no longer relevant memories would appear to be highly functional. Indeed, as I have argued, the basic memory system may be designed to favor retention of repeated scenes and experiences, and to discard those that are ephemeral, that appear only once or that do not reappear after a short period of time (Nelson, 1993). Infancy is highly changeable over time and unpredictable except in the short run; memory should be functionally adapted to this condition. Overall, the argument for a simple implicit and readily overwritten cognitive and memory system in infancy, during the period of extreme dependency, neurological maturation, and rapid growth within a socially protective environment, is convincing on the face of it.

As the infant/child becomes capable of greater mobility and interaction with both people and objects, there is room for greater independent exploration of the world, which enables the expansion of practical knowledge, as well as true social learning through the medium of imitation. Imitation becomes especially valuable toward the end of the first year and into the second as the complexities of life proliferate and new skills are tried out or urged upon the child. Imitation is, of course, essential to the task of acquiring the first elements of language. Words can be acquired only through the imitation of the sounds of others (although their meanings depend as well on interpretation of the intentions of others).

Postinfancy Memory Development

Does mimetic memory, which is based in imitation, as described earlier, differ from general event memory (based in perception and self-action)? Recall that Donald proposed that mimesis reflects a novel kind of representational ability, accessible to voluntary recall and transformations. Mimesis is typically thought of in terms of action memory and reproduction, but it operates through the perceptual system that provides for the retention of a pattern to be reconstructed and produced at a later point. The event knowledge of infancy is based on successive experiences of the same event and interactions within that event routine, whereas mimesis enables the retention of a single experience of a complex event. Mimesis thus allows loosening the constraints of what can be retained in long-term memory in terms of frequency of experience.

Delayed imitation studies of memory in later infancy have established the developmental course of this type of memory. In the delayed imitation paradigm, a researcher demonstrates a novel action or series of actions with a set of props, and at the recall session the infant/toddler is given the props and encouraged to carry out the previously observed actions. These studies typically involve two to three repetitions of an event sequence to be recalled at a later time (Bauer, Wenner, Dropik, & Wewerka, 2000). Such memory becomes increasingly accurate and is retained longer—more than a year by the end of the second year (Bauer et al., 2000), indicating evidence of declarative memory. By age 2, children are able to repeat a sequence of actions after having been exposed only one time (Fivush, Gray, & Fromhoff, 1987). Whereas there is much to learn from the results of delayed recall studies with regard to the developmental course of memory over the first and second years, the distinction relevant to memory evolution and development that needs emphasis here is the acquisition, retention, and voluntary recall of a single episode after delay in contrast to the learning of a repeated event sequence. Thus, while young children continue to rely on event knowledge for the basic structure of life activities (as do adults), they are also capable of acquiring novel sequences through the mimetic capacity. That capacity also serves as a foundation for play, and for the variations on events displayed in pretend play and eventually in children's stories. These uses of mimesis appear to be unique to human children and adults. By the age of 2 years, toddlers give evidence of long-term memory—as long as 6 months or more—for specific events, or for information associated with specific people and places—through verbal means (Nelson & Ross, 1980).

Repeated event knowledge not only supports memory for specific happenings of a similar kind but over time also leads to the "degeneration" of specific knowledge, causing the child (and people in general) to rely on the default values of a familiar script rather than remembering the specifics of a particular event. These complications suggest that three aspects of memory need to be differentiated in early development. The first is reliance on general information derived from repeated experiences, whereas the second relates to the type of information derived, whether specific details or general gist (Brainerd & Reyna, 1990). Third is the mode of representation, whether mimetic or verbal, or both. Studies of delayed imitation could be expected to shed light on mimesis (and thus voluntary recall) as a specifically human memory ability, although thus far, there has been little research that bears on this issue. A study by Tomasello, Savage-Rumbaugh, and Kruger (1993) compared both immediate and delayed imitation in 18-month-old children, 30-month-old children, and two groups of chimpanzees and bonobos, one "enculturated" and one "mother-reared." The enculturated apes were exposed to conditions much like those of human children, including the learning of a symbolic communication system, as well as associating with conspecifics. Each child or non-human was shown a series of objects, for which the experimenter demonstrated two different actions and encouraged the subject to do the same thing. The results were clear in that the two groups of children and the enculturated apes performed similarly on immediate imitation, with the mother-reared apes performing at very low levels, significantly different from the others. On 48-hour delay trials, the enculturated apes actually performed better than the children and significantly better than the mother-reared animals. (However, because other studies have shown that even 9-month-old children may retain some part of the action in a delayed imitation test after 1 month, the poor performance of the children on the delayed test in this study is undoubtedly due to experimental artifacts.) The results of this study and two others that found evidence of delayed imitation in human-reared apes (Bering, Bjorklund, & Ragan, 2000; Bjorklund, Yunger, Bering, & Ragan, 2002) suggest that some aspects of mimetic capacities may be acquired from cultural learning, but they do not appear spontaneously in apes reared in their normal group environments. (See Bjorklund & Rosenberg, Chapter 3, this volume.) The skills involved appear similar to those of 1-year-old children, although the apes were much older (4–10 years). Whether the enculturated apes make use of these skills for purposes in everyday life is not known; for example, do they represent others' activities and attempt to reproduce them in the absence of the model as young children frequently do in play?

Episodic and Autobiographical Memory: Human Uniqueness and Its Cultural Basis

Can the mimetic capacity support what Tulving (1983) defined as episodic memory, a type of memory that he claims is unique to humans? Evidence in the previous section suggests that although mimesis might not appear ordinarily among other primates, given cultural training, it would emerge. Episodic memory might, like language, be unique to humans and be dependent upon cultural experiences for its emergence. The specific characteristic of episodic memory is its identification as located in a particular time and place, and involvement of the self in the experience; the latter constitutes its autonoetic character as self-knowing. There is considerable controversy over whether episodic memory of this kind exists in infancy and early childhood; Perner (2001), Povinelli, Landau, and Perilloux (1996) and Wheeler (2000) provide evidence and arguments that it does not. On the other hand, researchers on memory in infancy and early childhood tend to discount the distinction made between episodic memory and memory for episodes (e.g., Bauer et al., 2000). Episode memory can be interpreted simply as the memory for an event that happened one time, and, as previously noted, Donald views this as characteristic of primate cognition. Few have discounted the ability of apes to have such memory for a single episode, albeit it may not be recallable at will, that is, by self-cuing.

Episodic memory can be distinguished from memory for episodes on the following bases: it is recallable on a voluntary basis; it can be located as happening on a specific occasion in the past (not simply "known"); and it is characterized as a self-memory (again, not simply known). Of these, the first— voluntary recall—has been claimed for toddlers (and even infants of 9 months) on the basis that they can reconstruct the sequence of a series of actions observed to be carried out on a previous (months earlier) occasion. Although the conditions of the experience—the laboratory, the experimenter, the props—are the same as previously experienced and thus serve as salient cues for recall, it is claimed that the child must him- or herself call up the sequence of actions, thus exhibiting declarative memory. Whether one accepts this argument or not, it fails to speak to the other requirements of episodic memory—location in the past and self-experience. Theorists are divided on these issues. On the one hand, some (e.g., McDonough & Mandler, 1994) believe that the child's readiness to engage in the reconstruction of sequences that were observed in the past indicates both "pastness" and self-involvement. However, other researchers note that there is no evidence in the child's performance for either claim (e.g., Perner, 2001).

The issue of episodic memory devolves finally on the single issue of when and whether children place the self in time, that is, refer to past and future selves. This characteristic of human memory is basic to autobiographical memory, which does not emerge until the end of the preschool period, based on evidence of children's episode memory and of infantile amnesia in adults (Nelson & Fivush, 2004). Povinelli and his colleagues (1996) have provided convincing evidence that 3-year-old children fail to connect a video of themselves from a just-prior event with their own current self, thus implying that there does not exist continuity in time for the young child. The present appears to be a distinctive although changing event–space, illuminated by experiences from the past but not consciously located in the past. It is not until 4 or even 5 years of age that children begin to locate the self in events in the specific past and the future (Moore & Lemmon, 2001).

This is not to say that preschool children do not have memories of salient episodes from their lives; the research clearly shows that they do. Evidence comes from both reenactment studies, retelling of events staged in the laboratory, and salient personal experiences recounted with mothers or researchers (Fivush, Haden, & Reese, 1996). This evidence reveals that young children learn to reminisce, typically through talking about the past with parents, and through this practice acquire the discourse genre of "narrativizing" their personal memories (Nelson & Fivush, 2000, 2004).

The emergence of autobiographical memory is fostered by these social and cultural practices of engaging in talk about the past and making stories of personal experience. Autobiographical memory is socially and culturally framed within the culturally specific models of personhood (Leichtman, Wang, & Pillemer, 2003). It emerges during a period of early socialization of cultural forms and functions (the preschool period in Western societies), including the forms of narrative in stories, play, and media such as television. As Leichtman and her colleagues have documented in recent years, children in the United States tend to include more specific details in their accounts of personal memory and to orient their stories to self-involvement more than do children in Asian societies (Leichtman, Pillemer, Wang, Koresihi, & Han, 2000; Leichtman et al., 2003).

It is now possible to relate one of the most puzzling aspects of personal memory, the phenomenon of infantile or childhood amnesia, to this discussion of the evolution and development of human memory. "Childhood amnesia" is not, as the term seems to imply, lack of or disturbance of memory in childhood, but is rather a characteristic of adult autobiographical memory, the inability to recall episodic memories from early childhood. For most people, there are few and infrequent memories from the years prior to age 5 or 6, and none before the age of 3 years. (See Pillemer & White, 1989, for an overall view of the literature; see Howe, 2000, for a different perspective.) As Pillemer and White discussed, very early memories (those reported from the age of 3 years or younger) tend to be visual memories of single scenes that are sometimes hard to assign meaning to or interpret. Later memories, from age 6 and older, tend to be of whole events recalled with a narrative quality to their reconstruction in words.

These characteristics of childhood memories, and their infrequency prior to the school years, are consistent with the account of memory evolution and development presented here in the following way. Earliest memories in the form of generalized events, single episodes, and mimetic recall are functional for the individual in predicting action and interaction; they are functional in social life but are of little or no value as shareable "stories." When they cease to play a functional role in cognition or behavior, that is, when the conditions of life change, as they do for a rapidly growing and developing child, such memories tend to be overridden by more up-to-date accounts of how the world is organized. This situation is as true for adults as for small children, and it is likely to be true as well for the memory characteristics of other primates.

Episodic memory and talk about shared experiences differ from earlier memory in both structure and function. In terms of structure, autobiographical personal memory tends to be organized as more or less complete narratives about a coherent event with a beginning, end, and high point. Its function is dual, as many have recognized, serving both a social function of sharing experiences and the self-function of establishing a continuity of self from birth to the present (James, 1890/1950; see Bluck, 2003). These functions are characteristic of human social and cultural life.

Many have observed the central role that narrative plays in human cultures and some assert that narrative forms are one "natural kind" of human cognition (Bruner, 1990). This claim, of course, bears on whether we should attempt to account for autobiographical memory, infantile amnesia, and episodic memory in terms of the biological evolution of the human species or whether, as in Donald's theory, these may be accounted as "products" of human language and culture, through the process of cultural evolution. There seems little reason for assuming that narrative is an innate characteristic of the human mind, given its dependence on social and cultural experience, and variations observed in these across different cultures. The organization of experience in terms of events is, however, plausibly an inherent characteristic of the way that humans (and perhaps other primates) see the world. What cultural experience adds is the way that humans in a particular social milieu tend to construct stories from the events that they have experienced or imagined (see Nelson, 2003b, for further discussion).

Summary of the Relation of Evolution to Development of Memory

Donald's theory of cognitive and language evolution has provided the basis for considering the relation of memory evolution to the ontogenetic sequence in functional terms. To summarize this discussion, consider three hypotheses about the relation of memory development to the evolutionary sequence.

Hypothesis 1

Ontogeny recapitulates phylogeny: Event memory precedes mimesis, which precedes and is causally related to narrative memory, which precedes external memory. This sequence appears quite plausible (see Nelson, 1996), as the preceding discussion suggests. (See Table 14.2 for a summary of the developmental sequence.) Early infancy relies on basic memory processes—perceptual pattern recognition and procedural learning. This level is critical for all complex creatures to operate effectively in the world. For human infants, memory is robust over extended periods of time (weeks) by about 6 months for both perceptual information, such as faces and object categories, and for motor procedures related to specific contextual conditions learned over repeated trials or experiences (Rovee-Collier, 1997). Beginning in the latter half of the first year, this learning is supplemented by event memory, with clear evidence that infants have begun to accumulate "scripts" for familiar routines, which support their actions in the cultural arrangements of their lives, such as eating and sleeping routines, as well as baby games. Toward the end of the first year, infants demonstrate, through delayed imitation, long-term recall for specific actions associated with a one-time experience. Development in the neural basis of memory toward the end of the first year and into the second appears

TABLE 14.2. Developmental Sequence of Memory

Onset of memory kind	Memory type
First year	Perceptual representation (e.g., faces, prosody)
	Procedural (kicking)
	Event representations (peek-a-boo)
Second year	Mimetic representations: delayed imitation, words, etc.
3–5 years	Narrative representations—past talk
5 years +	Autobiographical memory

to be associated with these emerging skills (Carver & Bauer, 2001). From a DST perspective, emergence of changes in neural processes and related behavioral capacities reflects integrated biological and experiential developments. Any claim of human uniqueness on this dimension, however, must be qualified by the caution that future research may reveal that these neurological developments are not specific to human infants but are more general across primates.

Between ages 2 and 5 years, young children (in many cultures) both listen to narrative memory talk between adults and engage in such talk with parents and others, and increase in the specificity, elaboration, and narrative organization of their own verbal accounts of remembered events, including the characteristics of temporal organization, self-reference, and causal relations among episodes. These episodic reports mark the beginnings of autobiographical memory, which emerges from the systems integration of social and individual developmental processes (Nelson & Fivush, 2000, 2004). The influence of culture on memory becomes increasingly important during the preschool and early school years as children are called upon to remember culturally significant facts and pragmatic information. In summary, it appears that the emergence of different types of memory in childhood generally follows the emergence in the species suggested by Donald. However, whether that is a recapitulation of phylogeny in ontogeny remains in question, especially given the cultural dependence of most memory development in the postinfancy years.

Hypothesis 2

All levels postulated by Donald are available from the beginning of human life, maturing together over time, although becoming manifest in different ways at different points. Although Hypothesis 1 (ontogeny recapitulates phylogeny) appeared plausible, Hypothesis 2 seems in many ways to fit the evidence better, in that routine event knowledge and mimesis appear more or less together toward the end of the first year, followed closely by the beginnings of verbal skills that later enter into narrative and the beginnings of autobiographical memory. Moreover, many developmental theorists maintain that from the outset, children, even infants, organize domain knowledge in terms of theories, assumed in Donald's scheme to be a product of written forms of language.

The compression of the bases of cultural cognitive skills into infant mentality is a common move within developmental psychology today, but it leaves little room for development, and as argued earlier, it appears to burden the infant mind with unnecessary and unwarranted capacities. It also seems to be out of sync with the neural development of infancy and the functional demands of that period of life. As with the development of complex language, it is reasonable to claim that human cognition supports such acquisition, while still maintaining that the skills involved are not present at the beginning of life. These skills then remain to be developed in the context of human social and cultural contexts.

Hypothesis 3

Donald's Levels 1 (events) and 2 (mimesis) are "built-in" evolved human capacities that develop more elaborately in humans than other primates, and Level 2 may be dependent upon the availability of social and cultural interactions unique to human cultural contexts. Level 3 (narrative) depends on specific linguistic–social–discourse–narrative experience and is not achieved without specific experience in the cultural world. Level 4 (externally dependent theoretic) depends on specific, explicit, linguistic symbolic learning to use cultural symbols, although personal idiosyncratic systems may be devised as well.

Hypothesis 3 thus posits that Levels 1 and 2 are functional in later infancy, a heritage of evolutionary change prior to the emergence of *H. sapiens*. Specifically, imitation is assumed to be an early sign of the mimetic mode of representing, and it is well developed by the end of the first year. Event representations are also evident at this point, for example, in early scripts for familiar event routines. However, the early stages of language, word learning and simple combinations, seem to be part of mimetic development, that is, protosymbolic (Nelson, 2003a). Children typically do not acquire narrative organization of event memory until the end of the preschool years (Nelson & Fivush, 2000). Moreover, children do not typically use external memory until taught to do so in the school years, nor do they learn to use explicit strategies for remembering until late in the preschool and early school years. Representational use of written and graphic materials generally depends upon educational experience. Overall, the evidence seems most consistent with Hypothesis 3, with event knowledge and mimesis coming "online" toward the end of infancy, as basic modes of memory and cognition, while narrative language-based memory organization and externally supported theory-based organization of memory are successively developing modes that emerge with cultural learning and support.

Hypothesis 3 is obviously interrelated to the evolution of human language and culture. It is now quite widely accepted that, whatever prior roots in early hominid species language may have (imitation, mimesis, gestural symbols, protolanguage speech), fully complex and grammatical oral language—what I term representational language—became characteristic only of *H. sapiens* within the past 50,000 years, together with a rather sudden explosion of symbolic cultural artifacts (Bickerton, 1990; Deacon, 1997; Donald, 1991; Noble & Davidson, 1996). These unique cultural, cognitive, and communicative characteristics of the species cross the boundaries from biological to cultural constructions, and from biological to cultural evolution. But from a systems perspective, this is a false boundary inasmuch as biological evolution of the species made possible the cultural evolution that followed, which proceeds on a vastly faster time scale. The point of Donald's analysis is that the cognitive characteristics (and the consciousness) of modern humans are as much a product of cultural evolution as they are of strictly biological evolution. Complementary to this argument is Tomasello's (1999) analysis, that cultural evolution is made possible by the characteristic biological development of the human infant and child. This position also illustrates the developmental systems view in which the characteristic and reliable cultural contributions to development combine with neurological developments to produce uniquely human memory types.

CONCLUSIONS

Basic memory (perceptual and procedural) is adaptive for infancy and very early childhood during a period when it is necessary to lay down basic understandings of the perceptual world within which the individual lives, and to become an integral part of the social life and routines of the cultural world. During the first 2 years of life, the infant exists in a specifically human milieu, with all that that means in terms of its cultural and symbolic significance, but such existence is essentially private in the sense that the infant has no access to others' perspectives on the world, except through the interpretation of their behaviors. This position is similar to that of other animals, including other primates.

Through mimesis, the infant/child can begin to take on greater knowledge of other persons' positions and states, as well as begin to acquire the symbolic language that will open up access to others' perspectives and separate thoughts, providing a mirror to the self and a view to the past, as well as the present. Over time, the complex social world inducts the verbal child into new functions that take on the characteristic of new systems. These include lexical, grammatical, narrative, and taxonomic knowledge systems, critical to living in cultural environments. Becoming a distinctive self in a temporal social world is an important function served by new forms of memory systems.

From this perspective, human-specific memory functions are clarified. The puzzle of infantile amnesia may be solved through the realization of the different functions served by memory in different epochs of the child's life. The basic perceptual and procedural memory functions serve the first years of social and cognitive development but do not provide the distinctive view of the self that emerges later as the child becomes a member of the "community of minds" (Nelson, in press). However, the development of later, specifically human memory systems incorporates and builds on these early systems. The differentiation and elaboration of memory functions and the acquisition of new forms of memory as new functions come into play are conceptualized here as emerging systems reflecting the interdependence of individual cognitive, social, and cultural contributions.

NOTE

1. See also Arbib (2002) for an imitation account of the beginnings of language during the same period of evolution, based on mirror neurons.

REFERENCES

Arbib, M. A. (2002). The mirror system, imitation, and evolution of language. In C. Nehaniv & K. Dautenhahn (Eds.), *Imitation in animals and artifacts* (pp. 229–280). Cambridge, MA: MIT Press.

Bauer, P. J., Hertsgaard, L. A., & Dow, G. A. (1994). After 8 months have passed: Long-term recall of events by 1- to 2-year-old children. *Memory, 2,* 353–382.

Bauer, P. J., & Mandler, J. M. (1989). One thing follows another: Effects of temporal structure on one- to two-year-olds' recall of events. *Developmental Psychology, 25,* 197–206.

Bauer, P. J., Wenner, J. A., Dropik, P. L., & Wewerka, S. S. (2000). Parameters of remembering and forgetting in the transition from infancy to early childhood. *Monographs of the Society for Research in Child Development, 65*(4, Serial No. 263).

Bering, J. M., Bjorklund, D. F., & Ragan, P. (2000). Deferred imitation of object-related actions in human-reared juvenile chimpanzees and orangutans. *Developmental Psychobiology, 36,* 218–232.

Bickerton, D. (1990). *Language and species.* Chicago: University of Chicago Press.

Bjorklund, D. F. (1997). The role of immaturity in human development. *Psychological Bulletin, 122,* 153–169.

Bjorklund, D. F., & Bering, J. M. (2003). Big brains, slow development, and social complexity: The developmental and evolutionary origins of social cognition. In M. Brune, H. Ribbert, & W. Schiefenhoevel (Eds.), *The social brain: Evolutionary aspects of development and pathology* (pp. 133–151). New York: Wiley.

Bjorklund, D. F., & Pellegrini, A. D. (2002). *The origins of human nature: Evolutionary developmental psychology.* Washington, DC: American Psychological Association.

Bjorklund, D. F., Yunger, J. L., Bering, J. M., & Ragan, P. (2002). The generalization of deferred imitation in enculturated chimpanzees (*Pan troglodytes*). *Animal Cognition, 5,* 49–58.

Bluck, S. (Ed.). (2003). Autobiographical memory: Exploring its functions in everyday life [Special issue]. *Memory, 11*(2).

Boyce, W. T., & Ellis, B. J. (in press). Biological sensitivity to context: I. An evolutionary-developmental theory of the origins and functions of stress reactivity. *Development and Psychopathology.*

Brainerd, C. J., & Reyna, V. F. (1990). Gist is the grist: Fuzzy-trace theory and the new intuitionism. *Developmental Review, 10,* 3–47.

Bruner, J. S. (1990). *Acts of meaning.* Cambridge, MA: Harvard University Press.

Byrne, R., & Whiten, A. (Eds.). (1988). *Machiavellian intelligence.* Oxford, UK: Oxford University Press.

Campbell, R. L., & Bickhard, M. H. (1986). *Knowing levels and developmental stages.* Basel: Karger.

Carver, L. J., & Bauer, P. (2001). The dawning of a past: The emergence of long-term explicit memory in infancy. *Journal of Experimental Psychology, 130,* 726–745.

Deacon, T. W. (1997). *The symbolic species: The co-evolution of language and the brain.* New York: Norton.

Donald, M. (1991). *Origins of the modern mind.* Cambridge, MA: Harvard University Press.

Donald, M. (2001). *A mind so rare: The evolution of human consciousness.* New York: Norton.

Fivush, R., Gray, J. T., & Fromhoff, F. A. (1987). Two-year-olds talk about the past. *Cognitive Development, 2,* 393–410.

Fivush, R., Haden, C., & Reese, E. (1996). Remembering, recounting and reminiscing: The development of autobiographical memory in social context. In D. Rubin (Ed.), *Reconstructing our past: An overview of autobiographical memory* (pp. 341–359). New York: Cambridge University Press.

Gallistel, C. R. (1989). Animal cognition: The representation of space, time and number. In M. R. Rosenzwig & L. W. Porter (Eds.), *Annual review of psychology* (Vol. 40, pp. 155–189). Palo Alto, CA: Annual Reviews.

Gamble, C. (1994). *Timewalkers: The prehistory of global colonization.* Cambridge, MA: Harvard University Press.

Gottlieb, G. (1997). *Synthesizing nature–nurture: Prenatal roots of instinctive behavior.* Mahwah, NJ: Erlbaum.

Griffiths, P. E., & Gray, R. D. (2001). Darwinism and developmental systems. In S. Oyama, P. E. Griffiths, & R. D. Gray (Eds.), *Cycles of contingency: Developmental systems and evolution* (pp. 195–218). Cambridge, MA: MIT Press.

Howe, M. (2000). *The fate of early memories: Developmental science and the retention of childhood experience.* Washington, DC: American Psychological Association.

Hrdy, S. B. (1999). *Mother nature: A history of mothers, infants, and natural selection.* New York: Pantheon.

James, W. (1950). *The principles of psychology.* New York: Dover. (Original published in 1890)

Johnson, M. H., & Morton, J. (1991). *Biology and cognitive development: The case of face recognition.* Oxford, UK: Blackwell.

Jusczyk, P. W. (2000). *The discovery of spoken language.* Cambridge, MA: MIT Press.

Kadlubar, F. F., Berkowitz, G. S., Delongchamp, R. R., Wang, C., Breen, B. L., Tang, G., et al. (2003). The *CYP3A4*1B* variant is related to the onset of puberty, a known risk factor for the development of breast cancer. *Cancer Epidemiology, Biomarkers, and Prevention, 12,* 327–331.

Karmiloff-Smith, A. (1992). *Beyond modularity.* Cambridge, MA: MIT Press.

Keller, E. F. (2000). *The century of the gene.* Cambridge, MA: Harvard University Press.

Kuhl, P. K. (1991). Human adults and human infants show a "perceptual magnet effect" for the prototypes of speech categories, monkeys do not. *Perception and Psychophysics, 50,* 93–107.

Leichtman, M. D., Pillemer, D. B., Wang, Q., Koreishi, A., & Han, J. J. (2000). When Baby Maisy came to school: Mothers' interview styles and preschoolers' event memories. *Cognitive Development, 15,* 1–16.

Leichtman, M. D., Wang, Q., & Pillemer, D. B. (2003). Cultural variations in interdependence and autobiographical memory: Lessons from Korea, China, India, and the United States. In R. Fivush & C. Haden (Eds.), *Autobiographical memory and the construction of a narrative self: Developmental and cultural perspectives* (pp. 73–98). Mahwah, NJ: Erlbaum.

Mandler, J. M., & McDonough, L. (2000). Advancing downward to the basic level. *Journal of Cognition and Development, 1,* 379–405.

McDonough, L., & Mandler, J. M. (1994). Very long-term recall in infants: Infantile amnesia reconsidered. *Memory, 2,* 339–352.

Moore, C., & Lemmon, K. (Eds.). (2001). *The self in time: Developmental perspectives.* Mahwah, NJ: Erlbaum.

Nelson, K. (1983). The derivation of concepts and categories from event representations. In E. Scholnick (Ed.), *New trends in conceptual representation: Challenges to Piaget's theory?* (pp. 129–149). Hillsdale, NJ: Erlbaum.

Nelson, K. (1986). *Event knowledge: Structure and function in development.* Hillsdale, NJ: Erlbaum.

Nelson, K. (1993). The psychological and social origins of autobiographical memory. *Psychological Science, 4,* 1–8.

Nelson, K. (1996). *Language in cognitive development: The emergence of the mediated mind.* New York: Cambridge University Press.

Nelson, K. (2003a). Making sense in a world of symbols. In A. Toomela (Ed.), *Cultural guidance in the development of the human mind* (pp. 139–162). Westport, CT: Greenwood.

Nelson, K. (2003b). Self and social functions: Individual autobiographical memory and collective narrative [Special Issue on Functions of Autobiographical Memory (S. Bluck, Ed.)]. *Memory, 11,* 125–136.

Nelson, K. (in press). Language pathways into the community of minds. In J. W. Astington & J. A. Baird (Eds.), *Why language matters for theory of mind.* New York: Oxford University Press.

Nelson, K., & Fivush, R. (2000). Socialization of memory. In E. Tulving & F. Craik (Eds.), *Handbook of memory* (pp. 283–295). New York: Oxford University Press.

Nelson, K., & Fivush, R. (2004). Emergence of autobiographical memory: A social–cultural theory. *Psychological Review, 111,* 486–511.

Nelson, K., & Ross, G. (1980). The generalities and specifics of long term memory in infants and young children. In M. Perlmutter (Ed.), *Children's memory: New directions for child development* (Vol. 10, pp. 87–101). San Francisco: Jossey-Bass.

Noble, W., & Davidson, I. (1996). *Human evolution, language and mind.* New York: Cambridge University Press.

Oakley, D. A. (1983). The varieties of memory: A phylogenetic approach. In A. Mayes (Ed.), *Memory in animals and humans* (pp. 20–82). Workingham, UK: Van Nostrand Reinhold.

Oyama, S. (1985). *The ontogeny of information: Developmental systems and evolution.* New York: Cambridge University Press.

Oyama, S. (2000). *Evolution's eye: A systems view of the biology–culture divide.* Durham, NC: Duke University Press.

Oyama, S., Griffiths, P. E., & Gray, R. D. (Eds.). (2001). *Cycles of contingency: Developmental systems and evolution.* Cambridge, MA: MIT Press.

Parker, S. T., & McKinney, M. L. (1999). *Origins of intelligence: The evolution of cognitive development in monkeys, apes, and humans.* Baltimore: Johns Hopkins University Press.

Perner, J. (2001). Episodic memory: Essential distinctions and developmental implications. In C. Moore & K. Lemmon (Eds.), *The self in time: Developmental perspectives* (pp. 181–202). Mahwah, NJ: Erlbaum.

Pillemer, D. B., & White, S. H. (1989). Childhood events recalled by children and adults. In H. W. Reese (Ed.), *Advances in child development and behavior* (Vol. 21, pp. 297–340). New York: Academic Press.

Pinker, S., & Bloom, P. (1992). Natural language and natural selection. In J. H. Barkow, L. Cosmides, & J. Tooby (Eds.), *The adapted mind: Evolutionary psychology and the generation of culture* (pp. 451–494). New York: Oxford University Press.

Plotkin, H. C. (1988). An evolutionary epistemological approach to the evolution of intelligence. In H. J. Jerison & I. Jerison (Eds.), *Intelligence and evolutionary biology* (pp. 73–91). New York: Springer-Verlag.

Povinelli, D. J., Landau, K. R., & Perilloux, H. K. (1996). Self-recognition in young children using delayed versus live feedback: Evidence of a developmental asynchrony. *Child Development, 67,* 1540–1554.

Rovee-Collier, C. (1997). Dissociations in infant memory: Rethinking the development of implicit and explicit memory. *Psychological Review, 104,* 467–498.

Rovee-Collier, C., Hayne, H., & Columbo, J. (2001). *The development of implicit and explicit memory.* Amsterdam: Benjamins.

Rubin, D. C. (Ed.). (1986). *Autobiographical memory.* New York: Cambridge University Press.

Schacter, D. L. (1993). Understanding implicit memory: A cognitive neuroscience approach. In A. Collins, M. J. Conway, S. Gathercole, & P. Morris (Eds.), *Theories of memory* (pp. 387–412). Hillsdale, NJ: Erlbaum.

Schacter, D. L., & Moscovitch, M. (1984). Infants, amnesics, and dissociable memory systems. In M. Moscovitch (Ed.), *Infant memory: Its relation to normal and pathological memory in humans and other animals* (pp. 173–216). New York: Plenum Press.

Schacter, D. L., Wagner, A. D., & Buckner, R. L. (2000). Memory systems of 1999. In E. Tulving & F. M. I. Craik (Eds.), *The Oxford handbook of memory* (pp. 627–643). New York: Oxford University Press.

Schank, R. C. (1982). *Dynamic memory: A theory of reminding and learning in computers and people.* New York: Cambridge University Press.

Schank, R. C., & Abelson, R. P. (1977). *Scripts, plans, goals, and understanding.* Hillsdale, NJ: Erlbaum.

Spelke, E. S., Breinlinger, K., Macomber, J., & Jacobson, K. (1992). Origins of knowledge. *Psychological Review, 99,* 605–632.

Squire, L. R. (1992). Memory and the hippocampus: A synthesis from findings with rats, monkeys, and humans. *Psychological Review, 99,* 195–231.

Squire, L. R. (1995). Biological foundations of accuracy and inaccuracy in memory. In D. L. Schacter (Ed.), *Memory distortions: How minds, brains, and societies reconstruct the past* (pp. 197–225). Cambridge, MA: Harvard University Press.

Sun, R. (2002). *Duality of the mind: A bottom up approach toward cognition.* Mahwah, NJ: Erlbaum.

Thelen, E., & Smith, L. B. (1994). *A dynamic systems approach to the development of cognition and action.* Cambridge, MA: MIT Press.

Tomasello, M. (1999). *The cultural origins of human cognition.* Cambridge, MA: Harvard University Press.

Tomasello, M., & Call, J. (1997). *Primate cognition.* New York: Oxford University Press.

Tomasello, M., Kruger, A. C., & Ratner, H. H. (1993). Cultural learning. *Behavioral and Brain Sciences, 16,* 495–552.

Tomasello, M., Savage-Rumbaugh, S., & Kruger, A. C. (1993). Imitative learning of actions on objects by children, chimpanzees, and enculturated chimpanzees. *Child Development, 64,* 1688–1705.

Tulving, E. (1983). *Elements of episodic memory.* New York: Oxford University Press.

Turkewitz, G. (1993). The influence of timing on the nature of cognition. In G. Turkewitz & D. A. Devenny (Eds.), *Developmental time and timing* (pp. 125–142). Hillsdale, NJ: Erlbaum.

Wheeler, M.A. (2000). Episodic memory and autonoetic awareness. In E. Tulving & F. I. M. Craik (Eds.), *Oxford handbook of memory* (pp. 597–625). New York: Oxford University Press.

15

LANGUAGE EVOLUTION
AND HUMAN DEVELOPMENT

BRIAN MACWHINNEY

Language is a unique hallmark of the human species. Although many species can communicate in limited ways about things that are physically present, only humans can construct a full narrative characterization of events occurring outside of the here and now. Humans are also unique in their ability to fashion tools such as arrow points, axes, traps, and clothing. By using language to control the social coordination of tool making, humans have produced a material society that has achieved domination over all the creatures of our world and often over Nature herself. The religions of the world have interpreted our unique linguistic endowment as a Special Gift bestowed directly by the Creator. Scientists have also been influenced by this view of language, often attributing the emergence of this remarkable species-specific ability to some single, pivotal salutatory event in human evolution. I refer to this sudden evolutionary jump into true human language as linguistic saltation.

Linguistic saltationists (Bickerton, 1990; Chomsky, 1975; Hauser, Chomsky, & Fitch, 2002) tend to see language as a very recent evolutionary event. They can note that the divergence of our hominid ancestors from the Great Apes occurred over 6 million years ago (mya). However, evidence for distinctly human activities such as art, agriculture, writing, burial, pottery, and jewelry seldom goes back further than 40,000 years. Theorists such as Mithen (1996) have suggested that the crucial evolutionary development that led to the burst in creativity in the Neolithic was the emergence of human language as a method for integrating across cognitive modules. It seems quite likely that some aspect of language evolution played a major role in the recent creativity explosion. However, it would be a mistake to think that language could emerge suddenly in all its complex phonological and syntactic glory in the last 40,000 years without having been foreshadowed by major developments during the rest of our 6-million-year history. In particular, we know that 300,000 years ago there was a major expansion of the parts of the vertebrae that carry nerves for the intercostal muscles (MacLarnon & Hewitt, 1999). The intercostals are the muscles that control the pulmonic pulsing that drives human phonation. The expansion of these pathways indicates that we were developing a reliance on vocal communication as far back as 300,000 years ago. But it is also apparent that the language we produced at that time was not structured or complex enough to serve as a support for the development of material culture.

Language relies on far more physiological, social, and neural systems than just the intercostal muscles. It depends on systems for cortical control of vocalization, changes in group structure and affective relations, growth in cognitive abilities, neural pathways for information integration, and mechanisms for the formation of social hierarchies. The hominid lineage has undergone a remarkable series of physiological adaptations involving skeletal modifications to support upright posture, development of an opposing thumb, changes in the birth process (Hockett & Ascher, 1964), loss of hair (Morgan, 1997), adaptation of the gastrointestinal tract, increased innervation of the intercostal muscles (MacLarnon & Hewitt, 1999), loss of pronounced canine teeth, bending of the vocal tract, refinement of the facial musculature, freeing of the vocal folds, and sharpening of the chin. Each of these adaptations plays a role in supporting language. Beginning about 3 mya, a gradual tripling of brain size (Holloway, 1995) has brought massive changes in the interconnectedness of the frontal lobes, changes in the linkage of vocal production to motor and emotional areas, linkages of the visual areas to motor areas, and expansion of many older areas, including the cerebellum, basal ganglion, and thalamus. These various neurological developments have also provided a basis for a marked increase in humans' ability to produce actions through movement and sounds through vocalization. Alongside these changes in morphology and neurology, human society has undergone a parallel process of development involving the expansion of social groups, migrations first across Eurasia and then to the Americas, the refinement of warfare, the development of tools, and the emergence of language.

The concept of coevolution (Deacon, 1997; Givón, 1998) provides a useful framework for understanding how these various developments occurred in parallel. The theory of coevolution holds that changes in neurological and physiological structure facilitated advances in planning and communication. These advances in cognitive and communicative activities then provided an evolutionary environment that supported further neurological and physiological modifications. This notion of an evolutionary ratchet effect is fundamentally attractive. It depicts a species that is slowly and steadily moving toward fuller and fuller control over its environment. In this view, each new advance in ability should be accompanied by a greater control over the environment and a spread of habitat.

However, matters were apparently not so simple. The remarkable expansion of habitat to all of Africa and Eurasia by *Homo erectus* after 2 mya was not accompanied by any observable jump in the control of the material environment. Instead, it simply appears that these hominids achieved their success through group solidarity. As we noted earlier, the expansion of the vertebrae to support nerves for the intercostal muscles 300,000 years ago (MacLarnon & Hewitt, 1999) provides clear evidence of an emerging system of vocal communication. Yet despite the adaptive advantages that improved communication might have provided, the population of our direct ancestors was likely no more than 10,000 at a point some 70,000 years ago (Stringer & McKie, 1996). If the story of the human race is one of the continual successful coevolution of language and the brain, we have to ask ourselves how it is that a species with some advanced level of communicative abilities had such a narrow escape from complete extinction. At the same time, one could well argue that near extinction 70,000 years ago provided exactly the evolutionary pressure that led to the final emergence of modern language.

The next four sections outline how humans evolved to confront four major evolutionary challenges. Each of these major evolutionary changes played an important role in terms of providing cognitive and social bases for the development of language. This evolutionary analysis is designed to provide a basic account of the evolution of language in our species. In later sections, I turn to the specific impact of this evolutionary past on the shape of human childhood and the acquisition of language by the child.

BIPEDALISM

The advent of hominid bipedal gait stands as a remarkably clear evolutionary watershed in the late Eocene. Between 10 mya and 7 mya, Africa experienced a major tectonic event that led to the formation of the Great Rift Valley. This valley runs down the center of the continent, dividing the flat jungle of the West from the more arid plain of the East (Coppens, 1999). The rift valley encompasses vast bodies of water such as Lake Tanganyika and Lake Nyasa, as well as high mountain ranges with peaks such as Mt. Kilimanjaro. The rain shadow created by these mountains produces a major discontinuity in the climate of these two parts of sub-Saharan Africa.

Before the emergence of the rift, the great apes of Africa dwelled in the warm, lush forest of the Eocene that extended across the continent. With the advent of the rift during the Oligocene, the domain of the apes became restricted to the west of the continent, ending at the rift valley. Those apes that found themselves on the east side of the rift were forced to adapt to the loss of the jungle. The major competitors of the apes were the monkeys, who were better able to hide from predators in the short bush and scramble for pieces of food. The challenge to the apes of East Africa was to make use of the new, drier savannah habitat in a way that did not compete with the monkeys. They did this by adopting a bipedal gait. Instead of scampering about on four legs or even in a knuckle-walk posture, early hominids began to walk on their two hind legs. Australopithecines, such as *Australopithecus afarensis* (Coppens, 1999), were able both to climb trees and to walk with two legs on the ground. Other species, such as *Australopithecus anamensis*, adopted a more exclusively upright gait. The latter group included our direct ancestors.

Advantages of Bipedalism

Although we know that bipedalism was favored in the sparser habitat of East Africa, we do not understand exactly why it was so successful for many hominids. One account focuses on the fact that upright posture allows the animal to expose less body surface to the sun. Having less skin exposed to the sun decreases the impact of radiation and the need for cooling. A second factor must be the ability of the primate to use the forelimbs for other purposes, ranging from tool use to flea picking. A third factor is the defensive effect of greater height. Hunters in the *veldt* recognize the importance of always standing upright to convince lions, rhinos, and other animals of one's size to deter possible aggression (Kwa Maritane Guide, Pilanesberg Park, personal communication, July, 2000).

When we compare the great apes to the monkeys, we can see some other pressures that might have favored the move to an upright posture (Stanford, 2003). When chimps and gorillas are together in social groups, they move away from the four-legged knuckle-walk position to a sitting position. This allows them to maintain better eye contact with the others in their group. In the sitting position, they do not have to bend their neck up to maintain eye contact. The shift away from knuckle walking to an upright posture continues this emphasis on body positions that allow full eye contact.

Upright posture and full eye contact also provided room for the emergence of the first gestural signals between early hominids. As many have argued, it is likely that hominids went through a period of relying on some forms of gestural communication. It is clear that upright posture provides room for such a development. However, the evolutionary advantage of early gestures may have been overestimated, since the first bipedal primates had cognitive resources that were not yet greatly different from those of today's apes. Although we know that apes can learn and transmit a system of signs (Savage-Rumbaugh, 2000), there is little evidence that the level of sign use they display in natural contexts (Menzel, 1975) would provide any great evolutionary advantage.

The major evolutionary advantage of bipedalism is probably the fact that the forearms can then be used to hold tools and weapons (Coppens, 1995). This ability gave early hominids a clear advantage over monkeys in their search for food and defense against predators. Tools could be used to dig for roots, open termite hills, and even catch fish. Likely in response to such pressures, early hominids soon developed an opposing thumb that allowed for a stronger and more precise grasp. Because the arms were no longer needed for tree climbing, they could be committed in this way to object manipulation. Thus, this first coevolutionary period focused on the development of new systems for control of tools through the hands.

Bipedalism brought with it a series of evolutionary costs. It placed increased mechanical pressure on the neck, the spine, and all the joints of the legs. The reliance on the feet for walking made them less able to function for climbing. The lungs had to adapt to support the breathing needed for running. However, the most important of these costs involved the narrowing of the hips (Hockett & Ascher, 1964). Because early hominids did not have a significantly enlarged cranium, this was not a problem until perhaps 2 mya. However, after that time, brain expansion ran up against the earlier commitment to bipedalism, forcing a series of adaptations in female anatomy, parturition, and child rearing.

Tools and Imitation

The move to bipedalism opened up major cognitive challenges in terms of the control of the hands. Apes already have good control of reaching and basic object manipulation (Ingmanson, 1996). However, with both hands now always free for motion, humans were able to explore still further uses of their hands. Rizzolatti, Fadiga, Gallese, and Fogassi (1996) has shown that monkeys (and presumably other primates) have "mirror" neurons in the supplementary eye fields of premotor cortex that respond with equal force when an action such as "grabbing" is carried out either by the self or by the other, including a human. This mechanism provides a way of equating actions performed by the self with actions or postures performed by the other. These neurons are part of the dorsal visual system (Goodale, 1993) that allows us to represent the postural perspective of another in a way that is isomorphic with but nonidentical to our own postural perspective. This dorsal system for motor matching also connects to systems in motor cortex, cerebellum, and hippocampus that represent various postures and movements of the body. These systems then connect to frontal mechanisms for storage and perspective shifting that provide a way of using our own full body image to perceive the actions of others.

Although monkeys have basic neural mechanisms that allow them to map their body image onto those of conspecifics, they demonstrate much less free use of imitation than humans. The current analysis suggests that the first evolutionary support for imitation was in the context of learning tool use. Young hominids could learn to use branches and clubs by imitating their elders. They could acquire the ability to chip one stone against another to form primitive hand axes. The selectionist value of imitation of tool usage is clear.

The ability to imitate a series of actions requires construction of stored mental images of specific motor actions and postures. To plan the actions involved in chipping an axe, we must be able to call up an image of the desired product, and we must be able to sequence a long series of specific motions that are needed to locate good stones and devise methods for chipping edges. In this regard, the ability to construct a planned sequence of actions appears to be a unique property of hominids, as opposed to monkeys and apes. Students of primate tool use (Anderson, 1996; Visalberghi & Limongelli, 1996) have shown that chimpanzees and capuchin monkeys can use tools in a productive and exploratory way. However, they do not appear to make planful use of mental imagery to limit their search through possible methods of tool use. Instead, they apply all directly perceptible methods in hopes that one may succeed.

Because the move to a terrestrial environment was quite gradual (Corballis, 1999), hominids needed to provide neural control for the use of the hands in both the arboreal and terrestrial environments. The arboreal environment favors the development of a specific type of motor imagery. Povinelli and Cant (1995) have noted that increases in body weight for larger apes such as orangutans make it important to be able to plan motions through the trees. To do this, the animal needs a map of the self as it executes possible motor actions. The reflexes of this penchant for postural adaptation are still evident in the human enjoyment of dance, exercise, and sport. The pressures in the arboreal environment that had favored some limited form of brain lateralization were then carried over to the terrestrial environment (McManus, 1999). This ability to shift quickly between alternative environments required neural support for competing postural and affordance systems.

Bipedalism also put some pressure on another set of neural mechanisms. Because hominids ceased relying on trees for refuge, and because they were now ranging over a wider territory, they needed to develop improved means of representing spaces and distances. All species must have some way of representing their territory. However, hominids faced the task of representing a large, often changing territory in which they were both the hunters and the hunted. To do this, they needed to further elaborate earlier mechanisms for spatial encoding. The basic neural mechanisms for this are already well developed in many mammalian species, including primates (Menzel, 1973), canines, and felines. By linking newly developed systems for action imitation to earlier systems for spatial navigation, hominids could construct mental images of their bodies moving through space and time. However, instead of just predicting body position in the next few seconds, these mechanisms could be used to predict positions over longer periods of time. In addition, hominids could use the primate system of mirror neurons to track not only the posture of conspecifics but also their movements through space and time.

Holloway (1995) has presented evidence from endocasts (plaster casts of the interiors of skulls) indicating that there was, in fact, a major reorganization of parietal cortex after about 4 mya. This reorganization involved the reduction of primary visual striate cortex and the enlargement of extrastriate parietal cortex, angular gyrus, and supramarginal gyrus. Much of the evidence for Holloway's analysis comes from traces of the changing positions of the lunate sulcus and the intraparietal sulcus over time. According to Holloway, the areas that were expanded during these changes in the parietal cortex support three basic cognitive functions:

1. Processing in the dorsal (parietal) stream of the visual field is important for representing actions of the other in terms of one's own body image.
2. The association areas of parietal maintain a map of the environment for navigation in the new bipedal mode.
3. The supramarginal gyrus is involved in face perception. Expansion of this area would facilitate the development of social patterns and memory for social relations.

The first two of these functions are directly related to the developments that resulted from the adoption of bipedal gait. The third function may have played a large role during the next period, in which the focus of evolution was on social cohesion.

SOCIAL COHESION

The shift to bipedalism is clearly documented in the fossil record. However, fossils speak only indirectly about the evolution of primate social structures. Even basic facts about hominid group size are difficult to determine from the spotty fossil record. We do know, however, from studies of current primate groups, that larger groups provide better protection for group members, particularly the young. We also know that maintaining larger groups requires refinement of methods for social communication and food gathering. In this section, I explore the ways in which pressures toward larger group size led to the evolution of mechanisms for social cohesion. The developments discussed in the previous section lead directly to increases in individual fitness. For example, if a young hominid can use imitation to learn how to chip an axe, that individual will be more able to kill prey and to survive attacks from predators.

Evolutionary support for the development of social features tends to rely more heavily on mechanisms for mate selection. A prime case of this is imitation in both the auditory and visual modes. Individuals with high levels of imitative skill are likely to attract mates by entrancing their attention. Females who respond sexually to imitative (communicative) males will be likely to produce offspring who are themselves imitative, thereby following the selectional route of producing "sexy sons." At the same time, infants who respond imitatively to their mothers may receive better nurturing, thereby improving their chances for survival. As a tendency toward imitation spreads through a group, those individuals who are less capable of face-to-face imitation will receive less social support and will be dispreferred as mates. Although there will always be some ecological niches for individuals with low imitation ability, the general trend in the population will be toward continually improved imitation skill.

Vocal Support for Social Cohesion

As group size increases, there is increasing conflict for food, rank, control, and access to females. Dunbar (2000) argues that primates developed a large neocortex to deal with these tensions. However, other primate groups have been able to develop methods to maintain social cohesion that do not require radical changes in brain size (de Waal & Aureli, 1996). Moreover, hominids came under pressure to maintain large social groups well before there was a significant expansion in brain size. In particular, between 4.5 mya and 3.5 mya, the hominids in East Africa went through an expansion of their range and a proliferation of species. This proliferation was then followed by a period of tight competition with range contraction (Foley, 1999). During this period of range expansion and contraction, our ancestors did not improve their social organization simply by growing larger brains, although brain size did increase a bit, mostly allometrically (Holloway, 1995). Instead, as Nettle and Dunbar (1997) have argued, it is likely that the hominids of the Pliocene consolidated their group structure by a set of targeted neural–behavioral adaptations. Chief among these, I would argue, is the subordination of the vocal system to cortical control.

Our Pliocene ancestors probably possessed a set of vocal calls much like those used by other primates. It was not the emergence of new sounds that supported social cohesion, but the ability to use old sounds in new contexts. By calling up specific calls and gestures at will, our ancestors were able to use chatter to gain the attention of their compatriots to negotiate the basics of group relations. The fact that the great apes did not go through a parallel evolutionary process in West Africa can be attributed to the different requirements on group size in their arboreal habitat and the fact that they had not adopted bipedal gait and its resultant improvements in face-to-face communication.

One of the side effects of an increase of cortical control over vocalization might well be the ability of hominid groups to lock in patterns of vocal behavior that characterize the local group, as opposed to the wider hominid community. At first, these local forms of communication would not be sharply defined. However, as the mechanics for vocalization come increasingly under cortical control, it would become easier for a group to differentiate itself from others by unique vocal features that would transmit over a distance. Songbirds achieve this effect through species-specific processes of vocal learning (Konishi, 1995). In birds, dialects allow individuals and groups to maintain their territory against competitors. Hominids could achieve the same effect through differentiation of local patterns for speech and gesture.

Neural Modifications

Achieving neocortical control over the vocal–auditory channel required neuronal reorganization without a major increase in brain size. Ploog (1992) has shown that humans have more direct pyramidal connections between motor cortex and the speech and vocalization areas of the brainstem than do monkeys. Certain areas of the limbic system, such as the anterior thalamic limbic nuclei, have grown disproportionately large in humans. These nuclei serve the supplementary motor area and premotor and orbital frontal cortex. The expansion of these structures points to increased limbic input to the cortex, as well as input from the cortex to the limbic structures. Tucker (2001) shows that the basic adaptation here involved the absorption of the primate external striatum by the neocortex (Nauta & Karten, 1970).

In macaques (Jürgens, 1979), control of the vocal system relies on the periaqueductal gray matter of the lower midbrain. Additional midbrain regions can stimulate the periaqueductal gray, but the neocortex does not control or initiate primate vocalizations. In humans, on the other hand, electrical stimulation of both the supplemental motor area and the anterior cingulate of the frontal cortex can reliably produce vocalization. Primates make few attempts to structure local dialects or otherwise structure their call system through learning (Seyfarth & Cheney, 1999). Yerkes and Learned (1925) and others have tried to condition chimpanzee vocalizations in the laboratory and have failed. Human infants, on the other hand, rely at least in part on highly plastic cortical mechanisms to control vocalization. This allows them to pick up the sound patterns of their community through mere exposure. As a result, each hominid group can build a local vocal accent that is passed on to the next generation through mere exposure. Other aspects of communication, such as conversational sequencing (Trevarthen, 1984), may be more linked to modeling and imitation. However, this learning of conversational functions only occurs because the child is locked into the interaction by motivational forces that reward face-to-face vocalization (Locke, 1995).

Although primate vocalization is not under cortical control, it has an extremely direct connection to midbrain motivational areas (Pandya, Seltzer, & Barbas, 1988). Human language continues to rely on this underlying limbic architecture to provide emotional coloring to vocalization. As Tucker (2001) argues, the linkage of the vocal system to limbic mechanisms provides grounding in terms of arousal (brainstem and amygdala), motivation (basal ganglion), patterning (striatal–thalamic ciruits), and memory (limbic circuits). Humans also retain some direct links between audition and these limbic circuits, as evidenced in the directness of our responses to sounds such as infant cries or the growls of predators.

The linkage of vocalizations to cortical control allowed our ancestors to distinguish themselves from other hominids. It also allowed them to build up a system of face-to-face social interactions. MacNeilage (1998) has argued that the primate gesture of lip smacking is the source of the core CV (consonant–vowel) syllabic structure of human language. The CV syllable has the same motoric structure as lip smacking. Moreover, it is produced in an area of inferior frontal cortex close to that used for lip smacking and other vocal gestures. Primates use lip smacks as one form of social interaction during face-to-face encounters. However, even bonobos, the most social of all primates, do not maintain face-to-face conversations for the long periods that we find in human interactions. Obviously, one must go beyond a boring repetition of lip smacking to maintain a reasonable level of sustained face-to-face vocal contact. Increased cortical control of vocalization allowed our ancestors to begin the process of developing these elaborations. By linking its members into tight affiliative relations through face-to-face interaction, our ancestors achieved a form of social organization that allowed them to maintain large social groups for defense against other hominid groups.

The discussion so far has emphasize the role of auditory imitation. However, an equally compelling argument can be made for the importance of growth in visual imitation. To maximize the effectiveness of face-to-face interactions, hominids also needed to bring the production of facial gestures under cortical control. As in the case of the control of tool use through motor imagery, humans differ from monkeys (Myers, 1976) and apes (Gomez, 1996) in the extent to which the cortex can produce gestures upon demand.

In considering the role of face-to-face vocalization in hominid groups, we must not forget the possible divisive role played by aggressive males (Anders, 1994; Goodall, 1979). Hominid groups relied on aggressive males for their skills as hunters and their ability to defend the group against attack. However, groups also needed to provide ways to avoid the direction of male aggression toward other members of the group, particularly other males. We know that primates had already developed various methods for handling these conflicts, including exile for problematic males, the formation of master–apprentice relations, and development of male social groups. Within this already established social framework, males could also benefit from ongoing reaffirmation of their social status through face-to-face chat. By socializing young males into this productive use of language for social cohesion, mothers could also contribute to the stability of the group. Breakdowns in these processes could threaten the survival of the group and even the species.

This account has emphasized the importance of cortical control over the vocal apparatus. There is no evidence that there was a corresponding evolution of auditory abilities in hominids. The reason for this is that it appears that primates have already achieved a level of auditory processing ability sufficient to support analysis of all vocal communications (Hauser, Newport, & Aslin, 2001; Kuhl & Miller, 1978). There is currently no reason to believe that the human auditory system underwent any major adaptation in the last 6 million years. The linkage of vocal and facial expression to cortical control may seem like a fairly trivial neurological adaptation. However, it helped our ancestors through this period of intense competition between groups and set the stage for the major changes that were to come in the next period.

MIMESIS

By 2 mya, *Homo erectus* emerged victorious from the period of intense competition with other hominids. Recent analysis points to *Homo ergaster*, rather than *H. erectus* as the direct ancestor of *H. sapiens*. However, the details of the relations between *H. erectus* and *H. ergaster* are not yet clear. In this chapter, I refer to these two related populations as *H. erectus*, understanding that the details of this particular lineage may soon be revised.

During this period, the species had achieved some level of group solidarity through the social use of imitative vocalization and gesture. Beginning sometime before 2 mya, our ancestors were confronted with a third major evolutionary opportunity. Having committed themselves to face-to-face communication, and having elaborated their basic systems of social identification and imitation, the first groups of *H. erectus* were then able to elaborate new forms of symbolic communication in both vocal and gestural modalities. These new systems involved the spontaneous interaction of vocalizations, postures, and gestures in specific social and pragmatic contexts. Although the intertwining of these systems could serve admirably for maintaining shared attention and social cohesion, it would have proved difficult to link these spontaneous systems to a method for traditional transmission (Hockett, 1960). Vocalizations were just now coming under cortical control and had not yet been systematized in a way that would guarantee productivity and replicability. Gestural and postural patterns probably played a more central role. However, their iconic and situated nature may have served as a barrier to abstract systematization. To the degree that gestures could be made up "on the fly," there would be little evolutionary advantage supporting systematiziation.

Darwin (1877) thought it unlikely that a system such as language could have emerged directly from gesture. He believed that this would require the shifting of a function from one organ to another and then back again, as if flying had moved from the wing to the stomach and then back to the wing. However, there is no reason to think that Darwin would have excluded the possibility that gesture and vocalization underwent coevolution. Today, speech and gesture complement each other during communication (McNeill, 1985). Some messages are conveyed through speech, but others are conveyed through the hands and the posture. Still other messages are conveyed by changes in the tone of voice. It is likely that each of these channels of communication was also available to *H. erectus* and that they functioned in an interactive and complementary fashion, much as they do now.

Advantages of Mimesis

Donald (1991) has emphasized the central role of what he calls "mimesis" in the communicative world of *H. erectus*. Mimesis involves communication about actions, plans, feelings, and objects through iconic depiction of parts of those actions, states, and objects (see also Nelson, Chapter 14, this volume). The depiction may conjure up an image of an object by gesturing its shape or imitating its sound. Actions can be depicted by repetition of their central components. In general, mimesis achieves reference through partonymy, or mention of a part to express the whole. Mimesis can be expressed through signing, chant, song, drama, ritual, and basic forms of costume. To be maximally effective, these systems must occur within fixed social contexts that guarantee attention and some traditional form. As conventionalization advances, mimetic systems can support group solidarity, planning, and socialization in an increasingly structured way. Through conventionalized chant and dance, the male society can plan hunts and battles and reenact past struggles. At the same time, mothers can use song, sound play, and chant to hold the attention of their young children while socializing them into the practices of the community. Mimetic processes are linked to the emotional use of language that was elaborated during the previous evolutionary period. As a result, mimetic communications can be used to move people emotionally, preparing them for war, migration, or other major group activities.

It appears that mimesis was enormously successful in providing social cohesion and shared planning. As a result, H. erectus was able to expand its territory to all of Africa, eventually leading to the extinction of all other hominid species. It also allowed H. erectus to migrate successfully out of Africa to all parts of Asia, including the Middle East, China, and Indonesia. We should attribute this successful expansion to two basic processes. The first was an ability to eliminate competitors, particularly in Africa. To do this, erectus must have relied on group solidarity as a support for warfare. Second, to support the migration to new territories, erectus must have been extremely adaptive. This adaptivity could not have been grounded in some simple physical change. Instead, it must have resulted from a general improvement in cognitive capacity, particularly as reflected in group problem solving and adaptation.

MacWhinney (1999a) and Tomasello (1999) have developed parallel accounts of these changes that emphasize the importance of being able to take the perspective of another human being as an intentional agent. In both accounts, this ability is a precondition to the full successful use of language. Tomasello locates the emergence of this ability in the period after 200,000 years ago. However, like Donald (1991), MacWhinney sees the ability arising as early as 2 mya with ongoing developments during more recent periods. The account developed here emphasizes the initial role of social cohesion as an evolutionary support for communication. The movement to an upright position allowed us to engage more directly with our conspecifics both gesturally and vocally. The rise of cortical control over vocalization led to further improvements. However, to take full advantage of face-to-face communication, we needed to expand our image of the other. Supports for this include neural control of imitation (Decety, Chaminade, Grezes, & Meltzoff, 2002), face recognition (Moskovitch, Winocur, & Behrmann, 1997), and the construction of a full, projectable body image (Ramachandran & Hubbard,

2001). These new developments could rely on some parallel evolutions that had been occurring outside of the social realm. Because the movement to an upright posture freed the hands for increased use of tools, hominids derived additional evolutionary advantage from the formation of mental models of plans for tool usage and action schemas. These schemas relied on the development of a mental model for the self's activities. This same mental model could then eventually be projected onto the other, allowing hominids to develop increasingly sophisticated ideas about the future actions of others. However, without further support from language, this level of theory of mind construction could only go so far.

Neuronal Adaptations

The brain of *H. erectus* tripled in size during the period between 2 mya and 100,000 years ago. Some of this increase is allometrically related to the overall growth in stature during this period. Thus, it might be better to speak of a doubling in size, rather than a tripling in size. The brain expanded in size because the preconditions for a successful expansion were now all in place. In particular, previous evolution had already produced at least these five abilities:

1. The shift to bipedalism had freed the hands for gestural communication.
2. The freeing of the hands for tool use had led to further elaboration of primate mechanisms, such as "mirror" neurons, for representation of the actions of others.
3. During several millennia of migration and population movements across open ground and through the bush, our ancestors had developed systems for tracking their own spatial positions in the present, past, and future, as well as the spatial positions and perspectives of others.
4. Our ancestors could use their visual system to generate images of past actions and spatial configurations involving themselves and others.
5. During the period before 2 mya, our ancestors had developed a tight linkage of attention to vocalization processes during face-to-face interaction and imitation.

These developments provide preconditions for the evolution of mimesis. To further support mimesis, the brain needed to provide complete episodic storage for combinations of gesture and vocalization. It had to store whole chants or gestures as they expressed particular events of importance to individuals and the group. Some of these chants and gestures might have been rather extended. For example, there might have been a dance that represented the time of ripening of the mongongo nut or one that outlined the components of the hunt for the eland. At the same time, these larger mimetic sequences would be composed of smaller pieces that had achieved other cognitive–social grounding. For example, by pointing to a place in the area around the group's encampment, the dancer could signal the direction of a hunt. By holding his arm in a particular stance, the dancer could mime the attack on the game. These component gestures, movements of the body, and vocal chants could then be reused with other components in a relatively unsystematic fashion.

Unlike the evolutionary pressures of earlier periods, the storage and retrieval of conventionalized mimetic sequences cannot be achieved simply by linking up older areas or by reusing earlier connections. Instead, the brain must add new computational space to store the multitude of new visual and auditory images. In addition, the brain needs to expand the role of the frontal areas for storing and switching between perspectives. Because this system grew up in a haphazard way from earlier pieces of lip smacking, pointing, gesture, and rhythm, it would be difficult to extract a core set of elements from mimetic communications. Instead, patterns and forms must be learned and stored as holistic unanalyzed sequences. This Gestalt-like shape of early mimetic patterns corresponds well with the Gestalt-like cognitions that we develop through our interactions with objects (Gibson, 1977). For example, when we chop wood, there is a complete interpenetration of muscle actions, visual experiences, hand positions, and sounds. We can think of this as a single merged form such as I-hands-back-lift-axe-drop-split-chips-wood-cut. Mimetic forms have this same unanalyzed quality. This lack of analysis is not the result of chunking or automatization, since the Gestalt is not constructed by a system of combinatorial semantics. Instead, each chunk is a raw, unanalyzed whole that is fully grounded on direct action and perception. Because they are highly grounded on our direct perceptions and actions, they communicate in a basic way. However, they provide little support for cognitive organization.

The growth of the brain in response to these pressures was so rapid that it is typically assumed that it involved a single genetic mechanism. One such mechanism might involve regulatory genes (Allman, 1999) that control the development of structures in the fetus. Changes in the timing of the expression of these genes can lead to the observed across-the-board increase in size for the cortex and cerebellum that we see in *H. erectus*. However, the expansion of the cortex placed additional adaptive pressures on *H. erectus*. The bigger brain required a much greater level of caloric intake. This pressure could be met through changes in diet and modifications to the digestive system. A more fundamental pressure was the fact that increases in the size of the infant brain produce problems for the birth process. The width of the hips had narrowed in both men and women as a response to bipedalism. As long as the skull was not much larger than that found in the great apes, this did not cause major problems for the birth process. However, the expansion of the skull in *H. erectus* ran directly into this evolutionary barrier. To deal with this, the infant is born at a time when it is still fairly immature and the skull is relatively pliable. The increasingly organized shape of the society facilitates the survival of the child. In addition, women have had to sacrifice their ability to run quickly so that the hips could widen, permitting births with larger infant heads. The slowing of infant development not only helps in the birth process but also helps the child maintain cortical plasticity (Elman, Bates, Plunkett, Johnson, & Karmiloff-Smith, 1996; Julesz & Kovacs, 1995) even into adolescence, thereby further enhancing the ability of the group to construct accepted mimetic patterns.

SYSTEMATIZATION

By the end of the Pliocene, *H. erectus* had achieved dominance over its hominid competitors. There were no remaining hominid species in Africa, because *H. erectus* had eliminated its competitors either through warfare or resource competition, and had successfully migrated to Eastern Europe, Asia, and Indonesia. However, with the onset of the glaciations of the Pleistocene, our ancestors came under increasing pressure to adapt to the colder, drier environment. At this point, there was a contraction of territory back to Africa. We can talk about the emergence of *H. sapiens*, or modern man, as a new species beginning about 200,000 years ago. The analysis of mitochondrial DNA (Cann, 1995; Cavalli-Sforza, 1991; Templeton, 1992) allows us to trace the lineage of all current humans back to a single population and perhaps a single mother that lived in Africa about 200,000 years ago. Beginning from this time, modern people migrated again out of Africa to the Middle East and Europe. However, about 70,000 years ago, there was a near extinction that brought the number of our direct ancestors down to only 10,000 individuals worldwide. Of course, this population may well have coexisted with other hominids, such as the Neanderthals, who are not our direct ancestors.

After the recovery from this near extinction, humans went on to achieve major cultural and material breakthroughs in the Neolithic, including the remarkable cave paintings in Europe and the settling of Australia, the Americas, and Polynesia. The fact that the brain expansion of *H. erectus* was not enough by itself to trigger the emergence of material culture helps us to understand the shape of recent processes in human evolution. Instead, humans needed some way to systematize the growth in mimetic processes that had occurred during the Pliocene. The core of the new system involved the introduction of a set of phonological contrasts (Hockett & Altmann, 1973). To achieve accurate articulation of these contrasts, a further set of adaptions was needed for the serial ordering of actions and the precise articulation of sounds. These adaptations included loss of the canines, adaptation of the arytenoids, bending of the vocal tract (Lieberman, 1975), and shaping of the musculature of the tongue. Each of these modifications led to a separate and meaningful increment in our ability to articulate clearly a full inventory of phonetic contrasts. The complex and diverse nature of these modifications suggests that the phonetic revolution occurred not in a single leap, but gradually, across the period from 300,000 to 50,000 years ago. It is likely that those individuals who survived the evolutionary window 70,000 years ago were those who had made the greatest progress in terms of consolidating this phonological ability and the group planning that it facilitates. The fact that many children still show evidence of language disorders due to both neurological and physiological problems indicates that this process of systematization continues to unfold evolutionarily even today.

Selection for language-related proficiency is driven primarily by mate selection, with both women and men preferring mates who are able to imitate, articulate, and conceptualize effectively (Miller, 2001). Language can be used to construct the love and friendship that underlie many sexual relations, and to provide ongoing detection of cheating in these relations. At the same time, much of the evolutionary success of language-based courtship may derive from the use of language to deceive. By creating fictive mental images of faithfulness and pair-bonding, men can attain sexual favors from women, even without being truly faithful (Buss, 1999). Strategies of this type correspond to what we would now call "a smooth talker." An even greater advantage accrues to males who take on roles of charismatic group leader. For example, it is claimed that the rock star Jimi Hendrix fathered well over 100 children. Although such estimates may be difficult to verify, the ability of dominant males to secure larger numbers of females for reproduction is common in many species. What is unique in humans is the fact that the ability of a leader to achieve charismatic control is often achieved through activities such as political speaking, military display, and various forms of artistic expression.

Perspective, Lexicon, and Grammar

The development of smooth methods for articulatory planning opened up possibilities for the construction of a mental lexicon. By coding words into a compact set of contrastive features, *H. sapiens* was able to conventionalize, learn, store, and retrieve a virtually limitless set of names for things. However, by itself, the emergence of a lexicon is not enough to produce full human language. People also have to make use of a system for combining words into sentences. However, this basic combinatorial ability to control plans and strings of conventionalized actions had already been developing in a primitive form during the mimetic period with *H. erectus*. Thus, the flourishing of language after about 70,000 years ago involves a linking of the new lexical power with an older mimetic power. Like the older mimetic system, the new syntactic system relies heavily on the tracking of perspective. Elsewhere (MacWhinney, in press), I explain in detail how syntax and grammar emerge from the online tracking of perspective flow in sentences. This ability to track perspectives depends heavily on the imitative abilities that had been developing for nearly 3 million years, as well as the planning and mimetic abilities that had been developing for nearly 2 million years. However, when planning and mimesis are taken out of the concrete visual mode and constructed through the auditory mode, they place a greater load on abilities to construct and store alternative perspectives and mental models. Thus, it seems to me that the critical development between 70,000 and 40,000 years ago involved the growth of an ability to control perspective taking in the auditory mode. Those individuals who possessed this ability were able to rise to the top of Neolithic society as priests who could express a spiritual vision, and as leaders who could express a vision of conquest.

Advantages of the New System

With the power of a systematized lexicon, people could easily name and encode all of the important objects, properties, and actions in their environment. Having a full inventory of the physical world allowed early humans to use different animal and plant species for increasingly refined purposes. This new lexical richness became particularly powerful when it was embedded in the perspective-shifting system. Pinker and Bloom (1990) review some of the core linguistic constructs, such as tense, deixis, and transitivity supporting this expansion. For example, by forming complex locative descriptions, language was used to pinpoint the location of quarry sites for flints and other materials for stone weapons and tools. Master craftsmen used language to teach apprentices how to chip points, prepare hides for tanning, carve out wooden bowls, bind axes to poles with sinew, sew hides into tents, and tame pets. As tool making progressed, language was used to explain how, where, and when to plant and water seeds. By codifying these times and practices in verse and religion, the first agricultural systems were developed, and shortly thereafter, the first settled villages, such as Catalhöyük in Anatolia at about 9000 B.C. From these roots came the civilizations of the ancient Middle East, Egypt, and China, with their invention of writing, organized warfare, chariots, metallurgy, government, and increasingly formalized religion. Modern society has elaborated on this foundation with the creation of cities, books, bombs, law, medicine, and the Internet. All of these developments are consequences of the introduction of systematization for phonology and lexicon. However, this recent expansion would not have been possible without the major cognitive modifications of the preceding 6 million years of human evolution.

Neuronal Adaptations

Many of the adaptations required for smooth vocal production are quite peripheral (Lieberman, 1973), involving changes to the vocal tract, the structure of the larynx, muscle innervation, tongue support, and facial musculature. Some of these changes were under way before the Pleistocene; others have been more recent. To control this additional external hardware, the brain has needed to fine-tune its mechanisms for motor control. This fine-tuning does not require the type of brain expansion that occurred in *H. erectus*. Instead, it involves the linking of inferior frontal areas for motor control to temporal areas (Gabrieli, Brewer, Desmond, & Glover, 1997) for sequence storage. These linkages involve pathways that lie under the central sulcus. They constitute a functional neural circuit that implements a phonological loop for learning new words (Gupta & MacWhinney, 1997). The auditory shapes of words are stored in topological maps (Miikkulainen, 1990) in superior temporal auditory cortex and can be associated to visual images in inferior temporal areas.

Once *H. sapiens* had achieved an ability to produce, store, and learn a large vocabulary of phonologically organized forms, the remaining steps in the evolution of language were comparatively easy. Humans had already achieved a mimetic system for perspective taking and perspective switching. This system allowed listeners to mentally reenact the motions, rhythms, and chants of the speaker as they depicted movement between places and actions on objects. Once words became available, speakers and listeners could parse these single-package, Gestalt-like communications into their components. With words to name specific objects and participants, it was possible to separate out nouns from verbs. This adaptation to grammar required no particular new cognitive skill for nouns. However, for predicates such as verbs, it was important to store linkages between the overall configuration of the action and the specific uses with participants. In other words, children had to learn how to manage language in terms of item-based syntactic constructions (MacWhinney, 1975, 1982) and phrasal collocations, including "verb islands" (Tomasello, 2000). Neuronal processes for this level of control involve little in the way of new evolution. However, they place storage demands on the pathways between the temporal lexical areas and the frontal planning and sequencing areas.

As speakers build up longer and longer strings of propositions, they rely increasingly on frontal areas, such as dorsolateral prefrontal cortex (DLPFC) for the storage of one perspective that allows shifting to a secondary perspective. Shifts of this type are central in the processing of anaphors and gaps in argument structure. As I have shown (MacWhinney, 1999a), these various syntactic processes are grounded not on the construction of abstract syntactic trees, but on the direct processing of embodied perspectives of the type that were also important during the period of mimetic communication.

DEVELOPMENTAL CONSIDERATIONS

Having now reviewed the overall course of language evolution, we are in a position to assess linkages between evolution and the development of language in the infant and child.

Recapitulation

In this area, one theory that immediately suggests itself is the idea that language ontogeny in the child recapitulates language phylogeny in the species. In some regards, this may well be the case. For example, the cries of the newborn are driven exclusively by brainstem and midbrain mechanisms. It is not until well after the third month that infants begin to demonstrate some cortical control of vocalization. Although they have some imitative abilities soon after birth (Meltzoff, 1988), these abilities rise to important new levels toward the end of the first year (Bruner & Sherwood, 1976). We see major advances in lexical organization toward the end of the second year (Gershkoff-Stowe, Thal, Smith, & Namy, 1997) and a consolidation of articulatory abilities even later (Menn & Stoel-Gammon, 1995). Perhaps the final crown on the course of language development occurs during the acquisition of complex syntactic expressions to control perspective shifting lexically and syntactically (de Villiers & de Villiers, 1999). But the synchrony of these events is certainly not exactly that appearing in evolution. After all, children babble well before they walk, and we know that our ancestors became bipedal long before they achieved full cortical control of vocalization.

Traditional Transmission

It is perhaps more fruitful to ask a rather different set of questions about the role of language evolution in human development. Specifically, it seems important to focus on the fact that human language is transmitted traditionally from generation to generation. In order to achieve this cultural transmission, evolution needed to operate in detail on the relation between the child and the mother. In the terms of Bjorklund and Pellegrini (2000), we can say that the evolved psychological mechanism of language itself undergoes development during human childhood. The pivotal mechanism here is the linkage between the mother and the child, particularly in the first year (Locke, 1993). Although primate mothers are devoted to their young, they do not engage in the types of continual face-to-face vocal interaction that we see from human mothers. Few would doubt the central role of early mother–child bonding. However, in many cultures, after the first year, children are raised by cowives and older siblings. Thus, there is no universal requirement that the mother should be the only person teaching language to the child. Instead, much of language learning after the first year rests on the shoulders of children, who seem to soak up the speech patterns of those around them as if they were linguistic sponges. Of course, the ability to learn language does not terminate during childhood, since we can learn second languages well into adulthood, albeit with a noticeable foreign accent.

Demodularization

Language is grounded on the evolutionary achievements of the past 6 million years. However, once language is available as a method of cognitive representation, cognition itself is fundamentally altered. The most remarkable property of human language is that it has smooth and nearly immediate access to the entire brain. Through this ability to integrate across modalities and modules, language is able to overcome modularity and open up the mind to fully human consciousness. Language relies on the entire brain to achieve its complete cognitive simulation of experience in terms of objects, space, action, and social relations. Because it integrates these separate modules so thoroughly, it allows us to fully escape the modularity that is present in primates (Russon & Bard, 1996) and young children (Hermer-Vazquez, Moffet, & Munkholm, 2001). Without language, it may be possible to focus directly on the position of an object without regard to earlier orientations or the orientations of others. Without language, we can focus on an action without breaking it apart into its component participants. In order to achieve lexicalization, language forces us to analyze experience into its components (Gentner, 1982). Although language forces us to break our experiences into pieces, it provides ways of then recombining these pieces into much larger edifices. Moreover, narrative and discourse allow us to integrate our own experiences more fully with those of others. In this way, language bundles the whole of mental life into a single, more fully conscious, but relatively less grounded whole.

Because language is a human invention, the brain provides us with a great deal of latitude in the way it can be represented. As Wittgenstein (1953) observed, language is a like a well-pruned hedge. Externally, each hedge must look like the others. However, internally, each hedge can have a very different shape. This means that we should not be surprised to find large individual differences in the neuronal basis of higher level dynamic control for language. For example, children with large focal lesions to the left hemisphere areas that typically control language are able to achieve normal language functioning by using parallel areas in the right hemisphere (Booth, MacWhinney, & Harasaki, 2000). Several patterns of reorganization to damage have been identified for young children (MacWhinney, Feldman, Sacco, & Valdes-Perez, 2000), and similar reorganization certainly occurs in adults (Holland et al., 1985). In addition to the flexibility found in patients with brain lesions, there are important individual differences in the way that the brain organizes for language in normally developing speakers. In particular, it is likely that the process of cerebral lateralization operates in very different ways in different children, with some making a sharp separation between the functions of the two hemispheres (Beeman et al., 1994) and others allowing for more redundancy.

The Child's Construction of Social Reality

Although the emergence of systematization in *H. sapiens* required little or no expansion in brain size and only limited reworking of neural connectivity, it has had major consequences for the way in which we use our brains. Vygotsky (1962) showed how language begins as an external social phenomenon and is then internalized to provide the backbone of human cognition. Vygotsky attributed this internalization to the emergence of "inner speech" and compressed forms of reference and topicalization, but provided little additional detail regarding his proposal. Tomasello (1999) and MacWhinney (1999a) extended Vygotsky's analysis by linking language learning to the child's ability to treat others as intentional agents. This assumption of an intentional stance helps the child follow the meaning of the parent when learning new words. Tomasello also shows how intentionality allows the child to construct the representations underlying causal predications. Infants will extend intentionality even to inanimate objects, when they have eyes that represent a face (Gergely, Nádasdy, Csibra, & Bíró, 1997) or even when they do not but appear to have intention (Csibra, Gergely, Bíró, Koos, & Brockbank, 1999). Later, through fictive extensional processes (Lakoff, 1987; Talmy, 1988), children treat even inanimate objects as acting intentionally and causally.

This system of causal representation forms the basis for grammatical processes such as case marking, conflation, passivization, inverse, and causitivization. For example, when listening to the sentence, "The dog the man chased caught the ball," we begin by taking the perspective of the "dog" as the sentence subject. However, when we begin processing the relative clause, we shift our causal perspective to "the man," who then becomes the one who chases the dog. However, once the relative clause is finished, we need to return to the perspective of the dog that is catching the ball. In even such as simple example as this, we can see that the smooth production and comprehension of grammatical structures involves a continual shift between perspectives. In fact, I (MacWhinney, 1999a; in press) argue that grammar arose specifically for the purpose of representing these perspective shifts. It is difficult to imagine how *H. erectus*, without systematized methods for producing words, and without additional grammatical devices for marking perspective shifting, could have achieved anything close to the level of narrative flexibility that *H. sapiens* can achieve through fully grammaticized language.

By providing technical methods for encoding and decoding perspective shifts, grammar allows us to construct increasingly complex social relations. In these relations, we often need to take the perspective of the other and imagine how that person will react to a variety of possible actions that we might perform. In practice, we select the exact shape of a given utterance or action out of a much larger field of potential actions based largely on this act of social perspective taking. Would our utterances offend some particular individual? Would they violate some moral precept? Would we fail to properly articulate our position and therefore leave ourselves open to later misinterpretation? As we compute these various possible scenarios, we use the three lower levels of perspective taking (direct perception, space–time, causal action) to move about in a conceptual space that was constructed through linguistic interactions embedded in a social context. These processes allow us to construct enormously complex, systematic (Levi-Strauss, 1963) views of social structure. Yet the cognitive resources we are using are little more extensive than those available to *H. erectus*. Instead, through the construction of a method for creating new words, we have been able to reuse our mimetic resources to support the full articulation of human culture. In this sense, the appearance of modern language is a paradigm case of an emergent behavior (MacWhinney, 1999b).

Disorders of Communication

Genetic theory would lead us to believe that those adaptations that are most recent should be the ones that are least fully integrated into the human genome. Because the systematization of articulation in the interests of lexical structuring emerged relatively late in evolution, it is not surprising that we find extensive problems in these areas of motor control:

1. Stuttering: a process that involves problems in the activation and coordination of output processes based on individual lexical items.
2. Dysphagia: problems with chewing and swallowing that may reflect some instability in the rewiring of innervation of the vocal tract.
3. Articulation disorders: between the ages of 4 and 8, many children have problems articulating the exact shapes of words. Disorders such as lisping sometimes continue into adulthood.
4. Tongue curling: about 30% of the adult population cannot perform the type of tongue curling or the type of tongue bending needed to properly articulate sounds such as the retroflex stops of Hindi. There are similar problems with the articulation of one of the three Czech *r* sounds.

There is good reason to believe that these disabilities represent incomplete consolidation of recent evolutionary changes. If we then further parcel out cases of mental retardation, autism, fetal damage, and chromosomal abnormalities, we are left with a group of children who are said to have specific language impairment (SLI). The incidence of some form of SLI in the population is often estimated to be about 7%. In the clinic, language disorders are nearly four times more frequent in males than in females (Bishop, 1997). However, epidemiological studies have shown that the actual balance in the population is nearly equally distributed between the sexes (Leonard, 1998). Once we parcel out the children with primarily motor problems and those with serious nonlinguistic impairments, we are left with children who seem to have problems organizing the flow of syntax. Recent studies (Franks & Connell, 1996; van Der Lely & Stollwerk, 1996, 1997) have suggested that children with grammatical disorders have a specific problem with argument chains. Within the context of the current analysis, this could best be viewed as a deficit in the ability to switch perspective. Note that these children are able to shift perspective in simple clauses. It is the processing of complex and multiple-perspective shifts in grammar that causes them problems.

Although some children will display various forms of language disorders, these disorders are never so severe that they fully block the acquisition of human language. This is because the acquisition of language is protected by a system of multiple buffering. Some children may learn through analysis, others through auditory encoding, and still others through direct imitation. If one of these systems is partially blocked, the others can operate. Moreover, there is no human group that does not have language, and the core aspects of language learning, although they may differ somewhat in timing, are essentially universal. Some take this as evidence for a recent evolution of Universal Grammar. I would argue instead that it indicates the extent to which language capitalizes on our shared human nature.

CONCLUSIONS

The study of language evolution has made solid advances in recent years. New evidence from the fossil record, paleoclimatology, genetic analysis, neuroscience, infancy research, and cognitive grammar has fueled these advances. As the database of evidence regarding humans' last 6 million years continues to grow, we will be able to articulate increasingly precise ideas about the coevolution of language, brain, and social processes. Modern human children illustrate the ongoing and dynamic nature of this evolution. To learn language, they depend on systems of imitation, empathy, mimesis, play, articulation, lexicalization, and perspective switching that have developed across millions of years. At the same time, they use language during their own lifetimes to elaborate new cultural objects and ways of thinking.

REFERENCES

Allman, J. R. (1999). *Evolving brains.* New York: Scientific American Library.

Anders, T. (1994). *The origins of evil: An inquiry into the ultimate origins of human suffering.* Chicago: Open Court.

Anderson, J. (1996). Chimpanzees and capuchin monkeys: Comparative cognition. In A. E. Russon, K. A. Bard, & S. T. Parker (Eds.), *Reaching into thought: The minds of the great apes* (pp. 23–56). Cambridge, UK: Cambridge University Press.

Beeman, M., Friedman, R. B., Grafman, J., Perez, E., Diamond, S., & Lindsay, M. B. (1994). Summation priming and coarse coding in the right hemisphere. *Journal of Cognitive Neuroscience, 6,* 26–45.

Bickerton, D. (1990). *Language and species.* Chicago: University of Chicago Press.

Bishop, D. (1997). *Uncommon understanding.* Hove, UK: Psychology Press.

Bjorklund, D., & Pellegrini, A. (2000). Child development and evolutionary psychology. *Child Development, 71,* 1687–1708.

Booth, J. R., MacWhinney, B., & Harasaki, Y. (2000). Developmental differences in visual and auditory processing of complex sentences. *Child Development, 71,* 981–1003.

Bruner, J., & Sherwood, V. (1976). Peekaboo and the learning of rule structures. In J.

Bruner, A. Jolly, & K. Sylva (Eds.), *Play: Its role in development and evolution* (pp. 277–285). New York: Basic Books.

Buss, D. (1999). *Evolutionary psychology: The new science of mind.* Needham Heights, MA: Allyn & Bacon.

Cann, R. L. (1995). Mitochondrial DNA and human evolution. In J.-P. Changeux & J. Chavaillon (Eds.), *Origins of the human brain* (pp. 124–140). Oxford, UK: Clarendon.

Cavalli-Sforza, L. (1991, November). Genes, people, and languages. *Scientific American,* pp. 104–110.

Chomsky, N. (1975). *Reflections on language.* New York: Random House.

Coppens, Y. (1995). Brain, locomotion, diet, and culture: How a primate, by chance, became a man. In J.-P. Changeux & J. Chavaillon (Eds.), *Origins of the human brain* (pp. 4–12). Oxford, UK: Clarendon Press.

Coppens, Y. (1999). Introduction. In T. G. Bromage & F. Schrenk (Eds.), *African biogeography, climate change, and human evolution* (pp. 1–15). New York: Oxford University Press.

Corballis, M. C. (1999). Phylogeny from apes to humans. In M. C. Corballis & S. E. G. Lea (Eds.), *The descent of mind: Psychological perspectives on hominid evolution* (pp. 40–70). Oxford, UK: Oxford University Press.

Csibra, G., Gergely, G., Bíró, S., Koos, O., & Brockbank, M. (1999). Goal attribution without agency cues: The perception of pure reason in infancy. *Cognition, 72,* 237–267.

Darwin, C. (1877). A biographical sketch of an infant. *Mind, 2,* 292–294.

Deacon, T. (1997). *The symbolic species: The co-evolution of language and the brain.* New York: Norton.

Decety, J., Chaminade, T., Grezes, J., & Meltzoff, A. (2002). A PET exploration of the neural mechanisms involved in reciprocal imitation. *Neuroimage, 15,* 265–272.

de Villiers, J. G., & de Villiers, P. (1999). The comprehension of perception verbs by young deaf children. In M. Almgren, A. Barreña, M. Ezeizaberrena, I. Idiazabal, & B. MacWhinney (Eds.), *Research on child language acquisition* (pp. 321–344). Boston: Cascadilla.

de Waal, F. B. M., & Aureli, F. (1996). Consolation, reconciliation, and a possible cognitive difference between macaques and chimpanzees. In A. E. Russon, K. A. Bard, & S. T. Parker (Eds.), *Reaching into thought: The minds of the great apes* (pp. 80–110). Cambridge, UK: Cambridge University Press.

Donald, M. (1991). *Origins of the modern mind.* Cambridge, MA: Harvard University Press.

Dunbar, R. (2000). Causal reasoning, mental rehearsal, and the evolution of primate cognition. In C. Heyes & L. Huber (Eds.), *The evolution of cognition* (pp. 134–166). Cambridge, MA: MIT Press.

Elman, J., Bates, E., Plunkett, K., Johnson, M., & Karmiloff-Smith, A. (1996). *Rethinking innateness.* Cambridge, MA: MIT Press.

Foley, R. (1999). Evolutionary geography of Pliocene African hominids. In T. G. Bromage & F. Schrenk (Eds.), *African biogeography, climate change, and human evolution* (pp. 328–348). New York: Oxford University Press.

Franks, S. L., & Connell, P. J. (1996). Knowledge of binding in normal and SLI children. *Journal of Child Language, 23,* 431–464.

Gabrieli, J. D. E., Brewer, J. B., Desmond, J. E., & Glover, G. H. (1997). Separate neural bases of two fundamental memory processes in the human medial temporal lobe. *Science, 276,* 264–266.

Gentner, D. (1982). Why nouns are learned before verbs: Linguistic relativity versus natural partitioning. In S. Kuczaj (Ed.), *Language development: Language, culture, and cognition* (pp. 301–334). Hillsdale, NJ: Erlbaum.

Gergely, G., Nádasdy, Z., Csibra, G., & Bíró, S. (1997). Taking the intentional stance at 12 months of age. *Cognition, 56,* 165–193.

Gershkoff-Stowe, L., Thal, D. J., Smith, L. B., & Namy, L. L. (1997). Categorization and its developmental relation to early language. *Child Development, 68,* 843–859.

Gibson, J. J. (1977). The theory of affordances. In R. E. Shaw & J. Bransford (Eds.), *Perceiving, acting, and knowing: Toward an ecological psychology* (pp. 67–82). Hillsdale, NJ: Erlbaum.

Givón, T. (1998). On the co-evolution of language, mind and brain. *Evolution of Communication, 2,* 45–116.

Gomez, J. C. (1996). Ostensive behavior in great apes: The role of eye contact. In A. E. Russon, K. A. Bard, & S. T. Parker (Eds.), *Reaching into thought: The minds of the great apes* (pp. 131–151). Cambridge, UK: Cambridge University Press.

Goodale, M. A. (1993). Visual pathways supporting perception and action in the primate cerebral cortex. *Current Opinion in Neurobiology, 3,* 578–585.

Goodall, J. (1979). Life and death at Gombe. *National Geographic, 155,* 592–620.

Gupta, P., & MacWhinney, B. (1997). Vocabulary acquisition and verbal short-term memory: Computational and neural bases. *Brain and Language, 59,* 267–333.

Hauser, M., Chomsky, N., & Fitch, T. (2002). The faculty of language: What is it, who has it, and how did it evolve? *Science, 298,* 1569–1579.

Hauser, M., Newport, E., & Aslin, R. (2001). Segmentation of the speech stream in a non-human primate: Statistical learning in cotton-top tamarins. *Cognition, 78,* B53–B64.

Hermer-Vazquez, L., Moffet, A., & Munkholm, P. (2001). Language, space, and the development of cognitive flexibility in humans: The case of two spatial memory tasks. *Cognition, 79,* 263–299.

Hockett, C. F. (1960, September). The origin of speech. *Scientific American,* pp. 6–12.

Hockett, C. F., & Altmann, S. A. (1973). A note on design features. In T. A. Sebeok (Ed.), *Animal communication* (pp. 61–72). Bloomington: Indiana University Press.

Hockett, C. F., & Ascher, R. (1964). The human revolution. *Current Anthropology, 5,* 135–167.

Holland, A., Miller, J., Reinmuth, O., Bartlett, C., Fromm, D., Pashek, G., et al. (1985). Rapid recovery from aphasia: A detailed language analysis. *Brain and Language, 24,* 156–173.

Holloway, R. (1995). Toward a synthetic theory of human brain evolution. In J.-P. Changeux & J. Chavaillon (Eds.), *Origins of the human brain* (pp. 42–60). Oxford, UK: Clarendon Press.

Ingmanson, E. J. (1996). Tool-using behavior in wild *Pan paniscus*: Social and ecological considerations. In A. E. Russon, K. A. Bard, & S. T. Parker (Eds.), *Reaching into thought: The minds of the great apes* (pp. 190–210). New York: Cambridge University Press.

Julesz, B., & Kovacs, I. (Eds.). (1995). *Maturational windows and cortical plasticity.* Wesley, MA: Addison-Wesley.

Jürgens, U. (1979). Neural control of vocalization in nonhuman primates. In H. D. Steklis & M. J. Raleigh (Eds.), *Neurobiology of social communication in primates* (pp. 82–98). New York: Academic Press.

Konishi, M. (1995). A sensitive period for birdsong learning. In B. Julesz & I. Kovacs (Eds.), *Maturational windows and adult cortical plasticity* (pp. 87–92). New York: Addison-Wesley.

Kuhl, P. K., & Miller, J. D. (1978). Speech perception by the chinchilla: Identification functions for synthetic VOT stimuli. *Journal of the Acoustical Society of America, 63*, 905–917.

Lakoff, G. (1987). *Women, fire, and dangerous things.* Chicago: University of Chicago Press.

Leonard, L. (1998). *Children with specific language impairment.* Cambridge, MA: MIT Press.

Levi-Strauss, C. (1963). *Structural anthropology.* New York: Basic Books.

Lieberman, P. (1973). On the evolution of language: A unified view. *Cognition, 2*, 59–94.

Lieberman, P. (1975). *On the origins of language: An introduction to the evolution of human speech.* New York: Macmillan.

Locke, J. (1993). *The child's path to spoken language.* Cambridge, MA: Harvard University Press.

Locke, J. (1995). Development of the capacity for spoken language. In P. Fletcher & B. MacWhinney (Eds.), *The handbook of child language* (pp. 278–302). Oxford, UK: Blackwell.

MacLarnon, A., & Hewitt, G. (1999). The evolution of human speech. *American Journal of Physical Anthropology, 109*, 341–363.

MacNeilage, P. (1998). The frame/content theory of evolution of speech production. *Behavioral and Brain Sciences, 21*, 499–546.

MacWhinney, B. (1975). Pragmatic patterns in child syntax. *Stanford Papers and Reports on Child Language Development, 10*, 153–165.

MacWhinney, B. (1982). Basic syntactic processes. In S. Kuczaj (Ed.), *Language acquisition: Vol. 1. Syntax and semantics* (pp. 73–136). Hillsdale, NJ: Erlbaum.

MacWhinney, B. (1999a). The emergence of language from embodiment. In B. MacWhinney (Ed.), *The emergence of language* (pp. 213–256). Mahwah, NJ: Erlbaum.

MacWhinney, B. (Ed.). (1999b). *The emergence of language.* Mahwah, NJ: Erlbaum.

MacWhinney, B. (in press). The emergence of grammar from perspective. In D. Pecher & R. A. Zwaan (Eds.), *The grounding of cognition: The role of perception and action in memory, language, and thinking.* Mahwah, NJ: Erlbaum.

MacWhinney, B., Feldman, H. M., Sacco, K., & Valdes-Perez, R. (2000). Online measures of basic language skills in children with early focal brain lesions. *Brain and Language, 71*, 400–431.

McManus, I. C. (1999). Handedness, cerebral lateralization, and the evolution of language. In M. C. Corballis & S. E. G. Lea (Eds.), *The descent of mind: Psychological perspectives on hominid evolution* (pp. 194–217). Oxford, UK: Oxford University Press.

McNeill, D. (1985). So you think gestures are nonverbal? *Psychological Review, 92*, 350–371.

Meltzoff, A. N. (1988). Infant imitation and memory: Nine-month-olds in immediate and deferred tests. *Child Development, 59*, 217–225.

Menn, L., & Stoel-Gammon, C. (1995). Phonological development. In P. Fletcher & B. MacWhinney (Eds.), *The handbook of child language* (pp. 335–360). Oxford, UK: Blackwell.

Menzel, E. (1973). Chimpanzee spatial memory organization. *Science, 182,* 943–945.

Menzel, E. (1975). Purposive behavior as a basis for objective communication between chimpanzee. *Science, 189,* 652–654.

Miikkulainen, R. (1990). A distributed feature map model of the lexicon. In *Proceedings of the 12th Annual Conference of the Cognitive Science Society* (pp. 447–454). Hillsdale, NJ: Erlbaum.

Miller, G. (2001). *The mating mind: How sexual choice shaped the evolution of human nature.* New York: Anchor.

Mithen, S. (1996). *The prehistory of the mind: The cognitive origins of art, religion, and science.* London: Thames & Hudson.

Morgan, E. (1997). *The aquatic ape hypothesis.* London: Souvenir Press.

Moskovitch, M., Winocur, G., & Behrmann, M. (1997). What is special about face recognition? *Journal of Cognitive Neuropsychology, 9,* 555–604.

Myers, R. E. (1976). Origins and evolution of language and speech. *Annals of the New York Academy of Sciences, 280,* 745–757.

Nauta, W. J. H., & Karten, H. J. (1970). A general profile of the vertebrate brain, with sidelights on the ancestry of cerebral cortex. In G. C. Quarton, T. Melnechuck, & G. Adelman (Eds.), *The neurosciences* (pp. 7–26). New York: Rockefeller University Press.

Nettle, D., & Dunbar, R. (1997). Social markers and the evolution of reciprocal exchange. *Current Anthropology, 38,* 93–99.

Pandya, D. P., Seltzer, B., & Barbas, H. (1988). Input-out organization of the primate cerebral cortex. In H. Steklis & J. Irwin (Eds.), *Comparative primate biology: Neurosciences* (pp. 38–80). New York: Liss.

Pinker, S., & Bloom, P. (1990). Natural language and natural selection. *Behavioral and Brain Sciences, 13,* 707–784.

Ploog, D. W. (1992). Neuroethological perspectives on the human brain: From the expression of emotions to intentional signing and speech. In A. Harrington (Ed.), *So human a brain: Knowledge and values in the neurosciences* (pp. 3–13). Boston: Birkhauser.

Povinelli, D. J., & Cant, J. G. H. (1995). Arboreal clambering and the evolution of self-conception. *Quarterly Journal of Biology, 70,* 393–421.

Ramachandran, V. S., & Hubbard, E. M. (2001). Synaesthesia: A window into perception, thought and language. *Journal of Consciousness Studies, 8,* 3–34.

Rizzolatti, G., Fadiga, L., Gallese, V., & Fogassi, L. (1996). Premotor cortex and the recognition of motor actions. *Cognitive Brain Research, 3,* 131–141.

Russon, A. E., & Bard, K. A. (1996). Exploring the minds of the great apes: Issues and controversies. In A. E. Russon & K. A. Bard (Eds.), *Reaching into thought: The minds of the great apes* (pp. 1–22). New York: Cambridge University Press.

Savage-Rumbaugh, S. (2000). Linguistic, cultural and cognitive capacities of bonobos (*Pan paniscus*). *Culture and Psychology, 6,* 131–153.

Seyfarth, R., & Cheney, D. (1999). Production, usage, and response in nonhuman primate vocal development. In M. Hauser & M. Konishi (Eds.), *Neural mechanisms of communication* (pp. 57–83). Cambridge, MA: MIT Press.

Stanford, C. (2003). *Upright: The evolutionary key to becoming human.* New York: Houghton Mifflin.

Stringer, C., & McKie, R. (1996). *African exodus*. London: Pimlico.

Talmy, L. (1988). Force dynamics in language and cognition. *Cognitive Science, 12,* 59–100.

Templeton, A. R. (1992). Human origins and analysis of mitochondrial DNA sequences. *Science, 255,* 737–740.

Tomasello, M. (1999). *The cultural origins of human communication.* New York: Cambridge University Press.

Tomasello, M. (2000). Do young children have adult syntactic competence? *Cognition, 74,* 209–253.

Trevarthen, C. (1984). Biodynamic structures, cognitive correlates of motive sets and the development of motives in infants. In W. Prinz & A. F. Sanders (Eds.), *Cognition and motor processes* (pp. 327–350). Berlin: Springer.

Tucker, D. (2001). Embodied meaning: An evolutionary–developmental analysis of adaptive semantics. In T. Givón (Ed.), *The evolution of language* (pp. 51–72). Philadelphia: Benjamins.

van Der Lely, H., & Stollwerk, L. (1997). Binding theory and grammatical specific language impairment in children. *Cognition, 62,* 245–290.

van der Lely, H. K. J., & Stollwerk, L. (1996). A grammatical specific language impairment in children: An autosomal dominant inheritance? *Brain and Language, 52,* 484–504.

Visalberghi, E., & Limongelli, L. (1996). Acting and undertanding: Tool use revisited through the minds of capuchin monkeys. In A. E. Russon, K. A. Bard, & S. T. Parker (Eds.), *Reaching into thought: The minds of the great apes* (pp. 57–79). Cambridge: Cambridge University Press.

Vygotsky, L. (1962). *Thought and language.* Cambridge, MA: MIT Press.

Wittgenstein, L. (1953). *Philosophical investigations.* Oxford, UK: Blackwell.

Yerkes, R. M., & Learned, B. W. (1925). *Chimpanzee intelligence and its vocal expressions.* Baltimore: Williams & Wilkins.

16

THE EVOLUTIONARY HISTORY OF AN ILLUSION

Religious Causal Beliefs in Children and Adults

JESSE M. BERING

> We shall tell ourselves that it would be very nice if there were a God who
> created the world and was a benevolent Providence, and if there were a
> moral order in the universe and an after-life; but it is a very striking fact that
> all this is exactly as we are bound to wish it to be. And it would be more
> remarkable still if our wretched, ignorant and downtrodden ancestors had
> succeeded in solving all these difficult riddles of the universe.
> —FREUD (1928/1961, p. 42)

Although recently there have been a few voices of dissent, most evolutionists
tend to agree that religion is *not* an adaptation, at least not in the sense that
we might speak of mate retention or reciprocal altruism as adaptations. Perhaps more so than other important human activities, religion frequently is
denounced as being a by-product of some other capacity, whether this capacity is as general as consciousness or even a "big brain" (Gould, 1991), or more
specific capacities such as anthropomorphism (Guthrie, 1993) or agency
detection (Barrett, 2000). Alternatively, religious beliefs are treated as causal
epiphenomena—unimportant, posthoc explanations for adaptive behaviors
(e.g., "The devil made me do it") (e.g., Daly & Wilson, 1988). Theorists have
taken religion to mean quite different things, however; some writers emphasize ritualistic behaviors (McCauley & Lawson, 2002; Whitehouse, 2000),
whereas others speak of attributional or attachment styles (Kirkpatrick, 1998;
Lupfer, Tolliver, & Jackson, 1996); finally, others seem to refer to religion as
a generic category of superstitious activities (Dawkins, 1998). Such a confusion of terms has led to a confusion of theory. Investigating the "adaptive ori-

gins of religion" simply will not work: Just like any complex human behavioral trait, religion must be dissected into its critical parts (Atran, 2002; Boyer, 2001; Hinde, 1999). It is at this level that we will find adaptive mechanisms, should they exist.

An important point I wish to stress straightaway, therefore, is that I take existential meaning to be *the* essential pivot upon which religion, as either a sociocultural or a private phenomenon, necessarily revolves. The self can scarcely help but envision the unique events that it experiences as happening for some special reason—*that there are "lessons" or "messages" to be had in the random vicissitudes of human life.* In other words, natural asocial changes in the environment are treated as potential sources of social information. As such, here, I evaluate the possibility of an information-processing system that serves to lend communicative meaning to otherwise *meaningless* natural events and that such a system is a powerful causal force behind adaptive human behavior. Importantly, I view this system as having been specially designed through traditional routes of natural selection and contingent on ancient epigenetic pathways characterizing normal patterns of human development.

"IT MUST BE A SIGN FROM GOD": THE OVERGENERALIZATION OF PSYCHOLOGICAL CAUSATION

Scholarly approaches to religion have tended to support the position that supernatural beliefs are the result of epistemological limitations. This is best captured by the aptly titled *God-of-the-gaps hypothesis* (Coulson, 1955), the idea that what cannot be explained by mere human minds is attributed by default to the workings of the gods. Yet just why is not there a universal proclivity toward biological or mechanical explanations rather than intentional explanations when filling in such epistemic gaps—why is the latter necessarily *easier*? When we are diagnosed with a fatal illness, or when our car breaks down on a deserted road in the middle of a pounding rainstorm, why do we feel that uncompromising urge to blame God (or perhaps some other supernatural figure, such as a dead loved one) or to appeal to supernatural agents for help? Why is not our first emotional impulse not more "useful"—after all, would such affect not be better directed at searching for a cure for our fatal illness? Would we not be better off saddling our hostility in the wake of this inauspicious breakdown and calmly searching for the mechanical cause of our car's trouble? In addition, religious beliefs are by no means limited to naive folk. Individuals who have achieved high levels of scientific education and training may give very sophisticated, logical, and scientific causal explanations of events, all the while harboring attributions to some supernatural agent—seeing certain events as carrying a "deeper" meaning or happening for some special purpose.

This tremendous difficulty in ridding our minds of a "demon-haunted world" has been the source of great angst, even hostility, for some evolutionary biologists bothered by the laity's shallow knowledge of natural selection (Dawkins, 1986, 1998). In spirit, this antireligious verve was shared by the psychoanalytic theories of Freud (1928/1961), who believed that religious ideas were simple, irrational wish fulfillments. Along with a growing number of my colleagues, however, I believe strongly that this is the wrong way to go about dealing with the "problem" of religion. Without making any theological claims, it is simply stating an empirical truth to say that the mind is geared toward the idea of supernatural agents, or at least toward the notion of some abstract intentional agency that communicates messages (i.e., colloquially, "signs") in the guise of natural events. In this light, we might begin to reveal at least a central aspect of religion for what it truly is—a brain-based biological phenomenon that employs human cognitive mechanisms in understandable and organized ways. Like any other human psychological trait, the idea of supernatural agency should not be exorcised from human minds by scientists with sociopolitical agendas, but carefully studied as a way of understanding what it means to be human.

In this chapter, the conceptual issue I wish to explore is the evolution of supernatural agency; more properly, the evolutionary and developmental origins of the human cognitive capacity to explain certain events and experiences as having been caused by an abstract intentional agent (e.g., gods, spirits, demons, ancestral relatives, etc.). At what age do children begin to see the natural events inevitably spilling into their perceptual construals as something other than natural events—as *standing for* something else? Symbolic events can be those that occur in the *biological* (e.g., being diagnosed with cancer), *physical* (e.g., a rainbow on one's birthday), or *social* (e.g., running into a long-lost relative at the supermarket) domains (Bering, 2003). Why do individuals throughout the world step outside of proprietary causal domains, and seem to defer to a supernatural agent when accounting for the causes of such events? There is even evidence that self-proclaimed nonreligious individuals routinely appeal to some abstract intentional agency in accounting for the causes of ironic or life-altering events, for example, through fatalistic judgments or by claiming that a given event was or was not *meant to be* (Deridder, Hendriks, Zani, Pepitone, & Saffioti, 1999; Pepitone & Saffioti, 1997; Weeks & Lupfer, 2000). By all accounts, it requires a great deal of cognitive effort to view the world as devoid of meaning and intent; at an intuitive level, it may be altogether impossible to do so (McCauley, 2000). Even the atheist's God seems to bite through its muzzle from time to time.

This pattern of reasoning, I believe, is inexorably tied to several core areas of cognitive development, such as the formation of a sense of self, moral reasoning, and ontogenetic advances in social communication. As such, I argue that evolutionary scholars must look to children if they wish to discover *how* supernatural beliefs become conceptually organized in individual minds, and also to discover *why* individuals within certain ontogenetic periods may be more susceptible to such beliefs than those in other periods of the lifespan. In addition, I argue that human psychology is divisible into *adaptive systems* that are comprised of both "new" (i.e., human cognitive specializations, qualitatively distinct from the minds of other species because they diverged *after* hominids separated from the human–great ape ancestor) and "old" (i.e., cognitive mechanisms that humans share with other primate species as products of a common ancestry) psychological functions, and that this distinction can be found with regard to religion.

SOME IMPORTANT THEORETICAL POINTS CONCERNING THE ORIGINS OF SUPERNATURAL ATTRIBUTION

Among the most heated and controversial issues in evolutionary psychology is the debate surrounding the theoretical grounds for labeling various cognitive mechanisms *adaptations*, particularly those mechanisms that are seemingly side effects, or by-products, of more general psychological systems (Andrews, Gangestad, & Matthews, 2002; Buss, Haselton, Shackelford, Bleske, & Wakefield, 1998). Also at issue are those originally functionless characteristics that were apparently co-opted by environmental conditions impinging on human behavior *after* some critical period of evolutionary adaptedness, the time period envisioned to have molded the standard cognitive hardware of the human brain.

Despite having good reason to argue that any given trait confers selective advantages *now*, we may lack evidence that the environment in the ancestral past similarly favored organisms equipped with such traits, the *sine qua non* of evolutionary functionalism. As an insulin-dependent diabetic, I have discovered that other individuals are prone to affording me numerous advantages in competitive social situations, and these handicaps may very well have translated into fitness effects that I otherwise might not have had. Nevertheless, it would be quite unreasonable to claim that diabetes mellitus is an adaptation!

Because natural selection is not forward-looking, any given trait can be adaptive without being an adaptation; one of the important tasks of evolutionary psychologists has involved discriminating between just these two cases. Pundits have cited the ease by which so-called adaptationists have lapsed into "just so" stories, referencing evolutionary psychologists' tendency to invent clever teleological accounts of human psychological traits just as Rudyard Kipling did for his characters in his famous *Just So Stories*, such as the story of "The Elephant's Child," in which a young elephant originally in possession of a "mere-smear nose" had its small nostrum elongated by a crocodile to help it swat flies and to spank others with its new trunk.

In fact, evolutionary psychologists have set increasingly high standards for diagnosing psychological traits as adaptations and arguably are even more adamant in restricting this label to its proper domain than are their critics. As is the case for any rigorous empirical science, progress in the field of evolutionary psychology is dependent on an accumulation of diverse data, experimentally supported and continually shifting theoretical frameworks, and the critical evaluation of other researchers' work in narrow and specialized areas of study that oftentimes disagree staunchly as to the validity of various evolutionary and phylogenetic claims (see Andrews et al., 2002).

To some extent, the present topic (generally, "religion") has fallen prey to the opposite theoretical fallacy from the aforementioned case in which psychological traits displaying adaptive utility *now* are mistaken for psychological traits that were useful in the *ancestral past*. Rather, in the case of supernatural agency, psychological traits that likely displayed adaptive utility in the ancestral past, and given similar environmental conditions to those found in ancestral conditions therefore continue to be expressed, are mistaken for nonadaptive traits because their current expression is strongly influenced by different epigenetic processes. In other words, because most modern human minds are now shaped by a confluence of factors that were unheard of in the period of evolutionary adaptedness, investigative strategies that rely solely on reverse-engineering the modern mind are problematic. Although naturalistic explanations for life events may have been one mode of explanatory theorizing in the ancestral past, just as it is for modern hunter–gatherers, it is unlikely that in the absence of a sociocultural emphasis on naturalistic and scientific causality our ancestors were intuitive realists. Rather, in what follows, I argue that intentionality (i.e., "aboutness") was—*and is*—the default explanatory mode in the "existential domain" just as it is in the social domain, and that current social conditions favoring naturalistic explanations for life events conflict with the innate architecture of the developing mind. Nevertheless, such conditions have likely resulted in a cognitive profile somewhat distinct from that of our ancestors. In a word, advances in empirical science and the cultural recurrence of organized pedagogical infrastructures that are explicitly designed to communicate these advances to children have made modern minds less *superstitious* than they once were—at least in principle.

Although I would stop somewhere short of claiming that religion can be *reduced* to existential meaning, I view the capacity to search for reasons for having certain life experiences to be religion's most important psychological feature. The capacity to attribute psychological causes to otherwise random events, such as illness, death, drought, or famine, may be a distinctively human specialization, because it is enabled by an intentionality system, a system that may be altogether unique to humans. Reasoning that a supernatural agent intentionally brought about such events requires the general capacity to reason about mental states. One might believe, for instance, that he or she is diagnosed with cancer because God is *punishing* him or her for some long-forgotten sin; a rainbow on a child's birthday may be interpreted as her recently deceased grandfather's way of telling her that he is *enjoying* the festivities; and a woman might believe that she ran into her long-lost stepbrother at the supermarket because her deceased stepmother *wanted* her to reconcile with him. Although it is tempting to stop here and claim that supernatural attributions represent merely an interesting by-product of a theory of mind, which evolved solely to explain and to predict the actions of social others, I suspect that this is an inadequate interpretation. Having a theory of mind is a necessary, but not sufficient, condition for finding communicative meaning (i.e., "signs") in natural events.

Contributing to my suspicion are the following characteristics that are associated with such causal ascriptions: (1) Reporting that there is *communicative meaning* in natural events occurs cross-culturally, and is perhaps even universal; (2) recent evidence suggests that the capacity to find such meaning in events is *developmentally based*, and is not necessarily coemergent with a theory of mind in the social domain; (3) such attributions are *made in response to events*, and are instantiated in the absence of those sorts of behavioral cues (e.g., eye gaze, facial expressions) envisioned to offset and fine-tune traditional theory of mind modules or systems; (4) the event types that trigger supernatural attributions appear to possess *recurrent and predictable profiles* (e.g., unexpected occurrences or deviations from canonical scripts, ability to produce high-affect responses or counterfactual thoughts); and, (5) perhaps most important to evolutionary analysis, attributing life events to the intentions of supernatural agents may serve a *moral regulatory function*, endorsing cooperation between group members and encouraging the behavioral inhibition of socially proscribed actions.

Together, these characteristics, which I describe shortly in more detail, raise the possibility that the capacity (and drive) to find meaning in the occurrence of personal events and experiences is part of a complex system that is sufficiently rule-driven and regular to warrant an investigation into its adaptive origins. Of course, such a causal explanatory system may appear to operate by design, but to qualify as an adaptation, it must be demonstrated as having likely enhanced genetic success in the ancestral past, a task that can be approximated by subjecting modern human minds to carefully controlled experiments capable of disconfirming clearly stated evolutionary hypotheses. Although most of the critical experimental work in this area has yet to be done, I present some preliminary findings from my laboratory that indirectly speak to the ontogenetic unfolding of a human psychological system that may be devoted to seeing random natural events as communicative signs from supernatural agents. First, however, I present some recent findings of children's religious beliefs more generally.

THE RARITY OF "LITTLE ATHEISTS": A BRIEF DEVELOPMENTAL ACCOUNT OF RELIGIOUS BELIEFS

Not long ago, I encountered a well-educated, middle-aged woman who was distressed over her atheistic 6-year-old daughter. The woman, in her own words, was not "terribly religious" herself, but she did claim to believe that there was *"something, somewhere* that had an interest in their lives." What was especially disconcerting to this mother was that her young daughter was irreverent and perhaps even sacrilegious when it came to religious matters, and this had become very embarrassing for the entire family. Once they had attended a funeral, and when the pastor presiding over the services mentioned how pleased the dead man must be to look down from above and to see how many people cared about him, the young girl erupted in laughter. When the mother, mortified, asked her daughter what on earth was so funny, the little girl simply said that it was on behalf of the pastor's stupidity that she laughed: "doesn't he know that that man is dead?" she exclaimed wide-eyed, pointing at the coffin. "D-E-A-D!" Although the mother had never pondered the existence of life after death too deeply, she was flabbergasted at her daughter's seemingly callous feelings on the matter. Perhaps, thought the mother, it was her own lackadaisical attitude toward religion that had thrown her daughter's spiritual development "off track." She therefore began taking the little girl to the local church and enrolled her in Sunday school, only to observe the child, like "Zarathustra's spawn herself," standing atop one of the church's pews in the middle of a sermon and demanding from the congregation proof of "this God" of whom they all seemed to be so fond.

If the foregoing case seems hard to swallow, it is because this 6-year-old nonbeliever is a figment of my imagination. She does not exist; nor are we likely, I would argue, to discover her real-world counterpart. Atheists are probably far more plentiful in foxholes than in first-grade classrooms. My sole purpose for presenting this fictitious case was to help illustrate how deeply engrained are our expectations for young children's religious behaviors and beliefs. The story of this "little atheist" violates our expectations on several grounds. First, the child displayed inappropriate social conduct and, even worse, called the beliefs of the significant majority into question and thus marked herself as a social dissident. Second, although we may be accustomed periodically to encountering adolescents and adults with explicit, perhaps inflammatory, antireligious sentiments, our experiences with young children do not readily call to mind their tendency for intentional sacrilege. Third, if anything, our experiences with young children inform us that it is the mother's modest belief system that would be distressing to her young child; for instance, the story might have been intuitively more pleasing had the child asked her mother questions about where the dead man went after he died, or what God was supposed to look like, and so on. Finally, what might have struck readers as odd about the little atheist in the foregoing example is that she held the existence of God up to the same standards of evidence that she might for any verifiable entity. She demanded *proof*. We are said to "lose our faith" the older we get—not to acquire it with time. Furthermore, adults who have "lost their faith" are often derogated as unfortunate victims of their own skepticism, and regaining their sense of spiritual belief, their "childhood innocence," is popularly viewed as a vast improvement of their character. (Among many scientists, "spiritual growth" may be something of an oxymoron, but this is certainly not the case among most individuals.) In general, how many 6-

year-olds have we encountered that actively resisted the religious indoctrina-tion of adults, boldly declaring that belief in God is superstitious and belief in life after death, irrational?

In fact, a small corpus of new research findings suggests that young chil-dren are all too ready to endorse religious beliefs. Indeed, it may not even be a stretch to say that they are *prepared* to do so. For example, in a number of influential studies with both British and American children, Kelemen (2003, 2004; see also Evans, 2001) has shown that young children readily extend teleological–functional explanations not only to artifacts (e.g., chairs are *for sitting*) and biological entities (e.g., eyes are *for seeing*) but also to natural inanimate entities, such as rocks and clouds (e.g., rocks are *pointy so that ani-mals wouldn't sit on them and smash them*). This "promiscuous teleology" seems to suggest that young children come into the world equipped with a mind to detect intentional design, even where no such design may exist. Such findings have prompted Kelemen (2004) tentatively to label children "intuitive theists." Indeed, many children in teleology studies come to carry this abstrac-tion toward the postulation of an explicit agent who mindfully designed the properties of the natural world, mentioning God by name. Kelemen empha-sizes that ambient religiosity seems not so much at issue, given predomi-nant leanings among British adults toward naturalistic origins explanations: "[These British findings] . . . weigh against interpretations that promiscuous teleological intuitions are a simple reflection of the relatively pronounced cul-tural religiosity or 'religious exceptionalism' of the United States" (p. 296).

Barrett, Richert, and Dreisenga (2001) presented complementary evi-dence of an intuitive theism in young children. These authors argue that chil-dren's understanding of God's mental states *precedes* their understanding of other social agents' minds, because the former is represented as having infalli-ble knowledge (i.e., omniscience) and thus does not require a "full-blown" theory of mind. In Barrett et al.'s studies, children between the ages of 3 and 8 years were presented with two nonhuman agent puppets and one human: a monkey, a kitty cat, and a girl named Maggie. They were informed that one of these agents, the kitty cat, had a special property of perception that allowed it to see in the dark. Children were then shown a shoe box with a small opening at the top and asked to look inside; all children reported that they could see nothing. Once a flashlight illuminated the inside of the box through another opening, however, children revealed that there was in fact a red block inside. Children were then asked what each of the puppets would see if they were to look inside of the darkened box without the flashlight. In addition, they were asked what God would think the box contained. Consistent with previ-ous findings on the perspective-taking limitations of young children, the preschool-age children tended to report that Maggie would be able to see the block, despite the darkness; not until age 5 did children reason correctly that Maggie would not be able to see inside of the darkened box. These older chil-dren also generalized such perceptual limitations to the monkey, but reasoned that the kitty cat could in fact see the block. However, "without receiving any training from the experimenter, children at all ages tended to report that God would see the block, thereby supporting the claim that children do not represent God as just another person but rather understand God as a meaningfully different sort of agent with some nonhuman properties" (Barrett et al., 2001, pp. 59–60). Because "getting God right" does not require the capacity to attribute false beliefs to others, but rather only to generalize one's own knowledge to another agent, Barrett et al. concluded that "children may be better prepared to conceptualize the properties of God than for understanding humans" (p. 60).

Such findings seem to provide a developmental mechanism of support for Pascal Boyer's (2001) claim that supernatural agents are nearly always represented as "full-access strategic agents." That is, they are envisioned as possessing knowledge of socially strategic information, having unlimited perceptual access to socially maligned behaviors that occur in private and therefore outside the perceptual boundaries of everyday human agents. Citing a wealth of anthropological evidence, Boyer argues that humans intuitively view culturally prevailing supernatural agents as "knowing what we're up to," despite the fact that we might pull off proscribed behaviors without other members of our social group being any the wiser. Importantly, what information happens to be strategic will vary as a function of both the sociocultural environment and specific social contexts; what is ghastly and sinful in one society, leading to severe social repercussions if detected, may be quite the norm in another. (I have more to say about this particular issue later on.) Likewise, what is irrelevant, uninteresting information for one person (e.g., why would God be interested in the fact that you are wearing a red-and-white-striped shirt?) may be strategic social information for another (e.g., you visited my home the other night, and the shirt is identical to the one missing from my bureau).

But just where do children get the idea of supernatural agents to begin with? Unfortunately (or fortunately!), because children are not raised in cultural vacuums, this is a perfectly confounded question. Although it may well be that children spontaneously construct their own pidgin religions in the absence of a steady diet of cultural religious concepts, there are simply no such societies in which explicit concepts of this sort are not part of the developmental histories of children. *All* children hear tales, whether in the spirit of absolute zealotry or mocking derision, whether through participation in a sober ritual or through their peers' word of mouth, of particular supernatural agents. *All* children are exposed to culturally specific religious ideas. You would find a lot of discrepancies among the responses of an average sample of American preschoolers asked who God is—this one might have gotten his information from his grandfather the rabbi; that one might have heard about God from watching football players on television huddled in prayer before the big game—but one thing is certain: You are not likely to find a single child who shrugs his shoulders, asking "Who?" Likewise, although there may well be cultural mechanisms by which particular supernatural agent concepts are transmitted to individual children's minds, for instance, through an intuitive attraction and enhanced memory for concepts that violate core ontological assumptions, such as a person who is invisible (e.g., an ancestral relative), or an inanimate object that has emotions (e.g., a statue of the Virgin Mary), it is hardly evident that children's cognitive systems would fail to generate supernatural agent concepts *anyway*, even without hearing *any* talk about religion. Taylor (1999) has shown, for instance, that children frequently create invisible friends that seem entirely of their own imagination.

When it comes to the development of afterlife beliefs, young children appear spontaneously to generate inferences about the continued existence of consciousness after death, and this may be fully independent of their particular religious training on the topic. In fact, the evidence in this area is inconsistent with an indoctrination model positing that children believe in life after death because of cultural influences that implant such beliefs in young, naive minds. Rather, children's afterlife beliefs actually *decrease* over time, and therefore over prolonged periods of socioreligious exposure to such concepts.

In a series of experiments by Bering and Bjorklund (2004; see also Bering, Hernández- Blasi, & Bjorklund, 2003), children between the ages of 4 and 12 years were presented with a puppet show in which an anthropomorphized mouse character was introduced in the context of a story (i.e., "the mouse is lost in the woods, trying to find his way home . . . "). Importantly, the narrative script included information about the mouse's occurrent psychological states, including *epistemic* (e.g., "the mouse is *thinking* about his mother"), *desire* (e.g., "the mouse *wants* to go home"), *emotional* (e.g., "the mouse is *sad* that he can't find his way home"), *perceptual* (e.g., "the mouse can *hear* the birds singing"), and *psychobiological* (e.g., "the mouse is *thirsty*") states. After children heard this story about the mouse, an alligator puppet lurking in the bushes crept out and ate the mouse. Children watched as the mouse was "eaten" by the alligator and were told that the mouse "is not alive anymore." Children were then asked a standardized, counterbalanced series of questions about the psychological status of the dead mouse. "Now that the mouse is not alive anymore, is he still *thinking* about his mother? [*wants* to go home? *sad* that he can't find his way home? etc.]." Responses to such queries were classified as reflecting either *continuity reasoning* (i.e., the child reasoned that the specific capacity for the psychological state in question, for example, the capacity to think, continued after death) or *discontinuity reasoning* (i.e., the child reasoned that the specific capacity for the psychological state in question discontinued after death).

The pattern of findings revealed a developmental trend whereby preschool-age children reason that dead agents possess a full complement of mental abilities after death; with increasing age, children become more likely to assert that psychobiological and perceptual states are "extinguished," while emotional, epistemic, and desire states continue (see Figure 16.1). Importantly, however, even preschoolers understand that biological functions cease to operate at death, with the majority, for instance, stating that once something is dead, it does not need to eat or drink—even that its brain stops working!

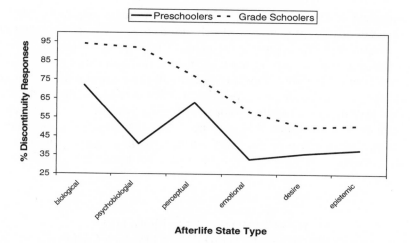

FIGURE 16.1. Percentage of participants within each age group who stated that biological imperatives and the different categories of psychological states stop at death. Each category consisted of several questions about the dead story character: *biological* (e.g., "Does his brain still work?"); *psychobiological* (e.g., "Is he still hungry?"); *perceptual* (e.g., "Can he see where he is?"); *desire* (e.g., "Does he want to go home?"); *emotional* (e.g., "Does he still love his mom?"); and *epistemic* (e.g., "Does he know that he's not alive?").

But they do not seem to tie this biological knowledge together with attendant subjective states until grade school; the same child who appears dumbfounded that an experimenter would be so naive as to ask whether a dead mouse would need to drink water ("of course not!") is one who avers with great sobriety that the dead mouse is still thirsty.

In a modified study with adults, even those individuals who classified themselves as "nonbelievers" found it difficult (as measured by their verbal judgments and response latencies) to deny a dead human character the capacity to experience emotions, to think or to have knowledge, and to have desires. Bering (2002) speculates that this may be a function of "simulation constraints": Since it is epistemologically impossible to know what it is "like" to be dead, the easiest thing to do is to put ourselves in the dead person's shoes. Yet because we have never consciously experienced the absence of consciousness, we end up imbuing dead people with minds very much like our own—with thoughts, desires, and emotions. On the other hand, because we *have* consciously experienced the absence of perceptual and psychobiological states (e.g., we know what it "feels like" not to see anything and to have our hunger sated), we are better able, when these simulations are combined with vitalistic knowledge, to reason that dead agents lack these "low-level" psychological capacities (but see commentary by Barrett, 2003; Boyer, 2003; Pyysiäinen, 2003).

Although it has found some initial support, the simulation constraint hypothesis of death representation clearly stands to be borne out by additional data. Nevertheless, the cognitive foundations of afterlife beliefs are particularly important for the current discussion. In a vast majority of societies, the spirits of dead people are believed to operate in the natural world, serving as the causative agents behind both positive and negative life events. If children's cognitive systems are naturally equipped to breed ghosts because of something like simulation constraints, this may help "set the stage" for supernatural attribution, because it provides them with ready-made agent concepts (e.g., specific ancestral relatives) that can be held accountable for life's little surprises.

DEVELOPMENTAL TRENDS: INFERRING COMMUNICATIVE INTENT IN THE OCCURRENCE OF RANDOM EVENTS

Believing that a supernatural agent *caused* some unexpected natural occurrence is one thing—trying to figure out *why* it did so is quite another. In a recent study, Bering and Baumann (2004) investigated the cognitive-developmental mechanisms that underlie children's ability to represent random events as "standing for" the intentions of a supernatural agent. Children between the ages of 3 and 7 years were asked to play a simple hiding game in which they were to guess the location of a hidden ball by placing their hand on one of two medium-size boxes. Only one of these boxes, they were told, contained the ball. The experimenter demonstrated by placing her hand, palm side down, on top of one box, and told the participants that "if you change your mind, then you can move your hand to the other box, like this—but wherever your hand is when I say 'Time's up!' is your final choice." Children were awarded prizes (i.e., stickers) if they chose the "correct" box, and received nothing for an "incorrect" response. In reality, however, there were two identical balls, one inside of each box, and "correct" responses were a function of children's hand movements during the course of each 15-second experimental trial (the particular box they happened to select was inconsequential).

After children displayed an understanding of the basic task demands of the game, they were shown a picture hanging on the inside of the laboratory door. The picture was a portrait of a friendly, make-believe (i.e., two-dimensional cartoon) female character wearing jewels and a crown. Children were told the following story about this "princess":

See this picture? This is a picture of *Princess Alice*. Isn't she pretty? Princess Alice is a magic princess. Do you know what she can do? She can make herself *invisible*. Do you know what invisible means? [Either, "That's right, it means you can't see her" or "It means you can't see her, even though she's there," depending on the child's response.] And guess what? Princess Alice is in the room with us right now. Where do you think she is? [If necessary, the experimenter then prompted the child by pointing to various areas of the room while asking, "Do you think she's over there, or over there? Remember, we can't see her."] And guess what else? Princess Alice really likes you and she's going to help you play the game. She's going to tell you when you pick the *wrong* box. I don't know how she's going to tell you, but somehow *she's going to tell you when you pick the wrong box.*

Children were then administered four "hiding game" trials, with the experimenter reminding the child prior to each trial about Princess Alice (i.e., "Now remember, Princess Alice will tell you if you choose the wrong box"). Two of these trials were identical to an initial training trial in which nothing out of the ordinary happened. Regardless of the location of the child's hand at the end of these control trials, the child was told that he or she had chosen the "correct" box and was awarded the prize. On the two counterbalanced probe trials, however, something unexpected (from the child's point of view) occurred in the laboratory as soon as the child's hand first made contact with one of the boxes. On such trials, an experimenter in an adjacent room either (1) used a remote-control device to make a table lamp directly in front of the child flash on and off twice in rapid succession (i.e., "ambiguous random event"), or (2) lifted a magnet on the opposite side of the closed laboratory door, causing the picture of Princess Alice suddenly to fall to the floor (i.e., "iconic random event"). Children received the prize on these probe trials only if they moved their hand to the opposite box in response to the random event (and kept it there). Following the study, children were then asked to provide verbal judgments about the causes of these unexpected occurrences.

Children's behavioral responses (i.e., whether they moved their hand to the opposite box) reflected a striking developmental pattern. Only 16% of the 3- and 4-year-olds in the study chose the "correct" box on either of the probe trials for the behavioral task. Although there were no significant differences between these preschoolers and slightly older children (5- to 6-year-olds), children in the middle age group were somewhat more prone (31%) to move their hands in response to the random events. Not until age 7, however, did children reliably choose the "correct" box on the probe trials: Nearly all (82%) children at this age moved their hand to the opposite box upon encountering at least one of the simulated random events in the laboratory.

Children's postexperiment verbal judgments revealed a similar developmental trend (see Figure 16.2). The youngest children provided mostly "nonagentive" verbal responses when asked why the lights flashed on and off and why the picture of Princess Alice fell—for instance, they shrugged their shoulders and said, "I don't know," or gave physical explanations (e.g., "Because it [the picture of Princess Alice] wasn't sticking very well"; 4 years, 8 months). Few preschoolers (18%) mentioned anything about Princess Alice when giving causal accounts of these events, let alone that she was trying to

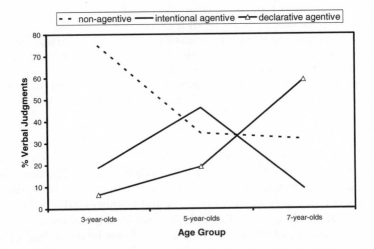

FIGURE 16.2. Verbal judgments of causes of "random" events by age group. *Nonagentive* included responses that did not explicitly mention the supernatural agent ("Princess Alice") said to be in the room (e.g., animistic cause, mechanical cause, no explanation). *Intentional agentive* meant that the child stated that the supernatural agent caused the event. *Declarative agentive* included responses in which the children stated that Princess Alice caused the event *and* that she did so in order to help them find the hidden object.

share information with them about the location of the hidden ball (6%). In contrast, the most frequent type of verbal judgment for the 5– and 6-year-olds was "intentional agentive," wherein 46% of children in this middle age group stated that Princess Alice caused the event, but upon follow-up questioning stated that they did not know why she did so, or stated that she just "wanted to" (e.g., "Princess Alice took [the picture] off." Why do you think she did that? "She thought it would look better in another place"; 5 years, 4 months). Only 19% of children in this age group claimed that either of the events occurred because Princess Alice was trying to help them find the ball. In contrast, this "declarative agentive" response type, in which the child stated that Princess Alice caused the event, and that she did so in order to help them find the ball, telling them that their hand was on the wrong box, was the most frequent type of causal reasoning among the 7-year-olds—65% of the oldest children in the study gave such verbal judgments (e.g., "It's another way of her [after attributing the picture falling to Princess Alice] not speaking, so that she doesn't have to talk to tell me that it's wrong"; 7 years, 6 months).

In other words, it was as if children in the middle age group merely saw Princess Alice as an invisible woman running around in the laboratory and "making things happen"—pulling the cord to the table lamp, knocking the picture off the wall—for no other purpose than to convey her presence in the room. The oldest children, in contrast, exploited her "antics" as a source of information; to them, the light turning on and off was analogous to her pointing to the correct box, and the picture falling off the door was treated as if it were Princess Alice saying, "No, not that one, the other one." For the youngest children, the picture falling was merely "the picture falling," and the light turning on and off was merely "the light turning on and off." Of course, it is not that preschoolers are skeptics—rather, they have not yet developed the cognitive skills necessary to be superstitious. Or have they?

Are Children Especially Sensitive to Supernatural Agency in the Moral Domain?

Additional work shows that when encountering unexpected events that are embedded in the moral domain, preschoolers indeed respond to such occurrences as if they were referentially meaningful. In a series of ongoing "Princess Alice" experiments, very young children who are primed with a supernatural agent concept and then led to disinhibit a socially undesirable response (i.e., cheating on a guessing game) respond to ambiguous random events as if they were imperative messages ("Stop that!") from the supernatural agent. In this study, children are shown a single, medium-size box and told that there is something *very* special inside that is just for them. The catch is that they must correctly guess the contents of the box in order to take the prize home with them; otherwise, they leave with nothing. (Of course, all children get the prize in the end; these instructions are for motivational purposes only.) Once children understand how the guessing game works, they are shown the picture of Princess Alice. As in the previous study, children are informed that Princess Alice has made herself invisible and is somewhere in the room with them. Unlike children in the previous study, however, children are told that "Princess Alice really likes good boys and girls. I bet she really likes you!"

Following this "introduction" to Princess Alice, children are then led back to the guessing game, where the experimenter promptly informs them that, before they get started with the game, she must tell their mother something important and has to leave the room briefly in order to do so. She instructs them to stay seated in their chair (directly in front of the mysterious box) until she returns: "But don't worry, you won't be alone, because Princess Alice will be in the room with you." In an adjacent room, a second experimenter observes the child alone in the room on a video monitor until either (1) he or she exhibits a "cheating" response, operationally defined as touching the handle or lid of the box as if to open it, or (2) for a period of 5 minutes, whichever comes first. If the child goes to "cheat," this second experimenter uses a remote control device to make a table lamp (toward which the child is facing) flash on and off. Following this event, the child is observed alone for another 30 seconds in order to see whether he or she will continue looking inside of the box, despite the unexpected event ("continuative response"), or withdraw his or her hand from the box in response to the unexpected event ("inhibitive response"). Otherwise, the experimenter simply returns to the room at the end of this 5-minute period and continues with the game.

Although sufficient data have not yet been collected for the critical between-subjects control condition (i.e., the experiment is conducted identically to the foregoing description but children do not receive supernatural priming—they hear nothing of "Princess Alice"), preliminary evidence suggests that even 2.5-year-olds display the inhibitive response after encountering the unexpected event in the midst of their cheating. Even these youngest children act as if they had been "caught red-handed" when the table lamp flashes on and off, hastily removing their hand from the forbidden box and refraining from actually looking inside. Some of these children display behavioral signs of dejection and fear. Moreover, many children spontaneously comment on the unexpected event as soon as the experimenter returns to the room. To quote one very excited and demonstrative 3-year-old girl upon the experimenter's entrance: "Princess Alice is real!"

ADAPTIVE SOLUTIONS
TO THE PROBLEM OF OTHER MINDS

Developmental research is beginning to yield important clues into the cognitive architecture that underlies religious causal beliefs in children. Presently it is unclear whether these mechanisms comprise an adaptive system whose component parts converged through selective processes, sowing the seeds of genetic prosperity for those individuals so equipped to imbue the natural world with symbolic meaning. In an effort to preempt the scorn of justifiably critical readers, therefore, I readily concede that the following evolutionary scenario is speculative and tentative. Although it is supported by the available data, these data fail to test directly evolutionary hypotheses; therefore, the model must remain a philosophical induction until such tests are performed. Nevertheless, we must begin to account for the strong influence of supernatural causal beliefs on human behavior if we are to understand religion as the natural and unmistakably human phenomenon that it is. The first step in this attempt must therefore be to acknowledge religious ideas as (potentially) *proximate causes* of human adaptive behaviors; supernatural beliefs are not merely epiphenomenally attendant with unconscious motives, as some evolutionary psychologists have claimed, but are often the "prime movers," the first-order causes, of adaptive behaviors. A woman who refrains from stealing a necklace from a jewelry store because she is convinced that her disapproving dead mother knows what she is up to might have just made a very adaptive decision; unbeknownst to her, there was a hidden camera in the ceiling aimed directly at her face. Take away this woman's belief in the afterlife, in the continuity of her mother's psychological prowess after her death, and her genetic fitness might be seriously compromised.

But I am getting ahead of myself. First, it is important to understand what I mean when I say that religious ideas can serve as proximate causes. A proximate cause both physiologically and psychologically directs the organism toward engaging in adaptive behavior (Mayr, 1961); in humans, it is the mechanism by which the organism gains representational access into the motives underlying its own behavior, as well as the engine by which the organism seeks to fulfill its adaptive goals. Thus, the proximate cause of sexual behavior is the analgesic effect of endorphins that are released into the cerebrospinal fluid at orgasm, elevating mood and reducing stress. Phenomenally, sexually mature individuals are driven toward reproductive activity for the subjectively pleasurable psychological and physiological effects. The *ultimate cause* of sexual behavior (and any other adaptive behavior) is the retention and propagation of one's genes in subsequent populations (Mayr, 1961). This ultimate cause, the heart of natural selection processes, is an unconscious determinant of adaptive behaviors: People are generally unaware of their genetically inspired motives for routine behaviors. Proximate causes are therefore the emotional manifestations of ultimate causes. For other species, it does not go beyond this; emotions gas-pedal overt behaviors, which either *are* or *are not* adaptive within particular ecological contexts. The adaptive behaviors of all species are therefore directly caused by proximate mechanisms that emerged phylogenetically through forces of natural selection.

Humans may be unique, however, in that their cognitive abilities permit them to reflect upon the causes of their own behaviors (Povinelli, Bering, & Giambrone, 2000; Tomasello & Call, 1997). Among cognitive developmentalists, this capacity is referred to as "metarepresentation"; it involves the representation of the self's private mental states (Perner, 1991). Traditionally, the field of evolutionary psychology has eschewed the explicit causal theories that are generated by people's metarepresentational processes as being mere epiphenomena (e.g., Daly & Wilson, 1988). The *American Heritage Dictionary* defines *epiphenomenon* as "a secondary phenomenon that results from and accompanies another." In psychological parlance, therefore, it would apply to the mental states that attend or arise from first-order causes but do not, in and of themselves, serve as first-order causes. Thus, if one claims to have murdered his neighbor because he was temporarily possessed by the devil, this explanation displays little causal relevance to most evolutionary psychologists. *It would be ignored.* This is because further investigation might reveal, for example, that the murderer suspected that his wife was romantically involved with the victim, a situation that set into motion an evolved affective–behavioral system designed for retaliatory aggression and perhaps even homicide. The perpetrator may very well believe that "The devil made me do it," but, again, most evolutionary psychologists would say that the behavior would have occurred anyway, even in the absence of such superstitious accounts, even if the person thought such ideas were foolish. The idea of the devil is merely a cultural construct that has ingratiated itself into this person's evolved psychological mechanisms. We could just as easily replace "the devil" with "the bad oysters I had for lunch" or "my troubled relationship with my mother"—no matter, all of these causal accounts are equally likely to be designated as epiphenomenal to the true proximate causes of jealousy-mediated mate retention and sexual competition.

I certainly agree that humans are, generally speaking, very poor at understanding the genetically motivated causes of their own behaviors. The conceptual caveat I would like to make to this proximate–ultimate distinction has not so much to do with individuals' knowledge of their selfish genes as with the human intentionality system "interfering" with more ancient proximate causal mechanisms. I view the intentionality system as a domain-general system that enabled humans to abstract unseen causal forces and to posit such forces as precipitates of observable events and behaviors. Causal constructs, whether they are in the *physical* (e.g., mass, gravity, connectedness), *psychological* (intentions, desires, beliefs), or *biological* (e.g., growth, death, sickness) domains, are intangible theoretical entities that permit individuals to predict, to explain, and to control both their own and others' behaviors, as well as the natural events unfolding around them. Although developmental psychologists have demonstrated children's intuitive knowledge in each of these core causal domains, the one that concerns us the most here is the psychological domain. Thus, when I speak of the "intentionality system" in this section, I am referring exclusively to the capacity to represent mental states as the unseen causes of behavior—the conceptualization of "mind" proper.

In accounting for the evolutionary origins of the human intentionality system, I assume strict *neurobiological continuity* over phylogenetic time (Gibson, 2003; Suddendorf & Whiten, 2001) but an equally strict *representational discontinuity* that has characterized hominid cognitive evolution only recently, at least within the past 5–7 million years, the time frame in which humans last shared a common ancestor with chimpanzees. At some point, the hominid brain, which is a continuation of form from the brains of ancestral primates, evolved a qualitatively distinct representational capacity allowing for the conceptualization of abstract causal states. Povinelli and his colleagues (Povinelli et al., 2000; Povinelli & Giambrone, 1999; Bering & Povinelli, 2003) have argued that the recent shared heritage between humans and great apes guarantees an ensemble of behavioral homologies, but that with the evolutionary emergence of a new representational system serving to register the unseen causes of these behaviors, humans began to "redescribe" these overt actions in terms of underlying mental states. Thus, because behaviors such as mate retention and retaliatory aggression have a deep evolutionary history, extant closely related species, such as *Pan troglodytes*, will probably exhibit similar behaviors. Such behaviors originated in the common ancestor of humans and chimpanzees, because they solved adaptive problems for this species. But, according to Povinelli, the overlap between human and chimpanzee behavior stops with morphological similarity in behavioral form. Unlike other great apes, only humans are capable of reasoning that behaviors associated with mate retention are caused by "jealousy" and those falling under the umbrella of retaliatory aggression are driven by "anger" or "shame." Of course, with such knowledge of underlying causal states, individuals become able to control others' behaviors by changing these mental states; for example, a woman might avert the homicidal behaviors of her jealous boyfriend by implanting a false belief in his head that she, in fact, has been consummately faithful.

Precisely when is uncertain, but sometime over the course of hominid speciation, therefore, the intentionality system grafted itself on top of ancient behavioral patterns and became capable of disrupting their occurrence. A key implication of Povinelli's argument is that once the ability to represent under-lying mental states evolved, humans were confronted with a new series of adaptive challenges that was unlike anything they or any other species had ever faced—they had to cope with the problem of *mind*. The question of whether people would rob banks if they were guaranteed never to get caught seems especially apt here. *They would*. What prevents them from doing so is that they decide that they are not likely to get away with it; people would find out. Other agents' minds are designed to gather and dispense with socially rel-evant information about the self (Baldwin & Moses, 1996), and this informa-tion can have deleterious effects on genetic fitness, because it often leads to negative social consequences (Bering & Shackelford, in press). Thus, it would be in one's genes' interests to refrain from selfishly indulging these very genes in behaviors that were adaptive before the intentionality system came along— *when one did not have to worry about what one knew*. Among large social groups, such a repertoire of previously adaptive behaviors that suddenly came into conflict with the intentionality system includes (among many others) sex-ual coercion, the appropriation of others' resources by physical force, overt aggression, the infanticide of unrelated or sickly offspring, and public promis-cuity. A chimpanzee eyeing another chimpanzee's prized parcel of bananas would not hesitate to steal the bunch, so long as the other was not around. Even if there were other chimpanzees watching the "theft" unfold, it makes no difference—who's going to tell? Modify the scenario to describe a man at the beach eyeing the wallet of another man, who has temporarily gone out for a swim in the ocean, and the problem of other minds presents itself. Every person on that beach is a potential "witness," a factor that, from a cost–benefit perspective, should make him think twice before pilfering the stranger's cash.

Generally speaking, these ideas are not novel. Nicholas Humphrey (1976) wrote of the social function of the human intellect nearly three decades ago, and Dunbar (1993; Dunbar & Spoors, 1995; see also Barkow, 1992) has writ-ten at length on the evolution of gossip and the role of language in the forma-tion of social groups. What is novel is the notion that intentionality was not, in and of itself, necessarily adaptive, but was instead a powerful selective force because it constituted entirely new adaptive problems for those so endowed. One of these problems was the rapid transmission of social information among group members, a process that would be detrimental to the self's genetic fitness should this information be negative. In previous work, Todd Shackelford and I (Bering & Shackelford, in press) have argued that "information-retention homicide" may be one adaptive solution to this problem. Individuals who have knowledge of others' social transgressions (eyewitnesses, defectors in mutual crimes, ex-confidantes, etc.) are more likely to be murdered than others, because the perpetrator is highly motivated to retain that damaging information from the social group. Another adaptive solution to the problem of information transmission might have been the evolution of a psychological system that rendered individuals highly susceptible to the illusion of supernatural agency.

Why Supernatural Agents Care about Our Sex Lives and Afterlives

Whether supernatural agency is an illusion, of course, is inconsequential to the system's adaptive value. Natural selection is pragmatic and is not concerned with attribution "errors." Humans appear strongly predisposed toward intentionality. As early as 12 months of age, infants appear sensitive to the goals and intentions of other agents (e.g., Gergely, Nádasdy, Csibra & Biró, 1995), and by their fourth birthdays, children have assumed a belief–desire psychology that enables them to represent epistemic states such as ignorance and knowledge, and to readily understand and explain actions in these terms (for reviews, see Wellman & Gelman, 1992; Flavell, 1999). The precise developmental mechanisms underlying these representational processes are the subject of some debate, for instance, whether a theory of mind module develops according to a maturational schedule, or whether an "incorrect" theory of mind is present at birth and simply refined with experiential input, but it is very clear that intentionality is canalized in human ontogeny (it will appear in all but the most impoverished conditions) and that it develops regularly and fairly rapidly.

As their social cognitive abilities emerge during development, children are simultaneously immersed in unique cultural environments where morality is chiefly determined by socioecological conditions. Although there is likely a common "moral grammar" underlying all children's development in this domain, the moral particulates of any given society are given shape by the demands of local environments. Diverse ecologies produce diverse behavioral strategies for maximizing genetic fitness; therefore, while there are general cross-cultural trends in the moral domain (e.g., proscriptions against "cheating" and "murder"), the criteria for moral transgressions will vary as a function of many complex environmental factors. What is considered "cheating" and "murder" is often quite different among cultural groups. For example, owing to a population surge and diminishing resources in ancient Greece, Aristotle argued in his *Politics* that "not only deformed children should be disposed of but that children born to unsuitably matched parents, particularly those over age for optimum breeding and those surplus to the needs of the state, should be destroyed as well" (Reynolds & Tanner, 1995, p. 88). Among Westerners, this moral dictum advocates the murdering of innocent children, but not so among most people at that time, and among contemporary groups suffering similar crises of unstable resources. Rather, for people living under such conditions, it may be considered immoral to allow such children to live. There are numerous other examples of cross-cultural differences in the moral domain, including the infanticide of disfigured offspring, sexual relations between adults and adolescents, marriage between first cousins, polygamy, ritualistic abuse of animals, and so on. There are sliding definitions of sin in that many proscriptions depend on the habitat into which one happens to be born.

What is important here is that children must learn about these variable cultural norms in the moral domain; although they are equipped to acquire this knowledge easily, it is not likely that children are born with an inherent sense of right and wrong at the level of moral particulates. Physical and psychological neotony will permit them sufficient slack in ontogeny to acquire behavioral norms, where adults are relatively permissive when it comes to the social transgressions of children (e.g., McCabe, 1984; Zebrowitz, Kendall-Tackett, & Fafel, 1991), but by adolescence, individuals are held accountable for their failure to conform to the moral prescriptions of the group and are subsequently punished. It is likely that all forms of punishment will lead to decrements in fitness, because social dissension leads to exclusion (either literally or symbolically, as in castigation) from group living. Consequently, rule breakers lose valuable reproductive opportunities by being labeled as such. Furthermore, because the genetic relatives of cheats and social dissidents are also ostracized, inclusive fitness is also negatively affected (see Bering & Shackelford, in press).

If a supernatural attribution system was ancestrally adaptive, it would be strange to speak of it as an *ontogenetic adaptation*, which implies that it would be limited to improving the genetic fitness of individuals occupying a definite period of cognitive development (Bjorklund & Pellegrini, 2002). With the exception, perhaps, of the first few years of life, individuals throughout the lifespan seem cognitively biased toward seeing "signs" and meaning in some categories of natural events. However, it may be the case that young children are particularly disposed toward the idea of supernatural agency because it facilitated the acquisition of culturally versatile moral rules and contributed to the development of behavioral inhibition. As the Princess Alice experiment on "cheating" seems to suggest, children who attribute unexpected occurrences to a supernatural agent may be more likely to inhibit socially unacceptable behaviors than children who ignore such "evidence" of supernatural agency. Ultimately, this might have led to meaningful gains in fitness effects because, under conditions where the self underestimates the likelihood of social detection by other group members, ambient natural events serve as an additional safeguard against others gaining knowledge of the self's social transgressions, prompting the child to inhibit those behaviors that evolved before the intentionality system and therefore still encouraged by its selfish genes. This particular form of causal reasoning requires that the child represents natural events as carrying an imperative ("Stop that!") message from a supernatural agent—it "knows what they're up to" and caused the event in question in order to tell them so. A light flashing on and off is not inherently negative, or a form of punishment per se, but when children are primed with knowledge of a supernatural agent, it becomes a source of adaptive information. This would be one mechanism by which superstitious behavior may have been advantageous at the level of the gene, perhaps more so than reasonable behavior.

A recent study by Roes and Raymond (2003) demonstrated that group size is positively correlated with the presence of "moralizing gods." According to these authors, "Cooperation between large numbers of people invariably means moral rules regulating relations between them and prescribing what is right and what is wrong, and with recurring threats [e.g., hostile neighboring societies, droughts], the moral rules should be imposed with authority. How better than by a moralizing god?" (p. 135). Similarly, Johnson and Krüger (2004) argue that the threat of supernatural punishment, whether in this life or in the hereafter, induces cooperation because religious beliefs often serve as literal truths: "The deterrent effect of supernatural punishment should not be underestimated, especially in the era of interest (pre-industrial human societies) when many natural phenomena remained inexplicable" (p. 164). Evolutionary biologists have long held that the advantages of group living significantly outweigh the disadvantages, yet conflicts will inevitably arise owing to the selfish genetic interests of individual group members. There should be strong selective pressure, therefore, for adaptive solutions to problems of group fission, and this may well come in the form of moralizing gods and the illusion of supernatural punishment. In this same vein, anthropological evidence reveals that funerary rights and the general deferential respect paid to the recently deceased likely have their origins in assuaging the discontent of troubled spirits, who, like anybody else, encountered social conflicts while they were alive and might have died without resolving them. Who, upon the death of a family member, friend, or even foe, has not regretted some unkind word or missed opportunity while the person was still alive? Our hostility toward our enemies wanes, our indifference to our acquaintances troubles us, our arrogance toward those we took advantage of haunts us at the moment we hear that these people have died. This immediate increase in subjective liking of the newly dead might be explained by an innate fear of supernatural punishment. In fact, it is somewhat difficult to explain otherwise.

But the system is also seemingly devoted to much more abstract forms of causal reasoning, where people routinely infer "lessons" and "meaning" in natural life events, events that appear to have less to do with punishment, and more to do with *cooperation* between the self and a supernatural agent. For example, the current Philippine president, Gloria Macapagal Arroyo, who holds a PhD in economics from the University of the Phillipines, is notorious for her strong religious beliefs. In a recent interview for *Time Asia* magazine (Schuman, 2003), Arroyo discusses how God communicates with her on a daily basis. Once, when she was scheduled to speak at an antidrug rally, her talk almost had to be cancelled because of a terrible rainstorm. But just as she stood up to speak, the rain suddenly stopped—a shift in weather that President Arroyo believed was a sign from God. Just days prior, a typhoon had forced her to cancel a return helicopter trip to her home, so she was forced to travel by car through the impoverished provinces back to Manila. She enjoyed the trip so much that the typhoon, too, was attributed to God. Such stories prompted the newspaper reporter, Michael Schuman, to comment that "Philippine President Gloria Macapagal Arroyo sees the hand of God everywhere" (p. 36). Indeed, Arroyo herself told Schuman that "God wanted me to be President at this very complex moment in our country's history" (p. 36).

This form of causal reasoning, in which random events are seen as communicative attempts by a supernatural agent to share socially strategic information with the self, was also demonstrated by the 7-year-olds (but not younger children) in the study by Bering and Baumann (2004). These children interpreted a flashing light and a falling picture as Princess Alice's way of telling them that they had chosen the wrong box when trying to find a hidden ball. The capacity to make this type of inference might demand second-order representational skills, which involves the attribution of recursive mental states. Previous research has shown that, unlike first-order theory of mind tasks (e.g., "I know that you know") children are not generally able to pass second-order theory of mind tasks (e.g., "I know that you know that I know") until they are around 6 or 7 years of age. In the current case, it would be something akin to "I *know* that Princess Alice *knows* that I *don't know* where the ball is." Therefore, reasoning that a random event such as a falling picture is "about" the child's false belief would be grounded in these higher order social-cognitive processes. If the self did not possess second-order representational abilities, in that it could not represent another agent as having knowledge of its own mental states, then random events could not be "about" these mental states. In other words, supernatural agents could not be envisioned as sharing information if they were not first represented as knowing that the self did not have this information. This is precisely what seemed to happen with the 5-year-olds in the study by Bering and Baumann, who believed that Princess Alice caused the picture to fall and the light to flash on and off, but had no idea why she did so other than that she "wanted to." Although highly speculative, one way in which this form of causal reasoning might have been ancestrally adaptive was in its ability to generate adaptive behaviors. If natural events are taken as evidence of the intentions and desires of powerful supernatural agents, and if these agents are represented as being personally invested in the self's genetic fitness (seeing God as concerned with one's political aspirations), reasoning in this manner may generate evolved affective–behavioral programs that promote adaptive behaviors.

PIECING IT ALL TOGETHER:
EPIGENETIC PATHWAYS TO AN ADAPTIVE SYSTEM
OF SUPERNATURAL AGENCY?

What the current perspective adds to the findings of Roes and Raymond (2003), and to the arguments of Johnson and Krüger (2004), is a rough sketch of the cognitive-developmental mechanisms by which this adaptive system that is designed to encourage group cohesion can actually operate. As evolutionary psychologists, we must explain not only the theoretical biology underlying adaptive processes, but we must also understand the cognitive hardware—the actual information-processing systems—that are designed to engage organisms in adaptive behaviors. Supernatural punishment can only be an effective deterrent insofar as individuals are capable of reasoning that negative life events are caused by supernatural agents who have explicit *reasons* for bringing about such events. Otherwise, negative life events are merely negative life events. Similarly, moralizing gods can only find their way into large social groups insofar as individuals are capable of envisioning these gods as enforcing their morals through the occurrence of positive and negative events. A moralizing god who fails to "communicate" with its followers would not be a very effective one.

We are making good progress in identifying the epigenetic pathways leading to this (possibly) adaptive cognitive system, but investigators still have a long way to go in uncovering all the psychological intricacies of meaning, morality, gods, and mortality. Nevertheless, if Freud (1928/1961) had had available to him the neo-Darwinian understanding of natural selection that is available to us today, he might have recanted his statement that "it would be . . . remarkable . . . if our wretched, ignorant and downtrodden ancestors had succeeded in solving all these difficult riddles of the universe" (p. 42). In a roundabout sort of way, they might have done just this.

ACKNOWLEDGMENTS

The following individuals provided useful comments and suggestions on earlier versions of this chapter: Joseph Bulbulia, Dominic Johnson, and Jason Slone.

REFERENCES

Andrews, P. W., Gangestad, S. W., & Matthews, D. (2002). Adaptationism: How to carry out an exaptationist program. *Behavioral and Brain Sciences, 25*, 489–553.

Atran, S. (2002). *In gods we trust: The evolutionary landscape of religion.* Oxford, UK: Oxford University Press.

Baldwin, D. A., & Moses, L. J. (1996). The ontogeny of social information gathering. *Child Development, 67*, 1915–1939.

Barkow, J. H. (1992). Beneath new culture is old psychology: Gossip and social stratification. In J. H. Barkow, L. Cosmides, & J. Tooby (Eds.), *The adapted mind: Evolutionary psychology and the generation of culture* (pp. 627–637). London: Oxford University Press.

Barrett, J. L. (2000). Exploring the natural foundations of religion. *Trends in Cognitive Sciences, 4,* 29–34.

Barrett, J. L. (2003). Epidemiological and nativist accounts in the cognitive study of culture: A commentary on Pyysiäinen's innate fear of Bering's ghosts. *Journal of Cognition and Culture, 3,* 226–232.

Barrett, J. L., Richert, R., & Driesenga, A. (2001). God's beliefs versus mother's: The development of nonhuman agent concepts. *Child Development, 72,* 50–65.

Bering, J. M. (2002). Intuitive conceptions of dead agents' minds: The natural foundations of afterlife beliefs as phenomenological boundary. *Journal of Cognition and Culture, 2,* 263–308.

Bering, J. M. (2003). Towards a cognitive theory of existential meaning. *New Ideas in Psychology, 21,* 101–120.

Bering, J. M., & Baumann, B. D. (2004). *Children's attributions of intentions to an invisible agent.* Manuscript submitted for review.

Bering, J. M., & Bjorklund, D. F. (2004). The natural emergence of reasoning about the afterlife as a developmental regularity. *Developmental Psychology, 40,* 217–233.

Bering, J., Hernández Blasi, C., & Bjorklund, D. F. (2003, April). *The role of metarepresentational–simulationist models in the development of death reasoning.* Paper presented at meeting of the Society for Research in Child Development, Tampa, FL.

Bering, J. M. & Povinelli, D. J. (2003). Comparing cognitive development. In D. Maestripieri (Ed.), *Primate psychology: Bridging the gap between the mind and behavior of human and nonhuman primates* (pp. 205–234). Cambridge, MA: Harvard University Press.

Bering, J. M., & Shackelford, T. (in press). The causal role of consciousness: A conceptual addendum to human evolutionary psychology. *Review of General Psychology.*

Bjorklund, D. F., & Pellegrini, A. D. (2002). *The origins of human nature: Evolutionary developmental psychology.* Washington, DC: American Psychological Association.

Boyer, P. (2001). *Religion explained: The evolutionary origins of religious thought.* New York: Basic Books.

Boyer, P. (2003). Are ghost concepts "intuitive," "endemic," and "innate"? *Journal of Cognition and Culture, 3,* 233–243.

Buss, D. M., Haselton, M. G., Shackelford, T. K., Bleske, A. L., & Wakefield, J. C. (1998). Adaptations, exaptations, and spandrels. *American Psychologist, 53,* 533–548.

Coulson, C. A. (1955). *Science and Christian belief.* Oxford, UK: Oxford University Press.

Daly, M., & Wilson, M. (1988). *Homicide.* Hawthorne, NY: Aldine de Gruyter.

Dawkins, R. (1986). *The blind watchmaker.* New York: Norton.

Dawkins, R. (1998). *Unweaving the rainbow: Science, delusion and the appetite for wonder.* Boston: Houghton Mifflin.

Deridder, R., Hendriks, E., Zani, B., Pepitone, A., & Saffioti, S. (1999). Additional cross-cultural evidence on the selective usage of nonmaterial beliefs in explaining life events. *European Journal of Social Psychology, 29*, 435–442.

Dunbar, R. I. M. (1993). Coevolution of neocortical size, group size and language in humans. *Behavioral and Brain Sciences, 16*, 681–735.

Dunbar, R. I. M., & Spoors, M. (1995). Social networks, support cliques, and kinship. *Human Nature, 6*, 273–290.

Evans, E. M. (2001). Cognitive and contextual factors in the emergence of diverse belief systems: Creation versus evolution. *Cognitive Psychology, 42*, 217–266.

Flavell, J. H. (1999). Cognitive development: Children's knowledge about the mind. *Annual Review of Psychology, 50*, 21–45.

Freud, S. (1961). *The future of an illusion.* New York: Norton. (Original work published 1928)

Gergely, G., Nádasdy, Z., Csibra, G., & Biró, S. (1995). Taking the intentional stance at 12 months of age. *Cognition, 56*, 165–193.

Gibson, K. R. (2003). Continuities between great ape and human behaviors. In A. Toomela (Ed.), *Cultural guidance in the development of the human mind: Advances in child development within culturally structured environments* (pp. 27–34). Westport, CT: Ablex.

Gould, S. J. (1991). Exaptation: A crucial tool for evolutionary psychology. *Journal of Social Issues, 47*, 43–65.

Guthrie, S. (1993). *Faces in the clouds: A new theory of religion.* New York: Oxford University Press.

Hinde, R. A. (1999). *Why gods persist: A scientific approach to religion.* London: Routledge.

Humphrey, N. K. (1976). The social function of the intellect. In P. P. Bates & R. N. Hinde (Eds.), *Growing points in ethology* (pp. 303–316). Cambridge, UK: Cambridge University Press.

Johnson, D. D. P., & Krüger, O. (2004). The good of wrath: Supernatural punishment and the evolution of cooperation. *Political Theology, 5*, 159–176.

Kelemen, D. (2003). British and American children's preferences for teleo-functional explanations of the natural world. *Cognition, 88*, 201–221.

Kelemen, D. (2004). Are children "intuitive theists"?: Reasoning about purpose and design in nature. *Psychological Science, 15*(5), 295–301.

Kirkpatrick, L. (1998). God as a substitute attachment figure. *Personality and Social Psychology Bulletin, 24*, 961–973.

Lupfer, M. B., Tolliver, D., & Jackson, M. (1996). Explaining life-altering occurrences: A test of the "God-of-the-gaps" hypothesis. *Journal for the Scientific Study of Religion, 35*, 379–391.

Mayr, E. (1961). Cause and effect in biology. *Science, 134*, 1501–1506.

McCabe, V. (1984). Abstract perceptual information for age level: A risk factor for maltreatment? *Child Development, 55*, 267–276.

McCauley, R. N., & Lawson, E. T. (2002). *Bringing ritual to mind.* New York: Cambridge University Press.

McCauley, R. N. (2000). The naturalness of religion and the unnaturalness of science. In F. C. Keil & R. A. Wilson (Eds.), *Explanation and cognition* (pp. 61–85). Cambridge, UK: Cambridge University Press.

Pepitone, A., & Saffioti, L. (1997). The selectivity of nonmaterial beliefs in interpreting life events. *European Journal of Social Psychology, 27*, 23–35.

Perner, J. (1991). *Understanding the representational mind.* Cambridge, MA: MIT Press.

Povinelli, D. J., Bering, J. M., & Giambrone, S. (2000). Toward a science of other minds: Escaping the argument by analogy. *Cognitive Science, 24,* 509–541.

Povinelli, D. J., & Giambrone, S. (1999). Inferring other minds: Failure of the argument by analogy. *Philosophical Topics, 27,* 161–201.

Pyysiäinen, I. (2003). On the "innateness" of religion. *Journal of Cognition and Culture, 3,* 218–225.

Reynolds, V., & Tanner, R. (1995). *The social ecology of religion.* New York: Oxford University Press.

Roes, F. L., & Raymond, M. (2003). Belief in moralizing gods. *Evolution and Human Behavior, 24,* 126–135.

Schuman, M. (2003, August 4). A time for prayer. *TIMEasia Magazine, 162,* 36–38.

Suddendorf, T., & Whiten, A. (2001). Mental evolution and development: Evidence for secondary representation in children, great apes, and other animals. *Psychological Bulletin, 127,* 629–650.

Taylor, M. (1999). *Imaginary companions and the children that create them.* New York: Oxford University Press.

Tomasello, M., & Call, J. (1997). *Primate cognition.* Oxford, UK: Oxford University Press.

Weeks, M., & Lupfer, M. B. (2000). Religious attributions and proximity of influence: An investigation of direct interventions and distal explanations. *Journal for the Scientific Study of Religion, 39,* 348–362.

Wellman, H. M., & Gelman, S. A. (1992). Cognitive development: Foundational theories of core domains. *Annual Review of Psychology, 43,* 337–375.

Whitehouse, H. (2000). *Arguments and icons.* Oxford, UK: Oxford University Press.

Zebrowitz, L. A., Kendall-Tackett, K., & Fafel, D. (1991). The influence of children's facial maturity on parental expectations and punishments. *Journal of Experimental Child Psychology, 52,* 221–238.

17

COGNITIVE DEVELOPMENT AND THE UNDERSTANDING OF ANIMAL BEHAVIOR

H. Clark Barrett

A 2-year old child at the forest edge encounters a strange object moving along a leaf. Elongated and green, the object changes shape in a fluid way, one end rising, bending, and contorting in the air as it reaches the edge of the leaf, then lowering back down and continuing its undulating motion along the leaf's edge. Some things about this thing the child does not understand: what it is called, what it eats, whether it is harmful. Other things are clear to the child, even at this age: The thing is alive; it is probably a "bug" of some kind, either worm or insect; when it moves, it moves with purpose, in the direction that its sensory apparatus takes it, lifting its head when it reaches the end of the leaf to sample its surroundings before moving on. None of these things is written in the movement or features of the object itself, but rather are inferred by the child. She observes the moving object from a distance, fascinated, and cannot help but try to figure out what this new creature is up to.

Parents and others who interact with young children frequently observe that they show an intense interest in animals. Children want to know what animals are called, how they are categorized, where they live, what they eat, how they stalk their prey, why they have stripes or whiskers or rattles on their tails, and so on. Most of us have encountered children whose expertise on these matters rivals or even outstrips our own: a child who knows the difference between a rainbow wrasse and a bluehead wrasse, or which of *Ceratosaurus* and *Hadrosaurus* was a predator. From a certain perspective, this is quite odd given that the kinds of activities that our children actually engage in during their day-to-day lives have little to do with live animals, at least wild ones. Children's interest in the details of animal biology and behavior is often, if not usually, far out of proportion to what the actual ecological usefulness of this information will be for them. Children in industrialized countries are very unlikely to encounter wild lions, jaguars, crocodiles, or sharks, and they are unlikely indeed ever to encounter a *Tyrannosaurus rex*. Why, then, are children's cognitive resources so devoted to an understanding of animals and their behavior?

An evolutionary developmental perspective might help to shed light on this question. As in evolutionary psychology in general, an evolutionary approach to children's understanding of animal behavior begins with the supposition that mechanisms shaping children's cognitive skills evolved to solve adaptive problems they faced in ancestral environments, and tries to deduce through a combination of the logic of adaptive design and empirical evidence what these mechanisms might be. Because encounters with animals loomed larger in children's lives in the past, it is perhaps not surprising to discover that animals loom large—perhaps "irrationally" so—in the minds of modern children. But an adaptationist perspective on this question implies and demands more than the mere observation that children should be interested in animals. It is a source of hypotheses about the design of the cognitive machinery and knowledge stores responsible for children's thinking about animals. While much was known about the cognitive development of children's understanding of animal behavior prior to widespread adoption of an evolutionary view, an evolutionary perspective not only helps us to organize what we already knew, but to point us in new directions that have only begun to be explored. In this chapter, I review our present state of knowledge about children's understanding of animal behavior, and attempt to organize this knowledge into a broad picture of how the cognitive system that children bring to bear in understanding animal behavior—what I refer to as the *agency system*—is organized.

MECHANISMS AND DOMAINS IN DEVELOPMENT

All of the mechanisms involved in acquiring and constructing knowledge and cognitive skills in children have evolved functions; the problem is merely discovering what they are. In the case of the cognitive development of the understanding of animal behavior, as for any domain of cognition, the underlying mechanisms can in principle be sorted into several categories: (1) those whose proper (evolved) function is specifically related to knowledge acquisition and inference about animal behavior per se; (2) those whose proper function is broader but is applied, in particular cases, to cognitive development of animal knowledge (mechanisms of working memory, object individuation mechanisms in the perceptual system, word parsing mechanisms, etc.); and (3) those that are being applied to problems specifically outside their proper, evolved domain (e.g., mechanisms evolved for making inferences about conspecifics that are then applied to nonhuman animals). Here, the distinction between *proper* domain and *actual* domain is relevant: A mechanism's proper or evolved domain is the set of inputs that the mechanism was designed by natural selection to process, whereas a mechanism's actual domain is the set of inputs that it actually processes (Sperber, 1994). For example, a mechanism designed to process information about living, animate agents might process information about automobiles, because they emit cues that satisfy the device's input conditions, even though they are not part of its proper domain (Barrett, 2001).

In the case of cognitive development of the understanding of animal behavior, all three kinds of mechanisms described earlier are involved. However, when trying to get a sense of how cognitive development in a particular domain is organized, it is useful to begin by asking: What are the adaptive problems associated specifically with this domain, and what kinds of mechanisms might have evolved to solve them? For some domains (e.g., chess), it may well be the case that there are *no* evolved mechanisms specific to that domain, and that problems in that domain are solved by mechanisms evolved for other purposes. For others (e.g., speech processing), there might well be mechanisms specific to that problem domain. Whether there are, of course, depends on factors such as whether or not the adaptive problem in question existed over sufficient periods of time and space during our evolution, whether the ability to solve it had an impact on fitness, and so on (Tooby & Cosmides, 1992). What about children's understanding of animal behavior? What are the relevant adaptive problems, and might we expect specialized cognitive machinery to solve them?

Before turning to this issue, it is important to note that "understanding of animal behavior" should not really be regarded as *a* domain. Rather, the mechanisms involved in development and deployment of knowledge about animal behavior are manifold, and each mechanism has its own proper domain. Whether any correspond strictly to the actual biological category *animal* or *nonhuman animal* is an empirical matter, and many certainly do not. For example, there are mechanisms whose proper function is to make inferences about animate *agents*, objects capable of goal-directed action, the proper domain of which includes any such object, including both human and nonhuman animals, but not *all* nonhuman animals (i.e., animals that do not exhibit goal-directed action, such as corals). Defined from a biological perspective, humans are, of course, animals; therefore, all of the mechanisms of social cognition are technically mechanisms whose proper function is the understanding of animal behavior. From this perspective, if one were to plot the ideal boundaries of domains in terms of sets of objects using Venn diagrams, one would draw concentric circles, with, for example, the circle representing animal-specific mechanisms completely containing the circle representing human-specific mechanisms. However, this tidy, logical nesting (all humans are animals; therefore, all inferences general to animals should also be applied to humans; all inferences about humans are also inferences about animals; etc.), while "philosophically correct," and indeed, phylogenetically correct, might not be reflected in the workings of the mind, which evolved not to satisfy the criteria of philosophers or biologists, but rather, the exigencies of survival and reproduction (Boyer & Barrett, in press).

Rather than conceiving of domains as sets of objects in the world or as categories defined by objective scientific criteria, domains should be conceived as input conditions for computational devices, where the inputs to a device include the information necessary to solve the computational problem to which it is dedicated (i.e., which it evolved to solve). We may well decide to describe some mechanisms or systems as having "animal behavior" as their proper domain, but this language is only permissible if we insist on cashing out the term "animal behavior" in terms of the specific triggering conditions and information inputs to the system (e.g., certain types of motion representation in the visual cortex, propositions referring to intentional agents) rather than the scientific or folk concepts to which the term "animal behavior" refers.

ANIMALS AS SELECTIVE AGENTS

On a priori grounds, why might we expect children to exhibit any understanding of animal behavior at all? In other words, why would there be any reliably developing aspects of cognition about animal behavior, or any mechanisms specifically dedicated to making inferences about it?

To begin with, it is certainly uncontroversial that nonhuman animals have been present in the environments that humans have inhabited over the course of evolutionary history. But this simple observation can be refined and expanded to produce a variety of insights about the adaptive problems that animals posed for children and adults in the past. When we look at modern foraging societies, we see that there are several ways in which humans regularly interact with animals. First, there are animals that pose a threat to humans, which can be subdivided into several categories. There are animals that prey on humans, such as tigers and leopards, animals that are dangerous because of their aggressive behavior, such as hippos and cape buffalo, and animals that are dangerous because of their formidable weapons of self-defense, such as poisonous spiders, snakes, and scorpions. These animals pose threats to humans today wherever their habitats overlap, and are likely to have done so in the past (Barrett, 1999; Kruuk, 2002).

The second way in which humans regularly interact with animals is as food. Hunting is a subsistence practice in existing preagricultural societies, is practiced by our closest evolutionary relatives, chimpanzees, and the archaeological record suggests that meat has been an important part of human and hominid diets for millions of years (Stanford, 1999). Humans and nonhuman animals may also have interacted in the past as competitors for food (Brantingham, 1998). Finally, there is the practice of keeping wild animals as pets or for food, practiced in many traditional societies today, and more recently, domestication, which is known to have shaped not only the morphology and physiology of domesticated species but also their cognitive skills (Hare, Brown, Williamson, & Tomasello, 2002), and may have also had an impact on human evolution.

Of these various modes of interaction with animals, the most important are likely to have been interactions with predators and other dangerous animals, and interactions with prey. For young children, interactions with dangerous animals, and decisions and behavior that influenced the likelihood of such interactions, are likely to have been of the greatest importance with respect to fitness. Interactions with prey, on the other hand, would have been less important for younger children than for older children. In traditional societies today, such as the Shuar of Ecuador, children begin to participate in subsistence activities involving prey (e.g., fishing) as young as age 4 or 5. However, such activities crescendo throughout childhood, and true hunting, in which knowledge of animal behavior is likely to play a major role, becomes important in later childhood. This suggests that there may be a difference in the developmental trajectories of predator knowledge and prey knowledge. Early acquisition of knowledge about prey behavior may serve more of a preparatory role, organizing knowledge for later use, whereas early acquisition of knowledge about the behavior of predators and other dangerous animals may have direct utility for children even at early ages. For example, even though a 4-year-old Shuar child might not be able to fend off an attacking anaconda in a direct encounter, knowledge that anacondas tend to hunt near riverbanks could have major fitness benefits for the child.

What kinds of cognitive problems would animals have posed for children in the past? In other words, what burdens would animals, be they predators, prey, or otherwise, have placed on children's developing information-processing capacities? Because of the adaptive importance of predator avoidance for children, I focus here on predators and other dangerous animals as examples, but the same logic applies to other categories of animal as well.

In principle, one can identify two broad classes of problem that animals (as well as any other category of things in the world) would have posed for children: problems of *prediction*, or inference, and problems of *knowledge acquisition*, or learning. Here, I use prediction and inference interchangeably to refer to the use of observed or known information (perceptual cues, propositional utterances or other representations, conceptual knowledge, etc.) to produce new representations—inferences, guesses, inductions—that were not previously known to be true. The major fitness-relevant problem with this class of cognitive operation is that the results are uncertain. I might infer or predict that a predator in a particular situation is not going to attack, and yet be wrong. Natural selection shapes the mechanisms responsible for such inferences and predictions as a result of their fitness outcomes, iterated over populations and generations, leading to mechanisms that are more likely to make correct inferences, or more specifically, fitness-promoting inferences (in general, correct inferences tend to promote fitness more than incorrect ones, but there are many possible correct inferences that would have no effect on fitness). The result of the evolutionary process is mechanisms that are increasingly predisposed to attend to, acquire, and use causally relevant information about animals, and to disregard or discount types of information that have tended to have poor predictive power over evolutionary time. Because predictive inferences make use of both databases of acquired information (knowledge) plus a variety of cognitive capacities that process this information, natural selection will act on the many systems evolved, so that they interface effectively and embody principles or rules that are "ecologically rational" in the sense of being well-fitted to the causal structure and statistical regularities of animal behavior (Gigerenzer & Todd, 1999; Tooby & Cosmides, 1992).

With these considerations in mind, let us examine the specific skills relevant to understanding animal behavior that one might expect natural selection to have favored in children. These range from the ability to distinguish things that behave (animals capable of movement) from things that cannot (nonmobile animals, plants, nonliving things), to the ability to sort and categorize animals for different purposes (e.g., to categorize animals into taxa based on relatedness, or into functional categories, such as predators), to knowledge about the ecology and behavioral dispositions of particular taxa, to the ability to predict animal behavior on the basis of inferences about goals, intentions, beliefs, and other internal states. Many of these skills, such as the ability to distinguish agents from nonagents, are not unique to humans. Others, such as the ability to predict behavior based on beliefs, may be uniquely present, or at least uniquely elaborated, in humans. Because the problem of understanding and predicting the behavior of predators and prey is composed of many subtasks, each with its own computational demands, the agency system is composed of multiple components, each of which I review in turn.

DISTINGUISHING ANIMALS FROM NONANIMALS: AGENCY DETECTION

In order to make inferences, organisms must make distinctions between different kinds of things in the world. At minimum, this is because there must be a fit between any given inference procedure and the target of inference, in order for inferences to be systematically correct. For example, applying the same kinds of inference to rocks or water that one applies to living things would often lead to systematically invalid inferences. Living things share properties that rocks, water, and other nonliving things do not. Moreover, an organism that failed to distinguish between its mother, a predator, and a rock, and to behave differently toward them, would soon be dead. This is why natural selection equips organisms with *intuitive ontologies:* means of sorting the world into kinds that share properties relevant for inference (Boyer & Barrett, in press).

A substantial literature in infant development suggests that basic ontological categories or distinctions emerge early in infancy (Spelke, Breinlinger, Macomber, & Jacobson, 1992; Wellman & Gelman, 1992). The category of things with which we are concerned here is animals, and specifically, of animals that "behave" (i.e., that exhibit goal-directed activity). From an evolutionary perspective, there are many benefits of distinguishing things that behave from those that do not. In the developmental literature, entities that are capable of acting in a goal-directed fashion (which are a subset of both living things and animals) are called *intentional agents*, or *agents* for short. A growing body of research has begun to explore agent-specific information-processing systems in the brain (Gergely, Nádasdy, Csibra, & Bíró, 1995; Johnson, 2000; Leslie, 1994; Rakison & Poulin-Dubois, 2001). From the perspective of these systems, the understanding of animal behavior is synonymous with the understanding of the behavior of agents (including humans): The various inference systems used for understanding animal behavior are restricted to this class of entities and to no other. Agency detectors can be regarded as filters that admit information about animals to cognitive processes further downstream and block information about nonagents (Kurzban, 1996). This implies that animals that do not behave, including dead animals, are dealt with by other systems (i.e., systems for handling inanimate objects and substances) (Barrett & Behne, in press).

Perhaps the most fundamental and phylogenetically ancient adaptive problem with respect to agents, then, is discriminating between things that are agents and things that are not. The costs of failing to make this discrimination are potentially quite large, and there may be asymmetries in costs of errors of different kinds, with failure to detect agency usually being more costly than mistaken attribution of agency (Guthrie, 1993; Haselton & Buss, 2000). One might therefore expect natural selection to have favored perceptual mechanisms that use reliable cues to agency to perform this discrimination task. Is there evidence for such mechanisms, and what cues do they use to discriminate agents from nonagents?

Self-Propelled Motion

The developmental literature suggests that there are several pathways to distinguishing agents from nonagents. Perhaps the most obvious feature that distinguishes agents from nonagents is the ability to move, or self-propelled motion, as opposed to motion caused by an external force. There is evidence that the brain contains motion detectors that distinguish between motion that has no obvious external cause, and motion caused by an external event such as a collision, and that uses self-propelled motion as a cue to agency. Early work by Michotte (1963) showed that a moving shape on a screen "colliding" with a stationary one that is then "launched" produces a strong perception of causality. A qualitative change in how causality is perceived occurs when the first shape does not contact the second one prior to launching, and even infants are surprised when there appears to be no direct transmission of force (i.e., when the object appears to react at a distance) (Leslie & Keeble, 1987). Since these initial studies, a variety of studies have shown that self-propelled, whole-body motion is an important cue to agency (Rakison & Poulin-Dubois, 2001; Scholl & Tremoulet, 2000). There are several important components to such motion, including simple initiation of motion in the absence of external cause (Leslie & Keeble, 1987, Premack, 1990), change of trajectory without apparent external cause (Tremoulet & Feldman, 2000), and apparent "goal-directedness" of the motion (Opfer, 2003). The latter has been of interest since classic studies by Heider and Simmel (1944), showing that adults spontaneously attribute goals and other intentional states to self-propelled shapes moving on a screen, and a variety of studies have since tried to quantify "goal-directedness" more precisely, exploring the cues that are used to infer what a moving agent is trying to do (see, e.g., Abell, Happé, & Frith, 2000; Blythe, Todd, & Miller, 1999; Gergely et al., 1995).

In addition to whole-body motion, other types of motion cues may be important cues to agency as well, such as changes in object shape in the absence of external cause, or "nonrigid transformations," such as breathing, postural changes, and so on (Gibson, Owsley, & Johnson, 1978; Johnson, Booth, & O'Hearn, 2001). An infant dishabituation study by Gergely et al. (1995) included breathing-like expansion and contraction of objects prior to whole-body movement, which may be a factor in triggering an agency mode of construal, although not strictly necessary (Csibra, Gergely, Bíró, Koós, & Brockbank, 1999). A variety of experiments have also shown that children and adults are able to identify both moving humans and nonhuman animals from point-light displays (i.e., from stimuli in which all cues are removed except points of light attached to limbs and other body parts) (Bertenthal & Pinto, 1994; Mather & West, 1993). These studies suggest that certain properties of the motions of animals, such as coordinated movements of limbs, oscillation around a center of gravity, and so on, can be used to distinguish animals (agents) from objects whose movement is not biological in nature.

Contingency and Distant Reactivity

Another feature that distinguishes agents from nonagents is the ability to engage in contingent and reciprocal interactions with other agents (Johnson, 2000). This may also be thought of as the reactivity of agents to distant external stimuli (i.e., distant reactivity) (Boyer & Barrett, in press). There are several ways in which such behavioral contingency might manifest itself. For example, agents might exhibit contingent whole-body motion trajectories, such as when a predator pursues its prey and modifies its trajectory to match that of the prey (Barrett, 1999). Contingent motions might take the form of contingent gestures, movements, or facial expressions, such as when one agent's gaze follows the gaze of another, or when one individual's fear evokes fear in another (Baron-Cohen, 1995). Contingency might also take the form of communicative interaction, such as when one agent makes a sound in response to a sound made by another (animal calls, human vocal utterances, etc.). A series of experiments by Johnson, Slaughter, and Carey (1998) suggests that even in infancy, contingent behavior is a powerful cue used to discriminate agents. Johnson et al. used a gaze-following paradigm to measure infants' categorization of objects as agents, in which following the "gaze" of a stimulus object was taken as an indication that the object had been categorized as an agent, and failure to follow gaze indicated that the object had not been so categorized. Johnson et al. found that triggering the agency system depended both on contingency of the object's behavior on that of the infant (in this case, beeping contingently in response to sounds produced by the infant) and presence of a face. These results were extended by a later study showing that imitation of goal-directed behavior and communicative gestures occurred only for objects that had a face *and* interacted contingently with the infant (Johnson et al., 2001). Interestingly, the objects in both studies were categorized as agents on the basis of face and contingency cues despite the fact that they did not look at all like people and only vaguely like animals (they were furry, oblong blobs). This suggests that from the perspective of the agency system, *agent* is synonymous with *behaving entity*, or *animal*, rather than with *human*, even in young infants (Johnson, 2000).

Morphology

Because the defining feature of agency is the ability to engage in goal-directed behavior, motion is of primary importance in agency detection. However, there may be other, nonmotion cues that are reliably correlated with agency. For example, as suggested in studies by Johnson et al. (2001), presence of a face or face-like cues, even static ones, may play a role in triggering the agency system. For example, the presence of eyes may be an important cue to agency (Baron-Cohen, 1995; Coss & Goldthwaite, 1995). In very young infants, a very simple stimulus array with eye, nose, and mouth spots arranged in the pattern of a face draws infant attention, whereas the same objects arranged in a different spatial pattern do not (Morton & Johnson, 1991).

Other morphological cues may also be important in distinguishing animals from nonanimals and perhaps in triggering the agency system, including asymmetry along one axis, the presence of four legs, a head, teeth, fur, and so on, though none of these proposals has been tested to date (Baron-Cohen, 1995; Premack, 1990). Some specific types of animals have characteristic features that can be used both to identify them as agents and to discriminate them from other kinds of agents. For example, snakes are a class of agents that have a particular morphology (shape), as well as a characteristic movement pattern, that can be used to identify them, and there may have evolved perceptual "templates" specifically for this class of agent (Öhman & Mineka, 2001). Evidence for such templates exists in other species that exhibit fear responses to predators despite being isolated from them for many thousands of years (Blumstein, Daniel, Griffin, & Evans, 2000). Other cues, for example, patterns of fur coloration for common predators such as leopards, might also be part of a recognition system (see Coss & Ramakrishnan, 2000). In humans, a variety of studies have shown that even infants are able to sort animals from nonanimals (e.g., vehicles) on the basis of static morphological cues (Mandler & McDonough, 1998; Quinn & Eimas, 1996).

PREDICTING AND INTERPRETING ANIMAL BEHAVIOR: THE AGENCY SYSTEM

From the perspective of natural selection, merely categorizing objects as agents or nonagents is not enough. The reason that there exist elaborate perceptual systems for discriminating agents from nonagents is that they allow organisms to respond differently to agents than to nonagents. In the presence of agents, an elaborate cognitive system is activated that brings to bear specialized judgment, inference, and decision-making skills tailored to the special properties of sentient, behaving things, including both humans and nonhuman animals. This cognitive system and its components are referred to here as the *agency inference system*, or the *agency system* for short.

The agency system, rather than being a single, undifferentiated system or "black box," is likely to have many components, each with its own proper domain, including some with domains that do not span the entire category of agents, and others that extend beyond it. In addition, there are systems that feed into and modulate the activity of the agency system, such as perceptual and emotional systems. In recent years, a variety of strands of research have begun to elucidate the design features of this system and its many components. Here, I specifically focus on processes of inference about animal behavior, offering one possible account of how the agency system is organized.

Any given inference about the behavior of animals is likely to make use of many kinds of information. Imagine, for example, a child who sees her cat sitting on the kitchen floor, looking up at the cabinet where the cat food is kept, and meowing. The child infers from this that the cat wants to be fed. This seems a simple inference, but when one tries to reconstruct the inferential processes that lead from perceptual inputs (the visual and auditory cues the cat is emitting) to the final inference, one realizes that the inferential chain must be a complex one that integrates perceptual information with internal representations in a chain of several steps to produce the inferential output. Subinferences leading to the inference that "the cat wants to be fed" might include the inference that the object in question is an agent, and a cat; that the cat is attending to, and perhaps referring to, the cabinet with its gaze and meows; that it knows or believes that there is food in the cabinet; that if it is referring to the food, it must be hungry; and so on. Clearly, many kinds of information must be integrated, and multiple mechanisms are involved.

In principle, one can identify at least three different types of inference that devices within an agency system might make: (1) inferences specific to particular *contexts* or *situations*, such as predator–prey interactions, social exchange, play, mating, behaviors such as sleeping, breathing, eating, and so on; (2) inferences specific to particular *categories* of agent, including taxonomic categories such as HUMAN, MAMMAL, BIRD, DOG, PARROT, and role categories such as PREDATOR, PREY, PARENT, FRIEND, MATE, and so on; and (3) inferences specific to *specific agents*, including agents for which a permanent "identity file" is maintained, which are mostly humans but sometimes also certain animals, as well as agents that are being tracked during the course of a specific interaction, such as *that dog that is watching me right now*, or *the mouse that just ran under the fridge*. Note also that inference devices not specific to the agency system must also interact with this system to produce complete inferences: For example, working memory may play a role in processing relevant information, systems for reasoning about objects and object permanence may be necessary to handle inferences about the position of agents in space, and so on.

Figure 17.1 shows one way in which the agency system can be conceptualized as an assemblage of mechanisms that carry out these various kinds of

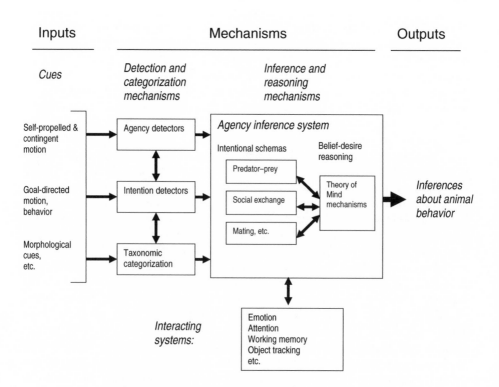

FIGURE 17.1. Components of the agency system.

functions to produce inferences about animal behavior. While there is often a tendency in cognitive science to think of mechanisms as organized hierarchically, it is at present an open question how these different mechanisms are organized with respect to each other (Figure 17.1 depicts one possibility). For our purposes, what matters is that each component of the agency system carries out a specific function and has its own proprietary domain (e.g., inferences specific to cats are not extended to dogs; inferences specific to predator–prey interactions are not extended to mating; etc.). Additionally, complete inferences about animal behavior (e.g., the cat wants to be fed) are likely to make use of more than one type of inference mechanism, including mechanisms not specific to the agency system per se. In the following sections, I review evidence for various subcomponents of the agency system.

CONTEXT-SPECIFIC INFERENCES: INTENTIONAL SCHEMAS

Since Dennett's (1987) influential volume on the intentional stance, it has come to be widely accepted that in understanding the behavior of agents (people and animals), both children and adults make use of intentional reasoning. To adopt the intentional stance with regard to an object is to assume implicitly that its behavior can be both explained and predicted as caused by unobservable internal states such as beliefs and desires, and that these states influence observable behavior in a manner that is directed towards some goal or intention. Currently, the term that is most widely used to refer to the inferential apparatus that instantiates the intentional stance in children and adults is "theory of mind" (*ToM*). Some authors prefer to reserve the term to refer only to types of inferences involving belief attribution (i.e., attribution of "epistemic" states, as opposed to inferences about nonepistemic states such as desires, which would not necessarily require the use of theory of mind) (see Baron-Cohen, 1995; Wellman, 1990). Although this distinction is an important one, here, I use the term "agency system" rather than "theory of mind" to refer to the set of inferential procedures involved in making inferences about intentional agents, because many of the types of inference discussed here do not require attribution of epistemic states (a capacity that some authors claim is unique to humans).

According to theorists of the intentional stance, in order to either explain or predict the behavior of an agent in a particular situation, it is necessary to attribute a goal to that agent, which in turn requires an inference from the agent's observed behavior. For example, to make sense of John's going to the refrigerator and opening it, we might attribute to John the goal of getting food, along with the desire-like state HUNGER, which (we assume), when present in an organism, leads it to attempt to achieve the goal of finding food. This set of inferences makes use of "theory-like" information about hunger. Each of us has a (mostly implicit) "theory" or "concept" of hunger—it might also be called a "hunger schema"—that contains inferential principles, such as *hunger is not present immediately following a meal* (i.e., a meal satiates hunger); *hunger increases with time since the last meal; the greater an organism's hunger, the more it will attempt to seek food;* and so on (encoded, of course, in a language of conceptual primitives or computational rules rather than in natural language, as depicted here). One might think of the "hunger schema" as a miniature conceptual structure or inference system, activated in certain conditions (e.g., when an organism is observed interacting with or seeking food), and with specific inferential outputs that are applied only in certain situations. As discussed below, there are likely to be many such schemas.

At what age do intentional schemas, and the ability to make inferences using them, develop? Gergely, Csibra, and colleagues (Gergely et al., 1995; Csibra et al., 1999) have demonstrated that from as early as 9 months of age, infants are able to use intentional schemas to make predictive inferences about the behaviors of agents. To demonstrate this, Gergely et al. (1995) used a dishabituation paradigm, which measures infants' surprise at events they were not expecting in order to assess predictive intuitions, as follows. Infants were "habituated" to a repeated display, in this case, a depiction of two objects on either side of a barrier, seen in side view. The objects displayed contingent behavior in the form of expansion and contraction, one object in response to the other. Following this, one object was seen to approach the barrier, "jump over" it, and finally reach the other object. Gergely et al. hypothesized that this sequence would lead infants to infer that the moving object had the goal of reaching the other object. In other words, something like an "approach schema" is activated. Part of this intentional schema, according to Gergely et al., is the assumption that an agent will take the shortest possible path to reach its goal. This assumption generates implicit predictions about the motion trajectory of an object, predictions that can then be violated. Gergely et al. demonstrated the existence of an approach schema in infants, and that this schema had been activated by the motion sequence just described, by observing infants' reactions to schema violations (i.e., violation of the assumption of shortest path to goal). When shown the identical "jumping" motion trajectory without an intervening wall, the infants dishabituated: They were surprised that the approaching agent would jump when no wall was present. In other words, they were surprised by the schema violation. In contrast, infants did not dishabituate when the agent approached the other agent in a straight line—consistent with the approach schema—despite the fact that the infants had not previously seen this particular trajectory.

These results are important because they establish that infants are not only capable of taking the intentional stance with regard to objects as early as 9 months of age (and perhaps earlier, if appropriate means of testing can be found) but also that the infants in this study used a *particular* schema to infer the likely behavior of an object (i.e., that it would take the shortest path because it was *trying* to reach, or had the *goal, intention,* or *desire* of reaching, the other object). One can further speculate that the schema involved is a social one rather than, for example, a predator–prey schema, because both agents "signaled" contingently toward each other prior to approach, and the approached agent did not attempt to flee or evade the approaching agent. In later work, Csibra, Bíró, Koós, and Gergely (2003) have also found an early-developing pursuit–evasion schema that may represent the initial stages of predator–prey understanding. Several other studies have documented the understanding of particular intentional interactions using motion stimuli (Scholl & Tremoulet, 2000).

Developmentally, the ability of 9-month-old infants to adopt the intentional stance with respect to particular objects is only the beginning of a long trajectory leading to full-blown theory of mind capacities, including the ability to engage in multilevel metarepresentational inferences that are present in older children and adults. A large and extremely rich literature in developmental psychology documents the emergence of theory of mind during childhood (for reviews, see Baron-Cohen, 1995; Mitchell & Riggs, 2000; Wellman, 1990). Because comprehensive reviews of this literature exist elsewhere, the large literature on theory of mind and its development is not reviewed here. This does not mean, however, that theory of mind abilities are not relevant to children's understanding of animal behavior. Indeed, as suggested earlier and argued by Johnson (2000) and others, many of the mechanisms involved in making mentalistic inferences about human behavior may have, as their proper domain, *all* intentional agents, including human and nonhuman animals.

Most current theories of ToM postulate some kind of content-general conceptual/inferential apparatus into which specific intentional contents, equivalent to what I am calling schemas, can be slotted (Fig 17.1). For example, Baron-Cohen's model of theory of mind involves four components: an Intentionality Detector (ID), an Eye Direction Detector (ED), a Shared Attention Mechanism (SAM), and a Theory of Mind Mechanism (ToMM) (Baron-Cohen, 1995; see also Chapter 18, this volume). Each of these mechanisms has a particular function: Note, for example, that the proposed function of ID is approximately the same as that of the set of mechanisms described in the earlier section on "agency detection." The function of ToMM is to handle representations involving epistemic states such as knowledge, belief, and pretense. Leslie (1994) proposes a similar system, though functionally differentiated along slightly different lines, with his ToMM system$_1$ being responsible for inferences regarding "agents and action," for example, inferences of the sort described earlier in the Gergely et al. (1995) experiments that do not require attribution of epistemic states, and ToMM system$_2$ being responsible for inferences about "agents and attitudes," for example, agents' beliefs about or representations of states of affairs in the world, or epistemic states.

Accounts involving relatively content-free inferential devices into which more content-specific information can be slotted presuppose, even if implicitly, the existence of something like intentional schemas, or at least quasi-theory-like information about specific intentional states and how they influence the behavior of organisms. It is important to note that simply "having an intentional stance" is useless without specific intentional or goal schemas of the sort described here. Having the intuition that John's refrigerator-opening behavior is caused by internal states—even with mechanisms like Baron-Cohen's ToMM or Leslie's ToMM$_2$, which contain a slot for John's belief about what is in the refrigerator—is useless unless one has principled knowledge about particular *kinds* of intentional states (in this case, hunger, or the intent to eat) and the behaviors and subgoals associated with them (food search, change in mood, etc.).

From an evolutionary perspective, it is not implausible to assume that the basic set of intentional schemas that is part of children's and adults' capacity to reason about animal and human behavior has been shaped by natural selection, albeit perhaps in skeletal forms that are then fleshed out by experience (see Mandler, 1992, for one such proposal). How many schemas might one expect, and which schemas would one expect to be reliably developing in the human cognitive architecture? Here, one expects conceptual structure to capture something of the causal structure of animal and human minds themselves, with a particular intentional schema for each internal state that has distinctive causal properties that influence behavior. Intentional states are likely to be something like "natural kinds" that recur across organisms, and that cohere due to causal regularities across different tokens or instantiations of the kind. For example, HUNGER is a state that leads organisms to act in particular goal-directed ways, and there are commonalities between organisms in how they behave when hungry. BELIEF is an epistemic state with variable contents that influence the goal-directed behavior organized by motivational states such as hunger and fear.

On this account, the inferential power of such conceptual primitives depends on causal links between the primitives in the system, ultimately leading to inferences about behavior: For example, *knowing* or *believing* that a predator is present leads to *fear*, which leads to escape *behavior*, with the *goal* or *intent* of avoiding capture. Individual conceptual primitives might be assembled into larger *interaction* or *situational schemas*, such as the approach schema (Gergely et al., 1995), the predator–prey schema (Barrett, 1999), or others involving mate choice, kin interactions, social exchange, and so on (Tooby & Cosmides, 1992, Fiske, 1991).

Consider, for example, the predator–prey schema. Barrett (1999) hypothesized that the recurrence of interactions with predators and prey over human evolutionary history would have selected for a reliably developing understanding of predator–prey interactions in the form of an inference system or schema containing inferential principles for predicting predator and prey behavior using the intentional stance. Such a system would play a role not only in guiding children's real-time decisions, for example, concerning where and when to play, but also would serve a preparatory function for later childhood, when foraging activities bring children into more frequent contact with predators and prey. Csibra et al. (2003) found evidence for early development of a pursuit–evasion schema. Later in childhood, this is elaborated into a full-blown conceptual schema that children use to reason about predator and prey behavior. In a study in which children were asked to play out an imaginary predator–prey interaction using animal models, children reliably attributed the goals of prey capture and predator evasion to predator and prey, respectively by age 4, and used these goals to accurately predict the responses of predator and prey to each others' behavior, as proposed by the predator–prey schema hypothesis. Identical results were found both for city-dwelling children in Berlin, Germany, and rural children among the hunter–horticulturalist Shuar of Ecuador (Barrett, 1999; in press). Furthermore, children understood that encounter with a predator can lead to death, and were able to make realistic judgments about the behavioral consequences of death (i.e., that the ability to act ceases at death) and that this is irreversible. These results were confirmed by a follow-up study (Barrett & Behne, in press).

Keenan and Ellis (2003) propose that there might be two distinct systems for dealing with predators and prey: a predator-avoidance system and a prey-capture system. Under this account, the predator-avoidance system develops early, whereas the prey-capture system develops relatively later, because the fitness benefits of the latter system do not accrue until later childhood, whereas predator avoidance is important even for young children. An asymmetry in development of the ability to reason from the perspective of predators versus prey was also suggested by Barrett (1999) and hinted at by results showing that young children more often infer malicious intent in predators than fear in prey (perhaps because it is more useful for a prey animal to infer the intentions of a predator than to infer its own intentions; therefore, children exhibit less uncertainty about predator intentions).

Whereas Barrett's (1999) predator–prey schema theory proposes that attribution of mental states is part of the design of early-developing systems for reasoning about predators and prey, Keenan and Ellis's (2003) theorizing about the predator-avoidance system does not explicitly address the mental states of predators and prey. Rather, Keenan and Ellis conceptualize the predator-avoidance system as constituting basic decision rules, such as "prey move away from predators," that, when activated by relevant content, function to reduce the probability of predation. As a result, Keenan and Ellis propose that activation of the predator-avoidance system generates fast, prepotent responding that can *impair* mental state reasoning in cases where, for example, children are asked to make inferences about prey moving toward a hidden predator about whose location the prey has a false belief but the child does not. The same impairment should not occur for prey stalking scenarios, argue Keenan and Ellis, because the prey-capture system has not yet developed in young children and thus does not generate comparable prepotent responding. Using the false belief task, a method that requires prediction of an agent's behavior on the basis of a belief whose content differs from that of the true state of the world (see Wellman, Cross, & Watson, 2001, for a recent review), Keenan and Ellis found that ability to correctly attribute false belief was significantly higher in playmate-avoidance conditions than in predator-avoidance conditions, when the false belief would lead to the protagonist approaching a hidden playmate or a hidden predator, respectively, and that activation of a prey-seeking scenario did not result in a similar impairment. These results are consistent with the proposal that activation of the predator-avoidance system interferes with the outputs of a mental state reasoning system, and that the predator-avoidance system develops earlier than a prey-capture system. It is also possible that children have difficulty with scenarios that require them to predict that a character will act to destroy itself, predator encounter being one such scenario. An important topic for future research will be to examine the nature of the underlying mechanisms involved in behavior prediction about predators and prey, to determine whether there are distinct mechanisms for predator and prey scenarios or a single system, and to determine the nature of the inputs and representational formats the system uses (e.g., whether predator and prey intentions and mental states are part of its proper domain).

DESCENT AND DESIGN IN THE UNDERSTANDING OF BEHAVIOR

In the study of children's understanding of animals, there has been considerable research on children's understanding of biological functions, such as growth, reproduction, breathing, and so on. These are design features of living things that, while not intentionally caused, are relevant to behavior. It is currently a matter of contention just how much the intentional stance is used by children to interpret biological functions such as these (see Carey, 1985; Inagaki & Hatano, 2002; Medin & Atran, 1999). Some researchers, such as Carey (1985), suggest that children's early understanding of biological functions in animals makes use, by analogical mapping, of children's understanding of intentionality, because children have no "autonomous" or core domain of biological understanding. Others, such as Inagaki and Hatano (2002), propose that children's early understanding of biological functions is "vitalist": that children implicitly or explicitly represent some "vital force" that is responsible for processes such as growth, but that is not under intentional control of the animal (agent) in question.

Barrett (2001; 2004) has argued that because two distinct processes shape the distribution of traits across organisms, inheritance of traits by descent and modification of traits by design, descent and design relationships may play distinct roles in the understanding of animal behavior. For example, taxonomic categories such as MAMMAL, BIRD, RODENT, or HUMAN might serve to constrain inferences about behavioral regularities common to members of the taxon but not shared by species or individuals outside the taxon (for reviews of studies of taxon-based inference, see Atran et al., 1999; Carey, 1985; Markman, 1989). Doing so is ecologically rational (Gigerenzer &

Todd, 1999), in that many traits, such as live birth, are shared within a taxon such as mammals due to descent from common ancestors. Other categories, such as PREDATOR, are ecological in nature, defined by particular goals or adaptive problems, and not confined to particular taxa. Predators in many taxa possess similar adaptations due to convergent evolution, and many inferences about behavior are better predicted by membership in the category PREDATOR than in a particular taxonomic category (e.g., traits that eagles and caimans have in common that sparrows do not have). Distinct descent and design modes of reasoning about behavioral and other traits appear to be present in children by early childhood (Gelman & Markman, 1986; Kelemen, 1999). In a recent study, Barrett (2004) found that Shuar children reason differently about properties shared by descent in closely related taxa and properties shared by design in convergently evolved but more distantly related predator taxa. Predators therefore appear to represent a special category of inductive inference, standing out against a general background of taxonomy-based inference that is relatively insensitive to the functionality of traits. These results are even more striking in light of Shuar children's relative lack of exposure to modern biology and Darwinism, suggesting an intuitive rather than explicitly educated basis for the observed patterns of inference.

ANTHROPOMORPHISM

It is often assumed that anthropomorphism is common in both children's and adults' thinking about animal behavior (Guthrie, 1993; Mitchell & Hamm, 1997). In its most common usage, "anthropomorphism" refers to the attribution of strictly human traits (usually psychological and behavioral traits) to nonhuman animals. A looser definition would be attribution of traits that are not *strictly* human to nonhuman animals, but this would render the etymology of anthropomorphism inappropriate, because it would not be, by definition, human-centered (e.g., consider attribution of breathing to nonhuman mammals; it is human but not strictly human). For this reason, anthropomorphism, as commonly conceived, implies mistaken attribution. There are several sources for the claim that children anthropomorphize. First, there is the notion, advanced by Piaget, that children are "animists": They see agency in the world where there is none, overattributing intentional causes to nonintentional phenomena. Piaget's proposal was that young children have no explanatory framework or causal stance other than the intentional one, and so apply it where it is unwarranted (but see Guthrie, 1993, for a different account of overattribution as a form of error management; Haselton & Buss, 2000). This proposal was later refined by Carey (1985), who argued that children use their intuitive psychology to understand and explain purely "biological" (i.e., nonintentional) phenomena, and moreover, that human psychology in particular is the source domain for children's inferences about nonhuman animals. Again, the central notion is that the possession of an intentional stance, along with the fact that children are intimately familiar with human motivations, thoughts, and feelings, gives children a single conceptual brush with which they paint the world of living things. One consequence of humans being the anchor point for children's inferences about animals, according to Carey, was her finding that rather than overattributing properties to animals, children tended to underattribute basic biological traits, such as eating, to animals that were perceived as dissimilar to humans. Although later studies cast doubt on the universality of these findings (Atran et al., 2001; Coley, 1995; Gutheil, Vera, & Keil, 1998), the general idea that children use humans as the source domain for inferences about animals retains an intuitive appeal. Indeed, it is widely held that adults do the same thing, not only in traditional cultures that do not have a formal, "non-anthropomorphic" vocabulary for describing animal behavior, but also even among highly trained scientists, who are often accused of anthropomorphically overattributing mental states and abilities to animals (Mitchell & Hamm, 1997).

Interestingly, Hebb (1946) observed that, among scientists working with chimpanzees, those who used "anthropomorphic" terms to describe chimps' behavior were often more successful at predicting their behavior than those who restricted themselves to nonanthropomorphic behavioral descriptions (e.g., "A got angry at B and attacked her" vs. "A moved to and hit B on the head"; see also Mitchell & Hamm, 1997). This fits with the observation that "intuitive psychology is still the most useful and complete science of behavior there is" (Pinker, 1997, p. 63). As German and Leslie (2000, p. 230) note, "It is striking to reflect that the best efforts of several generations of the brightest research scientists have done so little to improve upon the ideas that are grasped effortlessly by every untutored 4-year-old, mostly before they can add two and two." In other words, given that the proposed function of the intentional stance, the reason that it is a central part of our cognitive architecture to begin with, is to be able to predict the behavior of living things, it is not surprising that people spontaneously apply it to animals, and are more successful at predicting their behavior when doing so than when using more "objective" or supposedly uncolored scientific language.

The notion that follows from Hebb's (1946) observation is that far from being a mistake, as assumed in Piaget's notion of overextension, anthropomorphism may be a "good" thing to do, in that it can lead people to make correct inferences about animal behavior. In the anthropological literature, this has been proposed many times in regard to hunters' "personification" of animals in hunting societies (Blurton Jones & Konner, 1976; Liebenberg, 1990; Mithen, 1996). For example, Mithen (1996, p. 168) writes that anthropomorphism is

> universal among all modern hunters and its significance is that it can substantially improve prediction of an animal's behavior. Even though a deer or a horse may not think about its foraging and mobility patterns in the same way as Modern

Humans, imagining that it does can act as an excellent predictor for where the animal will feed and the direction in which it may move.

These descriptions all presuppose that what people are doing when they attribute mental states to animals is, in fact, anthropomorphizing. But is it? Remember that the definition of anthropomorphism is the extension of strictly human traits to nonhuman animals. If one were to say of a dog, for example, that it is hungry, it would be strange to call this "anthropomorphizing," because hunger is not a strictly human trait. It is often implicitly assumed that any use of the intentional stance or mentalistic inference with regard to animals is anthropomorphizing, but this in turn presupposes that the proper domain of the intentional stance is humans. As argued herein and by others (e.g., Johnson, 2000), the proper domain of many components of the agency system is likely to be *all* animals, or at least all animals capable of goal-directed activity, and only some subcomponents of the system are specific to humans (though these may be many).

The conception of the agency system depicted in Figure 17.1 allows for a cognitively precise definition of anthropomorphism. Each component in the system has a proper domain, defined as the class of inputs the device evolved to process. Some devices in the system, such as agency detection devices, evolved to discriminate any kind of agent from nonagents. Therefore, when such devices are triggered by any animal, human or otherwise, no anthropomorphism is occurring. Similarly, many of the intentional schemas, such as the HUNGER schema described earlier, are not specific to humans, so use of such schemas to make inferences about the behavior of, for example, a dog, would not be anthropomorphic. Anthropomorphism would occur when a mechanism whose proper domain is specifically humans—for example, a SOCIAL EXCHANGE schema (Tooby & Cosmides, 1992)—is activated by, or applied to, a nonhuman animal. According to the account presented here, each intentional schema is linked to the taxonomic inference system; there may be something like a "scope tag" (Cosmides & Tooby, 2000) that restricts the set of taxa to which that schema will normally be applied (e.g., HUNGER → all animals; SOCIAL EXCHANGE → humans only).

It may be that human-specific inferences are sometimes extended to nonhuman animals by mistake. A child might mistakenly think, for example, that the caterpillar that she is playing with is angry with her. But it might also be that human-specific inferences are sometimes extended to nonhuman animals in a "decoupled" or pretense mode (Cosmides & Tooby, 2000; Leslie, 1987), in which inferences can be entertained but are specially marked as being not literally true, and are therefore not allowed to propagate inferences through the system as they would if taken to be true. For example, a Koyukon hunter from Arctic North America may assert or believe that he is engaged in a social exchange relationship with the deer that he has just killed, thanking it and treating it with respect, so that it will reincarnate and return as another deer

(Nelson, 1983), but he is unlikely to believe or even consider all of the inferences that would logically follow if he were *literally* engaged in a social
exchange with the deer. For example, if the deer were actually willingly sacrificing itself to the hunter, it would be unnecessary to pursue it, there would be
no need for the hunter to conceal himself when approaching the deer, and so
on.

There are several pieces of evidence suggesting that peoples' thinking
about animal behavior may be more nuanced than a simple anthropomorphism account would have it. In a study of American adults, Mitchell and
Hamm (1997) examined subjects' willingness to make attributions of jealousy
and deception to humans and animals in different contexts. They found that
subjects' attributions of these states depended much more on contextual cues
than on the actual taxa involved. In other words, what led subjects to attribute a state such as jealousy were features of the situation, regardless of
whether the character being described was human or a nonhuman animal.
Although this is consistent with an anthropomorphism account of mental
state attribution, in that jealousy and deception might not actually occur in all
of the taxa examined (e.g., otters), it does not appear that subjects were basing
their judgments on similarity to humans, psychologically or otherwise (Mitchell & Hamm, 1997). Rather, jealousy is attributed when it seems to best
account for the behavior in question (aggression by a mate in the presence of a
rival). In this sense, the adults in this study did not show the pattern found by
Carey (1985) in children, with attributions declining as similarity to humans
decreased.

Even in children, the use of humans as a source domain for the attribution of properties might not be universal. In a study of Mayan children by
Atran et al. (2001), children did not show the human prototype effects
reported by Carey for American children, but rather, extended traits on the
basis of taxonomic relatedness. Gutheil et al. (1998), using a property extension task similar to that of Carey (1985), found that extensions of biological
properties to animals by young children became more adult-like (i.e., less
human-centered) when contextualized in terms of their function. Coley (1995)
found that patterns of attribution of psychological traits differ for different
kinds of animals, with some traits being more readily attributed to predators
and others to domestic animals. This suggests that even young children have
distinct mental models of what predators and nonpredators are like. This is
not easily explained on an anthropomorphism account, because different
kinds of psychological properties should not dissociate unless there is an
equivalent dissociation in humans. A study by Barrett (2004) is consistent
with this claim, showing that over 60% of mental state attributions to predators and prey by 3-year-olds, and over 80% of those by 4- and 5-year-olds,
were realistic and consistent with predictions of predator–prey schema theory
(e.g., "The lion wants to eat the zebra"), whereas only 1.5% of the total number of responses were "anthropomorphic" in the sense defined here (e.g.,

"The zebra wants to go to the hospital"). The study was conducted with both German and Shuar children, and the proportion of realistic, schema-consistent responses was high in both populations.

A recent study by Barrett (2003), examining attributions of psychological traits and states to prey animals by adult Shuar hunters in the Ecuadorian Amazon, supports the view that anthropomorphism is rare in the inferences that people use to actually predict animals' behavior. In the sample of Shuar hunters' attributions, the vast majority were realistic ones, both consistent with the predator–prey schema and of the sort that professional biologists would make, often referring to animals' sensory capacities and to whether or not they had detected the hunter. Interestingly, Shuar hunters appear to make use of mentalistic reasoning when explaining phenomena such as the use of imitative calls to attract animals; in this case, virtually all of the explanations of the animals' behavior attributed a belief to the animal, and specifically, the false belief that the call was being produced by a member of their own species. These findings are consistent with those of Blurton Jones and Konner (1976), Liebenberg (1990), and others, who have examined the kinds of reasoning hunters in traditional societies use when pursuing prey, and who report that hunters' knowledge of animal behavior and psychology is quite realistic and in some cases more accurate and detailed than that of Western zoologists studying the same animal taxa. Of course, both adults and children across societies frequently anthropomorphize, in contexts from fairy tales to cartoons. However, when they do so, I suggest that they are likely to be engaging either explicitly or implicitly in a form of pretense, or decoupled reasoning, in which a distinction between "real" and anthropomorphized behavior is maintained (Cosmides & Tooby, 2000; Leslie, 1987).

KNOWLEDGE ACQUISITION

The view of children's understanding of animal behavior developed here holds that children come equipped by natural selection with framework or skeletal cognitive systems that help to organize knowledge and inferences about animal behavior. For example, the evidence on agency detection reviewed earlier suggests that children do not have to learn certain basic distinctions between agents and nonagents, such as the fact that agents move in a goal-directed fashion and nonagents do not. Rather, this distinction is built implicitly into perceptual mechanisms that then are able to identify which things in the world *are* agents and which are not. Beyond the level of perceptual distinctions, natural selection may prespecify certain kinds of conceptual information as well, such as the concepts of BELIEF, DESIRE, and PRETEND (which might be extremely hard to learn through observation; German & Leslie, 2000; Leslie, 1987), and perhaps even more content-specific conceptual structures, such as the intentional schemas (hunger, predator–prey, etc.) hypothesized earlier. It might be that children do not have to learn what hunger is, only to identify when it is occurring; they might not have to learn *that* there are predators, only to identify which things in their environment *are* predators. From this perspective, learning is crucial, but evolved structures guide it.

For example, it is possible that the perceptual systems of children are designed so that animals are inherently appealing, and that their perceptual features have aesthetic properties for children that draw their attention, not as a matter of accident, but as a matter of the design of children's brains. In a Gibsonian sense, animals might have "affordances" that make them compelling objects for children, drawing their attention to them and thereby facilitating learning (Gibson, 1988). There might even be something like a "critical period" of intense interest in animals—marked by things like fascination with dinosaurs and such—that subsides by adulthood. Several studies suggest that the barrage of cues emitted by real animals can exert a very strong pull on children. For example, Kidd and Kidd (1987) compared the reactions of infants ages 6 months and up to real dogs and cats versus mechanical, battery-powered ones, and found that the interactivity of the real animals (nuzzling, making noises, etc.) made the real animals far more compelling than the artificial ones, consistent with findings of Johnson et al. (1998) regarding the importance of behavioral contingency. Nielsen and Delude (1989) compared the reactions of 9-month-olds to different kinds of animals, robot animals, and people, and found that the real animals evoked much more interest. And, as expected, several studies have shown that experience with real animals makes a difference in both the rate of acquisition and quality of children's knowledge about animals and their behavior (Inagaki & Hatano, 2002; Kellert, 1997).

Boyer (2001) has suggested that learning about animals is guided by a particular kind of skeletal cognitive structure that he calls an *animal template*. According to this proposal, when the child encounters a new animal, he opens a new, blank template for that animal: for example, WALRUS. Initially, the name and perceptual information for identifying the taxon are all that are present in the newly formed template. But the template has particular "slots" that are filled as relevant information is encountered: for example, the animal's habitat, its preferred diet, how it reproduces, and so on. Although a new token template must be created for each new animal the child learns about, the *type* of template is the same for all animals, and allows the child to "fill in" information that is true of all or most members of the ontological kind ANIMAL. For example, upon learning that there is a kind of animal called a WALRUS, a child may not initially know *what* walruses eat, but will infer, without being told, *that* walruses eat, and that they have a preferred diet. When this information becomes available (e.g., overheard in a conversation about walruses), the DIET slot in the WALRUS template will be filled. Similarly, the child will infer *that* walruses have a preferred habitat, even if he does not know at first whether it is land or sea, and *that* walruses reproduce, even if he does not know whether by laying eggs or live birth. These assumptions will not be made for artifacts, because the blank ARTIFACT template has different kinds of slots (not DIET, for example, but perhaps a slot for FUNCTION, which an animal template would not have). Boyer, Bedoin, and Honoré (2000) have provided initial experimental evidence that children do make unprompted assumptions about the kinds of traits that it is possible or not possible for a new, previously unknown animal to have (e.g., "turns black when angry" is possible, "is made of sand" is not).

One implication of Boyer's (2001) template model is that new token templates or files will be opened for each new taxon a child encounters, and the input necessary to open a new template may be fairly minimal. Possibly, simply overhearing an unfamiliar taxon name might be sufficient. Indeed, children might be predisposed from an early age to begin building taxonomies of the animals in their local environment. In modern environments, where information about extinct or nonexistent animals is abundantly available, children may construct taxonomies for these animals as well, if the available information about them satisfies the minimal input criteria for opening new templates. For example, children may acquire and maintain fairly encyclopedic knowledge databases about dinosaurs, even though the actual knowledge contained in these databases is ecologically useless (because dinosaurs do not exist). A recent study in England suggests that when information about real animals is impoverished, children may fill their taxonomic knowledge system with information about imaginary creatures. Balmford, Clegg, Coulson, and Taylor (2002) compared English children's knowledge of their local flora and fauna with their knowledge of the cartoon characters known as *Pokémon*, and found that the children's knowledge of Pokémon (e.g., ability to categorize individual exemplars) was greater than their knowledge of real local animal taxa.

There may be other learning mechanisms that help children to acquire knowledge that will be useful in negotiating encounters with animals. Steen and Owens (2001) have proposed that a particular form of pretend play, chase play, is an adaptation that allows children (and young of other mammals as well) to learn predator–prey skills without actually having to encounter a predator. Those features of chase play that make it entertaining, or compelling, are precisely what cause children to engage in interactions that will hone both cognitive and motor skills, and draw their attention to relevant features of chase play scenarios that will enable them to learn pursuit and evasion strategies. Barrett (1999) proposed that the predator–prey schema may play a similar role in drawing third-party attention to predator–prey interactions for the purposes of learning. It is far better to learn about predator–prey interactions by participating in safe simulations or by observing from a third-party perspective than to rely upon actual first-person encounters with predators as a source of information. In the case of third-party observation of predator–prey encounters, there is the additional advantage of being able to acquire detailed information about the attack strategies of particular predators, or escape strategies of prey, by observing the actual predators and prey themselves. The various triggering conditions for the predator–prey schema may therefore serve an attention-drawing function as well, and people may find third-party depictions of predator–prey interactions in documentaries or fictional films particularly compelling when observed from a distance, a proposal that I have called the "Jurassic Park hypothesis" to explain the popularity of films that are full of stimuli that would, at first glance, be expected to be highly aversive. Indeed, media aimed at both adults and children may be designed, either explicitly or implicitly, to trigger these attention-drawing mechanisms, whose evolved function is to guide learning, but that now provide the basis for entertainment (Steen & Owens, 2001).

CONCLUSIONS

Although much is known about children's understanding of animal behavior, much remains to be discovered. Living as many of us do in urban environments, where our food is packaged and the likelihood of encounter with animals of any kind other than pets, pigeons, and squirrels is minimal, it is easy to forget the importance that interactions with animals had in our evolution and in the daily lives of our ancestors. There may be hidden architecture for thinking about animals that psychologists have not yet imagined, much less discovered. In modern hunting cultures, the knowledge that adults possess about animal behavior is extraordinary, often rivaling or exceeding that of trained zoologists in certain aspects, and involving sophisticated, quasi-scientific chains of reasoning (Blurton Jones & Konner, 1976; Liebenberg, 1990). This knowledge is acquired and deployed by the same kinds of minds as those who live in nonhunting societies, which likely contain capacities for learning and thinking about the natural world that are never put to the test. In children, we see the beginning of a trajectory toward this kind of knowledge, even in Western industrialized societies where, by the time of adolescence, those activities that are important in our societies shift children's interests away from animals and the further development of skills that, in hunting societies, would continue to be elaborated and refined well into adulthood (Blurton Jones & Marlowe, 2002; Kaplan & Robson, 2002). At early ages, though, children have not yet realized that it really does not matter whether they know about lions, tigers, and bears; their interests have been shaped by a history of selection to solve survival problems, and these interests remain even when the survival problems have changed.

The view that I have proposed here is that humans have a multifaceted agency system that allows them to predict and understand both human and nonhuman animal behavior. In modern environments, the normal inputs to this system might be relatively impoverished, and in some cases, it might be pressed into service outside of its proper domain. It has often been remarked, for example, that we can use the intentional stance to understand things such as thermostats and computers (Dennett, 1987). But, given that many aspects of our mind are centered around interactions with the living world, from perceptual systems geared to appreciate and understand patterns that appear organic to an almost telepathic ability to interact contingently with other sentient agents, it may be that the artifacts that we create are themselves "evolving," with increasing technological sophistication, to mesh with these aspects of how our brains work. For example, computers are becoming more and more like contingently interactive agents, designed to behave and interact in ways that we intuitively grasp. It will be interesting to observe how our environments and lives will change as the diversity of real biological agents decreases and the diversity of artificial ones grows.

REFERENCES

Abell, F., Happé, F., & Frith, U. (2000). Do triangles play tricks?: Attribution of mental states to animated shapes in normal and abnormal development. *Journal of Cognitive Development, 15*, 1–20.

Atran, S., Medin, D. L., Lynch, E., Vapnarsky, V., Ek', E. U., & Sousa, P. (2001). Folkbiology doesn't come from folkpsychology: Evidence from Yukatek Maya in cross-cultural perspective. *Journal of Cognition and Culture, 1*, 3—42.

Balmford, A., Clegg, L., Coulson, T., & Taylor, J. (2002). Why conservationists should heed Pokémon. *Science, 295*, 2367.

Baron-Cohen, S. (1995). *Mindblindness: An essay on autism and theory of mind.* Cambridge, MA: MIT Press.

Barrett, H. C. (1999). Human cognitive adaptations to predators and prey. Doctoral dissertation, University of California, Santa Barbara.

Barrett, H. C. (2001). On the functional origins of essentialism. *Mind and Society, 3*, 1–30.

Barrett, H. C. (2003). *Hunting and theory of mind.* Paper presented at the Meetings of the Human Behavior and Evolution Society, Lincoln, NE.

Barrett, H. C. (2004). Descent versus design in Shuar children's reasoning about animals. *Journal of Cognition and Culture, 4*, 25–50.

Barrett, H. C. (in press). Adaptations to predators and prey. In D. M. Buss (Ed.), *Handbook of evolutionary psychology.* New York: Wiley.

Barrett, H. C., & Behne, T. (in press). Children's understanding of death as the cessation of agency: A test using sleep versus death. *Cognition.*

Bertenthal, B. I., & Pinto, J. (1994). Global processing of biological motions. *Psychological Science, 5*, 221–225.

Blumstein, D. T., Daniel, J. C., Griffin, A. S., & Evans, C. S. (2000). Insular tammar wallabies respond to visual but not acoustic cues from predators. *Behavioral Ecology, 11*, 528–535.

Blurton Jones, N., & Konner, M. J. (1976). Kung knowledge of animal behavior. In R. B. Lee & I. Devore (Eds.), *Kalahari hunter gatherers* (pp. 325–248). Cambridge, MA: Harvard University Press.

Blurton Jones, N. G., & Marlowe, F. W. (2002). Selection for delayed maturity: Does it take 20 years to learn to hunt and gather? *Human Nature, 13*, 199–238.

Blythe, P. W., Todd, P. M., & Miller, G. F. (1999). How motion reveals intention: Categorizing social interactions. In G. Gigerenzer & P. Todd (Eds.), *Simple heuristics that make us smart* (pp. 257–285). Oxford, UK: Oxford University Press.

Boyer, P. (2001). *Religion explained.* New York: Basic Books.

Boyer, P., & Barrett, H. C. (in press). Evolved intuitive ontology: Integrating neural, behavioural and developmental aspects of domain-specificity. In D. M. Buss (Ed.), *Handbook of evolutionary psychology.* New York: Wiley.

Boyer, P., Bedoin, N., & Honoré, S. (2000). Relative contributions of kind- and domain-level concepts to expectations concerning unfamiliar exemplars: Developmental change and domain differences. *Cognitive Development, 15*, 457–479.

Brantingham, P. J. (1998). Hominid–carnivore coevolution and invasion of the predatory guild. *Journal of Anthropological Archaeology, 17*, 327–353.

Carey, S. (1985). *Conceptual change in childhood.* Cambridge, MA: MIT Press.

Coley, J. D. (1995). Emerging differentiation of folkbiology and folkpsychology: Attributions of biological and psychological properties to living things. *Child Development, 66*, 1856–1874.

Cosmides, L., & Tooby, J. (2000). Consider the source: The evolution of adaptations for decoupling and metarepresentation. In D. Sperber (Ed.), *Metarepresentations: A multidisciplinary perspective* (pp. 53–116). New York: Oxford University Press.

Coss, R. G., & Goldthwaite, R. O. (1995). The persistence of old designs for perception. In N. S. Thompson (Ed.), *Perspectives in ethology: Vol. 11. Behavioral design* (pp. 83–148). New York: Plenum Press.

Coss, R. G., & Ramakrishnan, U. (2000). Perceptual aspects of leopard recognition by wild bonnet macaques (*Macaca radiata*). *Behaviour, 137*, 315–336.

Csibra. G., Bíró, S., Koós, O., & Gergely, G. (2003). One-year-old infants use teleological representations of actions productively. *Cognitive Science, 27*, 111–133.

Csibra, G., Gergely, G., Bíró, S., Koós, O., & Brockbank, M. (1999). Goal attribution without agency cues: The perception of "pure reason" in infancy. *Cognition, 72*, 237–267.

Dennett, D. (1987). *The intentional stance.* Cambridge, MA: MIT Press.

Fiske, A. P. (1991). *The structures of social life.* New York: Free Press.

Gelman, S. A., & Markman, E. M. (1986). Categories and induction in young children. *Cognition, 23*, 183–209.

Gergely, G., Nádasdy, Z., Csibra, G., & Bíró, S. (1995). Taking the intentional stance at 12 months of age. *Cognition, 56*, 165–193.

German, T. P., & Leslie, A. M. (2000). Attending to and learning about mental states. In P. Mitchell & K. Riggs (Eds.), *Reasoning and the mind* (pp. 229–252). Hove, UK: Psychology Press.

Gibson, E. J. (1988). Exploratory behavior in the development of perceiving, acting and the acquiring of knowledge. *Annual Review of Psychology, 39*, 1–41.

Gibson, E. J., Owsley, C. J., & Johnson, J. (1978). Perception of invariants by 5-month-old infants: Differentiation of two types of motion. *Developmental Psychology, 14*, 407–416.

Gigerenzer, G., Todd, P. M., & the ABC Research Group. (1999). *Simple heuristics that make us smart.* New York: Oxford University Press.

Gutheil, G., Vera, A., & Keil, F. C. (1998). Do houseflies think?: Patterns of induction and biological beliefs in development. *Cognition, 66,* 33–49.

Guthrie, S. (1993). *Faces in the clouds: A new theory of religion.* New York: Oxford University Press.

Hare, B., Brown, M., Williamson, C., & Tomasello, M. (2002). The domestication of social cognition in dogs. *Science, 298,* 1634–1636.

Haselton M. G., & Buss, D. M. (2000). Error management theory: A new perspective on biases in cross-sex mind reading. *Journal of Personality and Social Psychology, 78,* 81–91.

Hebb, D. O. (1946). Emotion in man and animal: An analysis of the intuitive processes of recognition. *Psychological Review, 53,* 88–106.

Heider, F., & Simmel, M. (1944). An experimental study of apparent behavior. *American Journal of Psychology, 57,* 243–259.

Inagaki, K., & Hatano, G. (2002). *Young children's naive thinking about the biological world.* New York: Psychology Press.

Johnson, S. C. (2000). The recognition of mentalistic agents in infancy. *Trends in Cognitive Science, 4,* 22–28.

Johnson, S. C., Booth, A., & O'Hearn, K. (2001). Inferring the unseen goals of a nonhuman agent. *Cognitive Development, 16,* 637–656.

Johnson, S. C., Slaughter, V., & Carey, S. (1998). Whose gaze will infants follow?: Features that elicit gaze-following in 12-month-olds. *Developmental Science, 1,* 233–238.

Kaplan, H., & Robson, A. (2002). The emergence of humans: The coevolution of intelligence and longevity with intergenerational transfers. *Proceedings of the National Academy of Sciences USA, 99,* 10221–10226.

Keenan, T., & Ellis, B. J. (2003). Children's performance on a false-belief task is impaired by activation of an evolutionarily-canalized response system. *Journal of Experimental Child Psychology, 85,* 236–256

Kelemen, D. (1999) Function, goals, and intention: Children's teleological reasoning about objects. *Trends in Cognitive Sciences, 3,* 461–468.

Kellert, S. R. (1997). *Kinship to mastery: Biophilia in human evolution and development.* Washington, DC: Island Press.

Kidd, A., & Kidd, R. (1987). Reactions of infants and toddlers to live and toy animals. *Psychological Reports, 61,* 455–464.

Kruuk, H. (2002). *Hunter and hunted: Relationships between carnivores and people.* Cambridge, UK: Cambridge University Press.

Kurzban, R. (1996). *Ontological filters.* Unpublished MA dissertation, University of California, Santa Barbara.

Leslie, A. M. (1987). Pretense and representation: The origins of "theory of mind." *Psychological Review, 94,* 412–426.

Leslie, A. M. (1994). ToMM, ToBy, and agency: Core architecture and domain specificity. In L. A. Hirschfeld & S. A. Gelman (Eds.), *Mapping the mind: Domain specificity in cognition and culture* (pp. 119–148). Cambridge, UK: Cambridge University Press.

Leslie, A. M., & Keeble, S. (1987). Do six-month-old infants perceive causality? *Cognition, 25,* 265–288.

Liebenberg, L. W. (1990). *The art of tracking: The origin of science.* Cape Town: David Philip.

Mandler, J. M. (1992). How to build a baby: II. Conceptual primitives. *Psychological Review, 99*, 587–604.

Mandler, J. M., & McDonough, L. (1998). Inductive inference in infancy. *Cognitive Psychology, 37*, 60–96.

Markman, E. M. (1989). *Categorization and naming in children.* Cambridge, MA: MIT Press.

Mather, G., & West, S. (1993). Recognition of animal locomotion from dynamic point-light displays. *Perception, 22*, 759–766.

Medin, D., & Atran, S. (1999). *Folkbiology.* Cambridge, MA: MIT Press.

Michotte, A. (1963). *The perception of causality.* London: Methuen.

Mitchell, P., & Riggs, K. J. (Eds.). (2000). *Children's reasoning and the mind.* New York: Psychology Press.

Mitchell, R. W., & Hamm, M. (1997). The interpretation of animal psychology: Anthropomorphism or behavior reading? *Behaviour, 134*, 173–204.

Mithen, S. J. (1996). *The prehistory of the mind: The cognitive origins of art, religion and science.* Cambridge, UK: Cambridge University Press.

Morton, J., & Johnson, M. H. (1991). Conspec and Conlearn: A two-process theory of infant face recognition. *Psychological Review, 98*, 164–181.

Nelson, R. K. (1983). *Make prayers to the raven: A Koyukon view of the northern forest.* Chicago: University of Chicago Press.

Nielsen, J. A., & Delude, L. (1989). Behavior of young children in the presence of different kinds of animals. *Anthrozoös, 3*, 119–129.

Öhman, A., & Mineka, S. (2001). Fear, phobias and preparedness: Toward an evolved module of fear and fear learning. *Psychological Review, 108*, 483–522.

Opfer, J. E. (2003). Identifying living and sentient kinds from dynamic information: The case of goal-directed versus aimless autonomous movement in conceptual change. *Cognition, 86*, 97–122.

Pinker, S. (1997). *How the mind works.* New York: Norton.

Premack, D. (1990). The infant's theory of self-propelled objects. *Cognition, 36*, 1–16.

Quinn, P. C., & Eimas, P. D. (1996). Perceptual cues that permit categorical differentiation of animal species by infants. *Journal of Experimental Child Psychology, 63*, 189–211.

Rakison, D. H., & Poulin-Dubois, D. (2001). Developmental origin of the animate–inanimate distinction. *Psychological Bulletin, 127*, 209–228.

Scholl, B., & Tremoulet, P. (2000). Perceptual causality and animacy. *Trends in Cognitive Sciences, 4*, 299–308.

Spelke, E. S., Breinlinger, K., Macomber, J., & Jacobson, K. (1992). Origins of knowledge. *Psychological Review, 99*, 605–632.

Sperber, D. (1994). The modularity of thought and the epidemiology of representations. In L. A. Hirschfeld & S. A. Gelman (Eds.), *Mapping the mind: Domain specificity in cognition and culture* (pp. 39–67). Cambridge, UK: Cambridge University Press.

Stanford, C.B. (1999). *The hunting apes: Meat-eating and the origins of human behavior.* Princeton, NJ: Princeton University Press.

Steen, F., & Owens, S. (2001). Evolution's pedagogy: An adaptationist model of pretense and entertainment. *Journal of Cognition and Culture, 1*, 289–321.

Tooby, J., & Cosmides, L. (1992). The psychological foundations of culture. In J. H. Barkow, L. Cosmides, & J. Tooby (Eds.), *The adapted mind: Evolutionary psy-*

chology and the generation of culture (pp. 19–136). Oxford, UK: Oxford University Press.

Tremoulet, P., & Feldman, J. (2000). Perception of animacy from the motion of a single object. *Perception, 29,* 943–951.

Wellman, H. M. (1990). *The child's theory of mind.* Cambridge, MA: MIT Press.

Wellman, H. M., Cross, D., & Watson, J. (2001). Meta-analysis of theory-of-mind development: The truth about false belief. *Child Development, 72,* 655–684.

Wellman, H. M., & Gelman, S. A. (1992). Cognitive development: foundational theories of core domains. *Annual Review of Psychology, 43,* 337–375.

18

THE EMPATHIZING SYSTEM

A Revision of the 1994 Model
of the Mindreading System

SIMON BARON-COHEN

Origins of the Social Mind as a book title is very broad, and in my chapter I focus specifically on "empathizing." This is defined as the drive to identify another person's emotions and thoughts, and to respond to these with an appropriate emotion. The chapter has three main aims: (1) to challenge my own earlier model of development (Baron-Cohen, 1994), (2) to consider the evidence for sex differences in empathizing, and (3) to outline the relevance of these first two aims for our understanding of the neurodevelopmental condition of autism.

A NEUROCOGNITIVE DEVELOPMENTAL MODEL:
A 10-YEAR REVISION

The Mindreading System

My 1994 model attempted to specify the neurocognitive mechanisms that comprise the "mindreading system" (Baron-Cohen, 1994, 1995). Mindreading is defined as the ability to interpret one's own or another agent's actions as driven by mental states. The model was proposed in order to explain (1) ontogenesis of a theory of mind, and (2) neurocognitive dissociations that are seen in children, with or without autism. The model is shown in Figure 18.1 and contains four components: ID, or the Intentionality Detector;

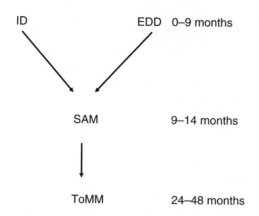

FIGURE 18.1. Baron-Cohen's (1994) model of mindreading. ID, Intentionality Detector; EDD, Eye Direction Detector; SAM, Shared Attention Mechanism; ToMM, Theory of Mind Mechanism.

EDD, or the Eye Direction Detector; SAM, or the Shared Attention Mechanism; and ToMM, or the Theory of Mind Mechanism. Full details of these components are given in the earlier publications; here, I briefly review their functions and justifications.

ID and EDD build "dyadic" representations of simple mental states. ID automatically interprets or represents an agent's self-propelled movement as a desire or goal-directed movement, a sign of its agency, or an entity with volition (Premack, 1990). For example, ID interprets an animate-like moving shape as "it wants x" or "it has goal y." EDD automatically interprets or represents eye-like stimuli as "looking at me" or "looking at something else"; that is, EDD picks out the fact that an entity with eyes can perceive. Both ID and EDD developmentally occur prior to the other two mechanisms, and are active early in infancy.

SAM is developmentally more advanced and comes online at the end of the first year of life. SAM automatically interprets or represents whether the self and another agent are (or are not) perceiving the *same* event. SAM does this by building "triadic" representations. For example, whereas ID can build the dyadic representation, "Mother *wants* the cup," and EDD can build the dyadic representation, "Mother *sees* the cup," SAM can build the triadic representation, "Mother *sees that I see* the cup." As is apparent, triadic representations involve embedding or recursion. (A dyadic representation ["I see a cup"] is embedded within another dyadic representation ["Mum sees the cup"] to produce this triadic representation.) SAM takes its input from ID and EDD, and triadic representations are made out of dyadic representations. SAM typically functions in infants from 9 to 14 months of age, and allows "joint attention" behaviors such as protodeclarative pointing and gaze monitoring (Scaife & Bruner, 1975).

ToMM is the jewel in the crown of the 1994 model of the mindreading system. It allows an *epistemic* mental states to be represented (e.g., "Mother *thinks* this cup contains water" or "Mother *pretends* this cup contains water"), and it integrates the full set of mental state concepts (including emotions) into a theory. ToMM develops in children between 2 and 4 years of age and allows pretend play (Leslie, 1987), understanding of false belief (Wimmer & Perner, 1983), and understanding of the relationships between mental states (Wellman, 1990). An example of the latter is the seeing-leads-to-knowing principle (Pratt & Bryant, 1990), where the typical 3-year-old can infer that if someone has *seen* an event, then he or she will *know* about it.

The model shows the ontogenesis of a theory of mind in the first 4 years of life and justifies the existence of four components on the basis of developmental competence and neuropsychological dissociation. In terms of developmental competence, joint attention does not appear possible until 9–14 months of age, and joint attention appears to be a necessary but not sufficient condition for understanding epistemic mental states (Baron-Cohen, 1991; Baron-Cohen & Swettenham, 1996). There appears to be a developmental lag between acquiring SAM and ToMM, suggesting that these two mechanisms are dissociable. In terms of neuropsychological dissociation, congenitally blind children can ultimately develop joint (auditory or tactile) attention, using the amodal ID rather than the visual EDD route. Children with autism appear able to represent the dyadic mental states of seeing and wanting but show delays in shared attention (Baron-Cohen, 1989b) and in understanding false belief (Baron-Cohen, 1989a; Baron-Cohen, Leslie, & Frith, 1985)—that is, in acquiring SAM and ultimately ToMM. It is this specific developmental delay that suggests that SAM is dissociable from EDD.

One reason for evolutionary psychologists' interest in the mindreading model is the central role that theory of mind, and social cognition more broadly, have been proposed to play in human evolution. A number of theorists, beginning with Humphrey (1976), have proposed that a potent selection pressure for the rapid evolution of complex cognition and representational thought in the line that lead to *Homo sapiens* was having to cooperate and compete with conspecifics (e.g., Alexander, 1979; Dunbar, 1998; Geary, 2005; see Bjorklund & Rosenberg, Chapter 3, this volume). Theory of mind in all modern human groups has its basis in understanding that one's actions and the actions of others are based on what one knows and what one wants, what Wellman (1990) referred to as *belief–desire reasoning*. For example, detecting cheaters or negotiating contracts have as their basis the folk psychology reflected in belief–desire reasoning.

The 1994 mindreading model provided specific mechanisms for the development of belief–desire reasoning and also a model for how theory of mind may have evolved. Consistent with the perspective of evolutionary psychology (Tooby & Cosmides, 1992), the 1994 model postulated domain-specific mechanisms, the product of natural selection that deal with specific problems faced by our ancestors. Some of these mechanisms (e.g., ID and EDD) are likely to be shared by many species of animal with brains, whereas others are likely to be unique to humans (e.g., SAM and ToMM). Importantly, hypotheses about the evolution of these abilities can be evaluated empirically by assessing the skills associated with these different mechanisms in extant species. Although findings from the primate literature are controversial (Povinelli & Bering, 2002; Suddendorf & Whiten, 2001), there is little evidence that human's closest living relative, chimpanzees (*Pan troglodytes*), can pass false-belief tasks, and thus seem not to possess ToMM (Bjorklund & Pellegrini, 2002; Call & Tomasello, 1999; Tomasello & Call, 1997). Mother-raised chimpanzees also seem not to engage in shared attention, suggesting they do not possess (or do not use) SAM. There is even debate about whether, in chimpanzees, EDD has all the functions that it has in *Homo sapiens*. For example, Povinelli and his colleagues (Povinelli & Eddy, 1996; Reaux, Theall, & Povinelli, 1999) reported that chimpanzees were just as likely to make food requests of a human caretaker whose eyes were obstructed (e.g., by wearing a blindfold, by having a bucket over her head) as a sighted caretaker, indicating that they are not aware that "eyes possess knowledge." Other research, however, in a food competition paradigm with a conspecific, reached the opposite conclusion (Hare, Call, Agentta, & Tomasello, 2000; Hare, Call, & Tomasello, 2001). Although it seems clear that chimpanzees possess some social-cognitive abilities, as reflected, for instance, in their transmission of what some observers have called "culture" from one generation to the next (Whiten et al., 1999), they seem not to have fully developed the more advanced components of the mindreading system (ToMM, SAM) suggesting that these are late-evolving mechanisms, fully developed only in *Homo sapiens* (or perhaps in earlier members of the *Homo* line).

The Empathizing System

Ten years on, the 1994 model of the mindreading system is still broadly able to explain the pattern of developmental and clinical data, as outlined earlier. However, to my mind, it is in need of minor but important revision because of certain omissions and too narrow a focus. The key omission is that information about *affective* states, available to the infant perceptual system, has no dedicated neurocognitive mechanism. In Figure 18.2, the revised model is shown and now includes a new fifth component: TED, or The Emotion Detector. But the concept of mindreading (or theory of mind) itself I find too narrow, in that it makes no reference to the affective state in the observer *triggered by* recognition of another's mental state. This is a particular problem for any account of the distinction between autism and psychopathy. For this reason, the model is no longer of "mindreading" but is of "empathizing," and the revised model also includes a new sixth component, TESS, or The Empathizing SyStem. (TESS is spelled as it is to playfully populate the mindreading

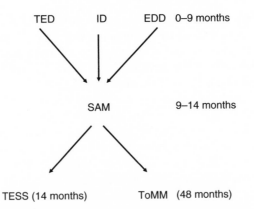

FIGURE 18.2. Baron-Cohen's (2004) model of empathizing. TED, The Emotion Detector; TESS, The Empathizing SyStem; other abbreviations as in Figure 18.1.

model with apparently anthropomorphic components.) Whereas the 1994 mindreading system was a model of a passive *observer* (because all the components had simple decoding functions), the 2004 Empathizing System is a model of an observer impelled toward *action* (because an emotion is triggered in the observer, which typically motivates the observer to *respond* to the other person). Both of these new additions are elaborated and justified further below.

Like the other infancy perceptual input mechanisms of ID and EDD, the new component of TED can build dyadic representations of a special kind, namely, it can represent *affective* states. An example would be "Mother—is *unhappy*" or even "Mother—is *angry*—with me." Formally, we can describe this as *agent–affective state–proposition*. We know that infants can represent affective states from as early as 3 months of age (Walker, 1982). As with ID, TED is amodal, in that affective information can be picked up from facial expression or vocal intonation, "motherese" being a particularly rich source of the latter (Field, 1979). Another's affective state is presumably also detectable from their touch (e.g., tense vs. relaxed), which implies that congenitally blind infants should find affective information accessible through both auditory and tactile modalities. TED allows the detection of the basic emotions (Ekman & Friesen, 1969), though it should be noted that questions have been raised about the use of the term "basic" in relation to emotion recognition (Baron-Cohen, Golan, Wheelwright, & Hill, 2003).

When SAM becomes available at 9–14 months of age, it can receive inputs from any of the three infancy mechanisms, ID, EDD, or TED. Here, we focus on how a dyadic representation of an affective state can be converted into a triadic representation by SAM. An example would be that the dyadic representation, "Mother is unhappy," can be converted into a triadic representation "I am unhappy that Mother is unhappy" or "Mother is unhappy that I am unhappy," and so on. Again, as with perceptual or volitional states, SAM's triadic representations of affective states have this special embedded, or recursive, property.

TESS, in the 2004 model, is the real jewel in the crown. This is not to minimize the importance of ToMM, which has been celebrated for the last 20 years in research in developmental psychology (Leslie, 1987; Whiten, 1991; Wimmer & Perner, 1983). ToMM is of major importance in allowing the child to represent the full range of mental states, including epistemic ones (such as false belief), and is important in allowing the child to pull mentalistic knowledge into a useful theory with which to predict behavior (Baron-Cohen, 1995; Wellman, 1990). But TESS allows more than behavioral explanation and prediction (itself a powerful achievement). TESS allows an empathic reaction to another's emotional state. And relevant to the evolutionary focus of this book, TESS carries with it the adaptive benefit of ensuring that organisms feel a drive to help each other.

To see the difference between TESS and ToMM, consider this example: *I see you are in pain.* Here, ToMM is needed, to interpret your facial expressions and writhing body movements in terms of your underlying mental state (pain). But now consider this further example: *I am devastated—that you are in pain.* Here, TESS is needed, since an appropriate affective state has been triggered in the observer by the emotional state identified in the other person. And where ToMM employs M-Representations (Leslie, 1995) of the form *agent–attitude–proposition* (e.g., "Mother—believes—Johnny took the cookie"), TESS employs a new class of representations, which we can call E-Representations of the form *Self-Affective state–[Self-Affective state–proposition]* (e.g., "I feel sorry that—Mom feels sad about—the news in the letter") (Baron-Cohen, 2003). The critical feature of this E-Representation is that the self's affective state is *appropriate to* and *triggered by* the other person's affective state. Thus, TESS can represent

> *I am horrified—that you are in pain*, or
> *I am concerned—that you are in pain*, or
> *I want to alleviate—that you are in pain*,

but it cannot represent

> *I am happy—that you are in pain.*

At least, it cannot do so if TESS is functioning normally. One could imagine an abnormality in TESS leading to such inappropriate emotional states being triggered, or one could imagine them arising from other systems (e.g., a competition system or a sibling-rivalry system), but these would not be evidence of TESS per se.

Before leaving this revision of the model, it is worth discussing why the need for this has arisen. First, emotional states are an important class of mental states to detect in others, yet the earlier model focused only on volitional, perceptual, informational, and epistemic states. Second, when it comes to pathology, it appears that in autism TED may function (Baron-Cohen, Spitz, & Cross, 1993; Baron-Cohen, Wheelwright, & Jolliffe, 1997; Hobson, 1986), at least in terms of detecting basic emotions, although this may be delayed. Even high-functioning people with autism or Asperger syndrome have difficulties both in ToMM (when measured with mental-age-appropriate tests) (Baron-Cohen, Joliffe, Mortimore, & Robertson, 1997; Baron-Cohen, Wheelwright, Hill, Raste, & Plumb, 2001; Happe, 1994) and TESS (Attwood, 1997; Baron-Cohen, O'Riordan, Jones, Stone, & Plaisted, 1999; Baron-Cohen, Richler, Bisarya, Gurunathan, & Wheelwright, 2003; Baron-Cohen & Wheelwright, 2004; Baron-Cohen, Wheelwright, Stone, & Rutherford, 1999). This suggests that TED and TESS may be fractionated.

In contrast, the psychiatric condition of psychopathy may entail an intact TED and ToMM, alongside an impaired TESS. The psychopath (or sociopath) can represent that *you are in pain*, or that *you believe—that he is the gas-man*, thereby gaining access to your house or your credit card. The psychopath can go on to hurt you or cheat you, without having the appropriate affective reaction to your affective state. In other words, he or she does not *care* about your affective state (Blair, Jones, Clark, & Smith, 1997; Mealey, 1995). Lack of guilt or shame or compassion in the presence of another's distress is diagnostic of psychopathy (Cleckley, 1977; Hare et al., 1990). Separating TESS and ToMM thus allows a functional distinction to be drawn between the neuro-cognitive causes of autism and psychopathy.

Developmentally, one can also distinguish TED from TESS. We know that at 3 months of age, infants can discriminate facial and vocal expressions of emotion (Trevarthen, 1989; Walker, 1982) but not until about age 14 months can they respond with appropriate affect (e.g., a facial expression of concern) to another's apparent pain (Yirmiya, Kasari, Sigman, & Mundy, 1992) or show "social referencing." Clearly, this account is skeletal in not specifying how many emotions TED is capable of recognizing. Our recent survey of emotions identifies 412 discrete emotion concepts that the adult English language user recognizes (Baron-Cohen, Golan, et al., 2003). How many of these are recognized in the first year of life is not clear. It is also not clear exactly how empathizing changes during the second year of life. We have assumed that the same mechanism that enables social referencing at 14 months of age also allows sympathy and the growth of empathy across development. This is the most parsimonious model, though it may be that future research will justify further mechanisms that affect the development of empathy.

In the second half of this chapter, I consider the development of empathizing in more detail, particularly focusing on normal sex differences. This is not only relevant to evolutionary theories of sexual dimorphism, but also to the "extreme male brain" (EMB) theory of autism.

SEX DIFFERENCES IN EMPATHIZING
AND SYSTEMIZING

Empathizing allows one to *predict* a person's behavior, and to care about how others feel. In this section, I review the evidence that, on average, females spontaneously empathize to a greater degree than do males. But I want to broaden the discussion to another psychological process, "systemizing," because this will help us understand normal sex differences and autism. Systemizing is the drive to analyze the variables in a system, to derive the underlying rules that govern the behavior of a system. Systemizing also refers to the drive to construct systems. Systemizing allows you to *predict* the behavior of a system, and to control it. I also review the evidence that, on average, males spontaneously systemize to a greater degree than do females (Baron-Cohen, Wheelwright, Griffin, Lawson, & Hill, 2002).

Empathizing has already been considered in relation to TESS. But systemizing is a new concept and needs a little more definition. By a "system" I mean something that takes inputs and deliver outputs. When you systemize, you use "if–then" (correlation) rules. The brain zooms in on a detail (or parameter) of the system and observes how this varies; that is, it treats a feature as a variable. Typically, the person actively manipulates this variable (hence the English word, "systematically"). The brain notes the effect(s) of operating on this one input in terms of its effects elsewhere in the system (the output). The key data structure or representation used in systemizing has the following form: [input–operation–output]. We can call these S-Representations. If I do x, a changes to b. If z occurs, p changes to q. Systemizing therefore needs an exact eye for detail.

There are at least six kinds of system that the human brain can analyze or construct:

- *Technical* systems (e.g., a computer, a musical instrument, a hammer)
- *Natural* systems (e.g., a tide, a weather front, a plant)
- *Abstract* systems (e.g., mathematics, a computer program, or syntax)
- *Social* systems (e.g., a political election, a legal system, a business)
- *Organizable* systems (e.g., a taxonomy, a collection, a library)
- *Motoric* systems (e.g., a sports technique, a performance, a musical technique)

Systemizing is an inductive process. You watch what happens each time, gathering data about an event from repeated sampling, often quantifying differences in some variables within the event and their correlation with variation in outcome. After confirming a reliable pattern of association, generating predictable results, you form a rule about how this aspect of the system works. When one exception occurs, the rule is refined or revised. Otherwise, the rule is retained.

Systemizing works for phenomena that are indeed ultimately lawful, finite, and deterministic. The explanation is exact and its truth value is defeasible ("The light went on because switch A was in the down position"). Systemizing is of almost no use when it comes to predicting the moment-by-moment changes in a person's behavior. To predict human behavior, empathizing is required. Systemizing and empathizing are wholly different kinds of processes.

Although systemizing and empathizing are in one way similar processes that allow us to make sense of events and make predictions, they are in another way almost the opposite of each other. Empathizing involves an imaginative leap in the dark, in the absence of much data ("Maybe she didn't phone me because she was feeling hurt by my comment"). The causal explanation is at best a "maybe," and its truth may never be provable. Systemizing is our most powerful way of understanding and predicting the law-governed inanimate universe. Empathizing is our most powerful way of understanding and predicting the social world. Ultimately, empathizing and systemizing depend on independent regions in the human brain (Baron-Cohen, Ring, et al., 1999; Ring et al., 1999).

The Main Brain Types

I argue that systemizing and empathizing are two key dimensions in defining the male and female brain. We all have both systemizing and empathizing skills. One can envisage five broad types of brain immediately.

- Individuals in whom empathizing (E) is more developed than systemizing (S). For shorthand, E > S (or Type E). This is what we call the female brain.
- Individuals in whom systemizing is more developed than empathizing. For shorthand, S > E (or Type S). This is what we call the male brain.
- Individuals in whom systemizing and empathizing are both equally developed. For shorthand, S = E. This is what we call the "balanced brain" (or Type B).
- Individuals with the extreme of the male brain. For shorthand, S >> E. In their case, systemizing is hyperdeveloped, while empathizing is hypodeveloped; that is, they may be talented systemizers but at the same time they may be "mind-blind" (Baron-Cohen, 1995). Later, we look at individuals on the autistic spectrum to see if they fit the profile of being an extreme of the male brain.
- Finally, we postulate the existence of the extreme of the female brain. For shorthand, E >> S. These people have hyperdeveloped empathizing skills, while their systemizing is hypodeveloped—they may be "system-blind."

The evidence reviewed below suggests that not all men have the male brain, and not all women have the female brain. Expressed differently, some women have the male brain, and some men have the female brain. The central claim of this chapter is only that *more* males than females have a brain of Type S, and *more* females than males have a brain of Type E. The evidence for these profiles is shown below. In the final section, I highlight the role of culture and biology in these sex differences.

The Female Brain: Empathizing

What is the evidence for female superiority in empathizing? In the studies summarized here, sex differences of a small but statistically significant magnitude have been found.

1. *Sharing and turn taking.* On average, girls show more concern for fairness, while boys share less. In one study, boys showed 50 times more competition, while girls showed 20 times more turn-taking (Charlesworth & Dzur, 1987).

2. *Rough-and-tumble play or "roughhousing"* (wrestling, mock fighting, etc.). Boys show more of this than do girls. Although there is a playful component, it can hurt or be intrusive, so lower empathizing is needed to carry it out (Maccoby, 1999).

3. *Responding empathically to the distress of other people.* Girls from age 1 year old show greater concern than boys through more sad looks, sympathetic vocalizations, and comforting. More women than men also report frequently sharing the emotional distress of their friends. Women also show more comforting, even of strangers, than do men (Hoffman, 1977).

4. *Using a "theory of mind."* By age 3 years old, little girls are already ahead of boys in their ability to infer what people might be thinking or intending (Happe, 1995). This sex difference appears in some but not all studies (Charman, Ruffman, & Clements, 2002).

5. *Sensitivity to facial expressions.* Women are better at decoding nonverbal communication, picking up subtle nuances from tone of voice or facial expression, or judging a person's character (Hall, 1978).

6. *Questionnaires measuring empathy.* Many of these find that women score higher than men (Davis, 1994).

7. *Values in relationships.* More women value the development of altruistic, reciprocal relationships, which, by definition, require empathizing. In contrast, more men value power, politics, and competition (Ahlgren & Johnson, 1979). Girls are more likely to endorse cooperative items on a questionnaire and to rate the establishment of intimacy as more important than the establishment of dominance. Boys are more likely than girls to endorse competitive items and to rate social status as more important than intimacy (Knight, Fabes, & Higgins, 1989).

8. *Disorders of empathy* (e.g., psychopathic personality disorder, or conduct disorder). These disorders are far more common among males (Blair, 1995; Dodge, 1980).

9. *Aggression, even in normal quantities, can only occur with reduced empathizing.* Here, again, there is a clear sex difference. Males tend to show far more "direct" aggression (pushing, hitting, punching, etc.), while females tend to show more "indirect" (or "relational," covert) aggression (gossip, exclusion, bitchy remarks, etc.). Direct aggression may require an even lower level of empathy than indirect aggression. Indirect aggression requires better mindreading skills than does direct aggression, because its impact is strategic (Crick & Grotpeter, 1995).

10. *Murder is the ultimate example of a lack of empathy.* Daly and Wilson (1988) analyzed homicide records dating back over 700 years, from a range of different societies. They found that "male-on-male" homicide was 30–40 times more frequent than "female-on-female" homicide.

11. *Establishing a "dominance hierarchy."* Males are quicker to establish these. This in part may reflect their lower empathizing skills, because often a hierarchy is established by one person pushing others around, to become the leader (Strayer, 1980).

12. *Language style.* Girls' speech is more cooperative, reciprocal, and collaborative. In concrete terms, this is also reflected in girls, being able to keep a conversational exchange with a partner going for longer. When girls disagree, they are more likely to express their different opinion sensitively, in the form of a question, rather than an assertion. Boys' talk is more "single-voiced discourse" (the speaker presents his own perspective alone). The female speech style is more "double-voiced discourse" (girls spend more time negotiating with the other person, trying to take the other person's wishes into account) (Smith, 1985).

13. *Talk about emotions.* Women's conversation involves much more talk about feelings, while men's conversation with each other tends to be more object- or activity-focused (Tannen, 1991).

14. *Parenting style.* Fathers are less likely than mothers to hold their infant in a face-to-face position. Mothers are more likely to follow through the child's choice of topic in play, while fathers are more likely to impose their own topic. And mothers fine-tune their speech more often to match what the child can understand (Power, 1985).

15. *Face preference and eye contact.* From birth, females look longer at faces, and particularly at people's eyes, whereas males are more likely to look at inanimate objects (Connellan, Baron-Cohen, Wheelwright, Ba'tki, & Ahluwalia, 2001).

Females have also been shown to have better language ability than males. It seems likely that good empathizing would promote language development (Baron-Cohen, Baldwin, & Crowson, 1997) and vice versa, so these may not be independent.

The Male Brain: Systemizing

The relevant domains in which to look for evidence of sex differences in systemizing would include any that are in principle rule-governed. Thus, chess and football are good examples of systems, while faces and conversations are not. Systemizing involves monitoring three things: input–operation–output. The operation is what one did to the input, or what happened to the input, to produce the output. What kind of evidence is there?

1. *Toy preferences.* Boys are more interested than girls in toy vehicles, weapons, building blocks and mechanical toys, all of which are open to being "systemized" (Jennings, 1977).

2. *Adult occupational choices.* Some occupations are performed almost entirely by males. These include metalworking, weapon making, manufacturing musical instruments, or the construction industries, such as boat building. The focus of these occupations is on constructing systems (Geary, 1998).

3. *Maths, physics, and engineering.* All require high systemizing and are largely male-dominated disciplines. The Scholastic Aptitude Math Test (SAT-M) is the math part of the test administered nationally to college applicants in the United States. Males, on average, score 50 points higher than females on this test (Benbow & Stanley, 1983). By the time one looks at those people scoring above 700, the sex ratio is 13:1 (men to women) (Geary, 1996).

4. *Constructional abilities.* If one asks people to put together a three-dimensional (3D) mechanical apparatus in an assembly task, on average men score higher. Boys are also better at constructing block buildings from two-dimensional (2D) blueprints. Lego bricks can be combined and recombined into an infinite number of systems. Boys show more interest in playing with Lego. Boys as young as age 3 are also faster at copying 3D models of outsized Lego pieces, and older boys, from age 9, are better at imagining what a 3D object will look like if it is laid out flat. They are also better at constructing a 3D structure from just an aerial and frontal view in a picture (Kimura, 1999).

5. *The Water-Level Task.* Originally devised by Swiss child psychologist Jean Piaget, in this task, the subject is shown a bottle, tipped at an angle, and then asked to predict the water level. Women more often draw the water level aligned with the tilt of the bottle, and not horizontal, as it should be (Wittig & Allen, 1984). We can think of this as involving systemizing, because one has to predict the output after performing an operation on the input.

6. *The Rod and Frame Test.* If a person's judgement of vertical is influenced by the tilt of the frame, he or she is said to be "field dependent": His or her judgement is easily swayed by extraneous input in the surrounding context. If not influenced by the tilt of the frame, he or she is said to be "field independent." Most studies show that females are more field dependent (i.e., women are relatively more distracted by contextual cues, rather than considering each variable within the system separately). They are more likely than

men to say (erroneously) that the rod is upright if it is aligned with its frame (Witkin, Dyk, Faterson, Goodenough, & Karp, 1962).

7. *Good attention to relevant detail is a general feature of systemizing.* It is not the only factor, but it is a necessary part of it. Attention to relevant detail is superior in males. A measure of this is the Embedded Figures Test. On average, males are quicker and more accurate in locating the target from the larger, complex pattern (Elliot, 1961). Males, on average, are also better at detecting a particular feature (static or moving) (Voyer, Voyer, & Bryden, 1995).

8. *The Mental Rotation Test.* Here, again, males are quicker and more accurate. This test involves systemizing, because one has to treat each feature in a display as a variable that can be transformed (e.g., rotated) and predict how it will appear (the output) (Collins & Kimura, 1997).

9. *Reading maps.* This is another everyday test of systemizing, because one has to take features from 3D input and predict how it will appear when transformed to two dimensions. Boys perform at a higher level than girls. Men can also learn a route in fewer trials, just from looking at a map, correctly recalling more details about direction and distance. This suggests they are treating features in the map as variables that can be transformed into three dimensions. If you ask boys to make a map of an area that they have only visited once, their maps have a more accurate layout of the features in the environment. Girls' maps include more serious errors in the location of important landmarks. Boys tend to emphasize routes or roads, whereas girls tend to emphasize specific landmarks (the corner shop, etc.). These two strategies—using directional cues versus landmark cues—have been widely studied. The directional strategy is an instance of understanding space as a geometric system, and the focus on roads or routes is an instance of considering space in terms of another system, in this case, a transport system (Galea & Kimura, 1993).

10. *Motoric systems.* If asked to throw or catch moving objects (target-directed tasks) such as playing darts or intercepting balls flung from a launcher, males tend to be better. Equally, if men are asked to judge which of two moving objects is traveling faster, on average they are more accurate than women (Schiff & Oldak, 1990).

11. *Organizable systems.* People in the Aguaruna tribe (northern Peru) were asked to classify 100 or more examples of local specimens together into related species. Men's classification systems had more subcategories (i.e., they introduced greater differentiation) and more consistency between each other. The criteria that the Aguaruna men used to decide which animals belonged together more closely resembled the taxonomic criteria used by Western (mostly male) biologists (Atran, 1994). Classification and organization involves systemizing, because categories are predictive. The more fine-grained the categories, the better the system of prediction will be.

12. *The Systemizing Quotient.* This questionnaire has been tested among adults in the general population. It has 40 items asking about the person's

level of interest in a range of different systems that exist in the environment (including technical, abstract, and natural systems). Males score higher than females on this measure (Baron-Cohen et al., 2003).

13. *Mechanics.* The Physical Prediction Questionnaire (PPQ) is based on an established method for selecting applicants for engineering. The task involves predicting which direction levers will move when an internal mechanism (of cog wheels and pulleys) of one type or another is involved. Men score significantly higher on this test compared to women (Lawson, Baron-Cohen, & Wheelwright, 2004).

Culture and Biology

At 1 year old, boys show a stronger preference to watch a video of cars going past (predictable mechanical systems), than to watch a film showing a human face. Little girls showed the opposite preference. Little girls also show more eye contact than do boys by 1 year of age (Lutchmaya & Baron-Cohen, 2002). Some argue that even by this age, socialization might have caused these sex differences. Although there is evidence for differential socialization contributing to sex differences, this is unlikely to be a sufficient explanation. This is because among *1-day-old* babies, boys look longer at a mechanical mobile (a system with predictable laws of motion) than at a person's face (an object that is next to impossible to systemize), and 24-hour-old girls show the opposite profile (Connellan et al., 2001). These sex differences are therefore present very early in life. This raises the possibility that, although culture and socialization may partly determine whether one develops a male brain (stronger interest in systems) or a female brain (stronger interest in empathy), biology may also partly determine this. There is ample evidence for both cultural and biological influence (Eagly, 1987; Gouchie & Kimura, 1991). For example, the amount of eye contact a 1-year-old child makes is inversely related to his or her level of *prenatal* testosterone (Lutchmaya, Baron-Cohen, & Raggett, 2002a, 2002b). The evidence for the biological basis of sex differences in the mind is reviewed elsewhere (Baron-Cohen, 2003).

Evolution and Social Development

From an evolutionary perspective, sex difference in empathizing and systemizing are likely to have been shaped by sexual selection and follow, at least in part, from sex differences in reproductive strategies. Female superiority in empathizing would not only facilitate development of stable social relationships, garner social support, and increase sensitivity to the needs of others (all of which are important for child rearing), but it would also be adaptive in negotiating the more subtle dominance hierarchies that develop among girls and women (e.g., relational aggression) (Geary, 1998). Selection pressures were thus especially likely to have favored empathizing skills in women. Conversely, high levels of empathy were unlikely to have been selected for in males. Too much empathy may impede success in rough-and-tumble play and other aggressive activities in male peer groups that function to prepare boys for later, within-group dominance striving, and intergroup competition and aggression. In addition, the evolutionary significance of male superiority in systemizing has long been discussed in terms of hunting and warfare and associated sex differences in use of tools, weaponry, and navigation of 3D space (Geary, 1998). (See Pellegrini & Archer, Chapter 9, this volume, for further discussion of the evolutionary–developmental bases of sex differences in social behavior.)

AUTISM: AN EXTREME FORM OF THE MALE BRAIN

Autism is diagnosed when a person shows abnormalities in social development and communication, and displays unusually strong obsessional interests from an early age (American Psychiatric Association, 2000). Asperger syndrome (AS) has been proposed, as a variant of autism, in children with normal or high IQ who develop speech on time. Today, approximately 1 in 200 children has one of the "autistic spectrum conditions," which include AS (Frith, 1991). Autism spectrum conditions affect males far more often than females. In people with high-functioning autism or AS, the sex ratio is at least 10 males to every 1 female. These conditions are also strongly heritable (Bailey, Bolton, & Rutter, 1998) and neurodevelopmental. There is evidence of structural and functional differences in regions of the brain (e.g., the amygdala being abnormal in size, and this structure not responding to cues of emotional expression) (Baron-Cohen et al., 2000).

The extreme male brain (EMB) theory of autism was first informally suggested by Hans Asperger in 1944. He wrote: "The autistic personality is an extreme variant of male intelligence. Even within the normal variation, we find typical sex differences in intelligence. . . . In the autistic individual, the male pattern is exaggerated to the extreme" (Asperger, 1944). This is Uta Frith's translation in 1991. In 1997, this controversial hypothesis was resurrected (Baron-Cohen & Hammer, 1997a). We can test the EMB theory empirically, now that we have definitions of the female brain (E > S), the male brain (S > E), and the balanced brain (E = S).

Evidence for the Extreme Male Brain Theory

To reiterate, the EMB theory predicts that females will perform better on tests of empathizing (E), males will perform better on tests of systemizing (S), and that people with autism spectrum conditions will show impaired E alongside intact or even superior S. Initial tests of this theory have proven positive (Baron-Cohen, 2000). Some of the convergent lines of evidence are summarized here.

Impaired Empathizing

1. *Mindreading.* Girls are better than boys on standard theory of mind tests, and children with autism or AS are even worse than normal boys (Happe, 1995). They have specific delays and difficulties in the development of mindreading (i.e., in making sense of and predicting another's feelings, thoughts, and behavior). Autism has been referred to as a condition of "mindblindness" (Baron-Cohen, 1995).

2. *The Empathy Quotient* (EQ). On this self-report questionnaire, females score higher than males, and people with AS or high-functioning autism (HFA) score even lower than males (Baron-Cohen, Richler, et al., 2003; Baron-Cohen & Wheelwright, 2004).

3. *The "Reading the Mind in the Eyes" Test.* Females score higher than males on this subtle test of emotion recognition, but people with AS score even lower than males (Baron-Cohen, Jolliffe, Mortimore, & Robertson, 1997).

4. *The Complex Facial Expressions Test.* Females score higher than males on this test of a range of emotional expressions, but people with AS score even lower than males (Baron-Cohen, Wheelwright, et al., 1997).

5. *Eye contact.* Females make more eye contact than do males, and people with autism or AS make less eye contact than males (Lutchmaya, Baron-Cohen, & Raggett, 2002b; Swettenham et al., 1998).

6. *Language development.* Girls develop vocabulary faster than boys, and children with autism develop vocabulary even more slowly than males (Lutchmaya et al., 2002a).

7. *Pragmatics.* Females tend to be superior to males in terms of chatting and the pragmatics of conversation, and it is precisely this aspect of language that people with AS find most difficult (Baron-Cohen, 1988).

8. *The Faux Pas Test.* Females are better than males at judging what would be socially insensitive or potentially hurtful and offensive, and people with autism or AS have even lower scores on tests of this than do males (Baron-Cohen, O'Riordan, et al., 1999).

9. *The Friendship Questionnaire* (FQ). This assesses empathic styles of relationships. Women score higher on the FQ than males, and adults with AS score even lower than normal males (Baron-Cohen & Wheelwright, 2003).

Superior Systemizing

1. *Islets of ability.* A proportion of people with autism spectrum disorders have "islets of ability." The more common domains in which these occur are mathematical calculation, calendrical calculation, syntax acquisition, music, or memory (e.g., for railway time table information to a precise degree)

(Baron-Cohen & Bolton, 1993). In the high-functioning cases, this can lead to considerable achievement in mathematics, chess, mechanical knowledge, and other factual, scientific, technical, or rule-based subjects. All of these are highly systemizable domains. Most of them are also domains where males in the general population have a greater interest.

2. *Attention to detail.* Autism also leads to extrafine attention to detail. For example, on the Embedded Figures Task (EFT), males score higher than females, and people with AS or HFA score even higher than males. The EFT is a good measure of detailed local perception, a prerequisite for systemizing (Jolliffe & Baron-Cohen, 1997). On visual search tasks, males exhibit better attention to detail than do females, and people with autism or AS have even faster, more accurate visual search skills (O'Riordan, Plaisted, Driver, & Baron-Cohen, 2001).

3. *Preference for rule-based, structured, factual information.* People with autism are strongly drawn to structured, factual, and rule-based information. A male bias for this kind of information is also found in the general population.

4. *Tests of intuitive physics.* Males score higher than females in solving these physics problems, and people with AS score higher than males (Baron-Cohen, Wheelwright, Scahill, Lawson, & Spong, 2001).

5. *Toy preference.* Boys prefer constructional and vehicular toys more than do girls (Maccoby, 1999), and clinical reports suggest that children with autism or AS have this very strong toy preference.

6. *Collecting.* Boys appear to engage in more collecting or organizing of items (e.g., CDs) than do girls (and this would benefit from a careful study); clinical accounts suggest that people with autism show this to an even greater extent.

7. *Obsessions with closed systems.* Individuals with autism are often naturally drawn to predictable things, such as computers. Unlike people, computers do follow strict laws. Computers are closed systems; all the variables are well-defined within the system, are knowable, predictable, and, in principle, controllable. Other individuals with autism may not make computers their target of understanding but may latch on to a different, equally closed system (such as bird migration or train spotting) (Baron-Cohen & Wheelwright, 1999). Again, such interests in the general population are more often associated with males (Baron-Cohen, 2003).

8. *The Systemizing Quotient.* As mentioned earlier, males score higher on this instrument, and people with autism and AS score even higher than normal males (Baron-Cohen, Richler, et al., 2003).

9. *The Autism Spectrum Quotient* (AQ). Males in the general population score higher than females, and people with AS or HFA score highest of all (Baron-Cohen, Wheelwright, Skinner, Martin, & Clubley, 2001).

The above evidence points to people with autism showing an extreme male profile, as defined earlier, but to what might this be due?

Family–Genetic Evidence

Familiality of talent. Fathers and grandfathers of children with autism (on both sides of the family) are overrepresented in occupations such as engineering, which require good systemizing but in which a mild impairment in empathizing (as has been documented) would not necessarily be an impediment to success (Baron-Cohen & Hammer, 1997b; Baron-Cohen, Wheelwright, Stott, Bolton, & Goodyer, 1997). There is a higher rate of autism in the families of those talented in fields such as maths, physics, and engineering, as compared to those talented in the humanities (Baron-Cohen et al., 1998). These latter two findings suggest that the extreme male cognitive style is in part inherited.

CONCLUSIONS AND FUTURE RESEARCH

In this chapter, I have introduced the first major revision to the 1994 model of the mindreading system by adding two neurocognitive mechanisms (the Emotion Detector and the Empathizing SyStem). I have also explained the need for taking a broader view, as the new model does of empathizing. One of the key benefits of this is that we can distinguish between two types of condition, autism versus psychopathy.

We have also considered the relevance of sex differences in both empathizing (female advantage) and systemizing (male advantage), and in terms of the EMB theory of autism. In Figure 18.3, these sex differences, and the extremes, are shown in a model that assumes empathizing and systemizing are two independent dimensions. Future research will need to test an alternative model: There is a trade-off such that the better one scores on one dimension, the worse one scores on the other. This would suggest a single mechanism (e.g., fetal testosterone?) may be involved in both. This is currently being tested.

We know something about the neural circuitry of empathizing (Baron-Cohen, Ring, et al., 1999; Frith & Frith, 1999; Happe et al., 1996) but at present, we know very little about the neural circuitry of systemizing (Ring et al., 1999). It is expected that research will begin to reveal the key brain regions.

Finally, in terms of the focus of this book on the origins of the social mind, it is my hope that with the new model of empathizing, one benefit of delineating these separable components will be not only to test for their neurological dissociability from one another but also to consider the adaptive importance of each component. It is apparent that each of these mechanisms would have conferred unique advantages on the individual, such that each could be the result of natural selection. Testing evolutionary hypotheses is, of course, notoriously difficult, but naturally occurring developmental conditions (e.g., autism and psychopathy) may provide a fruitful window into their neurological independence.

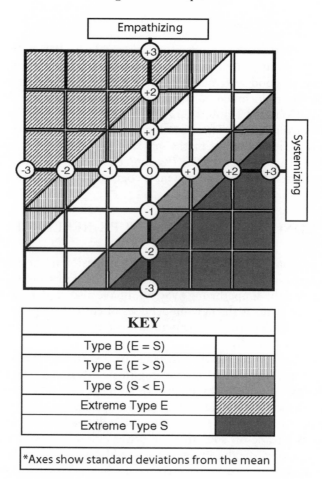

FIGURE 18.3. A model of empathizing and systemizing.

ACKNOWLEDGMENTS

The following agencies supported my work during the writing of this chapter: the Medical Research Council (UK) and the James S. McDonnell Foundation. Parts of this chapter are based on work published elsewhere (Baron-Cohen, Hill, Golan, & Wheelwright, 2002). I am grateful to Johnny Lawson for producing Figure 18.3.

REFERENCES

Ahlgren, A., & Johnson, D. W. (1979). Sex differences in cooperative and competitive attitudes from the 2nd to the 12th grades. *Developmental Psychology, 15,* 45–49.
Alexander, R. D. (1979). *Darwinism and human affairs.* Seattle: University of Washington Press.

American Psychiatric Association. (2000). *Diagnostic and statistical manual of mental disorders (4th ed., text rev.)*. Washington DC: Author.

Asperger, H. (1944). Die "Autistischen Psychopathen" im Kindesalter. *Archiv fur Psychiatrie und Nervenkrankheiten, 117*, 76–136.

Atran, S. (1994). Core domains versus scientific theories: Evidence from systematics and Itza-Maya folkbiology. In L. A. Hirschfeld & S. A. Gelman (Eds.), *Mapping the mind: Domain specificity in cognition and culture.* New York: Cambridge University Press.

Attwood, T. (1997). *Asperger's syndrome.* London: Jessica Kingsley.

Bailey, A., Bolton, P., & Rutter, M. (1998). A full genome screen for autism with evidence for linkage to a region on chromosome 7q. *Human Molecular Genetics, 7*, 571–578.

Baron-Cohen, S. (1988). Social and pragmatic deficits in autism: Cognitive or affective? *Journal of Autism and Developmental Disorders, 18*, 379–402.

Baron-Cohen, S. (1989a). The autistic child's theory of mind: A case of specific developmental delay. *Journal of Child Psychology and Psychiatry, 30*, 285–298.

Baron-Cohen, S. (1989b). Perceptual role taking and protodeclarative pointing in autism. *British Journal of Developmental Psychology, 7*, 113–127.

Baron-Cohen, S. (1991). Precursors to a theory of mind: Understanding attention in others. In A. Whiten (Ed.), *Natural theories of mind.* Oxford, UK: Blackwell.

Baron-Cohen, S. (1994). The mindreading system: New directions for research. *Current Psychology of Cognition, 13*, 724–750.

Baron-Cohen, S. (1995). *Mindblindness: An essay on autism and theory of mind.* Cambridge, MA: MIT Press/Bradford Books.

Baron-Cohen, S. (2000). The cognitive neuroscience of autism: Implications for the evolution of the male brain. In M. Gazzaniga (Ed.), *The cognitive neurosciences* (2nd ed.). Cambridge, MA: MIT Press.

Baron-Cohen, S. (2003). *The essential difference: Men, women and the extreme male brain.* London: Penguin.

Baron-Cohen, S., Baldwin, D., & Crowson, M. (1997). Do children with autism use the Speaker's Direction of Gaze (SDG) strategy to crack the code of language? *Child Development, 68*, 48–57.

Baron-Cohen, S., & Bolton, P. (1993). *Autism: The facts.* Oxford: Oxford University Press.

Baron-Cohen, S., Bolton, P., Wheelwright, S., Short, L., Mead, G., Smith, A., & Scahill, V. (1998). Does autism occurs more often in families of physicists, engineers, and mathematicians? *Autism, 2*, 296–301.

Baron-Cohen, S., Golan, O., Wheelwright, S., & Hill, J. (2003). *Mindreading: The interactive guide to emotions.* London: Jessica Kingsley.

Baron-Cohen, S., & Hammer, J. (1997a). Is autism an extreme form of the male brain? *Advances in Infancy Research, 11*, 193–217.

Baron-Cohen, S., & Hammer, J. (1997b). Parents of children with Asperger syndrome: What is the cognitive phenotype? *Journal of Cognitive Neuroscience, 9*, 548–554.

Baron-Cohen, S., Hill, J. J., Golan, O., & Wheelwright, S. (2002). Mindreading made easy. *Cambridge Medicine, 17*, 28–29.

Baron-Cohen, S., Joliffe, T., Mortimore, C., & Robertson, M. (1997). Another advanced test of theory of mind: Evidence from very high functioning adults with autism or Asperger syndrome. *Journal of Child Psychology and Psychiatry, 38*, 813–822.

Baron-Cohen, S., Leslie, A. M., & Frith, U. (1985). Does the autistic child have a "theory of mind"? *Cognition, 21*, 37–46.

Baron-Cohen, S., O'Riordan, M., Jones, R., Stone, V., & Plaisted, K. (1999). A new test of social sensitivity: Detection of faux pas in normal children and children with Asperger syndrome. *Journal of Autism and Developmental Disorders, 29*, 407–418.

Baron-Cohen, S., Richler, J., Bisarya, D., Gurunathan, N., & Wheelwright, S. (2003). The Systemising Quotient (SQ) : An investigation of adults with Asperger syndrome or high functioning autism and normal sex differences. *Philosophical Transactions of the Royal Society, Series B* [Special issue on "Autism: Mind and Brain"], *358*, 361–374.

Baron-Cohen, S., Ring, H., Bullmore, E., Wheelwright, S., Ashwin, C., & Williams, S. (2000). The amygdala theory of autism. *Neuroscience and Behavioural Reviews, 24*, 355–364.

Baron-Cohen, S., Ring, H., Wheelwright, S., Bullmore, E. T., Brammer, M. J., Simmons, A., & Williams, S. (1999). Social intelligence in the normal and autistic brain: An fMRI study. *European Journal of Neuroscience, 11*, 1891–1898.

Baron-Cohen, S., Spitz, A., & Cross, P. (1993). Can children with autism recognize surprise? *Cognition and Emotion, 7*, 507–516.

Baron-Cohen, S., & Swettenham, J. (1996). The relationship between SAM and ToMM: The lock and key hypothesis. In P. Carruthers & P. Smith (Eds.), *Theories of Theories of Mind*: Cambridge, UK: Cambridge University Press.

Baron-Cohen, S., & Wheelwright, S. (1999). Obsessions in children with autism or Asperger syndrome: A content analysis in terms of core domains of cognition. *British Journal of Psychiatry, 175*, 484–490.

Baron-Cohen, S., & Wheelwright, S. (2003). The Friendship Questionnaire (FQ): An investigation of adults with Asperger syndrome or high functioning autism, and normal sex differences. *Journal of Autism and Developmental Disorders, 33*, 509–517.

Baron-Cohen, S., & Wheelwright, S. (2004). The empathy quotient (EQ): An investigation of adults with Asperger syndrome or high functioning autism, and normal sex differences. *Journal of Autism and Developmental Disorders, 34*, 163175.

Baron-Cohen, S., Wheelwright, S., Griffin, R., Lawson, J., & Hill, J. (2002). The exact mind: Empathising and systemising in autism spectrum conditions. In U. Goswami (Ed.), *Handbook of cognitive development*. Oxford: Blackwell.

Baron-Cohen, S., Wheelwright, S., Hill, J., Raste, Y., & Plumb, I. (2001). The "Reading the Mind in the Eyes" test revised version: A study with normal adults, and adults with Asperger syndrome or high-functioning autism. *Journal of Child Psychiatry and Psychiatry, 42*, 241–252.

Baron-Cohen, S., Wheelwright, S., & Jolliffe, T. (1997). Is there a "language of the eyes"? Evidence from normal adults and adults with autism or Asperger syndrome. *Visual Cognition, 4*, 311–331.

Baron-Cohen, S., Wheelwright, S., Scahill, V., Lawson, J., & Spong, A. (2001). Are intuitive physics and intuitive psychology independent? *Journal of Developmental and Learning Disorders, 5*, 47–78.

Baron-Cohen, S., Wheelwright, S., Skinner, R., Martin, J., & Clubley, E. (2001). The Autism Spectrum Quotient (AQ): Evidence from Asperger Syndrome/High Functioning Autism, Males and Females, Scientists and Mathematicians. *Journal of Autism and Developmental Disorders, 31*, 5–17.

Baron-Cohen, S., Wheelwright, S., Stone, V., & Rutherford, M. (1999). A mathematician, a physicist, and a computer scientist with Asperger syndrome: Performance on folk psychology and folk physics test. *Neurocase, 5,* 475–483.

Baron-Cohen, S., Wheelwright, S., Stott, C., Bolton, P., & Goodyer, I. (1997). Is there a link between engineering and autism? *Autism: An International Journal of Research and Practice, 1,* 153–163.

Benbow, C. P., & Stanley, J. C. (1983). Sex differences in mathematical reasoning ability: More facts. *Science, 222,* 1029–1031.

Bjorklund, D. F., & Pellegrini, A. D. (2002). *The origins of human nature: Evolutionary developmental psychology.* Washington, DC: American Psychological Association.

Blair, R. J. (1995). A cognitive developmental approach to morality: Investigating the psychopath. *Cognition, 57,* 1–29.

Blair, R. J., Jones, L., Clark, F., & Smith, M. (1997). The psychopathic individual: A lack of responsiveness to distress cues? *Psychophysiology, 34,* 192–198.

Call, J., & Tomasello, M. (1999). A nonverbal false belief task: The performance of children and great apes. *Child Development, 70,* 381–395.

Charlesworth, W. R., & Dzur, C. (1987). Gender comparisons of preschoolers' behavior and resource utilization in group problem-solving. *Child Development, 58,* 191–200.

Charman, T., Ruffman, T., & Clements, W. (2002). Is there a gender difference in false belief development? *Social Development, 11,* 1–10.

Cleckley, H. M. (1977). *The mask of sanity: An attempt to clarify some issues about the so-called psychopathic personality.* St Louis: Mosby.

Collins, D. W., & Kimura, D. (1997). A large sex difference on a two-dimensional mental rotation task. *Behavioral Neuroscience, 111,* 845–849.

Connellan, J., Baron-Cohen, S., Wheelwright, S., Ba'tki, A., & Ahluwalia, J. (2001). Sex differences in human neonatal social perception. *Infant Behavior and Development, 23,* 113–118.

Crick, N. R., & Grotpeter, J. K. (1995). Relational aggression, gender, and social-psychological adjustment. *Child Development, 66,* 710–722.

Daly, M., & Wilson, M. (1988). *Homicide.* New York: Aldine de Gruyter.

Davis, M. H. (1994). *Empathy: A social psychological approach.* Boulder, CO: Westview Press.

Dodge, K. (1980). Social cognition and children's aggressive behaviour. *Child Development, 51,* 162–170.

Dunbar, R. I. M. (1998). The social brain hypothesis. *Evolutionary Anthropology, 6,* 178–190.

Eagly, A. H. (1987). *Sex differences in social behavior: A social-role interpretation.* Hillsdale, NJ: Erlbaum.

Ekman, P., & Friesen, W. (1969). The repertoire of non-verbal behavior: Categories, origins, usage, and coding. *Semiotica, 1,* 49–98.

Elliot, R. (1961). Interrelationship among measures of field dependence, ability, and personality traits. *Journal of Abnormal and Social Psychology, 63,* 27–36.

Field, T. (1979). Visual and cardiac responses to animate and inanimate faces by term and preterm infants. *Child Development, 50,* 188–194.

Frith, C., & Frith, U. (1999). Interacting minds—a biological basis. *Science, 286,* 1692–1695.

Frith, U. (1991). *Autism and Asperger's syndrome.* Cambridge, UK: Cambridge University Press.

Galea, L. A. M., & Kimura, D. (1993). Sex differences in route learning. *Personality and Individual Differences, 14,* 53–65.

Geary, D. (1996). Sexual selection and sex differences in mathematical abilities. *Behavioural and Brain Sciences, 19,* 229–284.

Geary, D. C. (1998). *Male, female: The evolution of human sex differences.* Washington, DC: American Psychological Association.

Geary, D. C. (2005). *The origin of mind: Evolution of brain, cognition and general intelligence.* Washington, DC: American Psychological Association.

Gouchie, C., & Kimura, D. (1991). The relationship between testosterone levels and cognitive ability patterns. *Psychoneuroendocrinology, 16,* 323–334.

Hall, J. A. (1978). Gender effects in decoding nonverbal cues. *Psychological Bulletin, 85,* 845–858).

Happe, F. (1994). An advanced test of theory of mind: Understanding of story characters' thoughts and feelings by able autistic, mentally handicapped, and normal children and adults. *Journal of Autism and Development Disorders, 24,* 129–154.

Happe, F. (1995). The role of age and verbal ability in the theory of mind task performance of subjects with autism. *Child Development, 66,* 843–855.

Happe, F., Ehlers, S., Fletcher, P., Frith, U., Johansson, M., Gillberg, C., et al. (1996). Theory of mind in the brain: Evidence from a PET scan study of Asperger syndrome. *NeuroReport, 8,* 197–201.

Hare, B., Call, J., Agentta, B., & Tomasello, M. (2000). Chimpanzees know what conspecifics do and do not see. *Animal Behaviour, 59,* 771–785.

Hare, B., Call, J., & Tomasello, M. (2001). Do chimpanzees know what conspecifics know? *Animal Behaviour, 61,* 139–151.

Hare, R. D., Hakstian, T. J., Ralph, A., Forth-Adelle, E., et al. (1990). The Revised Psychopathy Checklist: Reliability and factor structure. *Psychological Assessment, 2,* 338–341.

Hobson, R. P. (1986). The autistic child's appraisal of expressions of emotion. *Journal of Child Psychology and Psychiatry, 27,* 321–342.

Hoffman, M. L. (1977). Sex differences in empathy and related behaviors. *Psychological Bulletin, 84,* 712–722.

Humphrey, N. K. (1976). The social function of intellect. In P. P. G. Bateson & R. A. Hinde (Eds.), *Growing points in ethology.* Cambridge, UK: Cambridge University Press.

Jennings, K. D. (1977). People versus object orientation in preschool children: Do sex differences really occur? *Journal of Genetic Psychology, 131,* 65–73.

Jolliffe, T., & Baron-Cohen, S. (1997). Are people with autism or Asperger's syndrome faster than normal on the Embedded Figures Task? *Journal of Child Psychology and Psychiatry, 38,* 527–534.

Kimura, D. (1999). *Sex and cognition.* Cambridge, MA: MIT Press.

Knight, G. P., Fabes, R. A., & Higgins, D. A. (1989). Gender differences in the cooperative, competitive, and individualistic social values of children. *Motivation and Emotion, 13,* 125–141.

Lawson, J., Baron-Cohen, S., & Wheelwright, S. (2004). Empathising and systemising in adults with and without Asperger syndrome. *Journal of Autism and Developmental Disorders, 34,* 301–310.

Leslie, A. (1995). ToMM, ToBy, and agency: Core architecture and domain specificity. In L. Hirschfeld & S. Gelman (Eds.), *Domain specificity in cognition and culture.* New York: Cambridge University Press.

Leslie, A. M. (1987). Pretence and representation: The origins of "theory of mind." *Psychological Review*, 94, 412–426.

Lutchmaya, S., & Baron-Cohen, S. (2002). Human sex differences in social and non-social looking preferences at 12 months of age. *Infant Behaviour and Development*, 25, 319–325.

Lutchmaya, S., Baron-Cohen, S., & Raggett, P. (2002a). Fetal testosterone and vocabulary size in 18- and 24-month-old infants. *Infant Behavior and Development*, 24(4), 418–424.

Lutchmaya, S., Baron-Cohen, S., & Raggett, P. (2002b). Fetal testosterone and eye contact in 12 month old infants. *Infant Behavior and Development*, 25, 327–335.

Maccoby, E. (1999). *The two sexes: growing up apart, coming together*. Cambridge, MA: Harvard University Press.

Mealey, L. (1995). The sociobiology of sociopathy: An integrated evolutionary model. *Behavioral and Brain Sciences*, 18, 523–599.

O'Riordan, M., Plaisted, K., Driver, J., & Baron-Cohen, S. (2001). Superior visual search in autism. *Journal of Experimental Psychology: Human Perception and Performance*, 27, 719–730.

Povinelli, D. J., & Bering, J. M. (2002). The mentality of apes revisited. *Current Directions in Psychological Science*, 11, 115–119.

Povinelli, D. J., & Eddy, T. J. (1996). Factors influencing young chimpanzees' (*Pan troglodytes*) recognition of attention. *Journal of Comparative Psychology*, 110, 336–345.

Power, T. G. (1985). Mother–and father–infant play: A developmental analysis. *Child Development*, 56, 1514–1524.

Pratt, C., & Bryant, P. (1990). Young children understand that looking leads to knowing (so long as they are looking into a single barrel). *Child Development*, 61, 973–983.

Premack, D. (1990). The infant's theory of self-propelled objects. *Cognition*, 36, 1–16.

Reaux, J. E., Theall, L. A., & Povinelli, D. J. (1999). A longitudinal investigation of chimpanzee's understanding of visual perceptioin. *Child Development*, 70, 275–290.

Ring, H., Baron-Cohen, S., Williams, S., Wheelwright, S., Bullmore, E., Brammer, M., et al. (1999). Cerebral correlates of preserved cognitive skills in autism: A functional MRI study of embedded figures task performance. *Brain*, 122, 1305–1315.

Scaife, M., & Bruner, J. (1975). The capacity for joint visual attention in the infant. *Nature*, 253, 265–266.

Schiff, W., & Oldak, R. (1990). Accuracy of judging time to arrival: Effects of modality, trajectory and gender. *Journal of Experimental Psychology, Human Perception and Performance*, 16, 303–316.

Smith, P. M. (1985). *Language, the sexes and society*. Oxford, UK: Blackwell.

Strayer, F. F. (1980). Child ethology and the study of preschool soical relations. In H. C. Foot, A. J. Chapman, & J. R. Smith (Eds.), *Friendship and social relations in children*. New York: Wiley.

Suddendorf, T., & Whiten, A. (2001). Mental evolution and development: Evidence for secondary representation in children, great apes and other animals. *Psychological Bulletin*, 127, 629–650.

Swettenham, J., Baron-Cohen, S., Charman, T., Cox, A., Baird, G., Drew, A., et al. (1998). The frequency and distribution of spontaneous attention shifts between social and non-social stimuli in autistic, typically developing, and non-autistic developmentally delayed infants. *Journal of Child Psychology and Psychiatry*, 9, 747–753.

Tannen, D. (1991). *You just don't understand: Women and men in conversation.* London: Virago.

Tomasello, M., & Call, J. (1997). *Primate cognition.* New York: Oxford University Press.

Tooby, J., & Cosmides, L. (1992). The psychological foundations of culture. In J. Barkow, L. Cosmides, & J. Tooby (Eds.), *The adapted mind* (pp. 19–136). New York: Oxford University Press.

Trevarthen, C. (1989). The relation of autism to normal socio-cultural development: The case for a primary disorder in regulation of cognitive growth by emotions. In G. Lelord, J. Muk, & M. Petit (Eds.), *Autisme et troubles du développement global de l'enfant.* Paris: Expansion Scientifique Francaise.

Voyer, D., Voyer, S., & Bryden, M. (1995). Magnitude of sex differences in spatial abilities: A meta-analysis and consideration of critical variables. *Psychological Bulletin, 117,* 250–270.

Walker, A. S. (1982). Intermodal perception of exptessive behaviours by human infants. *Journal of Experimental Child Psychology, 33,* 514–535.

Wellman, H. (1990). *Children's theories of mind.* Bradford, MA: MIT Press.

Whiten, A. (1991). *Natural theories of mind.* Oxford, UK: Blackwell.

Whiten, A., Goodall, J., McGrew, W. C., Nishida, T., Reynolds, V., Sugiyama, Y., et al. (1999). Cultures in chimpanzees. *Nature, 399,* 682–685.

Wimmer, H., Hogrefe, J., & Perner, J. (1988). Children's understanding of informational access as a source of knowledge. *Child Development, 59,* 386–396.

Wimmer, H., & Perner, J. (1983). Beliefs about beliefs: Representation and constraining function of wrong beliefs in young children's understanding of deception. *Cognition, 13,* 103–128.

Witkin, H. A., Dyk, R. B., Faterson, H. F., Goodenough, D. G., & Karp, S. A. (1962). *Personality through perception.* New York: Harper & Row.

Wittig, M. A., & Allen, M. J. (1984). Measurement of adult performance on Piaget's water horizontality task. *Intelligence, 8,* 305–313.

Yirmiya, N., Kasari, C., Sigman, M., & Mundy, P. (1992). Empathy and cognition in high-functioning children with autism. *Child Development, 63,* 150–160.

19

FOLK KNOWLEDGE AND ACADEMIC LEARNING

David C. Geary

The field of evolutionary psychology is growing in prominence and influence despite the reluctance of many social scientists to apply evolutionary principles to understanding human behavior (Segerstrale, 2000). Included among the phenomena that are now studied from this perspective are developmental activities and processes, and with this, the emergence of the subfield of evolutionary–developmental psychology (Bjorklund, 1997; Bjorklund & Pellegrini, 2002; Freedman, 1974; Geary & Bjorklund, 2000). One focus of theory and research in this subfield is on the relation between children's evolved cognitive and motivational biases and the demands of academic learning (Geary, 1995, 2001, 2002a; Rozin, 1976). In this chapter, I present an overview of a framework I am developing to understand the relation between evolved abilities and the nonevolved academic competencies that are built through instructional practices. The former are called biologically primary abilities, and the latter, biologically secondary abilities. In the first section, I present a taxonomy of primary cognitive domains (see also Geary, 2005; Geary & Huffman, 2002), and in the second, I discuss some of the ways in which these evolve cognitive and associated motivational and developmental systems may be related to academic learning and the construction of secondary abilities.

TAXONOMY OF PRIMARY COGNITIVE ABILITIES

In the first section, I set up the basic theoretical frame for conceptualizing the function and evolution of primary abilities. In the second and third sections, I present a taxonomy of primary abilities and place these abilities in a developmental context.

Motivation to Control

There is consensus among psychologists that humans have a basic motivation to achieve some level of control over relationships, events, and resources that are significant in their lives (Fiske, 1993; Heckhausen & Schulz, 1995; Thompson, Armstrong, & Thomas, 1998). There is no consensus as to whether this motivation to control has evolved. Nonetheless, it is necessarily true that any motivational disposition will evolve if it contributes to the ability to achieve control of the resources that covary with survival and reproductive outcomes, and if individual differences in the trait are heritable. My thesis here and elsewhere is that the human motivation to control is indeed an evolved disposition and is implicitly—sometimes explicitly—focused on attempts to control social relationships and control the forms of biological (e.g., food) and physical (e.g., territory) resources that tended to covary with survival and reproductive prospects during human evolution, and the variants of these resources that are of importance in the local ecology and social group (Geary, 1998, 2005).

I am not arguing that people always have a conscious and explicit goal to control other individuals and resources in their environment; often they do not. What I am proposing is that selection pressures (e.g., social competition) will operate such that behavioral biases will evolve that focus on securing social and ecological resources, and that these biases covaried with survival or reproductive outcomes during the species' evolutionary history. The biases result from the activity of an array of brain, cognitive, and affective mechanisms that process the corresponding information patterns (e.g., movement patterns of prey species) and guide behavioral activities toward these features of the social and ecological world. In other words, one way of organizing brain, cognitive, affective, and behavioral systems under a single principle is to cast them as reflecting a fundamental motivation to control within-species and between-species (e.g., prey capture, or predator avoidance) behavioral dynamics and to gain control of resources that have tended to covary with evolutionary outcomes. With respect to humans, the Darwin and Wallace (1858, p. 54) conceptualization of natural selection as a "struggle for existence" becomes additionally a struggle with other human beings for control of the resources that support life and allow one to reproduce.

Figure 19.1 shows the affective, psychological, and cognitive mechanisms and underlying modular systems that support control-related behavioral strategies. The details of the affective and psychological systems are described elsewhere (Geary, 2005). Briefly, the functions of the affective systems are to generate social displays, such as facial expressions, and form a conscious awareness of corresponding feelings, such as fear or happiness (Damasio, 2003). These regulate social and other behavioral dynamics, and provide the individual with feedback as to how the current or simulated future situation might affect his or her well-being. The psychological system is defined, in part,

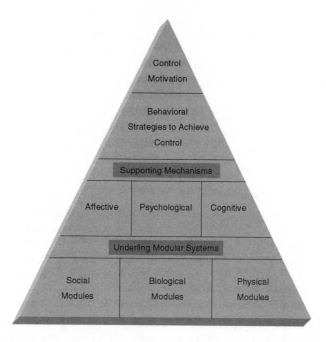

FIGURE 19.1. The apex and following section represent the proposal that human behavior is basically driven by a motivation to control the social, biological, and physical resources that have tended to covary survival and reproductive outcomes during human evolution. The midsection shows the supporting affective, psychological (e.g., attributional biases), and cognitive (e.g., working memory) mechanisms that support the motivation to control and operate on the modular systems shown at the base.

by the ability to form an explicit and conscious representation of the self (Tulving, 2002), and the ability to create a self-centered mental simulation of the "perfect world." A perfect world is one in which the individual is able to organize and control social (e.g., mating dynamics), biological (e.g., access to food), and physical (e.g., shelter) resources in ways that would have enhanced the survival or reproductive options of the individual and kin during human evolution. The evolved function of the simulation is to enable the use of problem solving, reasoning, attributions, and so forth, to devise behavioral strategies that can be used to reduce the difference between one's current situation and this perfect world.

The mental simulation of a perfect world requires the ability to decouple cognitive systems from engagement of the actual world (Cosmides & Tooby, 2000), and then use these systems to either re-create a previous episode, simulate a potential future episode, or create a more abstracted and decontextualized representation of social dynamics or other aspects of the world

(Alexander, 1989). Following Johnson-Laird (1983), and others (Deacon, 1997; Kosslyn & Thompson, 2000), the representations are built from more modular, biologically primary systems and are typically language-based, visuospatial, or some combination of the two. The mental reconstitution of a past episode allows the individual consciously and explicitly to evaluate the dynamics of the episode (e.g., "What did he mean when he said . . . ?"), and to plan and rehearse behavioral strategies for anticipated future episodes that involve the same person or theme. Mental simulations can also involve abstractions of common features or themes across episodes.

The creation of psychological simulations is dependent on working memory resources and is driven by executive control (Baddeley, 1986; Moscovitch, 1994) and associated brain regions in the prefrontal cortex. Working memory and executive functions, in turn, are the cognitive component in the middle section of Figure 19.1. The modular systems at the base of the figure are predicted to process evolutionarily significant forms of information (e.g., facial features) associated with domains of resource control; specifically, social (conspecifics), biological (e.g., other species that serve as food or medicine), and physical (e.g., demarcating the group's territory) resources. The modular systems are components of folk psychology, folk biology, and folk physics, respectively (Atran, 1998; Brothers & Ring, 1992; Carey & Spelke, 1994; Gelman, 1990; Humphrey, 1976; Povinelli & Preuss, 1995; Pinker, 1997). These represent forms of information, such as the shape of a human face or specific facial expression, that have been relatively invariant throughout human evolution. The associated brain and cognitive systems automatically and implicitly process this information and through affective mechanisms bias behavioral responding.

There are other forms of information that also have an evolutionary history but can vary from one situation to the next, as in complex social dynamics. The cognitive (e.g., working memory), psychological (e.g., simulated perfect world), and supporting brain systems at the level above the modules in Figure 19.1 are also evolved but function to cope with such conditions, that is, dynamics that fluctuate across generations and within lifetimes. The explicit representation of a psychological simulation in working memory allows people to anticipate these fluctuations and allows the use of problem solving and reasoning to generate and rehearse potential behavioral strategies to cope with the situation. Although not the evolved function of these explicit cognitive and psychological systems, their operation may be the key to understanding the mechanisms involved in creating secondary competencies from evolved, primary domains. I touch on this issue in the Academic Learning section, and provide more complete analyses and discussion elsewhere (Geary, 2005).

Primary Domains

As I just noted, evolutionarily significant patterns of information largely coalesce around the domains of folk psychology, folk biology, and folk physics. Although there appear to be other primary abilities that are of educational relevance (e.g., numerical information; Geary, 1995, 2001), my position is that the domains shown in Figure 19.2 capture the essential primary abilities that are common to all people; of course, individual differences in these abilities (e.g., sensitivity to facial expressions) are expected. The defining features of modules and the extent to which modular competencies are the result of inherent constraint or patterns of postnatal experience are vigorously debated (Finlay, Darlington, & Nicastro, 2001; Gallistel, 2000; Pinker, 1994; Tooby & Cosmides, 1995), the details of which are beyond the scope of this treatment (Geary, 2005; Geary & Huffman, 2002). It is, however, assumed that these competencies emerge through an epigenetic process, specifically, interaction between inherent constraint and patterns of developmental experience (Bjorklund & Pellegrini, 2002; Geary & Bjorklund, 2000).

Most of the time, primary knowledge is implicit; that is, it is represented in the organization of primary brain systems and the corresponding long-term memories; the latter represent the types of information (e.g., shape of a human face) to which the brain and perceptual systems respond. Conscious, explicit representations result when more automatic, primary systems do not result in a desired outcome or do not allow for easy explanation of the current situation (Geary, 2005). These are situations that appear to result in automatic attentional shifts to representations of the self, the goal, and features of the situation that are thwarting achievement of the goal (Botvinick, Braver, Barch, Carter, & Cohen, 2001). As I describe in the section Folk Knowledge and Academic Learning, the attentional shifts result in the representation of the information in working memory, and thus make this information available for use in control simulations.

Folk Psychology

Folk psychology is defined as the affective, cognitive, psychological, and behavioral systems that are common to all people and enable them to negotiate social interactions and relationships. For instance, even infants preferentially orient their attention and much of their behavior toward other people, and behave in ways (e.g., smile or cry) that result in parental engagement in the relationship (Freedman, 1974). The attentional and behavioral biases of infants and parents are guided by the implicit (below conscious awareness) operation of folk psychology systems. From an evolutionary perspective, the cognitive systems should function to process and manipulate (e.g., categorize) the forms of social information that have covaried with survival and reproduction during human evolution. The associated domains involve the self, relationships and interactions with other people, and group-level relationships and interactions. These dynamics are supported by the respective modular systems corresponding to self, individual, and group, shown in the bottom and leftmost sections of Figure 19.2.

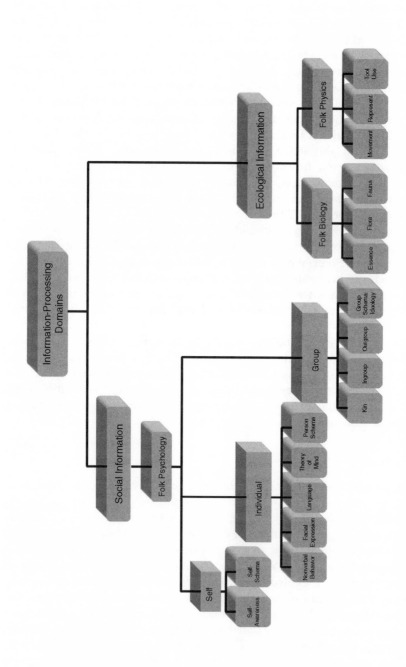

FIGURE 19.2. Evolutionarily salient information-processing domains and associated cognitive modules that compose the domains of folk psychology, folk biology, and folk physics.

Self. Self-related cognitions include awareness of the self as a social being (Tulving, 2002), and a self-schema (Markus, 1977). The self-schema is a long-term memory network of information that links together knowledge and beliefs about the self, including positive (accentuated) and negative (discounted) traits (e.g., friendliness), episodic memories, self-efficacy in various domains, and so forth. Whether implicitly or explicitly represented, self-schemas appear to regulate goal-related behaviors, specifically, where one focuses behavioral effort and whether or not one will persist in the face of failure (Sheeran & Orbell, 2000). Social regulation results from a combination of implicit and explicit processes that influence social comparisons, self-esteem, valuation of different forms of ability and interests, and the formation of social relationships (Drigotas, 2002). For instance, when evaluating the competencies of others, people focus on attributes that are central features of their self-schema, and prefer relationships with others who provide feedback consistent with the self-schema. Athletes implicitly compare and contrast themselves to others on dimensions that involve physical competencies, whereas academics focus more on intellectual competencies (Fiske & Taylor, 1991). People value competencies on which they excel and discount competencies for which they are at a competitive disadvantage (Taylor, 1982).

Person. The person-related competencies function to enable the monitoring and control of dyadic interactions, and the development and maintenance of one-on-one relationships. Caporael (1997) and Bugental (2000) described universal patterns of dyadic interaction and individual relationships, including parent–child attachments and friendships, among others. There are, of course, some differences across these dyads, but all of them are supported by the person-level sociocognitive modules shown in Figure 19.2. These modules include those that support the reading of nonverbal behavior and facial expressions, language, and theory of mind (Baron-Cohen, 1995; Pinker, 1994; Rosenthal, Hall, DiMatteo, Rogers, & Archer, 1979). The latter represents the ability to make inferences about other people's intentions, likely future behavior, and so forth.

The person schema is a long-term memory network that includes representations of the other persons' physical attributes (age, race, sex), memories for specific behavioral episodes, and more abstract trait information, such as individuals' sociability (e.g., warm to emotionally distant) and competence (Schneider, 1973). It seems likely that the person schema will also include information related to other modular systems, such as theory of mind, as well as the person's network of social relationships and kin (Geary & Flinn, 2001). The former would include memories and trait information about how the person typically makes inferences (e.g., tends to attribute hostile intentions to others, the *hostile attribution bias*), responds to social cues, and their social and other goals.

Group. A universal aspect of human behavior and cognition is the parsing of the social world into groups (Alexander, 1979; Premack & Premack, 1995). The most consistent groupings are shown in Figure 19.2 and reflect the categorical significance of kin, the formation of ingroups and outgroups, and a group schema. The latter is an ideologically based social identification (e.g., nationality, religious affiliation). The categorical significance of kin is most strongly reflected in the motivational disposition of humans to organize themselves into families of one form or another in all cultures (Brown, 1991). In traditional societies, nuclear families are typically embedded in the context of a wider network of kin (Geary & Flinn, 2001). Individuals within these kinship networks cooperate to facilitate competition with other kin groups over resource control and manipulation of social relationships. As cogently argued by Alexander (1979), coalitional competition also occurs beyond the kin group, is related to social ideology, and is endemic throughout the world (Horowitz, 2001). As with kin groups, competition among ideology-supported groups is over resource control.

Basically, individual- and group-level cooperative relationships and conflicts of interest are invariably generated as each individual attempts to gain control of social relationships and the biological and physical resources that covary with survival or reproductive prospects in the local ecology and culture (Alexander, 1979; Chagnon, 1988; Horowitz, 2001; Irons, 1979; Keeley, 1996). People develop cooperative relationships to the extent that social influence, resource control, and other issues that are of significance in their lives require such relationships.

Folk Biology and Folk Physics

Humans living in traditional societies use the local ecology and other species to support their survival and reproductive needs. The associated activities are supported by, among other things, the folk biological and folk physical modules shown in the rightmost sections of Figure 19.2 (Geary, 1998, 2005; Geary & Huffman, 2002). The folk biological modules support the categorizing of flora and fauna in the local ecology, especially species used as food, medicines, or in social rituals (e.g., Berlin, Breedlove, & Raven, 1973). Folk biology also includes systems that support an understanding of the *essence* of these species (Atran, 1998). Essence is knowledge about growth patterns and behavior that facilitates hunting and other activities involved in securing and using these species as resources (e.g., food). Physical modules are for guiding movement in three-dimensional space, mentally representing this space (e.g., demarcating the ingroup's territory), and for using physical materials (e.g., stones, metals) for making tools (Pinker, 1997; Shepard, 1994). The associated primary abilities support a host of evolutionarily significant activities, such as hunting and the use of tools as weapons or to secure biological resources (e.g., stone hammers to break open bones and secure high-fat marrow).

Attributional and Inferential Biases

Inferential and attributional biases are also integral features of folk knowledge, and are part of the psychological component of the motivation to control (Geary, 2005). Social attributional biases that favor members of the ingroup and derogate members of outgroups are well known (Stephan, 1985) and facilitate coalitional competition (Horowitz, 2001). The essence associated with folk biology allows people to make inferences (e.g., during the act of hunting) about the behavior of members of familiar species, as well as about the likely behavior of less familiar but related species (Atran, 1998; see also Barrett, Chapter 17, this volume). Attributions about causality in the physical world have also been studied. For instance, children and adults have natural, naïve conceptions about motion and other physical phenomena (Clement, 1982; Kaiser, McCloskey, & Proffitt, 1986; Kaiser, Proffitt, & McCloskey, 1985; Spelke, Breinlinger, Macomber, & Jacobson, 1992).

It is often the case that naïve notions and attributional and inferential biases associated with folk knowledge are inaccurate from a scientific perspective, as elaborated in the Academic Learning and illustrated in the Folk Physics sections below. Although such inaccuracies are important from an educational perspective, they are irrelevant from an evolutionary perspective. Selection will operate on attributional and inferential biases that facilitate resource control, whether or not the biases are accurate from a scientific perspective. Indeed, many attributional and inferential biases result in judgments that are generally accurate enough for coping with many everyday situations (Stanovich, 1999), although they often do not result in the most logical conclusions (Tversky & Kahneman, 1974).

Development

A long developmental period is associated with the risk of dying before the age of reproduction; thus, an extended childhood would only evolve if there were benefits that outweighed this risk (Stearns, 1992). Mayr (1974) suggested that one function, and the presumed adaptive benefit, of delayed maturation is the accompanying ability to refine the competencies that covaried with survival and reproductive outcomes during the species' evolutionary history (see Flinn & Ward, Chapter 2, this volume). The corresponding assumption here is that one function of human childhood is to flesh out the cognitive, affective, and psychological systems that comprise folk knowledge, such that these systems are adapted to social conditions (e.g., level of warfare) and the biological (e.g., types of species) and physical (e.g., terrain) nuances of the local ecology (Bjorklund & Pellegrini, 2002; Geary, 2002b, 2005; MacDonald, 1992).

Play, social interactions, and exploration of the environment and objects appear to be the mechanisms through which these emerging competencies are practiced, refined, and adapted to local conditions. In theory, these child-initiated activities are intimately linked to cognitive and brain development, in that these activities result in the environmental experiences that are an integral part of the epigenetic processes that result in adult competencies (Greenough, 1991; Scarr & McCarthy, 1983). In other words, children are inherently motivated to attend to and seek out experiences and engage in activities that will lead to the adaptation of inherent but often skeletal folk knowledge, such that the associated cognitive, affective, psychological, and behavioral systems are adapted to the nuances of the local ecology (Gelman, 1990). These child-initiated activities and associated inherent biases in motivational, cognitive, and brain systems will be focused on recreating the experiences that lead to the refinement of the competencies that covaried with survival and reproduction during human evolution.

For instance, the strong bias of human infants to attend to human faces, movement patterns, and speech reflects, in theory, the initial and inherent organizational and motivational structure of the associated folk psychological modules (Freedman, 1974). These biases re-create the microconditions (e.g., parent–child interactions) associated with the evolution of the corresponding modules (Caporael, 1997), and provide the experiences needed to adapt the architecture of these modules to variation in parental faces, behavior, and so forth (Gelman & Williams, 1998). It allows your infant to discriminate your voice from the voice of other potential parents, with only minimal exposure to your voice. Indeed, when human fetuses (gestation age of about 38 weeks) are exposed *in utero* to human voices, their heart-rate patterns suggest that they are sensitive to and learn the voice patterns of their mother, and discriminate her voice from that of other women (Kisilevsky et al., 2003).

Boys' group-level competition (e.g., team sports) provides another example with the early formation of competition-based ingroups and outgroups, and the coordination of social activities that may provide practice for primitive group-level warfare in adulthood (Geary, 1998; Geary, Byrd-Craven, Hoard, Vigil, & Numtee, 2003). These natural games may provide the practice needed for the skilled formation and maintenance of social coalitions in adulthood, and result in the accumulation of memories for associated activities and social strategies. In other words, and in keeping with the comparative analyses of Pellis and colleagues (e.g., Pellis & Pellis, 1998), these games may be more strongly related to learning the skills of other boys and acquiring the social competencies for coordinated group-level activities, as contrasted with learning specific fighting behaviors, such as hitting. My assumption is that these activities, and the accompanying effects on brain and cognition, are related to the group-level social selection pressures noted earlier, and provide experience with the dynamics of forming ingroups and outgroups.

As another example, sociodramatic play appears to be an important vehicle for elaborating children's social competencies, such as learning the implicit scripts that choreograph many social interactions. Beginning around age 3, children practice social scripts in the context of their play (Rubin, Fein, &

Vandenberg, 1983). Initially, this type of play involves using dolls or other toys to act out everyday social experiences (e.g., dinner). The use of toys allows the child to practice coordinating social interactions at an age when he or she does not yet have the competencies do to so effectively with other children. Later, particularly between the ages of 4 and 6 years, children rehearse and then expand on these scripts with groups of other children (Rubin et al., 1983). Thus, from ages 3 to 6, children's play activities involve increasingly complex patterns of social interaction. The fantasy element of sociodramatic play might also be involved in the development of the psychological component of the motivation to control. More precisely, the fantasy component of this form of play might provide practice at using mental simulations to rehearse social strategies (Geary, 1998).

ACADEMIC LEARNING

From an evolutionary perspective, the folk knowledge and inferential and attributional biases that define primary abilities are not sufficient for academic learning in modern society, but, at the same time, are the foundation from which biologically secondary academic competencies are likely to be built. The implications for academic learning are multifold and thus I can only touch on a few of these (Geary, 1995, 2001, 2002a, 2005). In the first section, I provide several examples of the relation between folk knowledge and academic competencies, and in the second section, I discuss the relation between the motivation to control and the motivation to learn in school. The mechanisms through which primary systems are modified to create academic competencies are not known, but in the third section, I suggest that these mechanisms might be related to the cognitive and psychological systems that support the ability to cope with fluctuating conditions. In the final section, I outline a few instructional implications.

Secondary Competencies

When approached from an evolutionary perspective, schools are predicted to emerge in societies in which scientific, technological, and intellectual advances result in a gap between folk knowledge and the academic (e.g., need to read) demands of the society (Geary, 2002a). One of the corresponding goals of schooling should be to narrow this gap; specifically, to ensure that children learn the biologically secondary competencies needed to function successfully (e.g., obtain gainful employment) in the society. In the following sections, I provide examples of how folk knowledge may be related to the learning of secondary abilities. In the first section, I illustrate the construction of novel academic competencies (reading and writing) from primary domains, and in the second and third sections, I illustrate the relation between folk knowledge and scientific knowledge in biology and physics.

Folk Psychology

Following Rozin's (1976) lead, my hypothesis is that the invention of written symbols emerged from the motivational disposition to communicate with and influence the behavior of other people (e.g., morals in the Bible); thus, writing–reading is predicted to be dependent on folk psychological communication systems. More precisely, learning to read and write involves co-opting primary folk psychological systems: "Co-optation" is defined as the adaptation (typically through instruction) of evolved cognitive systems for culturally specific uses (Geary, 1995, 2002a; Rozin, 1976; Rozin & Schull, 1988). The first issue that must be addressed concerns whether or not reading–writing can in fact be linked to folk psychological systems. I emphasize reading, because more is known about learning to read than to write.

Although the research is not definitive, it is consistent with the hypothesis that the acquisition of reading-related abilities (e.g., word decoding) involves the co-optation of primary language and language-related modular systems, among others (e.g., visual scanning), as originally proposed by Rozin (1976). Wagner, Torgesen, and Rashotte (1994) found that individual differences in the fidelity of kindergarten children's phonological processing systems, which are basic components of the language domain, are strongly predictive of the ease with which basic reading abilities (e.g., word decoding) are acquired in first grade (Bradley & Bryant, 1983). Children who show an explicit awareness of basic language sounds are more skilled than other children at associating these sounds with the symbol system of the written language. In further support of the co-optation hypothesis, Pugh and his colleagues (1997) found that the brain and cognitive systems that are engaged during the processing of phonemes are also engaged during the act of reading.

It is also likely that reading comprehension engages related modular systems, including theory of mind and the person schema, at least for literary stories, poems, dramas, and other genres that involve human relationships (Geary, 1998). This is because comprehending the gist of these stories involves making inferences about the nuances of social relationships, which, by definition, engages theory of mind. Characters within stories typically have personalities, behavioral styles, and so forth—information that could be used to create a person schema for these individuals (e.g., Sherlock Holmes). It is also of interest that some of the more popular forms of literature are focused on interpersonal relationships and dynamics, and reproductive relationships in the case of the romance novel (e.g., Whissell, 1996). The self-schema would be engaged to the extent the individual identifies with the protagonist or antagonist of the story.

Folk Biology

As stated earlier, folk biology represents the evolved ability to develop classification systems of flora and fauna, and mental models of the essence of these species (Atran, 1998). Although folk biological knowledge almost certainly provided the foundation for the emergence of the scientific classification system of Western biology, this folk knowledge is rudimentary in comparison to the vast knowledge of modern-day biological science. As an example, people, even young children, infer that living things have innards that differ from the innards of nonliving things, and that offspring will have the same appearance and essence as their parents (Carey & Spelke, 1994; Coley, 2000; Gelman, 1990). The scientific study of "innards" is, of course, anatomy and physiology, and the study of "essence" is behavioral ecology. The latter involves the scientific study of animal behavior in natural environments, and "essence" represents knowledge of, for instance, the behavior of hunted animals and where in the ecology they are most likely to be found (Atran, 1998).

Not only is the gap between folk biology and the knowledge base of the biological sciences widening at a rapid pace but also the inferential biases of this folk system may sometimes interfere with the comprehension of scientific models of biological phenomena. The most fundamental of these are the principles of natural selection independently discovered by Darwin and Wallace (1858). Two of the crucial features of natural selection are that (1) it acts on *individual differences* in those traits (e.g., size at birth) that are related to survival prospects and (2) results in changes in those traits *across* generations. Yet inferential biases in folk biology may conspire to make these basic mechanisms difficult to comprehend. First, one inferential bias results in a focus on similarities across members of the same, and related, species (see Atran, 1998). This bias facilitates the functional goal of being able to predict the behavior (e.g., growth patterns) of these plants and animals, as related to procuring food and medicine. At the same time, the focus on within-species similarities runs counter to the insight that within-species individual differences, or variability, provide the grist for evolutionary selection. Second, folk biological knowledge is also implicitly focused on the behavior of flora and fauna at different points in a single lifespan (e.g., maturity of a plant, relative to when it is best to harvest) and not the cross-generational time scale over which natural selection occurs.

In summary, people are biased to think about and understand the biological world in ways that are at odds with the principles of natural selection. Darwin, in fact, did not recognize the extent of within-species variability in natural environments, and thus the ease with which natural selection can operate in these environments, until his extensive work in the 1850s on barnacles (Desmond & Moore, 1994), 15 or so years after his initial insights on natural selection (Ospovat, 1981). One educational implication is that children need exposure to variation within species, and instruction on how these individual differences are related to survival prospects and mate choice, if they are to fully understand the mechanisms of natural selection.

Folk Physics

As noted earlier, people have a naïve understanding of certain physical phenomena (Piaget, 1927/1930, 1946/1970), and the initial emergence of physics as a domain of explicit intellectual activity was likely to have been based on this folk knowledge. As an example, when asked about the forces acting on a thrown baseball, many people infer a force propelling it forward, something akin to an invisible engine, and a force propelling it downward. The downward force is, of course, gravity, but there is in fact no force propelling it forward, once the ball leaves the player's hand (Clement, 1982). The concept of a forward force, called "impetus," is similar to pre-Newtonian beliefs about motion prominent in the 14th–16th centuries. The idea is that the act of starting an object in motion, such as throwing a ball, imparts to the object an internal force—"impetus"—that keeps it in motion until the impetus gradually dissipates. Even though adults often describe the correct trajectory for a thrown object, their explanations reflect this naïve understanding of the forces acting upon the object.

Although "impetus" is in fact a fictional force, it is a reasonable explanation of most everyday situations. Nevertheless, this and other naïve conceptions about the workings of the physical world interfere with learning the scientific principles associated with mechanics, as well as many other principles, such as those representing centrifugal force and velocity (Clement, 1982; McCloskey, 1983). Moreover, as with biology, the knowledge base of the physical sciences is exponentially larger than the knowledge base of folk physics, and in some cases (e.g., quantum mechanics) the accompanying conceptual models bear little resemblance to the naïve concepts of folk physics. Educational implications are discussed below.

Folk Knowledge and Academic Learning

Rozin (1976) and Karmiloff-Smith (1992) proposed that one of keys to understanding the relation between primary abilities, such as language, and secondary abilities, such as reading, is the mechanism or mechanisms involved in making the implicit primary systems explicit—the individual is consciously aware of the information (e.g., a language sound)—and then rewriting them, so to speak, as a secondary competency. My goal is to integrate research on the relation between general intelligence and learning and with the cognitive mechanisms (e.g., working memory) that support control-related behavioral strategies (Geary, 2005). One reason is because the best predictor of the ease of learning secondary competencies is general intelligence, or g (Jensen, 1998): Walberg (1984) reviewed 3,000 studies of the relation between performance on academic achievement tests, which largely assess secondary abilities, and a variety of student attributes, (e.g., intelligence), home environment (e.g., television viewing), and classroom variables. By far, the best individual predictor of achievement was g, specifically IQ ($r = .7$). Moreover, the cognitive mechanisms that underlie g are likely to be engaged when primary abilities are rewritten as secondary abilities (Geary, 2005). These mechanisms include the central executive component of working memory and attentional control (e.g., Baddeley, 1986; Conway & Engle, 1994), as well as the supporting areas of the prefrontal cortex and anterior cingulate cortex (Duncan et al., 2000; Kane & Engle, 2002). These mechanisms also support control-related mental simulations.

The details of how these domain-general systems may be involved in academic learning and the co-opting of primary abilities for the construction of secondary competencies are described elsewhere (Geary, 2005). As an illustration of the basics, consider that the dorsolateral prefrontal regions are particularly important for explicitly representing goals and information to be manipulated in working memory (Duncan, 2001; Kane & Engle, 2002; Miller & Cohen, 2001; Shallice, 2002). These ends appear to be achieved by biasing, perhaps through attentional amplification (Dehaene & Naccache, 2001; Posner, 1994), the activation of posterior and subcortical pathways that represent the information needed for goal achievement. These posterior regions include those that support many of the primary modules, such as the processing of language sounds, that I described in the Primary Domains section. The result appears to be a simultaneous and synchronized activation of the dorsolateral prefrontal areas and the posterior brain regions engaged for the specific task.

To illustrate how the process may work: One of the basic academic competencies that supports learning how to read, phonemic decoding (Bradley & Bryant, 1983), requires an explicit awareness and representation in working memory of a basic language sound and the association of this sound, as well as blends of sounds, with corresponding visual patterns, specifically, letters and letter combinations. Attentional focus on the relation between the sound and the letter should, in theory, result in the amplification of the activity of the posterior brain regions that process this information and the simultaneous representation of both forms of information in working memory. The process should result in the synchronization of this posterior brain activity with activity in the dorsolateral prefrontal cortex and the formation of a learned association between the sound and letter. With practice, the association becomes represented in long-term memory and thus becomes implicit knowledge, presumably due to the formation or strengthening of neural links among these posterior regions (Garlick, 2002). When this is achieved, the association between the sound and letter, or letter combination and word sound, is automatically triggered when the letter string is processed during the act of reading and thus no longer engages the prefrontal cortex.

Academic learning also involves more complex activities, including problem solving, reasoning, and the understanding of complex intellectual and scientific principles. Elsewhere, I described how these processes may also engage the dorsolateral prefrontal areas and accompanying central executive and working memory systems (Geary, 2005). The psychological component of the motivation to control is also important for the formation of mental simulations of many phenomena and is likely engaged in the creation of many forms of secondary knowledge. For instance, Darwin and Wallace (1858) likely used mental simulations, as well as reasoning, problem solving, and so forth, in their construction of the principles of natural selection (see Geary, 2005). The point is that learning simple associations involved in phonemic decoding, and the more complex processes involved in scientific discovery and the creation of secondary knowledge, may involve many of the same cognitive and brain systems, specifically, the psychological and cognitive components of my motivation to control model.

Motivation to Learn

Another implication of the evolutionary approach is that children are innately curious about and motivated to engage actively in and explore social relationships and the biological and physical world. These are biases directed toward information and activities associated with fleshing out folk knowledge and adapting these brain and cognitive systems to local conditions, as I noted earlier (Gelman, 1990; Gelman & Williams, 1998; Geary, 1995). However, if the activities that promote the fleshing out of folk knowledge differ from the activities that promote academic learning, then a motivational mismatch will arise between children's preferred activities and effective instructional activities. In other words, the motivation to engage in activities related to folk knowledge will often conflict with the need to engage in activities that will lead to the mastery of academic competencies (see Geary, 1995, 2001, 2002a).

For instance, if social competition over resource control generated selection pressures that contributed to human cognitive and social evolution, then children should have a strong and inherent motivational bias to engage in activities that will re-create the forms of social cooperation and competition that were important during human evolution (Caporael, 1997). The finding that a universal aspect of children's (and adults') self-directed activities are social and typically involve a mix of cooperative and competitive endeavors is consistent with this prediction (Baumeister & Leary, 1995). Competition over friends, called relational aggression, is one example (Feshbach, 1969). A corollary prediction is that a burning desire to master algebra or Newtonian physics will not be universal, or even common.

There are, of course, many individuals who pursue learning in secondary domains and engage in secondary activities on their own initiative, but this follows from the assumption that most activities, primary and secondary, can be categorized as related to social, biological, or physical interests (Geary, 2002a). From this perspective, scholars in the humanities and social sciences are predicted, and appear, to be fundamentally motivated to understand human social relationships, and biologists and physicists, to be motivated to understand the biological and physical worlds, respectively (Roe, 1956). The difference between scholars in these domains and other people is predicted to be related to several dimensions of human individual differences, including the cognitive systems underlying g (i.e., working memory and attentional control; Jensen, 1998), certain dimensions of personality (e.g., open mindedness;

Stanovich, 1999), a touch of psychopathology (Simonton, 2003), and the willingness to engage in the long and often tedious training required to master the academic discipline (Ericsson, Krampe, & Tesch-Römer, 1993). It is individuals at the extreme end of all of these distributions—which makes them very rare—who generate a disproportionate number of scholarly, scientific, and technological advances (Simonton, 1999).

There may also be individual differences in the degree of inherent elaboration of folk psychological, biological, and physical systems, and these in turn may contribute to the foci on one domain or another and the degree to which secondary knowledge dependent on these domains can be developed. Baron-Cohen and his colleagues found that at least some highly successful mathematicians and physical scientists appear to have an enhanced understanding of folk physics but a poor understanding of aspects of folk psychology (Baron-Cohen, Wheelwright, Stone, & Rutherford, 1999). When an enhanced intuitive understanding of folk physics and an enhanced motivation to engage in associated activities is combined with high *g*, the result can be advances in the associated scientific or scholarly domain. Newton's social isolation and near obsessive focus on physical phenomena (e.g., optics; White, 1998) and Linnaeus's obsession with creating an explicit taxonomy of flora (e.g., Lindroth, 1983) are but two examples: Linnaeus created the binomial rules (e.g., based on similarities in the shape of flower petals) for the scientific classification of species and was the first to use this taxonomic system. The result of the work of Newton and Linnaeus was scientific revolutions in physics and biology, respectively, and a significant widening of the gap between folk knowledge and these emerging scientific disciplines.

For most people, however, the motivational disposition will be expended on rather more mundane activities. These activities are predicted to be largely social in nature, based on a social-competition model of human evolution (Alexander, 1987; Geary, 2005), but can involve more secondary activities. The motivation to engage in secondary activities is predicted to be related to evolutionary themes embedded in the content of the activity and not directed toward secondary learning per se. To illustrate, reading is a biologically secondary activity, but many people choose to read. The motivation to read is probably driven by the content of the activity rather than by the process itself. As I noted earlier, the content of many stories and other secondary activities reflects evolutionarily relevant themes (e.g., social relationships), and it is interest in these themes that motivates engagement in the activity.

In any case, the point is that children's inherent motivational dispositions and activity preferences are likely to be at odds with the need to engage in the activities, such as the drill and practice needed to learn mathematical procedures, that promote academic learning. This does not preclude self-initiated engagement in secondary activities, but it does lead to the prediction that children's natural curiosity and preferred mode of learning (e.g., play and exploration) will not always be sufficient for acquiring secondary competencies.

Instructional Implications

Considerable debate has been expended on attempts to understand the acquisition of academic competencies (Hirsch, 1996; Loveless, 2001). Almost none of the associated research programs have been informed by evolutionary considerations and, as a result, fail to explain even basic observations, such as why children learn language more readily than they learn how to read and write. The difference in the ease of acquiring language as contrasted with reading and writing is readily understandable from the evolutionary perspective: The inherent cognitive systems and child-initiated activities that foster the adaptation of primary abilities, such as language, to local conditions will not be sufficient for the acquisition of secondary abilities, such as reading and writing. In the two sections below, I discuss related instructional implications.

Folk Knowledge and Instruction

If folk knowledge and inferential biases sometimes run counter to related scientific concepts, then this folk knowledge will impede the learning and adoption of these scientific concepts or procedures. To illustrate, most people make judgments about the relative risk of various activities based on how easily they can remember examples of mishaps associated with those activities. This memory-based heuristic probably works rather well in environments in which the inferential bias evolved (Gigerenzer & Selten, 2001), that is, environments in which memories for risk-related accidents can only be accrued through personal experience or folk tales based on experiences in similar environments. However, this risk heuristic often leads to poor probability and risk judgments in modern societies. This is because mass media create memories for events individuals have not actually experienced, but these memories sometimes affect people as if they had actually experienced the event. Most people can remember many disturbing plane crashes but have not personally experienced these crashes. They were exposed to them through television (Lichtenstein, Slovic, Fischhoff, Layman, & Combs, 1978). The result is that many people overestimate the very small risk associated with flying. Statistical and mathematical methods provide a much more accurate and reliable method of risk assessment, but reliance on this evolved heuristic appears to interfere with the learning and use of formal statistics to make risk assessments (Brase, Cosmides, & Tooby, 1998).

Similar biases and instructional impediments have been noted for physics (Clement, 1982; Hunt & Minstrell, 1994). One counter to these biases is to set up demonstrations or experiments that create results that are contrary to folk intuitions, as Hunt and Minstrell (1994) have done for teaching basic concepts in high school physics. Prior to performing such an experiment, the teacher piques interest in the principles involved by asking for predictions, with the students discussing their reasons for their predictions. The demonstration is then performed, and the teacher and students discuss the results and their implications. This method appears to facilitate the understanding, retention, and transfer of biologically secondary concepts. When the students make predictions and discuss their reasons for the predictions, they are making their existing knowledge explicit. In making predictions, the students rely on their folk beliefs about physical systems, which are often incorrect or only useful in very limited specific situations. In order for incorrect (or incomplete) beliefs to be changed, the student must be made explicitly aware of them. By comparing predictions based on folk beliefs and those based on scientific knowledge to experimental outcomes, the utility of the latter becomes apparent.

Folk knowledge and inferential biases may, at other times, facilitate the acquisition of secondary abilities. As an example, a relationship between spatial abilities and mathematics, especially geometry, has been posited for thousands of years. Geometry can be defined as the study of space and shape (Devlin, 1998), and the movement and representation modules (i.e., primary spatial abilities) associated with folk physics may provide an intuitive understanding of certain features of geometry (Geary, 1995). Basically, there is order and structure to the physical universe, and many of the spatial abilities of humans, and other species, reflect the evolution of primary systems that are sensitive to this order (Gallistel, 1990; Shepard, 1994). The associated competencies include the ability to navigate in the world and generate a mental map of this world, as well as more basic skills, such as the ability to track moving objects. Nearly all of this knowledge of the physical world is implicit. Some aspects of this intuitive knowledge appear to form the foundation for some aspects of Euclidean geometry. Euclid's first principle—a line can be drawn from any point to any point; that is, a line is a straight line—reflects the intuitive understanding that the fastest way to get from one place to another is to "go as the crow flies," that is, to go in a straight line. At the same time, there is little reason to believe that other aspects of academic geometry, such as theorems, are as intimately related to spatial knowledge.

It follows that the goals of instructional research will include identifying folk knowledge and inferential biases that relate to academic competencies and then determining instructional approaches that disabuse students of folk knowledge that runs counter to scientific concepts and capitalize on folk knowledge (often implicit) that can be used to teach academic concepts. The latter often involves making implicit knowledge formalized and explicit; Euclid's first principle is an explicit and formalized representation of an implicit aspect of folk physics. As I described earlier, making the implicit explicit requires attentional focus and the representation of the information in working memory, which implies that direct instruction of some secondary knowledge may be the most efficient method of teaching this information.

Motivation

Surveys of the attitudes and preferences of schoolchildren indicate that most of these children value achievement in sports more than achievement in any academic area (Eccles, Wigfield, Harold, & Blumenfeld, 1993). The result is not surprising. When children are allowed to self-direct their activities, they typically engage in some type of social discourse. Boys, for instance, spontaneously organize their social activities around group-level competition, such as team sports (Lever, 1978). Geary and colleagues (1998; Geary et al., 2003) interpreted this child-initiated activity as a reflection of an evolved motivational disposition that results in the practice of group-level warfare, and a refinement of the supporting group-level social modules, such as the formation of ingroups and outgroups, and coordination of the activities of ingroup members as related to competition with an outgroup. Time spent in these preferred, child-initiated activities is time that cannot be spent engaged in the types of activities that promote the acquisition of secondary competencies.

The first instructional implication is that universal education will be dependent to a large degree on the social and cultural valuation of school-based competencies (Stevenson & Stigler, 1992). In other words, the need to learn many academic competencies comes from the demands of the wider society and not the inherent interests of children. Social and cultural supports, such as spelling bees, social and parental valuation of school achievement, and so forth, are thus likely to be needed to support children's investment in school learning. A second implication is that schooling and instructional activities must to some degree organize the behavior of children such that they engage in activities—effective instructional activities—in which they otherwise would not engage. In essence, instructional materials, lesson plans, and teachers must organize and guide children's academic learning, because it cannot be assumed that children's "natural curiosity" will result in an interest in all academic domains or result in the motivation to engage in the activities that will foster the mastery of these domains.

CONCLUSIONS

An evolutionary approach to cognition and development provides a much needed anchor for conceptualizing academic learning and for guiding instructional research and practice. An evolutionarily informed science of academic development is in fact the only perspective that readily accommodates basic observations that elude explanation by other theoretical perspectives (Geary, 1995). It follows logically from the evolutionary approach that children will easily learn the language of their parents and competencies in the other primary domains shown in Figure 19.1, and do so without formal instruction. However, years later, many of these children will have difficulty learning to read and write, and difficulty in many other academic domains, even with formal instruction. The differences in the ease of learning these primary and secondary competencies follow readily from the evolutionary perspective.

More precisely, much of the learning associated with primary domains occurs automatically and effortlessly, because the brain and mind of children have been designed by selections pressures for learning in these domains; specifically, adapting inherent but skeletal brain and cognitive systems to the nuances of the local social, biological, and physical ecologies (Geary & Huffman, 2002; Gelman, 1990). Learning in secondary domains, in contrast, requires co-opting the brain and cognitive systems that define this folk knowledge, and adapting them for uses for which they were not designed. The process of adapting these systems is academic learning and is effortful because it requires sustained attentional control and working memory resources, as I described earlier (see also Geary, 2005). I am not arguing that the issues outlined here and elsewhere (Geary, 1995) are the final word on the relation between evolved social and cognitive biases and academic development. Rather, they should be viewed as the blueprint for conceptualizing academic development and guiding instructional theory and research. There is much to be learned about the specifics of folk knowledge and associated inferential biases, and still more to be learned of their relation to academic learning.

REFERENCES

Alexander, R. D. (1979). *Darwinism and human affairs.* Seattle: University of Washington Press.

Alexander, R. D. (1987). *The biology of moral systems.* Hawthorne, NY: Aldine de Gruyter.

Alexander, R. D. (1989). Evolution of the human psyche. In P. Mellars & C. Stringer (Eds.), *The human revolution: Behavioural and biological perspectives on the origins of modern humans* (pp. 455–513). Princeton, NJ: Princeton University Press.

Atran, S. (1998). Folk biology and the anthropology of science: Cognitive universals and cultural particulars. *Behavioral and Brain Sciences, 21,* 547–609.

Baddeley, A. D. (1986). *Working memory.* Oxford, UK: Oxford University Press.

Baron-Cohen, S. (1995). *Mindblindness: An essay on autism and theory of mind.* Cambridge, MA: MIT Press/Bradford Books.

Baron-Cohen, S., Wheelwright, S., Stone, V., & Rutherford, M. (1999). A mathematician, a physicist and a computer scientist with Asperger syndrome: Performance on folk psychology and folk physics tests. *Neurocase, 5,* 475–483.

Baumeister, R. F., & Leary, M. R. (1995). The need to belong: Desire for interpersonal attachments as a fundamental human motivation. *Psychological Bulletin, 117,* 497–529.

Berlin, B., Breedlove, D. E., & Raven, P. H. (1973). General principles of classification and nomenclature in folk biology. *American Anthropologist, 75,* 214–242.

Bjorklund, D. F. (1997). The role of immaturity in human development. *Psychological Bulletin, 122,* 153–169.

Bjorklund, D. F., & Pellegrini, A. D. (2002). *The origins of human nature: Evolutionary developmental psychology.* Washington, DC: American Psychological Association.

Botvinick, M. M., Braver, T. S., Barch, D. M., Carter, C. S., & Cohen, J. D. (2001). Conflict monitoring and cognitive control. *Psychological Review, 108,* 624–652.

Bradley, L., & Bryant, P. E. (1983). Categorizing sounds and learning to read—a causal connection. *Nature, 301,* 419–421.

Brase, G. L., Cosmides, L., & Tooby, J. (1998). Individuation, counting, and statistical inference: The frequency and whole-object representations in judgment under uncertainty. *Journal of Experimental Psychology: General, 127,* 3–21.

Brothers, L., & Ring, B. (1992). A neuroethological framework for the representation of minds. *Journal of Cognitive Neuroscience, 4,* 107–118.

Brown, D. E. (1991). *Human universals.* Philadelphia: Temple University Press.

Bugental, D. B. (2000). Acquisition of the algorithms of social life: A domain-based approach. *Psychological Bulletin, 126,* 187–219.

Caporael, L. R. (1997). The evolution of truly social cognition: The core configurations model. *Personality and Social Psychology Review, 1,* 276–298.

Carey, S., & Spelke, E. (1994). Domain-specific knowledge and conceptual change. In L. A. Hirschfeld & S. A. Gelman (Eds.), *Mapping the mind: Domain specificity in cognition and culture* (pp. 169–200). New York: Cambridge University Press.

Chagnon, N. A. (1988). Life histories, blood revenge, and warfare in a tribal population. *Science, 239,* 985–992.

Clement, J. (1982). Students' preconceptions in introductory mechanics. *American Journal of Physics, 50,* 66–71.

Coley, J. D. (2000). On the importance of comparative research: The case of folkbiology. *Child Development, 71,* 82–90.

Conway, A. R. A., & Engle, R. W. (1994). Working memory and retrieval: A resource-dependent inhibition model. *Journal of Experimental Psychology: General, 123,* 354–373.

Cosmides, L., & Tooby, J. (2000). Consider the source: The evolution of adaptations for decoupling and metarepresentation. In D. Sperber (Ed.), *Metarepresentations* (pp. 53–115). Oxford, UK: Oxford University Press.

Damasio, A. (2003). *Looking for Spinoza: Joy, sorrow, and the feeling brain.* Orlando, FL: Harcourt.

Darwin, C., & Wallace, A. (1858). On the tendency of species to form varieties, and on the perpetuation of varieties and species by natural means of selection. *Journal of the Linnean Society of London, Zoology, 3,* 45–62.

Deacon, T. (1997). *The symbolic species: The co-evolution of language and the brain.* New York: Norton.

Dehaene, S., & Naccache, L. (2001). Towards a cognitive neuroscience of consciousness: Basic evidence and a workspace framework. *Cognition, 79,* 1–37.

Desmond, A., & Moore, J. (1994). *Darwin: Life of a tormented evolutionist.* New York: Norton.

Devlin, K. (1998). *The language of mathematics: Making the invisible visible.* New York: Freeman.

Drigotas, S. M. (2002). The Michelangelo phenomenon and personal well-being. *Journal of Personality, 70,* 59–77.

Duncan, J. (2001). An adaptive coding model of neural function in prefrontal cortex. *Nature Reviews: Neuroscience, 2,* 820–829.

Duncan, J., Rüdiger, J. S., Kolodny, J., Bor, D., Herzog, H., Ahmed, A., et al. (2000). A neural basis for general intelligence. *Science, 289,* 457–460.

Eccles, J., Wigfield, A., Harold, R. D., & Blumenfeld, P. (1993). Age and gender differences in children's self- and task perceptions during elementary school. *Child Development, 64,* 830–847.

Ericsson, K. A., Krampe, R. T., & Tesch-Römer, C. (1993). The role of deliberate practice in the acquisition of expert performance. *Psychological Review, 100,* 363–406.

Feshbach, N. D. (1969). Sex differences in children's modes of aggressive responses toward outsiders. *Merrill–Palmer Quarterly, 15,* 249–258.

Finlay, B. L., Darlington, R. B., & Nicastro, N. (2001). Developmental structure in brain evolution. *Behavioral and Brain Sciences, 24,* 263–308.

Fiske, S. T. (1993). Controlling other people: The impact of power on stereotyping. *American Psychologist, 48,* 621–628.

Fiske, S. T., & Taylor, S. E. (1991). *Social cognition* (2nd ed.). New York: McGraw-Hill.

Freedman, D. G. (1974). *Human infancy: An evolutionary perspective.* New York: Wiley.

Gallistel, C. R. (1990). *The organization of learning.* Cambridge, MA: MIT Press/Bradford Books.

Gallistel, C. R. (2000). The replacement of general-purpose learning models with adaptively specialized learning modules. In M. S. Gazzaniga (Ed.), *The new cognitive neurosciences* (2nd ed., pp. 1179–1191). Cambridge, MA: MIT Press.

Garlick, D. (2002). Understanding the nature of the general factor of intelligence: The role of individual differences in neural plasticity as an explanatory mechanism. *Psychological Review, 109,* 116–136.

Geary, D. C. (1995). Reflections of evolution and culture in children's cognition: Implications for mathematical development and instruction. *American Psychologist, 50,* 24–37.

Geary, D. C. (1998). *Male, female: The evolution of human sex differences.* Washington, DC: American Psychological Association.

Geary, D. C. (2001). A Darwinian perspective on mathematics and instruction. In T. Loveless (Ed.), *The great curriculum debate: How should we teach reading and math?* (pp. 85–107). Washington, DC: Brookings Institute.

Geary, D. C. (2002a). Principles of evolutionary educational psychology. *Learning and Individual Differences, 12,* 317–345.

Geary, D. C. (2002b). Sexual selection and human life history. In R. Kail (Ed.), *Advances in child development and behavior* (Vol. 30, pp. 41–101). San Diego: Academic Press.

Geary, D. C. (2005). *The origin of mind: Evolution of brain, cognition, and general intelligence.* Washington, DC: American Psychological Association.

Geary, D. C., & Bjorklund, D. F. (2000). Evolutionary developmental psychology. *Child Development, 71,* 57–65.

Geary, D. C., Byrd-Craven, J., Hoard, M. K., Vigil, J., & Numtee, C. (2003). Evolution and development of boys' social behavior. *Developmental Review, 23,* 444–470.

Geary, D. C., & Flinn, M. V. (2001). Evolution of human parental behavior and the human family. *Parenting: Science and Practice, 1,* 5–61.

Geary, D. C., & Huffman, K. J. (2002). Brain and cognitive evolution: Forms of modularity and functions of mind. *Psychological Bulletin, 128,* 667–698.

Gelman, R. (1990). First principles organize attention to and learning about relevant data: Number and animate–inanimate distinction as examples. *Cognitive Science*, *14*, 79–106.

Gelman, R., & Williams, E. M. (1998). Enabling constraints for cognitive development and learning: Domain-specificity and epigenesis. In W. Damon (Series Ed.) & D. Kuhl & R. S. Siegler (Vol. Eds.), *Handbook of child psychology: Vol. 2. Cognition, perception, and language* (Vol. 2, pp. 575–630). New York: Wiley.

Gigerenzer, G., & Selten, R. (Eds.). (2001). *Bounded rationality: The adaptive toolbox*. Cambridge, MA: MIT Press.

Greenough, W. T. (1991). Experience as a component of normal development: Evolutionary considerations. *Developmental Psychology*, *27*, 14–17.

Heckhausen, J., & Schulz, R. (1995). A life-span theory of control. *Psychological Review*, *102*, 284–304.

Hirsch, E. D., Jr. (1996). *The schools we need: Why we don't have them*. New York: Doubleday.

Horowitz, D. L. (2001). *The deadly ethnic riot*. Berkeley: University of California Press.

Humphrey, N. K. (1976). The social function of intellect. In P. P. G. Bateson & R. A. Hinde (Eds.), *Growing points in ethology* (pp. 303–317). New York: Cambridge University Press.

Hunt, E., & Minstrell, J. (1994). A cognitive approach to the teaching of physics. In K. McGilly (Ed.), *Classroom lessons: Integrating cognitive theory and classroom practice* (pp. 51–74). Cambridge, MA: MIT Press.

Irons, W. (1979). Cultural and biological success. In N. A. Chagnon & W. Irons (Eds.), *Natural selection and social behavior* (pp. 257–272). North Scituate, MA: Duxbury Press.

Jensen, A. R. (1998). *The g factor: The science of mental ability*. Westport, CT: Praeger.

Johnson-Laird, P. N. (1983). *Mental models*. Cambridge, UK: Cambridge University Press.

Kaiser, M. K., McCloskey, M., & Proffitt, D. R. (1986). Development of intuitive theories of motion: Curvilinear motion in the absence of physical forces. *Developmental Psychology*, *22*, 67–71.

Kaiser, M. K., Proffitt, D. R., & McCloskey, M. (1985). The development of beliefs about falling objects. *Perception and Psychophysics*, *38*, 533–539.

Kane, M. J., & Engle, R. W. (2002). The role of prefrontal cortex in working-memory capacity, executive attention, and general fluid intelligence: An individual-differences perspective. *Psychonomic Bulletin and Review*, *9*, 637–671.

Karmiloff-Smith, A. (1992). *Beyond modularity: A developmental perspective on cognitive science*. Cambridge, MA: Bradford Books/MIT Press.

Keeley, L. H. (1996). *War before civilization: The myth of the peaceful savage*. New York: Oxford University Press.

Kisilevsky, B. S., Hains, S. M. J., Lee, K., Xie, X., Huang, H., Ye, H. H., et al. (2003). Effects of experience on fetal voice recognition. *Psychological Science*, *14*, 220–224.

Kosslyn, S. M., & Thompson, W. L. (2000). Shared mechanisms in visual imagery and visual perception: Insights from cognitive neuroscience. In M. S. Gazzaniga (Editor-in-Chief), *The new cognitive neurosciences* (2nd ed., pp. 975–985). Cambridge, MA: Bradford Books/MIT Press.

Lever, J. (1978). Sex differences in the complexity of children's play and games. *American Sociological Review, 43,* 471–483.

Lichtenstein, S., Slovic, P., & Fischhoff, B., Layman, M., & Combs, B. (1978). Judged frequency of lethal events. *Journal of Experimental Psychology: Human Learning and Memory, 4,* 551–578.

Lindroth, S. (1983). The two faces of Linnaeus. In T. Frängsmyr (Ed.), *Linnaeus: The man and his work* (pp. 1–62). Berkeley: University of California Press.

Loveless, T. (Ed.). (2001). *The great curriculum debate: How should we teach reading and math?* Washington, DC: Brookings Institute.

MacDonald, K. (1992). Warmth as a developmental construct: An evolutionary analysis. *Child Development, 63,* 753–773.

Markus, H. (1977). Self-schemata and processing information about the self. *Journal of Personality and Social Psychology, 35,* 63–78.

Mayr, E. (1974). Behavior programs and evolutionary strategies. *American Scientist, 62,* 650–659.

McCloskey, M. (1983). Intuitive physics. *Scientific American, 248,* 122–130.

Miller, E. K., & Cohen, J. D. (2001). An integration of theory of prefrontal cortex function. *Annual Review of Neuroscience, 24,* 167–202.

Moscovitch, M. (1994). Memory and working with memory: Evaluation of a component process model and comparisons with other models. In D. L. Schacter & E. Tulving (Eds.), *Memory systems 1994* (pp. 269–310). Cambridge, MA: MIT Press.

Ospovat, D. (1981). *The development of Darwin's theory: Natural history, natural theology, and natural selection, 1838–1859.* Cambridge, UK: Cambridge University Press.

Pellis, S. M., & Pellis, V. C. (1998). The structure–function interface in the analysis of play fighting. In M. Bekoff & J. A. Byers (Eds.), *Animal play: Evolutionary, comparative, and ecological perspectives* (pp. 115–140). Cambridge, UK: Cambridge University Press.

Piaget, J. (1930). *The child's conception of physical causality* (M. Worden, Trans.). New York: Harcourt, Brace, & World. (Original French edition published 1927)

Piaget, J. (1970). *The child's conception of movement and speed* (G. E. T. Holloway & M. J. Mackenzie, Trans.). London: Routledge & Kegan Paul. (Original French edition published 1946)

Pinker, S. (1994). *The language instinct.* New York: Morrow.

Pinker, S. (1997). *How the mind works.* New York: Norton.

Posner, M. I. (1994). Attention: The mechanisms of consciousness. *Proceedings of the National Academy of Sciences USA, 91,* 7398–7403.

Povinelli, D. J., & Preuss, T. M. (1995). Theory of mind: Evolutionary history of a cognitive specialization. *Trends in Neuroscience, 18,* 418–424.

Premack, D., & Premack, A. J. (1995). Origins of human social competence. In M. S. Gazzaniga (Ed.), *The cognitive neurosciences* (pp. 205–218). Cambridge, MA: Bradford Books/MIT Press.

Pugh, K. R., Shaywitz, B. A., Shaywitz, S. E., Shankweiler, D. P., Katz, L., Fletcher, J. M., et al. (1997). Predicting reading performance from neuroimaging profiles: The cerebral basis of phonological effects in printed word identification. *Journal of Experimental Psychology: Human Perception and Performance, 23,* 299–318.

Roe, A. (1956). *Psychology of occupations.* New York: Wiley.

Rosenthal, R., Hall, J. A., DiMatteo, M. R., Rogers, P. L., & Archer, D. (1979). *Sensi-*

tivity to nonverbal communication: The PONS test. Baltimore: Johns Hopkins University Press.

Rozin, P. (1976). The evolution of intelligence and access to the cognitive unconscious. In J. M. Sprague & A. N. Epstein (Eds.), *Progress in psychobiology and physiological psychology* (Vol. 6, pp. 245–280). New York: Academic Press.

Rozin, P., & Schull, J. (1988). The adaptive–evolutionary point of view in experimental psychology. In R. C. Atkinson, R. J. Herrnstein, G. Lindzey, & R. D. Luce (Eds.), *Steven's handbook of experimental psychology* (2nd ed., Vol. 1, pp. 503–546). New York: Wiley.

Rubin, K. H., Fein, G. G., & Vandenberg, B. (1983). Play. In P. Mussen & E. M. Hetherington (Eds.), *Handbook of child psychology: Socialization, personality, and social development* (4th ed., Vol. 4, pp. 693–774). New York: Wiley.

Scarr, S., & McCarthy, K. (1983). How people make their own environments: A theory of genotype→environment effects. *Child Development, 54,* 424–435.

Schneider, D. J. (1973). Implicit personality theory: A review. *Psychological Bulletin, 79,* 294–309.

Segerstrale, U. (2000). *Defenders of the truth: The battle for science in the sociobiology debate and beyond.* New York: Oxford University Press.

Shallice, T. (2002). Fractionation of the supervisory system. In D. T. Stuss & R. T. Knight (Eds.), *Principles of frontal lobe function* (pp. 261–277). New York: Oxford University Press.

Sheeran, P., & Orbell, S. (2000). Self-schemas and the theory of planned behaviour. *European Journal of Social Psychology, 30,* 533–550.

Shepard, R. N. (1994). Perceptual–cognitive universals as reflections of the world. *Psychonomic Bulletin and Review, 1,* 2–28.

Simonton, D. K. (1999). *Origins of genius: Darwinian perspective on creativity.* New York: Oxford University Press.

Simonton, D. K. (2003). Scientific creativity as constrained stochastic behavior: The integration of product, person, and process perspectives. *Psychological Bulletin, 129,* 475–494.

Spelke, E. S., Breinlinger, K., Macomber, J., & Jacobson, K. (1992). Origins of knowledge. *Psychological Review, 99,* 605–632.

Stanovich, K. E. (1999). *Who is rational?: Studies of individual differences in reasoning.* Mahwah, NJ: Erlbaum.

Stearns, S. C. (1992). *The evolution of life histories.* New York: Oxford University Press.

Stephan, W. G. (1985). Intergroup relations. In G. Lindzey & E. Aronson (Eds.), *Handbook of social psychology: Vol. II: Special fields and applications* (pp. 599–658). New York: Random House.

Stevenson, H. W., & Stigler, J. W. (1992). *The learning gap: Why our schools are failing and what we can learn from Japanese and Chinese education.* New York: Summit Books.

Taylor, S. E. (1982). The availability bias in social perception and interaction. In D. Kahneman, P. Slovic, & A. Tversky (Eds.), *Judgment uncertainty: Heuristics and biases* (pp. 190–200). Cambridge, UK: Cambridge University Press.

Thompson, S. C., Armstrong, W., & Thomas, C. (1998). Illusions of control, underestimations, and accuracy: A control heuristic explanation. *Psychological Bulletin, 123,* 143–161.

Tooby, J., & Cosmides, L. (1995). Mapping the evolved functional organization of mind and brain. In M. S. Gazzaniga (Ed.), *The cognitive neurosciences* (pp. 1185–1197). Cambridge, MA: Bradford Books/MIT Press.

Tulving, E. (2002). Episodic memory: From mind to brain. *Annual Review of Psychology, 53*, 1–25.

Tversky, A., & Kahneman, D. (1974). Judgment under uncertainty: Heuristics and biases. *Science, 185*, 1124–1131.

Wagner, R. K., Torgesen, J. K., & Rashotte, C. A. (1994). Development of reading-related phonological processing abilities: New evidence of bidirectional causality from a latent variable longitudinal study. *Developmental Psychology, 30*, 73–87.

Walberg, H. J. (1984). Improving the productivity of America's schools. *Educational Leadership, 41*, 19–27.

Whissell, C. (1996). Mate selection in popular women's fiction. *Human Nature, 7*, 427–447.

White, M. (1998). *Newton: The last sorcerer*. Reading, MA: Perseus Books.

INDEX

521